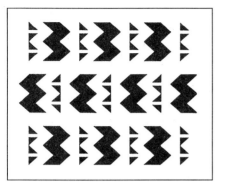

Student Study Guide to Accompany Ignatavicius, Workman, and Mishler

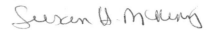

MEDICAL-SURGICAL NURSING

A Nursing Process Approach

Second Edition

ANNABELLE M. KEENE, MSN, RNC

ASSISTANT PROFESSOR
COLLEGE OF NURSING
UNIVERSITY OF NEBRASKA MEDICAL CENTER
OMAHA, NEBRASKA

JANE HOKANSON HAWKS, DNSc, RNC

ASSISTANT PROFESSOR
MIDLAND LUTHERAN COLLEGE
FREMONT, NEBRASKA

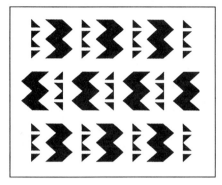

Student Study Guide to Accompany Ignatavicius, Workman, and Mishler

MEDICAL-SURGICAL NURSING

A Nursing Process Approach

Second Edition

W. B. SAUNDERS COMPANY

A Division of Harcourt Brace & Company

Philadelphia London Toronto Montreal Sydney Tokyo

W. B. SAUNDERS COMPANY
A Division of Harcourt Brace & Company
The Curtis Center
Independence Square West
Philadelphia, PA 19106

Cover Art: Georgia O'Keeffe, *Oriental Poppies,* 1928, Courtesy of the Collection Frederick R. Weisman Art Museum at the University of Minnesota, Minneapolis

Student Study Guide to Accompany Ignatavicius, Workman, and Mishler:
MEDICAL-SURGICAL NURSING
A Nursing Process Approach
Second Edition

Printed in the United States of America

ISBN 0-7216-4865-7

Last digit is the print number: 9 8 7 6 5 4 3 2 1

Preface

We have written the *Student Study Guide to Accompany Ignatavicius, Workman, and Mishler: Medical-Surgical Nursing,* Second Edition, to help you learn the content of your textbook.

In each chapter, you will find **Learning Objectives** to help you anticipate the contents and purposes of the chapter. Following the Learning Objectives, you will find a list of **Prerequisite Knowledge** items. These items identify topics that you may find helpful to review before you read each chapter or *as* you read each chapter. For more information on these topics, you may want to refer to your textbooks from courses in basic nursing or fundamentals of nursing, pharmacology, nutrition and diet therapy, and mathematics related to medication administration.

The organization of the questions in each *Student Study Guide* chapter follows that of your textbook. Initial questions in each chapter relate to either normal anatomy and physiology or to pathophysiology, etiology, and incidence or prevalence. For "Assessment" chapters, questions focusing on client assessment follow. For "Interventions" chapters, questions focusing on collaborative management follow and have the nursing process as their framework.

The questions in the *Student Study Guide* do not cover all of the content in your textbook; instead, their purpose is to help you learn to apply the nursing process. Questions draw on your understanding of ethics, the legal aspects of nursing, change, and growth and development—important "curricular strands" that you will encounter throughout your formal nursing education.

The *Student Study Guide* presents questions in various formats. Their purpose is to promote your recognition of information for which a nursing instructor might hold you accountable. Multiple-choice items have the additional purpose of giving you practice in handling the question format used in standardized testing, such as licensure or certification examinations.

For most of the questions in the *Student Study Guide,* we provide answers in an **Answer Key** at the back of the book. These answers allow you to quickly verify your responses. When an answer is detailed or involves more complex content, we refer you to the corresponding pages of your textbook for review. When a question requires complex application of knowledge—what is known as "critical thinking"—we ask you to submit your responses to (or discuss them with) your clinical instructor. For your convenience, we identify these **Critical Thinking Exercises** with a special symbol: **CT**.

New to this edition are **Case Studies,** which appear at the ends of most chapters. The Case Studies, which we have provided as another way of helping you develop your critical thinking skills, describe scenarios representing the more common medical-surgical problems discussed in the textbook. Specific questions about the scenarios then follow for you to address.

The Case Studies require higher level integration and application of information that appears in the textbook. Because of this, answers to the Case Studies do not appear in the *Student Study Guide.* Instead, we encourage you to review or discuss your answers to the Case Studies with your clinical instructor.

We hope that the *Student Study Guide* will help you to better understand and apply the nursing process to your medical-surgical nursing practice.

One final word: we gratefully acknowledge the contributions of Joyce M. Black, MSN, RNC, CPSN, to the first edition.

Annabelle M. Keene, MSN, RNC
Jane Hokanson Hawks, DNSc, RNC

Contents

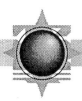

C H A P T E R 1

Concepts of Health and Illness

LEARNING OBJECTIVES

At the end of this chapter, the student will be able to

- Define *health* and *illness*
- Identify variables that affect health and illness
- Assess the illness experience
- Identify health promotion and maintenance behaviors
- Identify the three types of illness prevention

PREREQUISITE KNOWLEDGE

Nothing required

STUDY QUESTIONS

Definitions of Health and Illness

1. Identify factors that have influenced the definition of health.

   a. _____

   _____

   b. _____

   _____

   c. _____

   _____

2. Define *high-level wellness* in your own terms. Use a separate sheet.

3. Identify and define the three factors that are reflected in an individual's level of wellness.

   a. _____

   _____

   _____

   _____

   b. _____

   _____

   _____

   _____

   c. _____

   _____

   _____

4. Describe the concept of holistic health and its relationship to high-level wellness. Use a separate sheet.

5. Contrast the definitions of *disease* and *illness*. Use a separate sheet.

CT 6. Draw a diagram of a health–illness continuum. Using the diagram, place the following clients on the continuum and identify the rationale for their placement. Submit the completed exercise to the clinical instructor.

    a. A 30-year-old stable diabetic client

    b. A 20-year-old female drug addict with a $200/day habit

    c. A 64-year-old who recently suffered a compression fracture of the spine resulting from long-standing osteoporosis

    d. A 72-year-old independent widow who has no known health problems

    e. A 28-year-old single mother of 2-year-old twins and a 4-year-old child

    f. A 41-year-old husband and father who had an above-the-knee amputation 18 years ago

    g. A 45-year-old husband and father who has been a paraplegic for 16 years

    h. A 22-year-old full-time nursing student on a low budget who is living away from her parents for the first time

7. Identify 11 factors that affect an individual's health/illness levels and give an example of each. Use a separate sheet.

Assessment

Match the following characteristics (8–15) with their associated illness categories (a or b). Answers may be used more than once.

    ____ 8. permanent impairment

    ____ 9. self-limiting

    ____ 10. rapid onset

    ____ 11. residual disability

    ____ 12. rehabilitation

    ____ 13. short duration

    ____ 14. specific treatment

    ____ 15. exacerbation/remission cycle

    a. acute

    b. chronic

16. Identify changes occurring in an individual that indicate illness is present.

    a. _____

    _____

    b. _____

    _____

    c. _____

    _____

    d. _____

    _____

    e. _____

    _____

    f. _____

    _____

    g. _____

    _____

17. List the types of responses an individual may have when reacting to illness. Give an example of each.

    a. _____

    _____

    _____

    b. _____

    _____

    _____

    c. _____

    _____

18. Identify factors that may influence an individual's reaction to illness.

    a. _____

    _____

    b. _____

    _____

    c. _____

    _____

d. _____

_____

e. _____

_____

19. Describe the concept of *sick role,* including its defining characteristics. Use a separate sheet.

Match the following events (20–29) with their associated stages of illness (a–e). Answers may be used more than once.

_____ 20. acceptance of diagnosis

_____ 21. responsibilities relinquished

_____ 22. normal activities resumed

_____ 23. emotional response

_____ 24. validation of illness

_____ 25. focus on minor ailments

_____ 26. self-treatment

_____ 27. sick role relinquished

_____ 28. regressive behavior

_____ 29. sick role legitimized

a. experiencing symptoms

b. assuming the sick role

c. health care contact

d. dependent role

e. recovery and rehabilitation

30. Identify the factors that affect the family unit when one of its members is ill.

a. _____

_____

b. _____

_____

c. _____

_____

Prevention

Match the following examples of preventive health behavior (31–36) with their associated levels of intervention (a–c). Answers may be used more than once.

_____ 31. early diagnosis

_____ 32. return to highest level of wellness

_____ 33. immunizations

_____ 34. use of seat belts

_____ 35. prevention of severe disability

_____ 36. reduce risk of complications

a. primary

b. secondary

c. tertiary

37. List examples of health practices that an individual can use to promote health.

a. _____

_____

b. _____

_____

c. _____

_____

d. _____

_____

e. _____

_____

f. _____

_____

g. _____

_____

CRITICAL THINKING EXERCISES

Case Study: Effect of Illness on Family Units

Describe the effects that illness may have in the following family units. Identify factors that should be assessed.

1. A recently married (6 months) young couple in which the 22-year-old wife has chronic bowel disease. She eventually has surgery, resulting in an ileostomy.

2. A 72-year-old retired lawyer, married with three children. He suffers a severe, debilitating cerebral vascular accident (stroke).

3. A 67-year-old married retired office clerk. He has suffered from progressive Parkinson's disease for 10 years and his medication has become decreasingly effective. His wife works full time; they have no children.

4. An 18-year-old male high school student, active in sports and the oldest of three children. He suffers a severe sprain of the knee ligaments.

5. A 40-year-old married farmer with four children who suffers severe burns of both hands while working on farm machinery.

C H A P T E R 2

The Nursing Profession and the Role of the Medical–Surgical Nurse

LEARNING OBJECTIVES

At the end of this chapter, the student will be able to
- Define *nursing*
- Describe the role of the nurse
- List settings in which nurses practice
- Identify how nursing expands its own special body of knowledge

PREREQUISITE KNOWLEDGE

Prior to beginning this chapter, the student should review
- The history of nursing from a fundamentals course (optional)

STUDY QUESTIONS

Definitions of Nursing

1. Identify three sources of definitions of nursing.

    a. _____

    _____

    _____

    b. _____

    _____

    _____

    _____

    c. _____

    _____

    _____

2. Briefly explain why it is difficult to have one, unified definition of nursing. Use a separate sheet.

Roles of the Nurse

Match the following nursing activities (3–8) with their associated types of nursing functions (a or b). Answers may be used more than once.

_____	3. giving a back rub	a. collaborative
_____	4. collecting a specimen	b. independent
_____	5. assessing skin condition	
_____	6. ordering a progressive diet	
_____	7. administering medications	
_____	8. increasing client's activity schedule	

Match the following role characteristics (9–20) with their associated nursing roles (a–f). Answers may be used more than once.

____ 9. interprets information to client

____ 10. models behavior to improve conditions

____ 11. conducts health team conferences

____ 12. determines client's motivation level to learn

____ 13. performs collaborative functions

____ 14. plans continued care

____ 15. assesses home resources

____ 16. becomes politically active

____ 17. explains implications of client's decisions

____ 18. provides physical care

____ 19. arranges for posthospitalization care

____ 20. provides information

a. caregiver
b. discharge planner
c. educator
d. advocate
e. care coordinator or manager
f. change agent

21. List factors affecting the teaching–learning process.

a. _____

_____

b. _____

_____

c. _____

_____

d. _____

_____

_____

e. _____

_____

_____

Practice Settings

22. Identify settings in which nurses practice.

a. _____

_____

b. _____

_____

c. _____

_____

d. _____

_____

e. _____

_____

f. _____

_____

g. _____

_____

Professional Development

23. Briefly discuss the significance of nursing having its own special body of knowledge. Submit the completed exercise to the clinical instructor on a separate sheet.

24. Briefly discuss the importance of ongoing education in nursing. Use a separate sheet.

25. Identify the primary tasks of nursing research.

a. _____

_____

_____

b. _____

_____

_____

26. Briefly discuss the significance of communicating the results of nursing research. Use a separate sheet.

CHAPTER 3

The Nursing Process

LEARNING OBJECTIVES

At the end of this chapter, the student will be able to

- Define the *nursing process*
- Describe the methods of data collection used in assessment
- Describe the process of data analysis
- Describe the planning phase of the nursing process
- Describe the implementation phase of the nursing process
- Describe the evaluation phase of the nursing process
- Identify several nursing documentation systems

PREREQUISITE KNOWLEDGE

Prior to beginning this chapter, the student should review

- The problem-solving process
- The decision-making process
- Critical thinking
- Systems theory

STUDY QUESTIONS

Problem-Solving Approaches

1. Compare the steps of the nursing process with those of the scientific method of problem-solving by completing the following chart on a separate sheet.

Nursing Process	Scientific Method
a. assessment	
b. analysis	
c. planning	
d. implementation	
e. evaluation	

Assessment

2. Identify the purpose of the assessment step in the nursing process. Use a separate sheet.

3. Differentiate between *subjective* and *objective* data. Use a separate sheet.

4. List three techniques used by nurses to collect client data.

    a. _____

    b. _____

    c. _____

Match the following characteristics (5–13) with their associated technique of data collection (a–c). Answers may be used more than once.

_____ 5. logical, organized approach

_____ 6. exploring perceptions

_____ 7. nonverbal cues

_____ 8. establishing trust

_____ 9. exploring conflicting findings

_____ 10. recognizing pertinent data

_____ 11. objective assessment

_____ 12. communication skills

_____ 13. using a stethoscope

a. interview

b. observation

c. physical examination

14. Identify the instrument used to collect primary client data. _____

_____

Match the following examples of data (15–26) with their associated data category (a–c). Answers may be used more than once.

_____ 15. reports smoking five cigarettes per day

_____ 16. skin smooth, warm

_____ 17. indwelling catheter draining clear, amber urine

_____ 18. check dressing every shift

_____ 19. denies shortness of breath

_____ 20. has occasional leg cramps

_____ 21. elevate head of bed 45 degrees

_____ 22. walks with unsteady gait

_____ 23. turn prone twice a day

_____ 24. lung sounds clear on auscultation

_____ 25. father had heart attack at age 54

_____ 26. ambulate with assistance

a. subjective

b. objective

c. neither subjective nor objective

27. List three secondary sources of client data.

a. _____

_____

b. _____

_____

c. _____

28. Describe the difference in focus of a nursing history compared to a medical history. Use a separate sheet.

Analysis

29. Identify the purpose of the analysis step in the nursing process. Use a separate sheet.

30. Define, in your own words, the concept of *nursing diagnosis.* Submit the completed exercise to the clinical instructor on a separate sheet.

31. Identify the three parts of a nursing diagnosis statement.

a. _____

_____

b. _____

_____

c. _____

_____

32. Which one of the following statements about nursing diagnosis is correct?

a. The list of nursing diagnoses is comprehensive and complete.

b. A nursing diagnosis indicates a client health problem treatable by a nurse.

c. Nursing diagnoses refer to the nurse's problems while caring for an individual client.

d. Nursing diagnoses have been definitively refined and clinically validated.

33. Briefly discuss the significance of including the etiology in a nursing diagnosis statement. Submit the completed exercise to the clinical instructor on a separate sheet.

Planning

34. List the five components of the planning phase in the nursing process.

a. _____

_____

b. _____

_____

c. _____

_____

d. _____

_____

e. _____

_____

35. Briefly discuss the significance of priority setting in the nursing process. Use a separate sheet.

36. Which one of the following statements about priority setting is correct?

a. Priorities are stable once they have been established.

b. A potential problem is of higher priority than an actual problem.

c. Resource availability is unrelated to priority problem management.

d. Priority setting is a mutual process between client and nurse.

37. Briefly discuss the purpose of goal setting in the nursing process. Use a separate sheet.

38. List three criteria that goals should meet.

a. _____

_____

b. _____

_____

c. _____

_____

39. Which one of the following statements about the client care plan is correct?

a. It is a record of the client's problems, preferences, priorities, potential complications of his or her condition, and goals.

b. It includes actions performed exclusively by the nurse.

c. It is a means of communicating the nurse's problems regarding the client's care.

d. It requires few revisions regardless of the client's length of stay.

40. Which one of the following statements about defining evaluation criteria in the planning phase is correct?

a. Predetermined criteria give direction to the implementation phase of the nursing process.

b. Standards of care serve as guidelines for the analysis of client problems.

c. Evaluation of client goal attainment is independent of specific criteria.

Implementation

41. List the guidelines used by the nurse when selecting nursing interventions.

a. _____

_____

b. _____

_____

c. _____

_____

d. _____

_____

e. _____

_____

f. _____

_____

42. Identify the three types of skills the nurse uses during implementation, and give an example of each.

a. _____

_____

_____

b. _____

_____

c. _____

_____

_____

Evaluation

43. Briefly discuss the importance of the evaluation phase in the nursing process. Use a separate sheet.

44. Identify the four possible outcomes of the evaluation phase and their implications for further nursing actions. Use a separate sheet.

Documentation

45. List examples of nursing documentation systems.

a. _____

_____

b. _____

_____

c. _____

_____

46. Which one of the following statements about why the nurse follows facility policies for documenting in the client's chart is correct?

a. The chart is a confidential document.

b. The chart is the legal record of the client's care.

c. The chart is the primary data source used in an outcome audit.

CRITICAL THINKING EXERCISES

Case Study: The Use of Nursing Diagnoses

Nursing student J. B. was working on a cardiac and respiratory unit of a hospital. This was the second week of her clinical rotation. J. B.'s client was a 70-year-old man with chronic airflow limitation (CAL) and congestive heart failure (CHF). After completing his morning care, she wrote her SOAP notes in the chart without having her instructor check them first. Her first diagnosis was Ineffective Airway Clearance related to CAL; her second diagnosis was Decreased Cardiac Output related to CAL and CHF. The client's physician made rounds and read her notes. He came to talk to her about making medical diagnoses on his client, for which she was not trained. She explained by saying that she was new to writing nurse diagnoses and would consult her instructor to clarify them to reflect more of nursing and less of medicine. The physician told J. B. that he would be back on the ward in the afternoon and wanted her to explain how a medical diagnosis and a nursing diagnosis differed.

Address the following questions:

1. What are the major differences between a medical diagnosis and a nursing diagnosis?
2. What should J. B. explain to the physician when he returns?
3. How can nursing diagnoses assist in interdisciplinary client care?
4. Rewrite her nursing diagnoses so that they are more reflective of nursing practice.

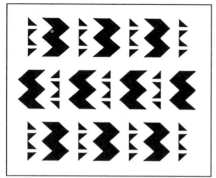

CHAPTER 4

Adult Development

LEARNING OBJECTIVES

At the end of this chapter, the student will be able to

- Describe various theories of adult development
- Discuss the biological theories of aging
- Describe the sociological theories of adult societal roles
- Discuss the psychological theories about adult personality changes
- Describe the physical, psychological, and social changes that affect young adults
- Describe the physical, psychological, and social changes of middle adulthood
- Describe the physical, psychological, and social changes of late adulthood

PREREQUISITE KNOWLEDGE

Prior to beginning this chapter, the student should review

- The principles of developmental psychology
- Normal growth and development
- The principles of sociology

STUDY QUESTIONS

Theories of Adult Development

1. Briefly discuss why there are multiple theories explaining adulthood. Use a separate sheet.

2. Which one of the following statements is true according to Erikson's "eight stages of man"?

   a. Identity confusion results from a positive self-concept.

   b. Mature young adults segregate their activities into the areas of work, leisure, and nurturing.

   c. Generativity focuses on one's physical or psychological decline.

   d. Dignity and acceptance of one's life indicate psychological well-being in the later years.

3. Which one of the following statements is true according to Peck's theory of the middlescence stage of adult development?

   a. Changes in body structure and function are accommodated by selecting alternative physical activities.

   b. Interpersonal relationships become more important than sexual relationships.

   c. Successful coping with common losses includes turning inward and avoiding new relationships.

   d. Mental flexibility puts the middle-aged adult at risk for developing psychological problems.

4. Which one of the following statements is true according to Peck's theory of old age?

   a. The major task at this stage is to develop a variety of meaningful diversional activities.

   b. Recapturing the past and self-pity are helpful in adjusting to this stage of life.

   c. The future is viewed as being limited and threatening.

   d. Sedentary activities are stressful and anxiety producing.

5. Which of the following statements is true according to Havighurst's theory of adult developmental tasks?

   a. The developmental task for the young adult is to disengage from some of his or her active roles.

   b. Responsibilities for middle-aged adults include discovering one's own identity.

   c. Later maturity adults adjust by regulating their roles to accomplish goals.

   d. Middle-aged adults must develop problem-solving abilities in order to make mature decisions.

Theories of Aging

Match the following definitions (6–11) with their related biologic theories of aging (a–f).

_____ 6. body wears out its parts until it ceases to function

_____ 7. organism is weakened from accumulation of successive stressful events over the life span

_____ 8. available energy supply becomes depleted and cannot be restored

_____ 9. cellular mutations result in foreign protein formation and resulting disease

_____ 10. inappropriate information is provided for normal cell function, resulting in mutagenesis

_____ 11. impaired control mechanisms result from a lowered oxygen supply

a. exhaustion
b. wear and tear
c. stress
d. genetic
e. single organ
f. autoimmune

12. Which one of the following statements reflects sociological theories of aging?

    a. Each role's demands are discrete and nonsequential.

    b. Earlier learning facilitates older adults' ability to learn new roles.

    c. Performance of socially valued role functions results in a meaningless future.

    d. Reduction of activities in the elderly results in enhanced self-esteem.

13. Which one of the following statements reflects psychological theories of aging?

    a. As individuals pass through the life span, they become increasingly similar to one another.

    b. Increased reflection indicates a decreasing interest in inner development.

    c. The last half of life is oriented toward biologic and social issues.

    d. Reflection stimulates personal growth, integration, and evolving identity.

Stages of Adulthood

Match the following physiological changes related to aging (14–25) with their corresponding age groups (a–c). Answers may be used more than once.

_____ 14. decreased respiratory excursion

_____ 15. menopause/climacteric occurs

_____ 16. decline in maximum motor function

_____ 17. muscular function at highest efficiency

_____ 18. prostate hypertrophy

_____ 19. eruption of third molars

_____ 20. loss of sweat glands

_____ 21. altered color perception

_____ 22. onset of graying and baldness

_____ 23. sleep interruptions

_____ 24. osteoporosis

_____ 25. progressive hearing loss

a. young adult
b. middle adult
c. late adult

Match the following descriptions of identity and self-concept issues (26–30) with their associated age groups (a–c). Answers may be used more than once.

_____ 26. erosion of psychological well-being

_____ 27. former goals questioned

_____ 28. sense of self is less influenced by others

_____ 29. need to be productive

_____ 30. potential developed more fully

a. young adult
b. middle adult
c. late adult

31. Which one of the following statements is true regarding sexuality throughout the life span?

    a. Contraceptive pills reduce dilemmas over sexual mores.

    b. Most men cannot produce sperm into old age.

    c. Widows and divorcees may lack available sexual partners.

    d. Young adults enter relationships indiscriminately.

32. Which one of the following statements is true about family structure for young adults?

    a. Learning to live intimately with another person is easy.

    b. Childbirth results in greater marital harmony.

    c. Role patterns and relationships stabilize.

    d. Social isolation may occur in a baby-centered family.

33. Which one of the following statements is true about family structure for middle-aged adults?

    a. A strong sense of self-identity enables a woman to adjust to an "empty nest."

    b. A shaky marriage is often strengthened after the children become independent.

    c. Caring for aging or aged parents requires minimal adjustments.

    d. Coping adequately with middlescent changes leads to dependency.

34. Which one of the following statements is true about family structure for older adults?

    a. Residence in a small rural town interferes with adjustment to widowhood.

    b. Grandparenting helps the older adult maintain ego integrity.

    c. Most families are unable to resolve problems with supporting their elders.

    d. Home health services for frail, dependent elderly people adequately meet the demand.

35. Which one of the following statements is true about work and leisure habits throughout the life span?

    a. Young adults must cope with multiple roles, which increases the availability of leisure time.

    b. Most adults continue in their chosen fields of work until retirement.

    c. Blue collar workers are less eager to retire due to good health.

    d. Maximum adjustment to retirement is characterized by decreasing one's level of activity.

36. Which of the following statements is true about health issues affecting young and middle-aged adults?

    a. Health maintenance behaviors in young adulthood have little effect on one's eventual health status.

    b. Depression occurs more often in middle-aged men because they experience more role changes.

    c. Health prevention practices during middlescence assist a person in retaining optimal health.

    d. Accidents are the leading cause of mortality in middle-aged adults.

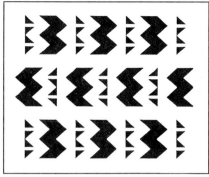

CHAPTER 5

Health Care of Older Adults

LEARNING OBJECTIVES

At the end of this chapter, the student will be able to

- Identify the subgroups of late adulthood (65 years of age or more) and their distribution in the health care system
- Discuss the health issues affecting the elderly
- Discuss the changes in mental health associated with old age
- Describe the economic concerns of the elderly

PREREQUISITE KNOWLEDGE

Prior to beginning this chapter, the student should review

- The principles of developmental psychology
- Normal growth and development
- The principles of sociology
- Health promotion behaviors

STUDY QUESTIONS

Health Issues

1. Which one of the following interventions is effective in reducing relocation stress in the elderly hospitalized client?

   a. Explain procedures and special tests in advance.

   b. Inform family members of the times allowed for visiting hours.

   c. Enforce hospital routines such as mealtimes and bathing schedules.

   d. Ask family members to take all personal belongings home for safe-keeping.

2. Identify the dimensions of wellness that should be evaluated when assessing the elderly.

   a. _____

   _____

   b. _____

   _____

   c. _____

   _____

   d. _____

   _____

   e. _____

   _____

3. Which one of the following statements is true about health issues affecting the elderly?

   a. Self-responsibility is promoted by adhering to stereotypes.

   b. Changes in smell and taste result in insufficient sodium intake.

   c. Role losses free the elderly to seek new supportive networks.

   d. Regular light exercise results in feelings of well-being.

4. Which one of the following statements is also true about health issues affecting the elderly?

   a. Relocation is often accompanied by feelings of powerlessness and depersonalization.

   b. The sense of environmental awareness is heightened, resulting in fewer injuries.

   c. Occurrence of adverse drug reactions is inversely related to the number of drugs taken.

   d. Effective learning about self-medicating is ensured by providing information.

5. Which one of the following interventions safely reduces the risk of falls in the hospitalized elderly client?

   a. applying vest restraints

   b. administering psychoactive medications

   c. raising bed side rails

   d. assisting the client to get up

Match the following physiological changes affecting drug use in older adults (6–13) with their associated pharmacodynamic actions (a–d). Answers may be used more than once.

_____ 6. increase proportion of adipose tissue

_____ 7. decreased gastric motility

_____ 8. reduced glomerular filtration

_____ 9. decreased liver enzyme activity

_____ 10. decreased total body water

_____ 11. decreased creatinine clearance

_____ 12. increased gastric pH

_____ 13. decreased cardiac output

a. absorption

b. distribution

c. metabolism

d. excretion

14. List the common types of adverse drug reactions that may occur in the elderly.

   a. _____

   b. _____

   c. _____

   d. _____

   e. _____

   f. _____

g. _____

h. _____

i. _____

j. _____

k. _____

l. _____

15. Identify common reasons why older adults make mistakes when self-administering medications.

   a. _____

      _____

      _____

      _____

   b. _____

      _____

      _____

      _____

   c. _____

      _____

      _____

16. Identify factors that deplete the elderly's resources for maintaining emotional well-being.

   a. _____

      _____

   b. _____

      _____

   c. _____

      _____

   d. _____

      _____

   e. _____

      _____

17. Differentiate between *dementia* and *depression* in the elderly. Use a separate sheet.

18. Which one of the following interventions is effective in helping reorient a client suffering from delirium?

   a. Apply wrist restraints as ordered by the physician.

   b. Reorient the client frequently using a calm voice.

   c. Remove personal items and store them safely away.

   d. Turn a radio on to a station that broadcasts popular music.

19. Which one of the following statements is true about elder abuse?

   a. The abuser is often a close family member.

   b. All older adults are vulnerable to being victims of elder abuse.

   c. Male adult children are usually the caregivers of their elderly parents.

   d. Physically independent older people tend to suffer abuse more often than dependent older people.

Economic Issues

20. Identify factors that contribute to the lack of economic self-reliance in the elderly.

   a. _____

   _____

b. _____

_____

c. _____

_____

d. _____

_____

e. _____

_____

f. _____

_____

Match the following governmental resources for supporting the elderly (21–24) with their associated funding programs (a–d).

_____ 21. nutrition sites

_____ 22. retirement income

_____ 23. rental assistance

_____ 24. health care insurance

a. Social Security Act

b. Medicare and Medicaid

c. Housing Program

d. Older Americans Act

CRITICAL THINKING EXERCISES

Case Study: Medication Use in the Elderly

A. L. is an 80-year-old client who is brought into the Emergency Department after fainting at home. His serum digoxin level is 2.3 ng/mL. A. L. is transferred to a medical nursing unit. The next day the nurse asks A. L. to tell her about his routine for taking his daily digoxin tablet. A. L. states that he was told to check his pulse every morning before taking a pill. He does this in his kitchen because "the clock on the wall has big numbers and I can see the second hand go around." The nurse asks A. L. how long he measures his pulse. A. L. replies, "I keep counting the beats until I get to 60. Sometimes it takes a long time! Then I take my heart pill."

Address the following questions:

1. Identify factors that may affect A. L.'s understanding of digoxin self-administration.

2. Devise a teaching plan to reinstruct A. L. about taking digoxin at home.

3. Discuss how the nurse can validate whether the teaching plan is effective.

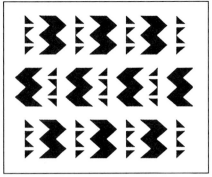

CHAPTER 6

Ethics

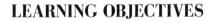

LEARNING OBJECTIVES

At the end of this chapter, the student will be able to

■ Define *ethics*

■ Contrast *utilitarianism* and *deontology* as ethical theories

■ Identify the basic principles that serve as a foundation for ethical decision making

■ Describe an ethical decision-making model

■ Describe resources nurses can use to resolve ethical dilemmas in nursing practice

■ Discuss issues of ethical concern for nurses

PREREQUISITE KNOWLEDGE

Prior to beginning this chapter, the student should review

■ The principles from an introductory course on ethics

■ Information on legal principles affecting nursing practice

■ The steps of the nursing process

STUDY QUESTIONS

Key Definitions

1. Check all of the following descriptions that apply when defining ethics.

_____ a. a branch of philosophy

_____ b. actual standards of conduct

_____ c. a science that studies the morality of human acts

_____ d. concerned with analyzing judgments and choices

_____ e. requires rationality and guiding principles

_____ f. consistent beliefs, attitudes, and values

_____ g. judges goodness and badness of human actions

_____ h. reflective thinking

2. Those who subscribe to the theory of deontology

a. treat all people equally

b. consider the social consequences of decisions

c. respect the dignity of clients

d. try to do the most good for all

19

Match the following definitions (3–9) with their ethical principles (a–d). Answers may be used more than once.

____ 3. without discrimina-
         tion or bias

a. non-maleficence

b. beneficence

____ 4. doing the most
         possible good

c. justice

d. autonomy

____ 5. right to know

____ 6. freedom of choice

____ 7. allocation of scarce
         resources

____ 8. lack of coercion

____ 9. avoiding harm

10. Which one of the following statements is true about women and moral reasoning according to Gilligan's work?

   a. Women's moral development stops at the conventional level.

   b. Women and men go through the same stages of moral development.

   c. Feminine moral development considers situations and relationships.

   d. A person's perspective on moral reasoning is determined by one's gender.

11. Which one of the following statements best defines *values*?

   a. Values direct how a person behaves.

   b. Values are constant and do not change.

   c. Values are imposed on a person by family and friends.

   d. Values determine whether an action is right or wrong.

Ethical Decision-Making and Resources

12. List the types of variables that influence ethical decision making by nurses. Give an example of each type.

   a. _____

   _____

   b. _____

   _____

   c. _____

   _____

13. Identify the common steps in normative ethical decision-making models.

   a. _____

   _____

   _____

   b. _____

   _____

   _____

   c. _____

   _____

   _____

   d. _____

   _____

   _____

14. List the difficulties nurses can have when faced with ethical decisions.

   a. _____

   _____

   _____

   b. _____

   _____

   _____

   c. _____

   _____

   _____

15. Which one of the following ethical resources would the nurse use when a client refuses to sign an operative permit?

   a. ANA's *Code for Nurses*

   b. the agency's Ethics Committee

   c. the ethics consultant

   d. the agency's policy manual

Ethical Issues

16. Give an example of each of the following ethical issues that concern nurses. Submit the completed exercise to the clinical instructor using a separate sheet.

Issue	Example
a. futility	
b. quality of life	
c. palliative care	
d. intentionality	
e. legal competency	
f. living will	
g. durable power of attorney	
h. verbal advance directive	
i. euthanasia	
j. placebo administration	
k. restraints	
l. confidentiality	
m. tube feeding	
n. unethical professional conduct	

17. Which one of the following statements about ethical reasoning corresponds to the assessment phase of the nursing process?

    a. consulting with ethical resources

    b. identifying the major ethical issues to resolve

    c. identifying all parties involved in the decision-making process

    d. determining whether the correct person made the ethical decision

CRITICAL THINKING EXERCISES

Case Studies: Too Many Daughters

C. R. and her husband live in a comfortable but not luxurious neighborhood. They are convinced that "zero population growth"—simply reproducing themselves and not having any more children—is the ethical principle to follow. But after two daughters are born, they try again because both have always dreamed of having a son as well. When their third daughter is born, they feel caught in an impossible dilemma, but then they hear about two new methods of "sex selection." Their physician explains that the odds of having a boy could be improved by partially separating Y (male) sperm from X (female) sperm and using mainly Y sperm for artificial insemination. This method would give them about a 70% chance of having a boy. Or more reliably, they could use amniocentesis to learn the sex of the fetus after the pregnancy has begun and abort the fetus if its sex is the "wrong" one. The couple choose the second course and, in time, a boy is born.

Address the following questions:

1. Is one of the two methods of "sex selection" ethically preferable?

2. What would be the parents' rights and responsibilities if tests showed that the fetus was female?

3. Assuming that it is ethical to allow abortion for unwanted children, then why not for unwanted genders?

4. Do parents have the right to choose the sex of their children? If so, and more boys are born than girls, what are the results for society?

5. Is the fetus allowed any rights?

Case Study: The Man Who Wanted To Die

J. G. is a 76-year-old man who is badly injured when a leaking propane gas line explodes. His son is killed in the accident. J. G. has second- and third-degree burns over 68% of his body; his eyes, ears, and most of his face are burned away. His hands require amputation due to the injury. After many months of skin grafts, he is susceptible to infections and he has to be bathed daily in a Hubbard tank. Although J. G. accepts treatment, he says he wants to die. Eventually he refuses treatment and insists on going home. His wife opposes his decision, and a psychiatrist agrees to see J. G. after getting the impression that he is irrational and depressed. J. G.'s competency is uncertain, and there is discussion of appointing a legal guardian who can authorize treatment. The psychiatrist finds J. G. to be bright, coherent, logical, and articulate. J. G. tells the psychiatrist, "I do not want to go on as a blind and crippled person." He wants his attorney to have him released from the hospital, by court order if necessary.

Address the following questions:

1. Are there circumstances in which a person has the right to refuse treatment?

2. Does J. G. have any responsibilities to others that should affect his decision? What are the responsibilities of the health care team to J. G.? To his wife? To his lawyer?

3. Are the rights of dying people different from those of the living? Is one of these rights the choice of whether to hasten the end of life?

4. Is there any justification for concealing medical facts from someone who is dying, especially the fact that death is imminent?

Case Study: What's A Nurse To Do?

K. O. is asked to work a double nursing shift because of a staffing shortage that day. She is usually assigned to a surgical nursing unit. K. O. is asked to float to the intensive care unit (ICU). She asks her head nurse and the nursing supervisor about the assignment. K. O. expresses concern about being uncomfortable in an area where she is unfamiliar and unsure. K. O. goes to the ICU because no one else is available. She reasons that the clients are better off with someone there rather than no one.

Address the following questions:

1. Is K. O.'s reasoning correct?

2. What are K. O.'s options in this situation?

3. What are the nursing supervisor's responsibilities in this situation? To K. O.? To the ICU? To the hospital?

4. There is one regular ICU staff nurse working in the unit when K. O. arrives. What are the nurse's responsibilities to K. O.? What are K. O.'s responsibilities to the ICU nurse?

During the course of the evening, K. O. fails to recognize and report electrocardiogram changes in a client in hepatic coma. The client suffers harm.

5. Is K. O.'s level of responsibility to this client equal to that of the ICU staff nurse? Or is it less because she is a "float" and unfamiliar with the client's diagnosis and treatment?

6. What is the ICU nurse's liability in this case?

(Also see Case Study: Lethal Dose in Chapter 14.)

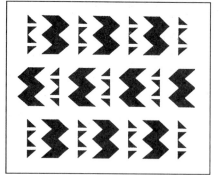

CHAPTER 7

Stress, Coping, and Adaptation

LEARNING OBJECTIVES

At the end of this chapter, the student will be able to

▮ Define *stress, appraisal, stressors, coping strategies,* and *adaptation*

▮ Compare and contrast theories about stress

▮ Compare and contrast theories of coping

▮ Identify the two outcomes of adaptation

▮ Provide care for the client or family that is stressed

PREREQUISITE KNOWLEDGE

Prior to beginning this chapter, the student should review

▮ General psychology as it relates to stress and adaptation

▮ The physiology of the stress response

▮ The effects of hospitalization on the individual and coping as reviewed in an introduction to nursing or fundamentals course

STUDY QUESTIONS

Key Definitions

Match the following terms associated with stress (1–5) with their definitions (a–e).

_____ 1. adaptation

_____ 2. appraisal

_____ 3. coping strategies

_____ 4. stress

_____ 5. stressor

a. approaches used by an individual to deal with anxiety-producing events

b. an event that leads to the appraisal of stress by an individual

c. an individual's reaction to an event that results in change or mastery and acceptance of stress

d. an individual's reaction to a threatening event in the environment

e. cognitive evaluation that an event is stressful

Stress Theories

6. Identify three prominent theories about stress.

   a. _____

   _____

   b. _____

   _____

   c. _____

   _____

7. List the three characteristics inherent in the general adaptation syndrome (GAS).

   a. _____

   _____

   b. _____

   _____

   c. _____

   _____

Match the following physiological events (8–15) with their associated GAS stages (a–c). Answers may be used more than once.

_____ 8. decreased production of adrenocorticotropic hormone (ACTH)

_____ 9. increased heart rate

_____ 10. decreased blood clotting time

_____ 11. secondary increase of ACTH secretion

_____ 12. release of glucose

_____ 13. specific adaptation activities occur

_____ 14. increased O_2/CO_2 exchange

_____ 15. occurrence of disease or death

    a. alarm stage

    b. stage of resistance

    c. stage of exhaustion

16. Complete the following exercise on the GAS response by filling in the blanks.

   a. A _____

   initiates the alarm reaction.

   b. The hypothalamus stimulates the

   _____

   _____

   to produce antidiuretic hormone (ADH).

   c. The hypothalamus also stimulates the release of _____

   from the anterior pituitary.

   d. The hypothalamus affects the sympathetic nervous centers and adrenal medulla causing release of _____

   and _____.

   e. The effects of ADH are to increase reabsorption of _____

   and _____

   and to decrease _____

   _____.

   f. The effects of ACTH on the adrenal cortex are to release _____

   and _____.

   g. The glucocorticoids produce increased

   _____

   and increased catabolism of _____

   and _____.

   h. The mineralocorticoids produce increased reabsorption of _____

   and _____ and

   excretion of _____.

   i. The combined effects of epinephrine and norepinephrine produce the

   _____

   _____ response.

   j. In the stage of resistance, _____

   levels return to baseline.

   k. If adaptation occurs during the stage of resistance, it helps lead to

   _____.

   l. Failure of adaptation mechanisms leads to

   _____

   _____.

17. List four examples of life events that are included in stress rating scales.

    a. _____

    b. _____

    c. _____

    d. _____

18. Identify the factor that demonstrates a stronger relationship to illness prediction than major life events.

    _____

    _____

19. List the appraisal factors that are related to the individual according to the transactional theory of stress.

    a. _____

    _____

    b. _____

    _____

    c. _____

    _____

20. List the five appraisal factors that are related to the event according to the transactional theory of stress.

    a. _____

    _____

    b. _____

    _____

    c. _____

    _____

    d. _____

    _____

    e. _____

    _____

Coping Theories

21. Identify which type of coping style (problem focused or emotion focused) the clients in the following situations are using.

    a. P. C. is a newly diagnosed, 50-year-old diabetic client who must learn to self-administer injections of insulin. She asks the nurse to leave several pamphlets so that she can read about the injection technique.

    b. M. W. is a 73-year-old client who must take antihypertensive medications three times a day. He misplaces his prescription and states, "I am feeling fine now. I don't need that medicine anymore."

    c. M. G. is a 28-year-old client who is infertile as a result of endometriosis. She makes an appointment with the clinic physician to discuss *in vitro* fertilization.

    d. D. H. is a 40-year-old client who injures his right shoulder in a fall while biking cross-country. He delays seeing a physician for treatment because he believes the injury to be minor.

    e. A. H. is a 68-year-old client who had a recent left above-knee amputation. He enjoys teasing staff and frequently jokes about operating a personal "taxi" service to shuttle busy staff with his wheelchair.

    f. L. N. is a 47-year-old client who is recovering from a myocardial infarction. He tells the nurse that he has bought an exercise bicycle and that he has also joined a walking club.

Match the following coping strategies (22–32) with their correct definitions (a–k).

_____ 22. avoidance

_____ 23. blaming one's self

_____ 24. denial

_____ 25. emphasizing the positive

_____ 26. fantasy

_____ 27. fatalism

_____ 28. hostility

_____ 29. humor

_____ 30. isolation

_____ 31. social support

_____ 32. tension reduction

a. accepting responsibility for an event

b. inducing relaxation

c. acceptance of what has happened without question

d. physical removal of one's self from a situation

e. assistance of family

f. hoping for a miracle

g. pretending a problem does not exist

h. looking on the bright side

i. reacting childishly

j. separating emotion from an event

k. making light of a situation

33. Briefly distinguish between event rehearsal and event review. Use a separate sheet.

Adaptation Theories

34. Briefly define the term *morale*. Use a separate sheet.

35. Briefly define the term *psychophysiologic disease*. Use a separate sheet.

36. List the three personality characteristics related to hardiness.

a. _____

_____

b. _____

_____

c. _____

_____

Collaborative Management

37. List aspects of the stress response that the nurse should assess in a hospitalized client. Give an example of each.

a. _____

_____

_____

b. _____

_____

_____

c. _____

_____

_____

d. _____

_____

_____

38. Briefly discuss the implications of having multiple nursing diagnoses for the client experiencing stress. Submit the completed exercise to the clinical instructor using a separate sheet.

Match the following interventions for promoting effective individual coping (39–47) with their associated etiological factors (a–i).

_____ 39. assisting with completion of a diet menu

_____ 40. explaining a diagnostic procedure

_____ 41. answering the call light promptly

_____ 42. encouraging verbalization of perceptions

_____ 43. allowing after-hours visitors

_____ 44. controlling background noise levels

_____ 45. encouraging self-care in activities of daily living (ADL)

_____ 46. arranging for pastoral visits

_____ 47. demonstrating the newborn's bath

a. fear
b. isolation from family
c. absence of social support
d. physical dependency
e. loss of control
f. changes in role
g. lack of knowledge
h. inaccurate stress appraisal
i. unnecessary stressors

48. List the four types of techniques that may assist the client to reduce the physical effect of stress on the body.

a. _____

_____

b. _____

_____

c. _____

_____

d. _____

_____

49. Briefly describe the overall effect that a client should experience when his or her stress and coping goals have been achieved.

_____

_____

_____

_____

50. List five common symptoms of "burnout" demonstrated by nurses.

a. _____

_____

b. _____

_____

c. _____

_____

d. _____

_____

e. _____

_____

_____

CRITICAL THINKING EXERCISE

Case Study: A Client Under Stress

J. S. is a 68-year-old male who is admitted to a nursing unit from the admissions department. This is his first hospitalization. En route, J. S. is taken to the radiology department. His clothing and personal belongings are brought to the unit by the transport aide. The nurse inventories J. S.'s belongings and takes his wallet and other valuables to a safety deposit box in the business office. When J. S. enters his room, he jumps out of the wheelchair and checks the bedside table and locker. When the nurse enters the room, J. S. is pacing the floor.

Address the following questions:

1. Identify the level of anxiety that J. S. is probably experiencing.

2. Which stressors are contributing to his anxiety level?

The nurse begins to interview J. S. for a health history. His eyes dart around the room and he answers questions with short, one-word responses. The nurse finds that she must repeat questions several times.

3. Formulate a tentative nursing diagnosis for J. S. based on the current data. Support the identified diagnosis with the etiological factors.

4. What would be the best actions for the nurse to take next?

5. J. S. is scheduled for a diagnostic test that requires his cooperation in maintaining certain positions. What does the nurse do to promote J. S.'s learning?

6. During the teaching/learning session, J. S. states, "My wallet is missing. I had over $2000 in it to pay for my hospital bill." What should the nurse do?

CHAPTER 8

Pain

LEARNING OBJECTIVES

At the end of this chapter, the student will be able to

- Define the experience of pain
- Identify the theories of the pain phenomenon
- Describe the anatomical and physiological basis of pain
- Describe pain perception, pain threshold, and pain tolerance
- Identify the psychosocial influences on pain
- Discuss nursing research findings on pain
- Distinguish between acute and chronic pain
- Identify assessment findings with acute and chronic pain
- Describe the characteristics of pain determined in the history
- Identify the objective data assessed during pain episodes
- List the nursing diagnoses directly and indirectly related to the client in pain
- Identify the goals for the client experiencing pain
- Describe pharmacologic measures to reduce acute pain
- Discuss nonpharmacologic measures to relieve acute pain
- Describe interventions for relief of chronic pain
- Discuss the physiological sequelae of opioid use
- Discuss the role of pain clinics in the treatment of chronic pain

PREREQUISITE KNOWLEDGE

Prior to beginning this chapter, the student should review

- The anatomy and physiology of the peripheral and central nervous systems
- The actions and side affects of opioid analgesics

STUDY QUESTIONS

Definitions of Pain

Match the following descriptions of the pain experience (1–8) with the authorship of the description (a–c). Answers may be used more than once.

_____ 1. stimulus indicating tissue damage

_____ 2. existing whenever the individual says it does

_____ 3. personal sensation of hurt

_____ 4. unpleasant sensory or emotional experience

_____ 5. definable only by the individual

_____ 6. whatever the individual says it is

_____ 7. response that protects from harm

_____ 8. described in terms of tissue damage

a. international definition

b. McCaffery

c. Sternbach

Pain Theories, Anatomy, and Physiology

Match the following pain-related concepts (9–13) with their associated theories (a–c). Answers may be used more than once.

_____ 9. pain conduction via rapid or slow fibers

_____ 10. transmission facilitated or inhibited

_____ 11. a unique discrete body sense

_____ 12. central summation

_____ 13. control at level of spinal cord

a. specificity
b. pattern
c. gate control

14. List the anatomical structures where painful stimuli can originate.

a. _____

_____

_____

b. _____

_____

_____

c. _____

_____

_____

15. Briefly explain the phenomenon of referred pain. Use a separate sheet.

16. Compare and contrast the characteristics of pain sensation originating in cutaneous, deep somatic, and visceral structures by completing the following chart on a separate sheet.

Origin	Localization	Intensity and Quality
a. cutaneous		
b. deep somatic		
c. visceral		

17. Briefly describe neuropathic pain: _____

_____

_____

_____

18. Identify the two types of nerve fibers responsible for transmitting pain stimuli and compare their structure and function by completing the following chart on a separate sheet.

Fiber	Structure	Function
a.		
b.		

19. Trace the route of pain from the peripheral stimulus to the cerebral cortex. Use a separate sheet.

Match the following definitions of concepts related to the pain experience (20–22) with their correct terms (a–c).

_____ 20. point at which individual feels and responds to pain

_____ 21. ability to endure the intensity of pain

_____ 22. awareness of the painful sensation

a. pain perception
b. pain threshold
c. pain tolerance

23. Identify two of the endogenous opiates and give their effects on the brain.

a. _____

_____

_____

b. _____

_____

_____

24. List the psychosocial variables that affect an individual's perception and response to pain. Use a separate sheet.

25. Define the term *psychosomatic pain.* Use a separate sheet.

26. Identify factors that may influence a nurse's ability to manage a client's pain episodes successfully. Use a separate sheet.

27. Compare acute and chronic pain by completing the following chart on a separate sheet. Submit the completed exercise to the clinical instructor.

	Acute	Chronic
a. etiology		
b. onset		
c. duration		
d. intensity		
e. localization		
f. characteristics		
g. emotional response		
h. physiologic response		

Collaborative Management

28. Briefly discuss why it is difficult for health care professionals to assess clients with chronic pain. Use a separate sheet.

29. List the subjective client data relevant to pain assessment. Use a separate sheet.

30. List the objective client data relevant to pain. Use a separate sheet.

31. Compare the advantages and disadvantages of using self-rating scales to measure pain. Use a separate sheet.

32. List the nursing diagnoses related to actual problems in clients experiencing pain.

    a. _____

    b. _____

33. List the nursing diagnoses clients with pain may have.

    a. _____

    b. _____

    c. _____

    d. _____

    e. _____

    f. _____

    g. _____

    h. _____

    i. _____

    j. _____

34. What is the goal for the client experiencing acute pain? _____

    _____

35. What are the goals for the client experiencing chronic pain?

    a. _____

    _____

    b. _____

    _____

36. What is the goal for the client experiencing cancer-related pain? _____

    _____

    _____

    _____

37. List four common classes of pharmacologic agents used to control pain and give an example of each.

    a. _____

    _____

    b. _____

    _____

    c. _____

    _____

    d. _____

    _____

38. Discuss the pitfalls of administering intermittent parenteral opioids on a prn schedule. Use a separate sheet.

39. Briefly discuss the rationale for using opioid adjuvants with opioid agents. Use a separate sheet.

40. List the assessments the nurse should make when caring for a client receiving opioid analgesics. Use a separate sheet.

41. Discuss the nurse's responsibilities in managing an epidural catheter inserted for analgesia. Use a separate sheet.

42. Briefly discuss why placebos are effective in clients who respond to them. Use a separate sheet.

43. Describe the advantages of patient-controlled analgesia (PCA). Use a separate sheet.

44. Identify the theoretical basis for the use of cutaneous stimulation as a pain relief intervention. Use a separate sheet.

45. List examples of cutaneous stimulation modalities used to manage pain.

    a. _____

    b. _____

    c. _____

    d. _____

    e. _____

46. Identify the limitations of cutaneous stimulation modalities in managing pain.

    a. _____

    _____

    _____

    b. _____

    _____

    _____

    c. _____

    _____

    _____

    d. _____

    _____

    _____

47. Compare the two types of transcutaneous electrical nerve stimulation (TENS) units by completing the following chart on a separate sheet.

	TENS	Pain Suppressor
a. type of pain		
b. local/systemic effects		
c. duration of use		
d. skin care		

48. Which of the following four statements is true about the strategy of distraction?

    a. Distraction is effective for acute and chronic pain relief.

    b. Distraction influences the cause of pain directly.

    c. Distraction may be used instead of other pain control measures.

    d. Distraction alters the perception of pain.

49. Which of the following statements about chronic pain management is true?

    a. Treatment begins with opioid agonists.

    b. Prn drug administration is preferred.

    c. Parental medications are preferred.

    d. Nonsteroidal anti-inflammatory agents (NSAIAs) are effective for managing mild pain.

50. Compare the advantages and disadvantages of using nonopioid agents for cancer pain management. Use a separate sheet.

Match the following classes of drugs (51–53) with their associated actions (a–c).

_____ 51. opioid agonists

_____ 52. opioid antagonists

_____ 53. antidepressants

    a. reverse the effects of morphine

    b. stimulate release of endogenous opiates

    c. bind to opiate receptor sites

Match the following definitions of physiological sequelae associated with opioid use (54–61) with their correct terms (a–c). Answers may be used more than once and more than one term may apply to each sequela.

_____ 54. persistent drug craving

_____ 55. withdrawal symptoms upon abrupt cessation

_____ 56. drug needed for normal tissue function

_____ 57. gradual resistance to opioid's effect

_____ 58. abuse for recreational purposes

_____ 59. adjustment of body to drug's adverse effects

_____ 60. higher doses needed to achieve pain relief

_____ 61. a common fear in clients

    a. physical dependency

    b. drug tolerance

    c. addiction

62. Which of the following statements about the adverse side effects of opioids is true?

    a. Bolus administration is less likely to produce central nervous system changes.

    b. Respiration may decrease with relaxation and pain relief.

    c. Opioid antagonists produce more respiratory depression than opioid agonists.

    d. Peripheral effects include vasoconstriction and elevated blood pressure.

Match the following descriptions (63–70) with their associated strategies for coping with pain (a–d). Answers may be used more than once.

_____ 63. massage to decrease muscle tension

_____ 64. physiological responses monitored

_____ 65. mental experience of sensations or events

_____ 66. altered state of consciousness

_____ 67. form of distraction

_____ 68. responses regulated using a variety of techniques

_____ 69. more effective when combined with other techniques

_____ 70. overall sense of reality lost

a. imagery
b. relaxation
c. hypnosis
d. biofeedback

71. Identify two purposes of acupuncture.

    a. _____

    _____

    b. _____

    _____

72. Briefly discuss the surgical procedure of rhizotomy in relationship to pain control. Use a separate sheet.

73. Discuss why pain clinics may refuse to treat clients suffering from chronic pain who receive financial disability payment or financial compensation from litigation, or who are involved in litigation for their pain-related problems. Submit the completed exercise to the clinical instructor on a separate sheet.

CRITICAL THINKING EXERCISES

Case Study: Acute Pain

T. O. is a 32-year-old man who fell 12 feet from a construction site. He is admitted to the hospital with a compression fracture of L-3 and L-4 and a fractured humerus. He has acute pain in his back, shooting down his legs, and in his arm. He can receive 10 mg of morphine every 3–4 hours for pain; his last does was at 7:30 a.m.

Address the following questions:

1. What is the physiological basis of his pain? Why does he have pain in his legs?

2. At 9:30 a.m. during his bath, he becomes very tense and complains of severe pain. What should be done for T. O.?

3. How can he be moved for his bath and his bed linen changed without increasing his pain?

4. The next morning he is given physician's orders to get up into a chair. How can he be ambulated to the chair without increasing his pain?

5. T. O. has required morphine every 3–4 hours for the past 3 days. What side effects should the nurse monitor for?

Case Study: Chronic Pain

R. U. is a 50-year-old woman involved in car accident 2 years ago. She has suffered with headaches and neck, shoulder, and back pain and spasms since that time. The pain has been nonprogressive, and physicians have ruled out physical causes of the pain. She has lost weight over the past 2 years and is currently taking two Percocet four times a day for pain relief, but recently it has not controlled the pain. She has not been able to return to work.

Address the following questions:

1. Describe three cognitive or behavioral strategies to decrease her pain.

2. How could opioids be tapered?

3. Discuss the advantages and disadvantages of giving her muscle relaxants.

4. Is R. U. a good candidate for a pain clinic? Why or why not?

Case Study: Cancer Pain

L. R. is a 62-year-old client admitted to the hospital with a diagnosis of terminal prostate cancer with metastasis to the spine and nerve entrapment of the spinal nerves. He had been at home under his wife's care until the pain became too severe for them to manage. He is ordered to have intrathecal morphine continuously at dosages needed to control his pain. His current needs for morphine are 1.5 mg every 10 minutes. He also receives prednisolone 7.5 mg T.I.D.

Address the following questions:

1. What side effects of these agents should the nurse observe for?

2. Mrs. R. says to the nurse, "My husband is going to be a drug addict if you keep giving him all of that stuff!" How should the nurse respond?

3. Should the nurse keep increasing the amount of opioid, or should other agents be used to control the pain?

4. L. R. says he wants to be dismissed and go to a foreign country for treatment of his cancer. He says that the treatment he is getting here is not helping him but that he has heard about a new treatment for cancer that involves large doses of vitamins. How should the nurse respond?

L. R.'s physician talks to him and his wife about surgical options for pain management. It is agreed that L. R. will have a trial nerve block and, if successful, a rhizotomy.

5. What is the purpose of a nerve block for L. R.? Why would the physician also recommend that a rhizotomy be done?

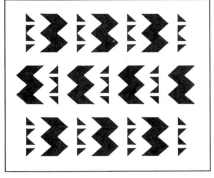

CHAPTER 9

Sensory Deprivation and Sensory Overload

LEARNING OBJECTIVES

At the end of this chapter, the student will be able to

■ Define *reception, perception, sensory deprivation,* and *sensory overload*

■ Discuss the central nervous system arousal mechanism

■ Describe the effects of hospitalization and placement in a long-term care facility on sensory overload and deprivation

■ Provide care for the client with sensory overload or deprivation

PREREQUISITE KNOWLEDGE

Prior to beginning this chapter, the student should review

■ Information related to aging, including sensory changes

■ The anatomy and physiology of the senses, sensory reception by the brain, the role of the reticular activating system, and the role of the central nervous system

STUDY QUESTIONS

Key Definitions

Match the following terms relating to the sensory process (1–5) with their correct definitions (a–e).

_____ 1. perception
_____ 2. reception
_____ 3. sensoristasis
_____ 4. sensory deprivation
_____ 5. sensory overload

a. result of an increase in environmental stimuli

b. impetus to maintain optimal level of sensory variation

c. result of a decrease in sensory input

d. ability to organize and comprehend incoming sensory stimuli

e. function of the sensory organs

Arousal Mechanism

6. Briefly discuss the role of the reticular activating system (RAS). Use a separate sheet.

7. Identify and describe two types of arousal mechanism disorders.

   a. _____

   _____

   _____

   b. _____

   _____

   _____

Sensory Deprivation and Sensory Overload

8. List the types of sensory deprivation and give an example of each.

   a. _____

   _____

   _____

   b. _____

   _____

   _____

   c. _____

   _____

   _____

   d. _____

   _____

   _____

   e. _____

   _____

   _____

   _____

   f. _____

   _____

   _____

   _____

9. List factors in the hospital setting that contribute to sensory deprivation.

   a. _____

   _____

   b. _____

   _____

   c. _____

   _____

   d. _____

   _____

   e. _____

   _____

10. Identify factors that affect the amount of sensory stimuli received by a client and give an example of each.

   a. _____

   _____

   b. _____

   _____

   c. _____

   _____

11. List the behavioral changes resulting from social isolation or confinement that have been identified by research.

   a. _____

   b. _____

   c. _____

12. List the behavioral changes in sensory-deprived healthy subjects that have been identified by research.

   a. _____

   b. _____

   c. _____

   d. _____

   e. _____

13. List four types of behavior changes observed in hospitalized clients that result from sensory deprivation. Give an example of each.

    a. _____

    _____

    b. _____

    _____

    c. _____

    _____

    d. _____

    _____

14. Describe the syndrome of critical care unit psychosis. Use a separate sheet.

15. Compare and contrast client behavior changes resulting from sensory deprivation versus sensory overload. Use a separate sheet.

Collaborative Management

16. List the subjective client data relevant to sensory input. Use a separate sheet.

17. List the objective client data relevant to sensory input. Use a separate sheet.

18. Identify four environmental factors the nurse should assess to determine the effect on a client's sensory processes.

    a. _____

    _____

    b. _____

    _____

    c. _____

    _____

    d. _____

    _____

19. Identify two etiologic factors that may contribute to sensory process alterations in the hospitalized client.

    a. _____

    _____

    b. _____

    _____

20. Compare and contrast the nursing interventions **CT** for sensory and perceptual alterations related to sensory overload versus sensory deprivation by completing the following chart on a separate sheet. Submit the completed exercise to the clinical instructor.

Stimulus	Deprivation	Overload
a. familiar objects		
b. time cues		
c. lighting levels		
d. teaching		
e. touch		
f. sound level		
g. rest periods		

21. List the expected outcomes for the nursing diagnosis of sensory and perceptual alterations.

    a. _____

    _____

    _____

    b. _____

    _____

    _____

    c. _____

    _____

    _____

CRITICAL THINKING EXERCISES

Case Study: Post-ICU Syndrome

B. T. is a 67-year-old male client who is transferred to a post-surgical nursing unit following a 5-day stay in the intensive care unit (ICU). Initially, he was hemodynamically unstable from shock and required vital signs monitoring every 15 minutes for 4 days and frequent interventions including suctioning and neurological assessment. Upon transfer to the medical nursing unit, B. T. is pale, has dark circles under his eyes, and looks fatigued. He states, "I hope I can get some rest here." After lunch, the nurse asks B. T. how well he ate. B. T. snaps, "I don't know; look for yourself."

Address the following questions:

1. Based on the above data, formulate a nursing diagnosis for B. T. and discuss the etiological factors.

2. What would be an appropriate reply for the nurse to make in response to B. T.'s comment about lunch?

3. Identify the assessments the nurse should perform to determine B. T.'s cognitive status.

B. T. continues to be irritable. He is on a regular diet and is to be ambulated at least twice a day. Vital signs are now monitored every 4 hours. Suctioning is no longer required. Pulmonary physical therapy treatments are ordered twice a day. A continuous intravenous infusion is in place, and cephalothin sodium (Keflin) 1 g is administered every 6 hours by intravenous piggyback.

4. Plan a schedule for B. T.'s treatments and interventions. Allow for rest periods and an optimal period of sleep during the night.

5. The intravenous solution is to infuse at a rate of 80 mL per hour. Calculate the drip rate for an administration set with a drip factor of 10 drops/mL.

6. The intermittent cephalothin sodium (Keflin) is diluted in 50 mL of D_5W and is to infuse over a 20-minute period. The piggyback administration set has a drip factor of 60 microdrops/mL. Calculate the drip rate required to administer a does of the antibiotic.

7. If all intravenous solutions are maintained at their specified rates of administration, what is the total volume of intravenous fluid B. T. receives in a 24-hour period?

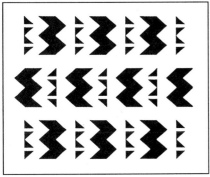

CHAPTER 10

Body Image

LEARNING OBJECTIVES

At the end of this chapter, the student will be able to

- Define the terms *body image, self-esteem,* and *self-concept*
- Describe factors that affect body image
- Describe Schilder's theory of body image
- Describe how body image changes throughout the life cycle
- Identify the effect of illness on body image
- Describe the adjustment response to body image changes
- Describe the effect of immobility, pain, alopecia, chronic illness, and eating disorders on body image
- Identify the effect of surgery on body image
- Use the nursing process to provide nursing care for the client with High Risk for or actual Alteration in Body Image

PREREQUISITE KNOWLEDGE

Prior to beginning this chapter, the student should review

- Information from general psychology as it relates to self-concept
- The principles of human growth and development as they relate to self-concept

STUDY QUESTIONS

Key Definitions

Match the following terms relating to self-ideation (1–3) with their correct definitions (a–c).

_____ 1. body image

_____ 2. self-concept

_____ 3. self-esteem

a. collection of feelings about one's self

b. an evaluation of one's self

c. internalized view of one's body

Factors Affecting Body Image

4. List four factors in the American culture that affect body image perception and give an example of each.

   a. _____

   _____

   b. _____

   _____

   c. _____

   _____

   d. _____

   _____

Theories of Body Image Development

Match the following body image changes (5–20) with their associated life cycle stages (a–h). Answers may be used more than once.

_____ 5. renewed interest in physical fitness

_____ 6. preoccupation with the body

_____ 7. increased fatigue

_____ 8. identifies feelings of discomfort

_____ 9. learns body concepts

_____ 10. development of secondary sexual features

_____ 11. focuses on physical appearance

_____ 12. begins to value body parts differently

_____ 13. stereotyping

_____ 14. use of hair dyes

_____ 15. feelings of worth-lessness

_____ 16. sexual identity begins to develop

_____ 17. influenced by one's occupation

_____ 18. verifies existence by touching

_____ 19. draws recognizable human figure

_____ 20. begins to trust feelings

a. infancy

b. toddlerhood

c. preschool years

d. middle childhood

e. adolescence

f. young adulthood

g. middle years

h. later years

Alterations in Body Image

21. Discuss the types of body image disturbances that may occur in clients with the following health problems: myocardial infarction; colostomy; prosthetic device; stroke; hypertension; amputation of a limb; diabetes mellitus; mastectomy; sudden hair loss; hearing loss. Submit the completed exercise to the clinical instructor on a separate sheet.

22. Briefly describe the effects of chronic illness on body image. Use a separate sheet.

Match the following descriptions of client behavior (23–30) with their associated stages of readjustment to altered body image (a–d). Answers may be used more than once.

_____ 23. passive dependency

_____ 24. adaptation of body image

_____ 25. refusal to believe a problem exists

_____ 26. mourning

_____ 27. anger and hostility

_____ 28. emotional growth

_____ 29. inability to make decisions

_____ 30. recognizing body change

a. psychologic shock

b. withdrawal

c. acknowledgment

d. integration

Match the following descriptions of client responses (31–35) with their associated stimuli (a–e).

_____ 31. fear of mutilation

_____ 32. unrealistic self-assessment

_____ 33. loss of independence

_____ 34. decreased self-esteem

_____ 35. isolation of a body part

a. immobility

b. pain

c. alopecia

d. surgery

e. obesity

Collaborative Management

36. List the historical client data relevant to body image. Use a separate sheet.

37. List the psychosocial client data relevant to body image. Use a separate sheet.

38. List the objective data relevant to body image. Use a separate sheet.

39. List the nursing diagnoses that are common in clients with body image disturbance.

a. _____

_____

b. _____

_____

c. _____

_____

40. Identify interventions the nurse uses to reduce anxiety in clients with actual or at high risk for disturbed body image.

    a. _____

    _____

    b. _____

    _____

    c. _____

    _____

    d. _____

    _____

41. A 24-year-old male law student sustains several deep lacerations and abrasions to the face from shattering glass. Discuss the short-term and long-term implications these injuries have for this individual. What interventions will assist him to reintegrate his body image and return to society? Submit the completed exercise to the clinical instructor on a separate sheet.

42. Briefly discuss why family members and significant others need support, as well as the client who has an altered body image. Use a separate sheet.

43. Dismissal planning for the client with altered body function includes which one of the following?

    a. discussion of long-term care needs

    b. warning that feelings of depression are abnormal

    c. assurance that daily routines will be similar at home

    d. referral to a support group after client has adjusted to being at home

CRITICAL THINKING EXERCISES

Case Study: Altered Body Image

M. M. is a 37-year-old client who has had a left radical mastectomy with a vertical incision. She returned to her room at 2:00 p.m., and it is now 8:00 p.m. A large compression dressing is in place, and a wound drain is connected to a closed suction bulb. M. M.'s husband is at her bedside. As the nurse enters the room, M. M. touches the dressing with her right hand and asks, "Is it gone?" Her husband looks at the nurse, gets up, and leaves the room.

Address the following questions:

1. What should the nurse do and say to M. M. at this time? What information does the nurse need so she can be the most therapeutic with M. M.?

After M. M. is comfortable and resting quietly, the nurse finds Mr. M. in the visitor's lounge. He is sitting with his head in his hands. The nurse sits next to him and tells him that he can return to the room. Mr. M. looks up and states, "I can't face her yet; I don't know what to say or do. It's so ugly!"

2. What should the nurse reply to Mr. M.?
3. What coping mechanism(s) is Mr. M. using?
4. Formulate a list of actual and potential nursing diagnoses for M. M. based on the known data.

Two day post-operatively the surgeon removes M. M.'s wound drain. During the procedure, M. M. keeps her head turned to the right. She asks the surgeon how the wound looks and when she can go home. Before he leaves, the surgeon tells M. M. that she is a candidate for breast reconstruction. M. M. later says to the nurse, "How can the doctor say that? A false breast can never replace the one I lost!"

5. What should the nurse do? What information would be beneficial to M. M. at this time?

Prior to dismissal, M. M. asks the nurse what can be done to help cover her scar.

6. What information can the nurse give to M. M.?

Six months after dismissal, M. M. returns to the same nursing unit. She is scheduled for left breast reconstruction the following day. M. M. is smiling and tells the nurse, "Well, I soon will be back to my old self again. I can't wait!"

7. What should the nurse reply?
8. What information does the nurse need to elicit from M. M. to determine if this is a realistic expectation?

CHAPTER 11

Human Sexuality

LEARNING OBJECTIVES

At the end of this chapter, the student will be able to

▌ Define *sexuality* and *sexual health*

▌ Identify factors that constitute sexual health

▌ Summarize research topics dealing with human sexuality

▌ Use appropriate interventions to promote clients' sexual health

PREREQUISITE KNOWLEDGE

Prior to beginning this chapter, the student should review

▌ The factors that influence sexuality and sexual health

STUDY QUESTIONS

Key Definitions

Match the following descriptions (1–8) with their associated sexuality concepts (a and b). Answers may be used more than once.

_____ 1. accurate knowledge of sexuality

_____ 2. inherited characteristics

_____ 3. social learning

_____ 4. awareness of attitudes toward sexual functioning

_____ 5. expression of attitudes, values, and behavior

_____ 6. congruency between gender assignment and identity

_____ 7. gender-associated attributes

_____ 8. freedom from impairment

a. human sexuality

b. sexual health

Theoretical Perspectives

9. Identify three aspects of human anatomy and physiology that are related to an individual's sexual health. Give an example of each.

a. _____

_____

_____

b. _____

_____

_____

c. _____

_____

_____

Match the following psychosexual behaviors (10–12) with their associated developmental stages (a–c).

_____ 10. adjustment to changes in sexual function

_____ 11. experimentation with explicit sexual activity

_____ 12. intimacy in relationships established

a. adolescence

b. early/middle adulthood

c. late adulthood

Match the following physiological responses (13–24) with their associated phases in the sexual response cycle(a–d). Answers may be used more than once.

_____ 13. ejaculatory inevitability

_____ 14. breast size increase

_____ 15. refractory period

_____ 16. nipple erection

_____ 17. state of prearousal

_____ 18. clitoris retraction

_____ 19. increased myotonia

_____ 20. vaginal lubrication

_____ 21. rhythmic contractions

_____ 22. increase in testicular size

_____ 23. detumescence

_____ 24. elevation of uterus and testes

a. excitement

b. plateau

c. orgasm

d. resolution

25. Identify variations in human sexual behavior and preference.

a. _____

b. _____

c. _____

d. _____

e. _____

26. Identify the sexual behavior variation that is considered to be a psychiatric disorder:

_____

CT 27. Discuss the changes in sexual function that occur in women and men during the aging process by completing the following chart on a separate sheet. Submit the completed exercise to the clinical instructor.

	Change
a. sexual arousal	
b. fertility	
c. vaginal lubrication	
d. ejaculatory volume	
e. need for intimacy	

28. Review Table 11-2 in the textbook, Effects of Illness on Adult Sexuality. Give an example illustrating how each of the following health problems may affect sexuality.

a. hospitalization: _____

_____

b. acute conditions: _____

_____

c. sexually transmitted diseases (STDs):

_____

_____

d. hypertension: _____

_____

e. arthritis: _____

_____

f. cancer: _____

_____

g. cardiovascular disease: _____

_____

h. diabetes mellitus: _____

_____

i. end-stage renal disease: _____

_____

29. Compare and contrast the effects of alcohol and other substances on sexuality during early-phase use versus late-phase abuse. Use a separate sheet.

30. Briefly discuss the effects an individual's attitudes and values have on his or her sexuality. Use a separate sheet.

31. List seven interpersonal skills that are essential to developing sexual relationships.

a. _____

_____

b. _____

_____

c. _____

_____

d. _____

_____

e. _____

_____

f. _____

_____

g. _____

_____

32. List attributes the nurse should possess to be able to assist clients with sexuality needs or problems and sexual health.

a. _____

_____

_____

b. _____

_____

_____

c. _____

_____

_____

d. _____

_____

_____

Collaborative Management

33. List the historical client data relevant to sexual health. Use a separate sheet.

34. List the psychosocial client data relevant to sexual health. Use a separate sheet.

35. List the objective client data relevant to sexual health. Use a separate sheet.

36. Identify etiological factors related to problems in sexual functioning.

a. _____

_____

b. _____

_____

c. _____

_____

d. _____

_____

e. _____

_____

37. Identify principles that direct the nurse in planning and implementing care for the client with a problem related to sexual dysfunction.

a. _____

_____

_____

b. _____

_____

c. _____

_____

d. _____

_____

_____

e. _____

_____

_____

38. What is ongoing behavior that a client and his or her partner should engage in while practicing the sensate focus technique?

_____

_____

CRITICAL THINKING EXERCISES

Case Study: Human Sexuality

In the following situations, identify the actual or potential nursing diagnoses related to human sexuality and develop plans for their nursing interventions.

1. A 50-year-old male client is admitted with uncontrolled hypertension related to noncompliance with taking his antihypertensive medications. He recently remarried. His prescriptions include methyldopa (Aldomet) 250 mg tid and hydrochlorothiazide (Esidrex) 25 mg qid. Develop a teaching plan.

2. A 35-year-old female client undergoes uterine dilation and curettage following the miscarriage of a planned pregnancy.

3. A 58-year-old male client has had a transurethral prostatectomy. He is concerned that the indwelling urinary catheter will have an effect on his future ability to have penile erections and successful intercourse.

4. An 18-year-old female client is being treated for second- and third-degree burns to the lower abdomen, labia, and upper thighs suffered when a deep-fat fryer overturned while she was cooking.

5.   A 26-year-old male client has epididymitis secondary to a mumps infection.

6. A 45-year-old female client, recently married, is in skeletal traction to her left lower extremity following an automobile accident.

7. A 22-year-old married man is being dismissed in a body cast following a spinal fusion. The cast will need to be worn for 12 weeks. Discuss options for sexual positions.

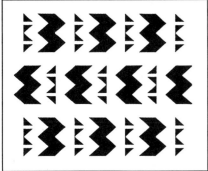

CHAPTER 12

Loss, Death, and Dying

LEARNING OBJECTIVES

At the end of this chapter, the student will be able to

▮ List the types of losses a person may experience

▮ Discuss the concepts of death and dying

▮ Identify responses to dying

▮ Discuss grieving

▮ Manage care for the grieving person

▮ Discuss the general features of hospice

▮ Compare and contrast the types of euthanasia

PREREQUISITE KNOWLEDGE

Prior to beginning this chapter, the student should review

▮ The concepts of stress, coping, and adaptation

STUDY QUESTIONS

Key Definitions

Match the following terms related to loss (1–4) with their correct definitions (a–d).

_____ 1. death

_____ 2. dying

_____ 3. grieving

_____ 4. loss

a. reaction to a loss

b. termination of life

c. the state of being without something one once had

d. a process leading to the end of life

5. Briefly describe the effect(s) the following types of loss may have on an individual.

a. loss of a loved one: _____

_____

_____

_____

b. loss of self: _____

_____

_____

_____

c. loss of objects: _____

_____

_____

_____

Dying, Death, and Grieving

6. Briefly explain, in your own terms, what is meant by the following sentence: "Medical and scientific advances have contributed to the longevity of life, but they have also contributed to the longevity of dying." Submit the completed exercise to the clinical instructor on a separate sheet. **CT**

7. List the traditional criteria used to determine whether death has occurred.

   a. _____

   _____

   b. _____

   _____

   c. _____

   _____

8. Briefly define the term *brain dead.* Use a separate sheet.

9. Contrast the term *persistent vegetative state* with the term *brain death.* Use a separate sheet.

10. Discuss the physiological significance of a definition of death that includes cessation of heartbeat as one of its criteria. Use a separate sheet.

11. Briefly discuss the ethical significance of having a clear definition of clinical death. Use a separate sheet.

12. List the stages identified by Kübler-Ross (1969) that individuals may experience in response to their own process of dying.

   a. _____

   b. _____

   c. _____

   d. _____

   e. _____

   f. _____

13. Briefly discuss the implications for nursing care that Kübler-Ross's and other researchers' findings have about the process of dying. Use a separate sheet.

14. Complete the following chart, on a separate sheet, by briefly defining and giving examples illustrating the identified pattern of living-dying.

Pattern	Example
a. peaks and valleys	
b. descending plateaus	
c. downward slope	
d. gradual slant	

15. Which of the following statements is correct about the grief response?

   a. It follows a predictable timetable.

   b. It is effective when the pain of loss can be faced.

   c. It occurs only in response to the death of a loved person.

   d. It follows progressive stages in all individuals.

16. Identify the goals for survivors of loss.

   a. _____

   _____

   _____

   _____

   b. _____

   _____

   _____

17. List the client data associated with grief. Use a separate sheet.

Match the following behaviors (18–29) with their associated phases of the grief response (a–e). Answers may be used more than once.

____ 18. resumption of life patterns	a. shock and disbelief
____ 19 lack of confidence	b. yearning, protest, anger, and guilt
____ 20. dreaming that the deceased person is alive	c. anguish, disorganization, and despair
____ 21. exhibiting the deceased person's mannerisms	d. indentification with the deceased person
____ 22. realization that loss is permanent	e. reorganization and restitution
____ 23. rejection of comfort measures	
____ 24. anger at the deceased person	
____ 25. transitory re-experiencing of pain	
____ 26. withdrawal from activities	
____ 27. fear of losing one's mind	
____ 28. crying and tearfulness	
____ 29. development of a new identity	

30. List the indications of high-risk bereavement. Use a separate sheet.

31. Identify groups of people at high risk for troublesome grief reactions. Use a separate sheet.

Collaborative Management

32. List the historical client data relevant to loss and death. Use a separate sheet.

33. List the psychosocial client data relevant to loss and death. Use a separate sheet.

34. List the objective client data relevant to loss and death. Use a separate sheet.

35. List the nursing diagnoses common to loss, death, or grief.

    a. _____

    _____

    b. _____

    _____

    c. _____

    _____.

Match the following interventions for grieving (36–40) with the examples of statements that best illustrate them (a–e).

_____ 36. offering physical or emotional support

_____ 37. facilitating expression of emotion

_____ 38. being realistic

_____ 39. avoiding explanations of the loss

_____ 40. teaching the family about physical signs of dying

a. "It's hard to understand why people have to die."

b. "Losing a loved one is painful."

c. "A support group meets regularly in your area."

d. "You can cry if it makes you feel better."

e. "Joe may have difficulty speaking and lie still most of the time."

41. Which one of the following interventions is correct when performing post-mortem care?

    a. Place the head of the bed at 30 degrees.

    b. Remove pillows from under the head.

    c. Leave a foley (indwelling) catheter in place in the bladder.

    d. Place pads under the hips and around the perineum.

42. Which one of the following interventions is correct in the unanticipated death of a client?

    a. Remove the body to the morgue or funeral home as soon as possible.

    b. Remove all tubes and lines from the body before significant others arrive.

    c. Leave all supplies, medications, or resuscitation equipment in the room for significant others to see.

    d. Allow the eyes to remain open so that a significant other may be the one to close them.

43. List interventions that may be helpful to dying clients and their significant others as they attempt to cope with fear. Use a separate sheet.

44. Identify which of the following apply when describing the concept of hospice.

    a. control of the disease process

    b. a special place

    c. control of symptoms

    d. ends with death

    e. palliative care in multiple settings

    f. care available 24 hours a day

    g. a philosophy of care

    h. makes terminal illness pleasant

    i. multidisciplinary approach

    j. support of family ends with client's death

    k. nonfragmented care

Match the following definitions of the types of euthanasia (45–48) with their correct terms (a–d).

_____ 45. refusal of heroic life-sustaining measures

_____ 46. intentionally committed act to shorten life

_____ 47. decided by someone other than the client

_____ 48. omission of life-sustaining measures

a. active

b. involuntary

c. passive

d. voluntary

49. Briefly present your opinion about suicide. **CT** Include in the discussion whether this act is ever justifiable. Submit the completed exercise to the clinical instructor on a separate sheet.

CHAPTER APPENDIX

To be effective therapeutically with dying clients, one must be aware of one's own mortality. The following exercise is designed to facilitate the student's understanding of his or her own mortality.

Personal Questionnaire: Perspectives on Dying

1. My first personal involvement with dying was with
   a. grandparent or great-grandparent
   b. parent
   c. brother or sister
   d. other family member
   e. friend or acquaintance
   f. stranger
   g. public figure
   h. pet

2. When I was young, the subject of dying was talked about in my family
   a. openly
   b. with some sense of discomfort
   c. only when necessary and then with an attempt to exclude me
   d. as though it were a taboo subject
   e. never that I can recall

3. My childhood concept of what happens after death is best described as
   a. heaven and hell
   b. the after-life
   c. a sleep
   d. cessation of all physical and mental activity
   e. mysterious and unknowable
   f. something other than the above
   g. no concept

4. Today, my concept of what happens after death is best described as
   a. heaven and hell
   b. the after-life
   c. a sleep
   d. cessation of all physical and mental activity
   e. mysterious and unknowable
   f. something other than the above
   g. no concept

5. My present attitudes toward dying have been most influenced by
   a. the death of someone else
   b. specific readings
   c. my religious upbringing
   d. introspection and meditation
   e. ritual (e.g., funerals)
   f. television, radio, or motion pictures
   g. the longevity of my family
   h. my health or physical condition

6. The role that religion has played in the development of my attitudes about dying is
   a. very important
   b. rather important
   c. somewhat important, but not major
   d. relatively minor
   e. nothing at all

7. I think about dying
   a. very frequently (at least once a day)
   b. frequently
   c. occasionally
   d. rarely (no more than once a year)
   e. very rarely or never

8. To me, death means
   a. the end; the final process of life
   b. the beginning of life after death
   c. a joining of the spirit with a universal cosmic consciousness
   d. a kind of endless sleep; rest and peace
   e. termination of this life but with survival of the spirit
   f. don't know

9. To me, the most disagreeable aspect of my death would be that I would
   a. no longer be able to have experiences
   b. be afraid of what might happen to my body
   c. be uncertain of what might happen to me if there is a life after death
   d. no longer be able to provide for my family
   e. cause grief to my relatives and friends
   f. not be able to complete all my plans and projects
   g. die painfully

10. I feel that the cause of most deaths
    a. results directly from the conscious efforts of the persons who die
    b. has a strong component of conscious or unconscious participation by the people who die (in their habits and use, misuse, nonuse, or abuse of drugs, alcohol, medicine, etc.)
    c. is not discernible; they are caused by events over which individuals have no control

11. I _____ believe that psychological factors can influence or even cause a person to begin dying.
    a. firmly
    b. tend to
    c. do and do not
    d. do not

12. When I think of dying or when circumstances make me aware of my own mortality, I feel
    a. fearful
    b. discouraged
    c. depressed
    d. purposeless
    e. resolved in relation to life
    f. pleasure in being alive

13. I feel the degree of effort that should be made to keep a fatally ill person alive is
    a. all possible effort
    b. reasonable for the person's age, physical condition, mental condition, and pain
    c. that after reasonable care has been given, a person ought to be permitted to die a natural death
    d. that a person should not be kept alive by elaborate artificial means

14. If my physician knew that I had a terminal disease, I _____ want him to tell me.
    a. would
    b. would not

15. If I had a terminal illness, I would _____ to talk to someone about my dying.
    a. want
    b. not want

16. I would most want to talk to _____ about my dying.
    a. spouse
    b. immediate family member
    c. relative
    d. clergyman
    e. physician
    f. nurse

17. I probably would feel _____ about talking with someone about my dying.
    a. embarrassed
    b. distressed
    c. willing
    d. at ease

18. If someone close to me had a terminal illness, I _____ want that person told.
    a. would
    b. would not

19. If someone close to me knew that he or she had a terminal illness and wanted to talk to me about dying, I would feel
    a. embarrassed
    b. distressed
    c. willing
    d. at ease

20. When I think of dying, I mostly fear
    a. a long-term illness
    b. a painful death
    c. that I'll be mentally disoriented
    d. physical disability
    e. having others take care of my personal needs
    f. what lies after death

21. The sight of a dead body is
    a. horrifying to me
    b. natural
    c. pleasant
    d. unsettling

22. When I'm notified of a funeral, I
    a. usually decline gracefully
    b. attend if at all possible
    c. dread it but usually go
    d. am happy to attend

23. When people talk about death in a social situation, I feel

    a. nervous

    b. like leaving the room

    c. interested in what they have to say

    d. generally disinterested

24. The fatal illness that I am most afraid of getting is

    a. heart disease

    b. cancer

    c. kidney failure

    d. overwhelming infection

    e. other (specify) _____

    _____

25. So far in my life, I feel that

    a. it has been satisfying

    b. I wish I could start over

    c. I have been very fortunate

    d. I have made some bad decisions

    e. I have been cheated out of lots of good things

    f. I have worked too hard

    g. I have wasted too much time

Reprinted with permission of Concept Media—*Perspectives on Dying*—Personal Questionnaire.

CRITICAL THINKING EXERCISES

Case Studies: Interventions for Grief

Discuss the following grief situations and how the nurse should intervene.

1. A 60-year-old male client is one day postoperative following an exploratory laparotomy. The surgeon found extensive inoperable cancer of the head of the pancreas. During morning rounds, the client asks the nurse, "What did the surgeon find?"

2. A student nurse is assigned to care for a 46-year-old female client who is terminally ill. The client has a daughter the same age as the student. Upon entering the client's room for the first time, the client states, "I don't want a student to take care of me. I want someone who knows what she is doing."

3. A nurse has been caring for a 74-year-old female client who reminds the nurse of her grandmother. Both the client and her family are fond of the nurse and often request that this particular nurse be assigned to care for the client, who is dying. One evening, the client dies while the nurse is working on another unit. The client's family requests that the nurse do the postmortem care; shortly after, a family member asks the nurse to come to the client's funeral.

4. A 28-year-old client is undergoing a spontaneous abortion and is admitted to a general medical nursing unit. This is the first pregnancy that the client has been able to carry beyond the first trimester. She has had two previous spontaneous abortions. The nurse answers the call light and the client asks for pain medication. She had been crying. While getting the injection, the client states, "This is so unfair, I would be a good mother."

5. A 52-year-old male client is 6 days postoperative following coronary artery bypass surgery. He was transferred to a general surgical nursing unit from the intensive care unit the previous day. During morning report, the client is found in bed, unresponsive, pulseless and not breathing, cyanotic, and cool. While awaiting the client's physician to pronounce the client dead, the client's wife is seen coming down the hall to her husband's room.

6. A 37-year-old female client has bilateral, inoperable breast cancer. She has had extensive treatment with chemotherapy and wants to go home after refusing further treatment. While packing her belongings, the client says to the nurse, "It will be so peaceful at home after this hospitalization. I've never been in so much pain."

C H A P T E R 1 3

Chronic and Disabling Conditions

LEARNING OBJECTIVES

At the end of this chapter, the student will be able to

- Describe chronic illness
- Differentiate the terms *impairment, disability,* and *handicap*
- Discuss the theories of rehabilitation
- Identify the settings for rehabilitation
- Identify the focus of the rehabilitation team
- Describe the assessment of the client undergoing rehabilitation
- Describe functional assessment tools
- Discuss psychological and vocational assessments
- Discuss management of the client with the nursing diagnosis of Impaired Physical Mobility
- Discuss management of the client with the nursing diagnosis of Self-Care Deficit
- Discuss management of the client with the nursing diagnosis of High Risk for Impaired Skin Integrity
- Discuss management of the client with the nursing diagnosis of Altered Patterns of Urinary Elimination
- Discuss management of the client with the nursing diagnosis of Constipation
- Discuss management of the client with the nursing diagnosis of Ineffective Individual Coping
- Describe home care preparation for the rehabilitated client

PREREQUISITE KNOWLEDGE

Prior to beginning this chapter, the student should review

- The anatomy and physiology of the neurologic, muscular, cardiac, and respiratory systems
- The techniques for urinary catheterization and bowel care
- The principles of bathing, transferring a client, range-of-motion (ROM), and ambulation techniques
- The hazards of immobility
- The concept of body image
- The concepts of loss and grieving
- The concept of adult development
- The concept of human sexuality

STUDY QUESTIONS

Key Definitions

1. List the characteristics of chronic illness.

   a. _____

   _____

   b. _____

   _____

   c. _____

   _____

   d. _____

   _____

   e. _____

   _____

2. Which of the following is *not* considered to be a chronic illness?

   a. arthritis

   b. coronary artery disease

   c. cancer

   d. skeletal fracture

   Match the following definitions (3–6) with their correct terms (a–d).

   _____ 3. process of learning to live with a disability

   _____ 4. an abnormality of a body structure or system function that is temporary or permanent

   _____ 5. disadvantage experienced due to a difference between performance and expectations

   _____ 6. consequence of an impairment

   a. disability
   b. handicap
   c. impairment
   d. rehabilitation

Theories

7. Briefly define *powerlessness:* _____

   _____

   _____

8. The nurse is caring for a paraplegic client who is hospitalized for treatment of ischial ulcers. He works late evenings as a disc jockey at a local radio station. Today, he needs to be bathed, sent to physical therapy for whirlpool treatment, and have his bladder catheterized every 6 hours. How could the theory of powerlessness be used to plan these activities?

   a. Schedule the whirlpool treatment in the physical therapy department later in the morning.

   b. Give him a bath right after breakfast, perform the catheterization, and send him to physical therapy.

   c. Ask the client when he wants to get a bath, have his bladder catheterized, and go to physical therapy.

   d. Complete the bath and catheterization procedures, working around the scheduled time for physical therapy.

9. Adaptation to a change requires

   a. independence

   b. inner energy

   c. discouragement

   d. interpretation

10. A 76-year-old female client had a left cerebrovascular accident (CVA) 2 weeks ago. She entered a rehabilitation setting on her physician's instructions. The nurse's notes indicate that the client is passive with the staff, saying, "I don't care; do whatever you want to do." The client moves about reluctantly. From these data, what can be inferred about the client's adaptation to her illness? The client

    a. may be having problems adapting and may need to be handled firmly so that complications do not occur.

    b. may be having problems adapting and more data should be collected before a conclusion can be reached.

    c. is not adapting to her condition due to the CVA's effects on her ability to reason rationally.

    d. is not adapting to her condition and is unable to be rehabilitated at this time.

11. Which of the following descriptions illustrates coping based on the definition of *coping* as an effort to manage, including anything a person does regardless of how well it works?

    a. denying the severity of illness by forcing oneself to do tasks impossible to perform

    b. seeking information to assist with managing a complex treatment schedule

    c. drinking alcoholic beverages to relax and decrease one's focus on illness

    d. all of the above.

CT 12. A 66-year-old retired coal miner lives with his wife at home. He has end-stage chronic airflow limitation (CAL). He is on continuous oxygen at 2 L per minute, receives six medications per day on varying schedules, and has inhalation therapy tid. Because he has dyspnea on exertion, the client is unable to perform his activities of daily living (ADL) without assistance. Discuss how the categories of coping tasks are evident in this client. What could the nurse do to assist this client with his coping? Submit the completed exercise to the clinical instructor on a separate sheet.

13. Identify the types of interventions (according to Orem) used by the nurse to assist a client's move toward health once a self-care deficit is identified.

    a. _____

    b. _____

    c. _____

    d. _____

14. Which of the following statements best reflects the comparison of self-concept changes between a client with bilateral arm burns and one who is receiving kidney dialysis for end-stage renal disease?

    a. The client with arm burns would have a more negative self-concept than the client on dialysis.

    b. The client on dialysis would have a more negative self-concept than the client with arm burns.

    c. There is no absolute way to predict the self-concept changes with illness.

    d. Both clients would have the same degree of negative self-concept change.

15. When assessing the family of a client with a chronic illness, data should include the client's

    a. strengths as an individual

    b. relationships with peers

    c. role and role functions in the group

    d. ability to communicate with the health care team

16. List the data included in an assessment of the family of a client with chronic illness. Use a separate sheet.

Rehabilitation and the Health Care System

17. Which of the following settings is *not* a setting for rehabilitation after hospitalization?

    a. board and care nursing home

    b. vocational rehabilitation center

    c. independent living center

    d. outpatient hospital rehabilitation center

18. Identify the two major purposes of the rehabilitation team.

    a. _____

    _____

    b. _____

    _____

Match the following members of the rehabilitation team (19–28) with their role descriptions (a–j).

____ 19. client

____ 20. nurse

____ 21. occupational therapist

____ 22. physical therapist

____ 23. physician

____ 24. psychologist

____ 25. recreational therapist

____ 26. social worker

____ 27. speech pathologist

____ 28. vocational counselor

a. assists with managing mobility problems

b. retrains clients with language or hearing problems

c. counsels about family or financial problems

d. assists with job placement or retraining

e. has final authority regarding treatment plan

f. assists with managing ADL

g. counsels about reactions to disability

h. leads the rehabilitation team

i. helps develop new hobbies or interests

j. coordinates team members

Assessment

29. List six categories of data that should be collective on all clients with a disabling or chronic illness.

    a. _____

    _____

b. _____

_____

c. _____

_____

d. _____

_____

e. _____

_____

f. _____

_____

30. List the data included in baseline assessment for the client entering a rehabilitation program. Use a separate sheet.

31. A client with decreased cardiac output is entering a rehabilitation program. Data collection should include whether the client

a. has shortness of breath with activity

b. has the ability to ambulate without angina

c. feels rested upon awakening from sleep

d. uses an antihistamine for pollen allergies

32. A 60-year-old man with cardiomyopathy is admitted to a rehabilitation facility. He is being admitted for medication management and strengthening. What data should be collected on admission? What data could be collected the following day? Submit the completed exercise to the clinical instructor on a separate sheet.

33. A client with tuberculosis is entering a rehabilitation program. Data collection should include whether the client

a. can endure activity without angina

b. is on fluid restriction

c. is able to manage his or her own toileting

d. knows the reason for taking his or her medications

34. A 52-year-old female client with CAL is transferred to a skilled extended care facility for further rehabilitation and ADL management. The client is oxygen dependent and has an order for continuous low-flow oxygen at 2 L per minute. What data should be collected upon admission? What data could be collected the following day? Submit the completed exercise to the clinical instructor on a separate sheet.

35. Gastrointestinal system assessment of the client who is entering a rehabilitation program should include

a. family and cultural background

b. baseline hemoglobin and hematocrit measurements

c. pre-illness habits of bowel elimination

d. manual dexterity, muscle control, and mobility

e. all of the above

36. A 27-year-old male client is being admitted to a  rehabilitation hospital with paraplegia. He was involved in a motorcycle accident 2 weeks ago and is now being dismissed from an acute care agency. The client is the father of two children ages 7 and 5 years. His wife works full-time as a waitress. What data should be collected upon admission? What data could be collected the following day? Submit the completed exercise to the clinical instructor on a separate sheet.

37. List the genitourinary system data relevant for the client who is entering a rehabilitation program. Use a separate sheet.

38. A client with a neurogenic bladder is to be taught how to perform intermittent self-catheterization. Which of the following is essential for the nurse to assess before beginning the teaching–learning sessions?

a. motor function of both upper extremities

b. whether a head injury had been sustained

c. perception of position sense and fine touch

d. all of the above

39. A 35-year-old woman with myasthenia gravis is admitted to a rehabilitation unit for assistance with strengthening exercises and ADL management. What data should be collected upon admission? What data could be collected the following day? Submit the completed exercise to the clinical instructor on a separate sheet.

40. List the data relevant to the musculoskeletal system for the client who is entering a rehabilitation program.

a. _____

_____

b. _____

_____

c. _____

_____

d. _____

_____

41. List the data relevant to the integumentary system for the client who has high risk for skin breakdown. Use a separate sheet.

42. List the data relevant to the integumentary system for the client with actual skin breakdown. Use a separate sheet.

43. Describe the purpose of functional assessment. Use a separate sheet.

44. Which of the following statements is correct about functional assessment tools?

    a. The PULSES Profile is used to evaluate care and develop data for longitudinal projection of an illness.

    b. The Katz Index of ADL is used to evaluate and classify functional capacity in chronically ill people.

    c. The Barthel Index is used to measure functional ability and mobility in the physically impaired.

    d. The Functional Independence Measure provides a general assessment for program evaluation.

45. List the theories and concepts that are used as a basis for understanding a client's psychological response to chronic illness and resulting disability.

    a. _____

    b. _____

    c. _____

    d. _____

    e. _____

    f. _____

    g. _____

46. Identify the purpose of vocational assessment:

    _____

    _____

Planning and Implementation

47. When assisting a client with a hemiparesis to transfer or ambulate, the nurse should instruct the client to

    a. lean the body weight backward

    b. use the weaker hand to assist

    c. lean the body weight on the nurse

    d. use the strong hand to assist

48. One of the earliest complications to occur with immobility is

    a. pressure sores

    b. renal calculi

    c. osteoporosis

    d. fractures

49. Which of the following statements is correct for ROM exercise? ROM exercises are performed

    a. for the knees, hips, elbows, and shoulders

    b. on each joint three times per session

    c. up to the point of pain or stiffness

    d. on each joint two times per day

50. When a client needs to increase musculoskeletal strength, which type of ROM exercise is indicated?

    a. active

    b. passive

    c. assisted

    d. resistive

51. Which of the following writing devices would be easiest to use by the client who has a weakened dominant hand?

    a. lead pencil

    b. wide magic marker

    c. crayon

    d. ballpoint pen

52. Energy conservation techniques include

    a. obtaining grooming equipment as it is needed

    b. scheduling physical therapy right after lunch

    c. providing a bed side commode for a hemiplegic client

    d. placing the bed controls on the client's weaker side

53. Which of the following clients is at greatest risk of developing a pressure sore?

    a. a 26-year-old woman who has had a tonsillectomy

    b. a 74-year-old woman who has had a bowel resection

    c. an 80-year-old man who has metastatic prostate cancer

    d. a 35-year-old man who is somnolent from a head injury

54. The use of mechanical pressure-relieving devices

    a. effectively eliminates the need to turn clients

    b. still requires repositioning clients regularly

    c. prevents pressure sores in debilitated clients

    d. has been shown to be ineffective against pressure sores

55. Intermittent catheterization is a method of bladder training best used for the client with the bladder pattern called

   a. reflex

   b. flaccid

   c. uninhibited

   d dysreflexia

56. The client who performs intermittent self-catheterization should use a sterile catheter when hospitalized because

   a. the clean technique is ineffective even when in the home setting

   b. the client is probably immunosuppressed and is prone to superinfections

   c. the risk of contracting a nosocomial infection is high in that environment

   d. the agency needs to be able to charge for the use of its supplies and nursing time

57. The practice of clamping in-dwelling urinary catheter drainage tubing increases the client's risk of

   a. bladder rupture

   b. ureterovesicular reflux

   c. kidney damage

   d. urinary tract infection

   e. all of the above

58. Which of the following medications would the client with a flaccid bladder most likely be given?

   a. dantrolene sodium (Dantrium)

   b. bethanechol chloride (Urecholine)

   c. flavoxate hydrochloride (Urispas)

   d. oxybutynin chloride (Ditropan)

59. Which of the following beverages should be included in the diet of the client with bladder dysfunction?

   a. lemonade

   b. orange juice

   c. prune juice

   d. ginger ale

60. Factors that should be assessed before initiating a bowel control regimen include

   a. the client's lifelong evacuation habits

   b. any use of stool softeners or laxatives

   c. the type, amount, and frequency of fluid intake

   d. the client's ability to perform the Valsalva maneuver

   e. all of the above

61. Which of the following clients is most likely to have a flaccid bowel dysfunction?

   a. a 28-year-old man with a crushed pelvis

   b. a 54-year-old man with Guillain–Barré syndrome

   c. an 18-year-old woman with a displaced cervical fracture

   d. a 68-year-old woman with a cerebrovascular accident

62. Digital stimulation of the rectum as a method of re-establishing bowel control is most successful in the client who has had

   a. a recent myocardial infarction

   b. chronic diarrhea resulting from radiation to the bowel

   c. constipation resulting from medications taken for pain control

   d. a spinal cord injury resulting from a diving accident

63. The drug of choice for long-term management of bowel dysfunction is

   a. castor oil

   b. senna (Senokot)

   c. glycerin suppository

   d. lactulose (Cephulac)

64. An example of a food that should be part of breakfast for the client with bowel dysfunction is

   a. raisins

   b. white bread

   c. cheddar cheese

   d. sausage links

65. Support systems for the client with a disability may include

   a. clergy member

   b. family members

   c. self-help groups

   d. all of the above

66. Which of the following statements best reflects the purpose of a disabled client going home on a leave of absence visit prior to being dismissed from a health care agency?

    a. The client may feel intense anxiety about going home and must prove to the health care team that independent living is once again possible.

    b. The client has specific goals for the leave of absence experience and needs to identify tasks or problems in the home setting that require further management.

    c. The pass for the leave of absence includes detailed, specific written instructions explaining all the steps for the various procedures that the client needs to perform or direct.

    d. The leave of absence experience forces the client to confront fears and anxieties about dismissal and provides an opportunity for demonstrating self-care capability.

CRITICAL THINKING EXERCISES

Case Study: Stroke Rehabilitation

F. S. is a 68-year-old female client who suffered a cerebral vascular accident (CVA) one week ago. She has a left hemiparesis and right-sided facial muscle weakness. F. S. also has difficulty with constipation and urinary incontinence. Prior to the CVA, F. S. was left-handed dominant for activities such as writing and eating. She has some problems with depth perception because the staff have reported that F. S. has placed her drinking glasses on the edge of the tray table rather than in the middle of it.

Address the following questions:

1. Based on the above data, what are the relevant nursing diagnoses for F. S.?

2. What problems should the nurse expect that F. S. will have with self-feeding and meeting her nutritional needs? What interventions may be helpful to F. S. when assisting her to compensate for these problems?

3. Identify the type of bowel and bladder pattern dysfunctions that F. S. most likely has.

4. Develop a plan of care that will assist F. S. in regaining control of her bowel and bladder functions.

F. S. is noted to be slumping over to her left side in the wheelchair. She had her left hand caught in the wheel, and when approached by the staff, F. S. thought that she was sitting upright, replying, "I'm OK."

5. What nursing diagnosis is used to describe specifically this problem? What interventions can be prescribed for it?

6. F. S. goes to physical therapy twice a day for ambulation and gait training. She has been fitted with a four-point cane and is to be ambulated on the nursing unit for toileting and mobilization. When attempting to assist her to ambulate to the bathroom, F. S. laughs until she cries and then sobs openly while in the bathroom. How can the nurse work with her emotional lability?

7. Describe what the nurse should do to assist F. S. with ambulation.

F. S. makes steady progress with the gait training and is able to feed herself with devices supplied by the occupational therapist. She is scheduled for dismissal to home in the care of her 70-year-old husband. They have no children or other family members who live close by. Their home is in a neighborhood of older single and duplex homes.

8. Discuss what should be done to prepare F. S. and her husband for dismissal.

9. What should be included in the home environment assessment?

10. What resources could be used to help the couple adjust to the transition from hospital to home?

CHAPTER 14

Fluid and Electrolyte Balance

LEARNING OBJECTIVES

At the end of this chapter, the student will be able to

- Define the *solvent–solute relationship*
- Compare *diffusion, osmosis,* and *active transport*
- Discuss the dynamics in the capillary that affect fluid volume
- Describe the role of aldosterone, antidiuretic hormone, and atrial natriuretic peptide in fluid balance
- Describe the composition and distribution of body water
- Discuss the electrolytes sodium, potassium, calcium, phosphorus, magnesium, and chloride
- Identify the changes in water and electrolyte balance with age
- Assess the client with potential or actual Fluid Volume Deficit or Excess

PREREQUISITE KNOWLEDGE

Prior to beginning this chapter, the student should review

- Fluid and electrolytes as reviewed in an anatomy and physiology course

STUDY QUESTIONS

Anatomy and Physiology Review

Match the following substances (1–6) with their correct category (a or b). Answers may be used more than once.

____	1. water	a.	solvent
____	2. sodium	b.	solute
____	3. potassium		
____	4. urea		
____	5. alcohol		
____	6. creatinine		

7. a. Using Figure 1a on the following page as the starting point, draw the process of osmosis in Figure 1b. Label the water levels and particle concentration on each side of the semipermeable membrane.

   b. Using Figure 2a on the following page as a starting point, draw the process of diffusion in Figure 2b. Label the water levels and particle concentration on each side of the semipermeable membrane.

8. Identify where the process of filtration occurs in the body:

   _____

   _____

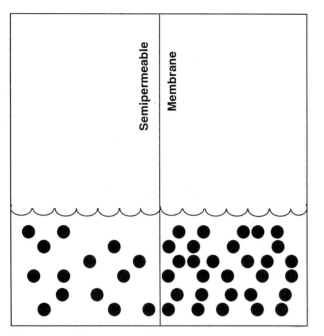

Figure 1a. Osmosis before

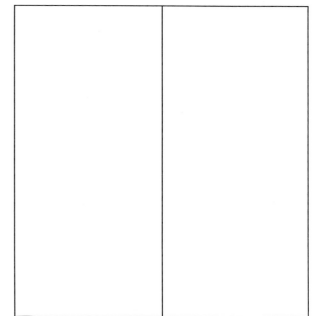

Figure 1b. Osmosis after

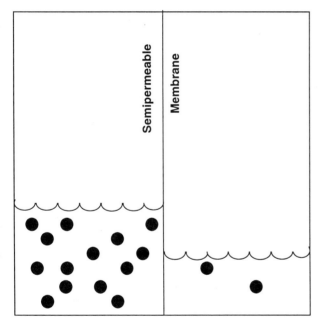

Figure 2a. Diffusion before

Figure 2b. Diffusion after

9. Which of the following examples best illustrates the principle of diffusion?

   a. water boiling at 212°F

   b. feeling cold when coming out of a swimming pool

   c. smelling smoke 12 feet away from a fire

   d. ice cubes floating in a glass of water

10. Explain facilitated diffusion as it occurs in type I diabetes mellitus. What problems might be experienced by a client with this disease? Use a separate sheet.

11. Discuss how osmosis differs from diffusion. Use a separate sheet.

12. What force results when a solute dissociates into ions and diffuses throughout a solution?

Match the following examples of intravenous solutions (13–16) with their osmotic properties (a–c). (Hint: body fluids are 0.9% salt.) Answers may be used more than once.

_____ 13. 1.5% salt

_____ 14. 0.9% salt

_____ 15. 0.45% salt

_____ 16. 0.02% salt

a. hypertonic

b. hypotonic

c. isotonic

17. Identify the form of solvent–solute movement that requires energy and give an example:

_____

_____

18. Identify the factors that determine blood flow at the capillary level.

a. _____

_____

b. _____

_____

c. _____

_____

19. Put the following five steps in order to illustrate the process of blood flow through a capillary.

_____ a. Osmosis pulls water from the tissues back into the capillary.

_____ b. Excess fluid that is not reabsorbed enters the lymphatic system.

_____ c. Plasma filters into the tissue spaces where pressure is lower.

_____ d. Blood enters the arterial end at 32 mm Hg pressure.

_____ e. The reabsorption force out of the tissue spaces exceeds the plasma hydrostatic pressure.

20. Which of the following substances creates colloid osmotic pressure in the capillaries?

a. albumin

b. plasma

c. salt

d. sugar

Match the following hormones (21–26) with their corresponding effects (a–f).

_____ 21. aldosterone

_____ 22. angiotensin I

_____ 23. angiotensin II

_____ 24. antidiuretic hormone (ADH)

_____ 25. atrial natriuretic peptide

_____ 26. renin

a. increases sodium and water loss in urine

b. stimulates release of aldosterone from the adrenal cortex

c. converts a substrate to angiotensin I

d. causes some vasoconstriction

e. increases reabsorption of sodium in the distal convoluted tubule

f. increases permeability to water in distal convoluted tubule and collecting duct

27. Which of the following clients would most likely have increased aldosterone secretion? One who

a. has excessive salt ingestion

b. has excessive water ingestion

c. loses both water and salt

d. loses potassium and water

Match the following compartments for body fluids (28–30) with their descriptions (a–c).

_____ 28. extracellular (ECF)

_____ 29. intracellular (ICF)

_____ 30. transcellular (TCF)

a. fluids found in the cell membrane

b. fluids located within special spaces

c. fluids located within the body's cells

31. Describe the two major functions of body fluids.

a. _____

_____

b. _____

_____

32. List three sources of body fluid intake and their respective amounts

a. _____

_____

b. _____

_____

c. _____

_____

33. What is the total amount of fluid intake for an average adult in a 24-hour period?

_____

34. List the factors that affect the renal tubules' ability to regulate fluid volume filtration.

a. _____

_____

b. _____

_____

c. _____

_____

d. _____

_____

35. Which of the following urine specific gravity readings indicates dehydration?

a. 1.005

b. 1.015

c. 1.025

d. 1.035

36. List the four usual routes of water loss from the body.

a. _____

b. _____

c. _____

d. _____

37. Identify causes of body water loss that may lead to a fluid imbalance.

a. _____

b. _____

c. _____

d. _____

e. _____

f. _____

g. _____

h. _____

38. List the factors that control electrolyte balance within the body.

a. _____

b. _____

Match the following electrolytes (39–44) with their descriptions (a–f).

_____ 39. sodium

_____ 40. potassium

_____ 41. calcium

_____ 42. phosphorus

_____ 43. magnesium

_____ 44. chloride

a. the free form is physiologically active

b. the cofactor in enzymatic reactions

c. important in calcium homeostasis

d. primarily responsible for ECF osmolarity

e. anion found in gastric acid

f. major cause of the normal resting membrane potential

45. Which of the following statements is correct about fluid and electrolyte changes associated with aging?

a. Nearly 60% of the body weight of an elderly person is water.

b. Renal function changes increase the risk of electrolyte imbalance.

c. Skin turgor is a reliable measure of body fluid levels.

d. Thirst sensation is the best indicator of body fluid balance.

Subjective Assessment

46. List the subjective client data relevant to fluid and electrolyte balance. Use a separate sheet.

47. Briefly discuss why psychosocial factors are important to an accurate fluid and electrolyte status assessment. Use a separate sheet.

Objective Assessment

48. List the objective client data relevant to fluid and electrolyte balance. Use a separate sheet.

49. Identify factors the nurse should be aware of when reviewing a client's laboratory results.

a. _____

_____

b. _____

_____

c. _____

_____

50. Calculate the total 24-hour intake and output for the following client in milliliters.

The client has a nasogastric feeding tube and is to receive continuous enteric feedings at 100 mL per hour. In addition, the nurse routinely instills 1/2 cup of free water every 6 hours. The client also receives medications via the tube every 4 hours followed by 2 oz of water. Prior to each administration of medication, the feeding tube is checked for placement and residual stomach volume. The residual volume has been 25 mL each time. Today, the client is to receive supplemental potassium chloride. The physician's order states, "40 mEq KCl dissolved in 1 cup water, give every 2 hours times four doses per NG tube today only." The client has six loose stools during the day with a volume of about 300 mL each. Urinary output is 200 mL per 8-hour shift.

CRITICAL THINKING EXERCISES

Case Study: Lethal Dose

S. P. is a 58-year-old male client admitted to the Emergency Department. He has a serum potassium level of 2.0 mEq/L. The physician orders the nurse to administer potassium by intravenous push to restore serum levels. The nurse refuses to give the drug because she knows that asystole is likely to result from a bolus injection of potassium. The physician tells the nurse to give the drug, stating he is responsible for the outcome.

Address the following questions:

1. Identify the ethical and legal principles involved in this situation. Which of these principles are in conflict?

2. What should the nurse do?

3. If the nurse administers the ordered drug and harm results to S. P., what is the nurse's liability? The physician's liability?

4. Is the hospital liable for the nurse's actions in question 3?

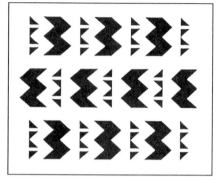

CHAPTER 15

Interventions for Clients with Fluid Imbalances

LEARNING OBJECTIVES

At the end of this chapter, the student will be able to

- Describe the three types of dehydration: isotonic, hypotonic, and hypertonic
- Use the nursing process to provide care for the client with dehydration
- Describe the three types of overhydration: isotonic, hypotonic, and hypertonic
- Use the nursing process to care for the client with potential or actual overhydration
- Identify the types of IV therapy administration
- List the principles for initiation of IV therapy
- Identify the nursing care for the client receiving IV therapy

PREREQUISITE KNOWLEDGE

Prior to beginning this chapter, the student should review

- Fluid and electrolytes as reviewed in an anatomy and physiology course
- Principles of infection transmission from a basic nursing, physiology, or microbiology course

STUDY QUESTIONS

Dehydration

Match the following sequelae (1–7) with their types of dehydration (a–c). Answers may be used more than once.

_____ 1. vascular volume deficit

_____ 2. cellular water loss

_____ 3. inadequate circulating volume

_____ 4. increased serum potassium

_____ 5. normal extracellular fluid (ECF) osmolarity

_____ 6. swelling of cells

_____ 7. normal vascular volume

a. isotonic
b. hypotonic
c. hypertonic

Match the following clinical problems (8–14) with their types of dehydration (a–c). Answers may be used more than once.

_____ 8. hyperventilation

_____ 9. diuresis

_____ 10. profound diuresis

_____ 11. chronic malnutrition

_____ 12. hemorrhage

_____ 13. very watery diarrhea

_____ 14. burn wounds

a. isotonic
b. hypotonic
c. hypertonic

15. List four factors that influence a client's fluid needs.

    a. _____

    b. _____

    c. _____

    d. _____

16. List the subjective client data relevant to dehydration. Use a separate sheet.

17. List the objective client data relevant to dehydration. Use a separate sheet.

18. Which of the following data would not be essential to collect in the initial assessment of a client with possible dehydration?

    a. height and weight

    b. known fluid loss

    c. history of contagious illness

    d. skin and mucous membrane turgor

19. Complete the following chart by indicating the rationale for the laboratory findings in the client with dehydration. Use a separate sheet.

Change	Rationale
a. blood urea nitrogen increased	
b. serum creatinine increased	
c. serum proteins increased	
d. hematocrit/hemoglobin increased	
e. urine specific gravity increased	
f. urine osmolarity increased	
g. urine volume decreased	

20. List the nurse's responsibilities in preventing dehydration. Use a separate sheet.

21. A 60-year-old male client is admitted with bleeding ulcers. He appears to be dehydrated because his intake is low due to pain. His mouth is dry and parched. Which of the following fluids should he be encouraged to consume?

    a. cola drink

    b. skim milk

    c. ice pops

    d. orange juice

22. Oral care for the alert client who is dehydrated includes

    a. offering oral hygiene immediately after meals or snacks

    b. rinsing the mouth every hour with plain tap water

    c. including foods such as meats with gravy in the diet

    d. limiting mouth care to brushing and flossing the teeth

23. Identify two reasons why commercial mouthwashes that contain alcohol are avoided for mouth care.

    a. _____

    _____

    b. _____

    _____

24. Which of the following statements best indicates that a dehydrated client who is being dismissed understands the plan of care?

    a. "I should drink some kind of liquid at least ever few hours or so."

    b. "If I start vomiting again, I'll want to call my doctor right away."

    c. "I plan to take my temperature once a day around 4:00 in the afternoon."

    d. "My friend can get a measuring cup for me to use when she shops next week."

Overhydration

25. The primary effect of isotonic overhydration is

    a. circulatory overload

    b. cellular edema

    c. renal shutdown

    d. Frank–Starling syndrome

26. Hypotonic overhydration results in

    a. increased ECF osmolarity

    b. decreased ECF hydrostatic pressure

    c. interstitial edema

    d. electrolyte concentration

27. Which of the following conditions may lead to overhydration?

    a. a 24-hour oral intake of 1500 mL in a normal adult

    b. adequate regulation of IV fluid therapy

    c. a low blood pressure with no renal perfusion

    d. the appropriate secretion of antidiuretic hormone (ADH)

28. List the subjective client data relevant to overhydration. Use a separate sheet.

29. List the objective client data relevant to overhydration. Use a separate sheet.

30. List the objective client data relevant to hypotonic overhydration.

    a. _____

    b. _____

    c. _____

    d. _____

    e. _____

CT 31. Using a pharmacology reference, identify specific nursing interventions for the medications listed in the following chart. Submit the completed exercise to the clinical instructor on a separate sheet.

Medication	Nursing Interventions
a. mannitol (Osmitrol)	
b. urea (Ureaphil)	
c. dexamethasone (Decadron)	
d. demeclocycline (Declomycin)	
e. furosemide (Lasix)	

Principles of Intravenous Therapy

32. Which one of the following venous access devices requires a special needle for use?

    a. Broviac catheter

    b. Groshong catheter

    c. Hickman catheter

    d. Mediport catheter

33. List four purposes of intravenous therapy.

    a. _____

    _____

    b. _____

    _____

    c. _____

    _____

    d. _____

    _____

34. List the principles and give the rationales to follow when selecting a peripheral intravenous site. Use a separate sheet.

35. Which one of the following pieces of equipment is not selected by the nurse when initiating intravenous therapy?

    a. tubing type

    b. type of fluid

    c. controller or pump

    d. size and type of cannula

36. Site preparation for IV therapy includes

    a. shaving excess hair from the area

    b. removing the client's identification bracelet

    c. cleansing the area with an iodophor pledget

    d. scrubbing the area using a back-and-forth motion

37. Identify three areas that the nurse assesses to maintain an IV infusion.

    a. _____

    b. _____

    c. _____

38. Give the preventive nursing interventions for the complications of intravenous therapy listed in the chart below. Use a separate sheet.

Complication	Nursing Interventions
a. infection	
b. tissue damage sites	
i. skin	
ii. veins	
iii. subcutaneous	
c. fluid and electrolyte imbalances	

39. A client is to receive 100 mL of 5% dextrose in 0.45% saline at 125 mL per hour. The administration tubing set has a drop factor of 15 gtt/mL. Calculate how many drops per minute the nurse should regulate the IV infusion.

    _____

    _____

CRITICAL THINKING EXERCISES

Case Study: Heat Exhaustion

A. K. is a 90-year-old woman who is admitted to a medical nursing unit with possible heat exhaustion. Her temperature on admission is 104°F and she is irritable and confused. Her blood pressure is 85/62. A. K.'s landlord had not seen her for two days, became concerned, and checked on her. He found A. K. lying on the floor in her apartment, "mumbling." A bottle of furosemide (Lasix) was found in A. K.'s purse.

Address the following question:

1. Based on the above data, identify the assessments the nurse should perform that would indicate whether a possible fluid and electrolyte imbalance exists.

Case Study: Fluid Imbalance

D. F. is an 85-year-old woman who just returned from surgery. An IV of 1000 mL of dextrose 5% in normal saline is infusing at 100 mL per hour. Upon entering the room 30 minutes later, the nurse notices that 500 mL of the solution has infused over the past 30 minutes. D. F. is complaining of difficulty breathing.

Address the following questions:

1. What should the nurse's immediate action be?
2. What imbalance might have occurred?
3. What nursing actions should be taken if D. F. has this imbalance?
4. How could this situation have been prevented?
5. Within the next 2 hours, D. F. urinates 700 mL of pale urine. Do these data indicate that the problem is resolving or worsening? Explain your answer.

C H A P T E R 1 6

Interventions for Clients with Electrolyte Imbalances

LEARNING OBJECTIVES

At the end of this chapter, the student will be able to

- Describe potassium imbalances: hypokalemia and hyperkalemia
- Use the nursing process to provide care for the client with altered potassium levels
- Describe sodium imbalances: hyponatremia and hypernatremia
- Use the nursing process to care for the client with altered sodium levels
- Describe calcium imbalances: hypocalcemia and hypercalcemia
- Use the nursing process to provide care for the client with altered calcium levels
- Describe phosphorus imbalances: hypophosphatemia and hyperphosphatemia
- Use the nursing process to provide care for the client with altered phosphorus levels
- Describe magnesium imbalances: hypomagnesemia and hypermagnesemia
- Use the nursing process to provide care for the client with altered magnesium levels

PREREQUISITE KNOWLEDGE

Prior to beginning this chapter, the student should review

- Fluid and electrolytes as reviewed in an anatomy and physiology course
- Normal nutrition requirements

STUDY QUESTIONS

Hypokalemia

1. *Hypokalemia* refers to a
   a. serum calcium level below 8.0 mg/dL
   b. serum potassium level below 5.0 mEq/L
   c. serum calcium level below 11.0 mg/dL
   d. serum potassium level below 3.5 mEq/L
2. Which of the following clinical signs best describes the effect of hypokalemia on the body?
   a. nervousness
   b. fidgeting
   c. weakness
   d. tremors

3. Which of the following clients is at risk for developing hypokalemia?

   a. a severely malnourished elderly man

   b. a man on high doses of furosemide (Lasix)

   c. a woman receiving massive blood transfusions

   d. a woman whose leg is crushed in a car accident

4. List the subjective client data relevant to hypokalemia. Use a separate sheet.

5. Elderly clients are at increased risk for developing hypokalemia mainly because they

   a. frequently require medications that predispose them to hypokalemia

   b. avoid taking laxatives to promote bowel movements and relieve constipation

   c. have an increased capacity for the kidney to concentrate urine

   d. tend to consume large volumes of fluids leading to water intoxication

6. List the objective client data relevant to hypokalemia. Use a separate sheet.

7. Which of the following laboratory data is frequently found in association with hypokalemia?

   a. decreased arterial blood PCO_2

   b. elevated blood glucose levels

   c. inverted urine sodium/potassium ratio

   d. increased urine potassium levels

8. Which of the following data are commonly seen in clients with hypokalemia?

   a. use of laxatives

   b. shallow respirations

   c. bounding pulses

   d. diet of baked foods

   e. postural hypotension

   f. tented T waves on ECG

   g. skeletal muscle spasms

   h. decreased sensation

   i. nausea and vomiting

   j. constipation

   k. concentrated urine

   l. poor concentration

9. Which of the following orders should the nurse clarify before implementing the order for the client who is hypokalemic?

   a. infuse D_5 1/4 normal saline and 40 mEq KCl at 100 mL per hour

   b. give KCl elixir 20 mEq ac qid

   c. hold furosemide today only

   d. give metoclopramide (Reglan) 10 mg ac PO

10. Which of the following foods is high in potassium?

    a. wheat bread

    b. poached eggs

    c. whole milk

    d. shelled nuts

11. Which of the following statements indicates that the client with hypokalemia who is being dismissed understands the plan of care?

    a. "My wife does all the cooking. She cooks everything until it's tender so that it's easier to chew."

    b. "When I take the liquid potassium in the evening, I'll eat a snack beforehand."

    c. "I usually have a bowl of corn flakes, orange juice, and a fried egg for breakfast."

    d. "I hate being stuck with needles all the time for blood. I'm sure glad to be going home."

Hyperkalemia

12. *Hyperkalemia* refers to a

    a. serum calcium level above 8.0 mg/dL

    b. serum potassium level above 3.5 mEq/L

    c. serum calcium level above 11.0 mg/dL

    d. serum potassium level above 5.0 mEq/L

13. Which of the following organs is the most sensitive to hyperkalemia?

    a. heart

    b. skeletal muscle

    c. gastrointestinal tract

    d. kidney

14. Which of the following statements explains the reason that hyperkalemia is uncommon?

    a. Symptoms do not develop until the serum electrolyte level is above 10 mEq/L.

    b. The kidney normally excretes any excess electrolyte at a fixed base rate.

    c. Few clients consume quantities of foods or liquids high in electrolytes.

    d. Hyperkalemia symptoms are indistinguishable from those of other conditions.

15. Which of the following is the most common cause of hyperkalemia in hospitalized clients?

    a. overuse of potassium-sparing diuretics

    b. failure to recognize acidosis in clients

    c. too rapid administration of IV fluids with potassium

    d. administering blood with an 18-gauge or larger needle

16. List the subjective client data relevant to hyperkalemia. Use a separate sheet.

17. List the objective client data relevant to hyperkalemia. Use a separate sheet.

18. Which of the following ECG changes would be typical in hyperkalemia?

    a. tall tented T waves

    b. narrow QRS complex

    c. tall P waves

    d. normal PR interval

19. Which of the following symptoms would be typical in hyperkalemia?

    a. decreased sensation in feet

    b. descending paralysis

    c. frequent, explosive diarrheal stools

    d. tachycardia and hypertension

20. Laboratory findings associated with hyperkalemia include

    a. increased hematocrit and hemoglobin levels in renal failure

    b. elevated serum electrolyte levels in water intoxication

    c. increased urine potassium level in renal failure

    d. decreased urine potassium level in renal failure

21. Which of the following interventions would be contraindicated in the emergency treatment of hyperkalemia?

    a. cation exchange enemas (Kayexalate)

    b. whole blood transfusions

    c. hemodialysis or peritoneal dialysis

    d. IV glucose and insulin

Hyponatremia

22. *Hyponatremia* refers to a

    a. serum sodium level below 135 mEq/L

    b. serum chloride level below 95 mEq/L

    c. serum sodium level below 145 mEq/L

    d. serum chloride level below 103 mEq/L

23. Which of the following statements is correct about the pathophysiology of hyponatremia?

    a. As the concentration of sodium falls in the ECF, it rises within the cell.

    b. Excitable membranes are more responsive during periods of hyponatremia.

    c. The nervous system tissues are the least affected by hyponatremia.

    d. Intracellular swelling may occur due to the shifts in osmotic pressure in the ECF.

24. Which of the following clients is at risk of developing hyponatremia?

    a. the diabetic client with a blood sugar of 130 mg/dL

    b. the febrile client with copious watery diarrhea

    c. the client with a massive systemic infection

    d. the client who is taking high doses of steroids

25. Which of the following complications commonly occurs with hyponatremia?

    a. prerenal failure

    b. increased intracranial pressure

    c. interstitial edema

    d. GI bleeding

26. List the subjective client data relevant to hyponatremia. Use a separate sheet.

27. List the objective client data relevant to hyponatremia. Use a separate sheet.

28. Laboratory findings associated with hyponatremia include

    a. decreased serum glucose

    b. increased total serum proteins

    c. decreased serum chloride levels

    d. normal hematocrit and hemoglobin

29. The nursing diagnosis of High Risk for Injury is commonly used in clients with hyponatremia. The etiology for this diagnosis is related to

    a. altered thought processes

    b. use of restraints

    c. headache

    d. hyponatremia

30. A client with hyponatremia reports an increasing incidence of headaches. Which of the following activities is permissible for this client?

    a. resting supine in bed

    b. straining to have a bowel movement

    c. applying ice caps to the forehead

    d. lifting objects from the floor

31. Which of the following foods is contraindicated for the client who is hyponatremic?

    a. cheese

    b. stewed tomatoes

    c. applesauce

    d. whole milk

Hypernatremia

32. *Hypernatremia* refers to a

    a. serum chloride level above 95 mEq/L

    b. serum sodium level above 135 mEq/L

    c. serum chloride level above 103 mEq/L

    d. serum sodium level above 145 mEq/L

33. Which of the following tissues is the most sensitive to changes in ECF sodium concentration?

    a. brain cells

    b. skeletal muscle

    c. cardiac muscle

    d. smooth muscle

34. Which two hormones are often used to correct for hypernatremia?

    a. aldosterone and serotonin

    b. ADH and epinephrine

    c. aldosterone and ADH

    d. ADH and Pitocin

Match the following clinical situations (35–42) with the types of hypernatremia (a–c). Answers may be used more than once.

_____ 35. severe diarrhea

_____ 36. presence of fever

_____ 37. profound diaphoresis

_____ 38. primary hyperaldosteronism

_____ 39. kidney disease of the proximal tubule

_____ 40. having one's arms restrained

_____ 41. multiple injections of sodium bicarbonate

_____ 42. severe vomiting

    a. inadequate water intake

    b. excess fluid loss

    c. excess sodium intake

43. List the subjective client data relevant to hypernatremia. Use a separate sheet.

44. List the objective client data relevant to hypernatremia. Use a separate sheet.

Match the following skin turgor data (45–47) with the types of hypernatremia (a–c).

_____ 45. skin turgor lasting longer than 6 seconds

_____ 46. skin turgor immediate return

_____ 47. skin turgor difficult to assess due to edema

    a. pure water loss

    b. excessive ECF loss

    c. ECF volume excess

48. Which of the following nursing diagnoses is most likely to appear in the plan of care for the client with hypernatremia?

    a. Diarrhea

    b. Altered Urinary Patterns

    c. Impaired Skin Integrity

    d. Altered Oral Mucous Membranes

49. Which of the following interventions would provide the hypernatremic client with a minimally stimulating environment?

    a. assigning a talkative roommate to improve orientation

    b. restricting television viewing to 4–6 hours per day

    c. limiting or restricting visitors, especially children

    d. moving the client to a private room near the nurses' station

Hypocalcemia

50. *Hypocalcemia* refers to a serum calcium level below

    a. 1.5 mEq/L

    b. 2.0 mEq/L

    c. 4.5 mEq/L

    d. 9.0 mEq/L

51. Which of the following clinical conditions is related to hypocalcemia?

    a. Cardiac muscle contraction is stimulated.

    b. Intestinal and gastric motility are increased.

    c. Peripheral nerve excitability is decreased.

    d. Bone density is increased markedly.

Match the following clinical conditions that predispose a client to hypocalcemia (52–62) with their etiologies (a–d). Answers may be used more than once.

_____ 52. alkalosis

_____ 53. pancreatitis

_____ 54. inadequate calcium intake

_____ 55. lactase deficiencies

_____ 56. parathyroidectomy

_____ 57. hyperphosphatemia

_____ 58. decreased serum protein

_____ 59. celiac disease

_____ 60. orthopedic surgery

_____ 61. calcium-binding medications

_____ 62. inadequate vitamin D intake

a. inhibited calcium absorption

b. decreased ionized calcium

c. endocrine disorder

d. other etiology

63. Which of the following clients is at greatest risk of developing hypocalcemia?

   a. a 70-year-old African-American woman with long-standing celiac disease

   b. a 45-year-old hypertensive Caucasian man on diuretic therapy

   c. a 50-year-old Caucasian woman with a recent ileostomy

   d. a 70-year-old African-American man on long-term lithium therapy

64. Preventive measures for hypocalcemia include

   a. increasing the daily dietary calcium intake to 500–1000 mg for clients at risk

   b. administering calcium supplements once per day following the morning meal

   c. applying a sun block and wearing protective clothing whenever outdoors

   d. administering calcium-containing IV fluids to clients receiving multiple blood transfusions

65. List the subjective client data relevant to hypocalcemia. Use a separate sheet.

66. List the objective client data relevant to hypocalcemia. Use a separate sheet.

67. Which of the following laboratory findings is associated with hypocalcemia?

   a. decreased serum phosphorus level

   b. increased total serum protein levels

   c. decreased arterial pH below 7.35

   d. increased urine levels of potassium

Match the following assessment findings (68–69) with their names (a or b).

_____ 68. muscle twitching when facial nerve is tapped in front of the ear

_____ 69. palmar flexion of the hand and fingers when blood pressure is checked

a. Trousseau's sign

b. Chvostek's sign

70. Which of the following findings would the nurse typically note when assessing the client with hypocalcemia?

   a. a history of nighttime leg cramps

   b. shortened ST segment on the ECG

   c. flank pain and urinary urgency

   d. severe muscle weakness

71. Which of the following medication orders should the nurse clarify before administering the drug to a client with hypocalcemia?

   a. magnesium sulfate 1 g intramuscularly (IM) every 6 hours for four doses

   b. aluminum hydroxide (Alternagel) 15 mL PO, tid

   c. calcium carbonate 1000 mg PO, ac tid

   d. calcium gluconate 500 mg IM "stat"

72. List four specific assessments that the nurse should perform for the client receiving IV calcium therapy.

   a. _____

   _____

   b. _____

   _____

   c. _____

   _____

   d. _____

   _____

73. Which of the following foods provides both calcium and vitamin D for the client who needs supplemental diet therapy for hypocalcemia?

   a. eggs

   b. cheese

   c. milk

   d. yogurt

74. Discuss the rationale for the use of drugs that decrease intestinal motility, such as kaolin (Kaopectate), and drugs that inhibit parasympathetic stimulation of the intestines in the treatment of calcium deficiency. Use a separate sheet.

75. Which of the following interventions would the nurse implement to reduce the risk for injury in the client with hypocalcemia?

    a. encourage activity by the client as tolerated

    b. massage the back muscles when giving a back rub

    c. move the client to a room near the nurses' station

    d. place oxygen and suction equipment at the bedside

Hypercalcemia

76. *Hypercalcemia* refers to a serum calcium level greater than

    a. 4.5 mEq/L

    b. 5.5 mEq/L

    c. 8.0 mEq/L

    d. 11.0 mEq/L

77. Which of the following statements is true about the pathophysiology of hypercalcemia?

    a. Hypercalcemia has little effect on blood clotting.

    b. Hypercalcemia can lead to increased bone strength.

    c. Cardiac and nerve tissues are sensitive to fluctuating calcium levels.

    d. Excess ECF calcium ions increase the responses of excitable tissues.

78. Which of the following conditions would increase bone resorption of calcium?

    a. renal failure

    b. lung cancer

    c. use of diuretics

    d. parathyroidectomy

79. What relationship does immobility have to hypercalcemia? _____

    _____

    _____

80. What relationship does hypervitaminosis have to hypercalcemia? _____

    _____

    _____

81. A preventive intervention for the client with hypercalcemia is

    a. restricting dietary calcium by eliminating milk products

    b. discouraging weight-bearing activity such as walking

    c. monitoring the client for fluid volume excess

    d. administering multivitamin tablets twice per day

82. List the subjective client data relevant to hypercalcemia. Use a separate sheet.

83. List the objective client data relevant to hypercalcemia. Use a separate sheet.

84. Which of the following findings would the nurse make when assessing the client with hypercalcemia?

    a. bradycardia

    b. paresthesia

    c. leg cramping

    d. hypoactive bowel sounds

85. Which of the following medication orders should the nurse clarify before administering the drug to the client with hypercalcemia?

    a. calcitonin (Calcimar) 250 IU, IV every day

    b. furosemide (Lasix) 20 mg, PO, bid

    c. ibuprofen (Motrin) 400 mg, PO, qid

    d. plicamycin (Mithracin) 1500 μg IV over 24 hours

86. Interventions for the client receiving calcitonin (Calcimar) include

    a. administering hydroxymagnesium aluminate (Riopan)

    b. encouraging bed rest while the medication is infusing

    c. storing the reconstituted medication at room temperature

    d. keeping parenteral calcium on standby for treating tetany

87. Develop a teaching/learning plan for the client 〖CT〗 with hypercalcemia for thrombus prevention. Submit the completed exercise to the clinical instructor on a separate sheet.

88. A preventive intervention for the client at risk of fracture related to decreased bone density is

    a. encouraging independent ambulation about the room

    b. using a lift sheet for moving the client up in bed

    c. reminding the client to shift position in bed frequently

    d. providing an overhead trapeze to assist position changes

Phosphorus Imbalances

89. The serum level of phosphorus exists in reciprocal balance to that of

    a. magnesium

    b. chloride

    c. calcium

    d. potassium

90. *Hypophosphatemia* refers to a serum level of phosphorus below

    a. 2.5 mg/dL

    b. 3.5 mg/dL

    c. 4.5 mg/dL

    d. 5.5 mg/dL

91. *Hyperphosphatemia* refers to a serum level of phosphorus above

    a. 2.5 mg/dL

    b. 3.0 mg/dL

    c. 3.5 mg/dL

    d. 4.5 mg/dL

Match the following clinical conditions (92–100) with their effects on serum phosphorus levels (a–b). Answers may be used more than once.

_____ 92. aggressive malignancy   a. hyperphosphatemia

                                    b. hypophosphatemia

_____ 93. malnutrition

_____ 94. alcoholism

_____ 95. hypoparathyroidism

_____ 96. inadequate vitamin D intake

_____ 97. hypocalcemia

_____ 98. respiratory alkalosis

_____ 99. renal disease

_____ 100. hyperparathyroidism

101. List objective client data relevant to hypophosphatemia. Use a separate sheet.

102. Interventions for the client with hypophosphatemia include

    a. aggressive treatment with parenteral phosphorus

    b. administering oral vitamin D and phosphorus supplements

    c. concurrent administration of calcium supplements

    d. eliminating beef, pork, and legumes from the diet

Magnesium Imbalances

103. The normal range of serum magnesium levels is

    a. 1.0–2.0 mEq/L

    b. 1.5–2.5 mEq/L

    c. 2.0–3.0 mEq/L

    d. 2.5–3.5 mEq/L

104. List four conditions that decrease intestinal absorption of magnesium.

    a. _____

    _____

    b. _____

    _____

    c. _____

    _____

    d. _____

    _____

105. List five conditions that increase renal excretion of magnesium.

    a. _____

    b. _____

    c. _____

    _____

    d. _____

    _____

    e. _____

    _____

106. List the objective client data relevant to hypo-magnesemia. Use a separate sheet.

107. The most significant assessment finding in the client with hypomagnesemia that does not occur in clients with other electrolyte imbalances is

    a. muscle spasms in legs

    b. paresthesia

    c. psychosis

    d. paralytic ileus

108. Interventions for the client with hypomagne-semia include

    a. administering intramuscular $MgSO_4$

    b. encouraging food such as fruits

    c. administering oral preparations of $MgSO_4$

    d. discontinuing diuretic therapy

109. List the objective client data relevant to hyper-magnesemia. Use a separate sheet.

110. Which of the following foods is limited in the diet to prevent hypermagnesemia?

    a. egg salad

    b. fruit compote

    c. ice milk

    d. spinach salad

CRITICAL THINKING EXERCISES

Case Study: Potassium Disturbance

A. N. is a client admitted for palpitations. His admission serum potassium level is 5.2 mEq/L. Yesterday, A. N. ate two eggs, bacon, and toast for breakfast. For lunch he had a fresh fruit salad, and for dinner he ate baked halibut, baked potatoes, a salad, and green beans. A. N. usually has a cola drink and salted peanuts for a snack. He uses a salt substitute regularly.

Address the following questions:

1. Identify the foods in his diet that may be contributing to his hyperkalemia.
2. Which EKG changes would be typical for a client such as A. N.?
3. Formulate relevant nursing diagnoses for A. N. based on the above data.

A. N. states that he has had abdominal cramping and several very loose diarrheal stools since yesterday. The physician orders a sodium polystyrene sulfonate (Kayexalate) retention enema to be given stat.

4. Discuss the etiology of A. N.'s symptoms.
5. Explain whether the nurse should clarify the physician's order before administering the enema.
6. A. N. is unable to retain the enema. What interventions should the nurse initiate to assist A. N. to retain the solution?
7. Eventually, A. N. recovers and is scheduled for dismissal. Develop a teaching–learning plan for him including information about his diet, self-monitoring of his pulse, and the need for regular follow-up care.

Case Study: Sodium Disturbance

The nurse is caring for W. G., an 81-year-old man who is admitted after a 3-day period of weakness. A CVA, or stroke, is suspected because he has right-sided weakness and difficulty speaking. He appears dehydrated, with a skin turgor of 5 seconds and a urine specific gravity of 1.028.

Address the following questions:

1. Discuss whether W. G.'s serum sodium would be elevated, decreased, or normal.
2. Develop a specific assessment plan for W. G.
3. Formulate relevant nursing diagnoses for W. G. based on the above data.

W. G. is filling out his menu for the next day. Since he is somewhat confused, the nurse reviews his food choices.

4. Which foods would not be advisable for W. G.? Which foods should be encouraged?
5. W. G. will be dismissed to home care. Develop a teaching–learning plan for him focusing on diet and safety.

Case Study: Fluid and Electrolyte Imbalance

K. G. is an 80-year-old female client who had a CVA, or stroke, 5 days ago. She has a long-standing history of furosemide (Lasix) diuretic therapy for fluid retention, which is continued during her hospitalization. It is difficult to get K. G. to drink and eat. She is becoming increasingly confused, irritable, weak, and hard to rouse.

Address the following questions:

1. Which fluid and electrolyte imbalances should the nurse assess for in K. G.?

2. Based on the above data, formulate relevant nursing diagnoses for K. G.

3. The physician orders a feeding tube to be inserted. The feeding tube keeps coiling in the back of K. G.'s throat during insertion. Discuss measures that can be used to promote passage of the tube.

4. What is the most accurate way to determine whether the tube is in the stomach?

5. The physician orders half strength Ensure at 100 mL per hour. At a calorie density of 0.5 calorie/mL, how many calories does this provide K. G. in a 24-hour period? Is this amount sufficient for her needs?

6. The furosemide (Lasix) is discontinued. What assessments should the nurse make to monitor K. G.'s fluid and electrolyte status?

7. K. G. is to receive digoxin (Lanoxin) 0.25 mg, hydrochlorothiazide and triamterene (Dyazide) 1 capsule, potassium (Kaochlor) 20 mEq, and a multivitamin this morning. K. G. chokes when she tries to swallow the medications. What can the nurse do to safely administer the drugs?

Four days after beginning the tube feedings, K. G.'s laboratory values are Na = 135 mEq/dL, K = 3.7 mEq/dL, Ca = 9.5 mEq/dL, urine specific gravity = 1.028, Hgb = 10.5, and hematocrit = 31.5. Her current weight is 95.4 pounds.

8. Which of these laboratory values are abnormal? Discuss why they have not improved.

9. What revisions are indicated in K.G.'s plan of care for the imbalances?

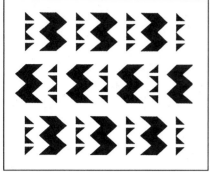

Acid–Base Balance

LEARNING OBJECTIVES

At the end of this chapter, the student will be able to

▪ Differentiate among acid, base, and buffer components in the body

▪ Describe how acid, base, and buffer components interact in the body to regulate acid–base balance

▪ Describe the roles that the chemical buffer system, lungs, and kidneys have in regulating acid–base balance

▪ Describe acid–base balance changes associated with aging

PREREQUISITE KNOWLEDGE

Prior to beginning this chapter, the student should review

▪ The principles of acid and base solutions from basic chemistry

▪ The normal anatomy and physiology of the lungs and kidneys

STUDY QUESTIONS

Anatomy and Physiology Review

Match the following definitions (1–9) with their correct terms (a–i).

_____ 1. hydrogen ion homeostasis

_____ 2. process in which an acid combines with a base to form a new substance

_____ 3. a solution in which the number and strength of acid and base components are in equilibrium

_____ 4. substance that liberates or donates a hydrogen ion

_____ 5. ability of the body to correct for changes in pH

_____ 6. largest source of buffers in the body

_____ 7. substance that binds free hydrogen ions in solution

_____ 8. substance that can act as either an acid or a base

_____ 9. difference in the electrical charge between the body's total anions and cations

a. acid

b. acid–base balance

c. anion gap

d. base

e. buffer

f. compensation

g. neutral

h. neutralization

i. proteins

10. Which of the following blood pH values is within normal limits?

a. 7.27

b. 7.37

c. 7.47

d. 7.57

11. List four changes in the body that would occur if the pH was not closely regulated.

    a. _____

    _____

    b. _____

    _____

    c. _____

    _____

    d. _____

    _____

12. Describe how a strong acid acts differently from a weak acid when it is dissolved:

    a. strong acid: _____

    _____

    b. weak acid: _____

    _____

13. When neutralizing an acid with a base, what product is usually formed?

    a. salt

    b. stronger acid

    c. weaker base

14. The Henderson–Hasselbalch equation is a formula used to

    a. analyze blood gases

    b. predict blood levels of CO_2

    c. determine blood pH

    d. calculate carbonic acid dissociation

15. The serum pH value is

    a. directly related to the concentration of carbon dioxide

    b. directly related to the concentration of hydrogen ions

    c. inversely related to the concentration of hydrogen ions

    d. inversely related to the concentration of bicarbonate

16. Which one of the following statements about pH is correct?

    a. A solution with a pH of 6.5 is a weak base and has more hydrogen ions than a solution with a pH of 6.9.

    b. A solution with a pH of 7.0 is neutral and has fewer hydrogen ions than a solution with a pH of 6.8.

    c. A solution with a pH of 7.5 is a weak acid and has fewer hydrogen ions than a solution with a pH of 7.8.

    d. A solution with a pH of 8.7 is a strong base and has more hydrogen ions than a solution with a pH of 8.5.

17. Draw a diagram on a separate sheet to represent each of the following conditions: acid–base balance, acid excess, base deficit, base excess, and acid deficit. Use the letter "A" to represent acid ions and "B" to represent base ions.

18. List five sources of hydrogen ions in the body that are by-products of normal metabolism.

    a. _____

    _____

    _____

    b. _____

    _____

    _____

    c. _____

    _____

    _____

    d. _____

    _____

    _____

    e. _____

    _____

    _____

19. Which of the following is the major extracellular fluid (ECF) buffer?

    a. carbon dioxide

    b. bicarbonate

    c. ammonium

    d. phosphate

20. Which of the following statements is correct about the role of chemical buffers in regulating acid–base balance?

    a. They are able to correct imbalances permanently.

    b. They are present in the body fluids and act immediately.

    c. They constitute the largest store of buffers in the body.

    d. They can correct underlying problems leading to imbalances.

21. The acid released by the lungs to regulate pH is

    a. bicarbonate

    b. phosphate

    c. hydrogen

    d. carbon dioxide

22. Which of the following statements is correct about the neural regulatory control of acid–base balance?

    a. Baroreceptors in the ECF are sensitive to bicarbonate.

    b. Chemoreceptors in the ECF are sensitive to carbon dioxide.

    c. Chemoreceptors in the brain are sensitive to carbon dioxide.

    d. Baroreceptors in the brain are sensitive to bicarbonate.

23. When the respiratory rate slows, pH

    a. rises

    b. falls

    c. is unchanged

24. The kidneys regulate pH by controlling

    a. urea

    b. bicarbonate

    c. carbon dioxide

    d hemoglobin

25. Ammonia, a normal by-product of protein metabolism, is converted to ammonium in the kidney by the addition of

    a. urea

    b. nitrogen

    c. hydrogen

    d. phosphate

26. List, in order of occurrence, the three regulatory mechanisms that the body uses to control acid–base balance.

    a. _____

    b. _____

    c. _____

27. Describe a situation in which the renal system is used to compensate for acid–base imbalance. Use a separate sheet.

28. Describe a situation in which the respiratory system is used to compensate for acid–base imbalance. Use a separate sheet.

29. Briefly compare full compensation with partial compensation. Use a separate sheet.

Changes with Aging

30. List the physiological changes that occur in the lungs with aging that contribute to the elderly's risk for acid–base imbalances.

    a. _____

    _____

    b. _____

    _____

    c. _____

    _____

31. List the physiological changes that occur in the kidneys with aging that contribute to the elderly's risk for acid–base imbalances.

    a. _____

    _____

    b. _____

    _____

32. Which of the following medications increases elderly clients' risk for acid–base imbalances?

    a. carbamazepine (Tegretol)

    b. conjugated estrogen (Premarin)

    c. furosemide (Lasix)

    d. metoclopromide (Reglan)

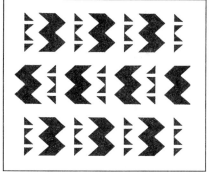

C H A P T E R 1 8

Interventions for Clients with Acid–Base Imbalances

LEARNING OBJECTIVES

At the end of this chapter, the student will be able to

▌ Compare and contrast acidemia with alkalemia, and acidosis with alkalosis

▌ Define the terms *base deficit* and *base excess*

▌ Describe the pathophysiology and etiology of acidemia

▌ List the etiologies of metabolic acidosis

▌ List the etiologies of respiratory acidosis

▌ Describe the management of the client with acidosis

▌ Describe the pathophysiology and etiology of alkalemia

▌ List the etiologies of metabolic alkalosis

▌ List the etiologies of respiratory alkalosis

▌ Describe the management of the client with alkalosis

PREREQUISITE KNOWLEDGE

Prior to beginning this chapter, the student should review

▌ The principles of acid–base balance

▌ The normal anatomy and physiology of the lungs and kidneys

▌ The principles of fluid and electrolyte balance

▌ The principles of intravenous (IV) therapy

STUDY QUESTIONS

Pathophysiology Review

1. Which of the following statements is correct about acid–base balance?

   a. Acidemia is a condition of excess bases compared with acids.

   b. Alkalemia is a condition of excess acids compared with bases.

   c. The normal range for the pH of the body is 7.25 to 7.35.

   d. A pH within normal range is critical to physiological functions.

2. List and describe two types of actions that lead to acid–base imbalances.

   a. _____

   _____

   _____

   _____

   b. _____

   _____

   _____

   _____

3. Describe the difference between acidosis and acidemia.

   acidosis: _____

   _____

   _____

   _____

   acidemia: _____

   _____

   _____

   _____

4. Describe the difference between alkalosis and alkalemia.

   alkalosis: _____

   _____

   _____

   _____

   _____

   alkalemia: _____

   _____

   _____

   _____

Match the following conditions (5–8) with their definitions (a–d).

_____ 5. acid excess

_____ 6. acid deficit

_____ 7. base excess

_____ 8. base deficit

a. relative increase in concentration and strength of acid components

b. relative increase in concentration and strength of base components

c. actual increase in concentration and strength of acid components

d. actual increase in concentration and strength of base components

Match the following pathological processes (9–18) with their resulting conditions (a or b). Answers may be used more than once.

_____ 9. increase in acid concentration

_____ 10. increase in base concentration

_____ 11. overelimination of acid components

_____ 12. overelimination of base components

_____ 13. overproduction of acids

_____ 14. overproduction of base components

_____ 15. underelimination of acids

_____ 16. underproduction of acid components

_____ 17. underproduction of base components

_____ 18. relative increase in base concentration

a. acidemia

b. alkalemia

19. List the major causes of acidemia and alkalemia.

   a. _____

   _____

   b. _____

   _____

   c. _____

   _____

20. Which of the following electrolyte balances is likely to be disrupted in acidemia?

   a. sodium

   b. potassium

   c. chloride

   d. calcium

21. Acidemia produces physical symptoms in the cardiac, neuromuscular, respiratory, and gastrointestinal systems. What is the physiological basis for these disruptions?

   a. Intracellular potassium is excreted into the extracellular fluid.

   b. The hydrogen ion concentration of excitable membranes is lowered.

   c. Excitable membranes are unable to generate or sustain action potentials.

   d. Hydrogen and potassium ions become bound in the serum and are inactivated.

22. Alkalemia produces physical symptoms in the central nervous, neuromuscular, and cardiac systems. What is the physiological basis for these disruptions?

 a. Excitable membranes are increasingly susceptible to depolarization.

 b. Potassium ions are retained inside the cells.

 c. Carbon dioxide diffusion and elimination are decreased.

 d. The hydrogen ion concentration of excitable membranes is increased.

23. Acidemia denatures and thus inactivates body protein. Which of the following examples illustrates this process?

 a. storing hard-boiled eggs in vinegar

 b. frying an egg over medium heat

 c. milk souring at room temperature

 d. broiling a steak over charcoal

Match the following clinical conditions of metabolic acidosis (24–35) with their causative mechanisms (a–f). Answers may be used more than once, and more than one answer may apply to each condition.

_____ 24. alcohol intoxication

_____ 25. aspirin poisoning

_____ 26. chronic pancreatitis

_____ 27. continuous diarrhea

_____ 28. dehydration

_____ 29. diabetic ketoacidosis

_____ 30. fever of 101°F

_____ 31. grand mal seizures

_____ 32. liver disease

_____ 33. myocardial infarction

_____ 34. starvation

_____ 35. renal failure

 a. excessive oxidation of fatty acids

 b. hypermetabolism

 c. excessive ingestion of acids

 d. underelimination of acids

 e. underproduction of bicarbonate

 f. overelimination of bicarbonate

36. The cause of respiratory acidosis is

 a. overexcretion of hydrogen and bicarbonate ions from the kidney

 b. underelimination of carbon dioxide from the lungs

 c. overelimination of carbon dioxide from the lungs

 d. underelimination of metabolic waste products from the GI tract

37. Which of the following conditions is *least* likely to result in respiratory depression?

 a. increased intracranial pressure

 b. airway obstruction

 c. general anesthesia

 d. myasthenia gravis

 e. hypokalemia

38. Inadequate chest expansion, which leads to respiratory acidosis, is most likely to be caused by

 a. lordosis

 b. emphysema

 c. prolonged bed rest

 d. first-trimester pregnancy

39. Clients at greater risk of airway obstruction include

 a. computer programmers

 b. garment workers

 c. school teachers

 d. stock brokers

40. Interference with alveolar–capillary diffusion results in

 a. carbon dioxide retention and acidemia

 b. hydrogen ion elimination and acidemia

 c. hydrogen depletion from water vapor loss

 d. aerobic metabolism and lactic acid build-up

41. One cause of metabolic alkalosis is

 a. aspirin poisoning

 b. overuse of antacids

 c. prolonged diarrhea

 d. potassium-sparing diuretics

42. Clients at greater risk of respiratory alkalosis include

 a. sky divers

 b. airline pilots

 c. house painters

 d. mountain climbers

Collaborative Management

43. List the subjective client data relevant to acidemia. Use a separate sheet.

44. List the subjective client data relevant to alkalemia. Use a separate sheet.

45. List the objective client data relevant to acidemia. Use a separate sheet.

46. List the objective client data relevant to alkalemia. Use a separate sheet.

Match the following assessment findings (47–58) with their associated conditions (a or b). More than one answer may apply to each.

_____ 47. bradycardia

_____ 48. comatose

_____ 49. dry, flushed skin

_____ 50. hypotension

_____ 51. Kussmaul's respirations

_____ 52. muscle twitches

_____ 53. muscle weakness

_____ 54. normal blood pressure

_____ 55. positive Trousseau's sign

_____ 56. seizure activity

_____ 57. tachycardia

_____ 58. weak peripheral pulses

a. acidemia

b. alkalemia

59. Arterial PO_2

    a. decreases in respiratory acidosis and alkalosis

    b. increases in metabolic acidosis and alkalosis

    c. increases in respiratory and combined acidosis

    d. is unchanged in all conditions of alkalosis

60. Serum potassium and calcium levels

    a. decrease in acidemia

    b. increase in acidemia

    c. decrease in alkalemia

    d. increase in alkalemia

61. The hallmark of metabolic acidosis is

    a. increased bicarbonate and normal carbon dioxide levels

    b. decreased bicarbonate and normal carbon dioxide levels

    c. increased bicarbonate and carbon dioxide levels

    d. decreased bicarbonate and carbon dioxide levels

62. The hallmark of chronic respiratory acidosis is

    a. elevated bicarbonate and increased arterial PCO_2 levels

    b. elevated bicarbonate and normal arterial PCO_2 levels

    c. decreased bicarbonate and normal arterial PCO_2 levels

    d. decreased bicarbonate and increased arterial PCO_2 levels

63. The hallmark of metabolic alkalosis is

    a. increased bicarbonate and normal arterial PCO_2 levels

    b. increased bicarbonate and rising arterial PCO_2 levels

    c. increased bicarbonate and decreased arterial PCO_2 levels

    d. decreased bicarbonate and falling arterial PCO_2 levels

64. The hallmarks of respiratory alkalosis include

    a. decreased bicarbonate and arterial PCO_2 levels

    b. increased bicarbonate and arterial PCO_2 levels

    c. decreased bicarbonate and normal arterial PCO_2 levels

    d. decreased bicarbonate and increased arterial PCO_2 levels

65. Both chronic respiratory acidosis and metabolic alkalosis are associated with the nursing diagnosis of Altered Thought Processes. Briefly compare the etiologies of these diagnoses on a separate sheet. Submit the completed exercise to the clinical instructor.

66. Discuss the rationale for administering inhalant bronchodilators prior to administering inhalant cortisol or mucolytic agents. Use a separate sheet.

67. The most effective way to administer oxygen to the client with chronic respiratory acidosis is by

    a. high-volume intermittent positive pressure

    b. low-flow oxygen (2 L per minute) via nasal prongs

    c. high-flow 40% oxygen via face mask

    d. hyperbaric pressure chamber

68. Which of the following assessments indicates that a client with chronic respiratory acidosis is responding favorably to treatment?

    a. nail beds pale, extremities cool

    b. respiratory stridor with inspiration

    c. expectorating clear, stringy mucus

    d. diffuse rales auscultated bilaterally

69. The diet of the client with chronic respiratory acidosis should include

    a. milk products

    b. raw fruits and vegetables

    c. chicken noodle soup (low sodium)

    d. carbonated soft drinks and juices

70. Provide rationales for the interventions initiated for the client with chronic respiratory acidosis by completing the following chart on a separate sheet.

Intervention	Rationale
a. Fowler's position	
b. side rails up	
c. low-level lighting	
d. postural drainage	
e. mucolytic agents	
f. small, frequent meals	
g. wall clock in room	

71. Discharge instructions for the client with chronic respiratory acidosis should include

    a. discussing how to plan for periods of increased activity

    b. teaching about a low-protein, low-carbohydrate diet

    c. demonstrating exercises to increase vital capacity

    d. encouraging participation in activities such as jogging

72. Interventions for the client with metabolic alkalosis include

    a. IV infusion of lactated Ringer's solution

    b. administration of bolus IV calcium gluconate

    c. side rails padded and kept in the "up" position

    d. allowance for visitors after visiting hours

CRITICAL THINKING EXERCISES

Case Study: Acid–Base Imbalance I

M. G. is a 55-year-old man with moderately severe chronic lung disease. He enters the hospital for abdominal surgery. His lung disease is stable, and preoperatively he was in compensated respiratory acidosis. After surgery his blood gases are pH = 7.30, $PaCO_2$ = 65 mm Hg, HCO_3 = 29 mEq/L, and PaO_2 = 60 mm Hg.

Address the following questions:

1. What acid–base imbalance exists in M. G. after surgery?
2. What are some etiologies of the disorder in M. G.?
3. Plan a postoperative care plan to improve M. G.'s acid–base problem.
4. Oxygen has been ordered at 2 L and he is reporting shortness of breath. With his PaO_2 level at 65 mm Hg, how much should the nurse increase his oxygen flow?

Case Study: Acid–Base Imbalance II

H. A. is a 25-year-old type I diabetic (IDDM). She has been seen in the Emergency Department (ED) many times in the past for hyperglycemia. She was admitted to the nursing unit after being seen in the ED with complaints of fatigue. Her breathing is rapid, almost as though she had been running. There is a sweet odor to her breath. Blood gases are drawn and reveal pH = 7.32, $PaCO_2$ = 20 mm Hg, HCO_3 = 24 mEq/L, and serum glucose = 625 mg/100 mL.

Address the following questions:

1. What acid–base imbalance exists in H. A.? Is it compensated? Or is it uncompensated?
2. How does her diabetes increase her risk of acidosis?
3. Why is her breathing rapid?

After H. A. is recovered from this acute episode, the nurse asks her how well she follows her diet. She replies that in her new job, she is limited to eating in the cafeteria or in fast-food restaurants. She thinks she may be taking in more calories than she can metabolize with her current dose of insulin.

4. What type of changes should H. A. make in her eating habits? Can she just increase her insulin to cover the additional calories? Would an increase in activity help? Explain your answer.
5. Develop a teaching/learning plan for H. A.'s diet and activity.

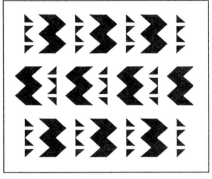

C H A P T E R 1 9

Interventions for Preoperative Clients

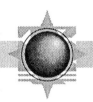

LEARNING OBJECTIVES

At the end of this chapter, the student will be able to

■ Define the term *perioperative period*

■ Describe how operations can be classified

■ Discuss the trends in surgical care

■ Describe the preoperative assessment and the rationale for collecting various types of data

■ Identify the common nursing diagnoses and client goals for the client undergoing surgery

■ Explain the purpose for and method of obtaining an operative permit

■ Describe the preparation of the client for surgery

■ Describe the usual client teaching about surgery

■ List the nursing interventions to reduce client and family anxiety

■ List nursing roles in immediate preparation of the client for surgery

PREREQUISITE KNOWLEDGE

Prior to beginning this chapter, the student should review

■ The principles of teaching and learning in client care

■ Normal laboratory values for hemoglobin, hematocrit, white blood cells (WBCs), red blood cells (RBCs), platelets, serum electrolytes, arterial blood gases, and urinalysis

■ The norms for vital sign measurements

STUDY QUESTIONS

Surgical Settings

1. Which of the following statements best reflects the meaning of the term *perioperative period?* Perioperative care is given

   a. in the operating room and immediately following surgery in the recovery room

   b. before, during, and after an operation

   c. in ambulatory surgery centers because of insurance regulations

   d. by the nursing staff on a medical–surgical care unit

Match the following types of operations (2–7) with their representative examples (a–f).

_____ 2. emergency

_____ 3. urgent

_____ 4. diagnostic

_____ 5. elective

_____ 6. cosmetic

_____ 7. palliative

a. biopsy of breast mass

b. removal of part of a bowel tumor

c. excision of cataract

d. external fixation of a closed femur fracture

e. face lift

f. stab wound to the chest

8. Which of the following statements demonstrates how regulations and reimbursement have affected perioperative client care?

   a. Ambulatory care centers are becoming less popular and decreasing in usage.

   b. A higher proportion of inpatient surgical procedures are urgent or emergency in nature.

   c. Postoperative infection rates have soared in clients having outpatient procedures.

   d. Elderly clients are hospitalized more frequently for all types of surgical procedures.

Collaborative Management

9. List the subjective client data relevant to the preoperative client. Use a separate sheet.

10. List the objective client data relevant to the preoperative client. Use a separate sheet.

11. Which of the following is the correct rationale for asking specific questions about a client's history?

    a. The client's age must be known so that the risk of postoperative complications can be determined.

    b. The use of tobacco products is assessed because more anesthetic is needed for clients who smoke.

    c. Medications used routinely are assessed because drug–drug interactions may occur.

    d. Previous surgeries are assessed because clients having had previous surgery require very little preoperative teaching.

12. A client reports being allergic to lobster. Which of the following precautions should the nurse take?

    a. No specific precautions are indicated.

    b. The client should be observed for rash after the skin is scrubbed with iodine soap.

    c. The client should be assessed for signs of malignant hyperthermia following surgery.

    d. The client should not be given any aminoglycosides.

13. A client's preoperative vital signs are as follows: temperature = 99.8°F (rectal), apical pulse = 92 and regular, respirations = 20 and regular, blood pressure = 162/92 in the left arm (sitting). Which of the following actions should the nurse take?

    a. Compare these values to previous vital signs and chart them. There is nothing reportable.

    b. Report the temperature and pulse immediately because the client probably has an infection.

    c. Report the temperature and blood pressure immediately to prevent postoperative stroke.

    d. Recheck the blood pressure after the client relaxes. If still elevated, report the blood pressure.

14. List two abnormal conditions for each of the following body systems that increase a client's risk from surgery and anesthesia.

    a. cardiovascular: _____

    _____

    _____

    b. respiratory: _____

    _____

    _____

    c. renal: _____

    _____

    _____

    d. neurological: _____

    _____

    _____

    e. nutritional: _____

    _____

    _____

    f. musculoskeletal: _____

    _____

    _____

    g. psychological: _____

    _____

    _____

15. A female client's preoperative laboratory results are as follows: RBCs = 4.8 million/mm^3, WBCs = 8.2/mm^3, hematocrit = 42 mL/dL, hemoglobin = 12.8 g/dL, platelets = 100,000/mm^3. This client

    a. has an insufficient blood volume to withstand a surgical hemorrhage

    b. is at increased risk of intraoperative or postoperative bleeding

    c. has an existing infection and needs immediate antibiotic therapy

    d. is at increased risk for developing an iron deficiency anemia

16. Preoperative diagnostic tests for the client over 40 years of age often include

    a. a chest x-ray to determine if the client is a smoker

    b. an IV pyelogram to determine kidney function

    c. an electrocardiogram to determine cardiac function

    d. an abdominal x-ray to determine if the bowel is empty

17. Which of the following statements is correct about surgical consent forms?

    a. The nurse clarifies any questions after preoperative sedation is given.

    b. The nurse's signature is to show witness to the client's signature.

    c. Consents are signed by clients only for major surgical procedures.

    d. Signed consents are required for every operation without exception.

18. Which of the following drugs would the nurse *not* withhold preoperatively?

    a. regular insulin

    b. furosemide (Lasix)

    c. docusate sodium (Colace)

    d. estrogen (Norinyl)

    e. digoxin (Lanoxin)

    f. calcium gluconate (Kalcinate)

    g. naproxen (Naprosyn)

    h. phenytoin sodium (Dilantin)

19. Which of the following problems does *not* result from prolonged enema administration?

    a. hypoglycemia

    b. hypokalemia

    c. hypotension

    d. dehydration

20. Nursing research has shown that infection can be reduced by performing the skin shave

    a. the night before surgery

    b. with the client's own razor

    c. immediately before the operation

    d. only on the head and perineal areas

21. Which of the following statements about the immediate postoperative period would be included in preoperative teaching for a client undergoing abdominal surgery?

    a. "You will be asked to breathe deeply 5 to 10 times every hour."

    b. "Lying flat on your back will decrease the pain after your surgery."

    c. "Pain medication will not be given for at least the first 8 hours after surgery."

    d. "As soon as you return to your room, you can have full liquids to drink."

22. Which of the following is an appropriate nursing intervention when preparing a client for surgery?

    a. Tell family members that they will be allowed in the operating room until the client is asleep.

    b. Explain to the client that deep breathing exercises will be taught after the operation.

    c. Put the client's rings in the hospital safe and tape the wedding band on his or her finger.

    d. Tape any dentures in a denture bag to the client's gown to go to the operating room.

23. Which of the following statements made by a client indicates that more teaching is needed about preoperative medication?

    a. "Here are my false teeth and watch."

    b. "I'm not supposed to smoke before surgery."

    c. "Let me go to the bathroom before I get that shot."

    d. "I'm not sleepy yet; you can leave those rails down."

24. List two examples of nursing interventions for reducing client and family anxiety in each of the following areas. Use a separate sheet.

    a. preoperative teaching

    b. communication

    c. rest

CRITICAL THINKING EXERCISES

Case Study: Preoperative Care

K. O. is a 55-year-old man who is scheduled for abdominal surgery in the morning under general anesthesia. He was admitted to a single room on the surgical nursing unit this afternoon. During the admission interview, K. O. tells the nurse that he has been on a liquid diet for 3 days.

Address the following questions:

1. What assessments should the nurse make to determine K. O.'s nutritional status and potential risk from the preoperative preparation and surgery?

2. Briefly discuss which of K. O.'s laboratory results the nurse should review and the rationale for doing so.

3. K. O. asks whether he can smoke in his room. The hospital permits smoking in patient rooms if there is no other roommate who will be bothered by the smoke. What should the nurse say to K. O.?

4. Develop a teaching–learning plan for K. O.'s postoperative care.

5. Mrs. O. visits her husband later in the evening. She asks whether she is permitted to come in early the next morning to be with her husband before the surgery. She is planning to take the day off from work to be there. What should the nurse tell Mrs. O.?

The next morning, the night shift nurse administers the preoperative injections. The preoperative medication orders for K. O. are as follows: atropine sulfate gr 1/4 IM, meperidine hydrochloride (Demerol) 75 mg IM, and promethazine hydrochloride (Phenergan) 25 mg IM. The nurse has on hand the following: atropine 0.4 mg/mL, Demerol 100 mg/mL, and Phenergan 25 mg/mL.

6. How many milliliters are given of each medication? What sites should the nurse use to administer the injections? Can any of the drugs be mixed together in the same syringe?

7. What information does the night nurse review on K. O.'s chart before medicating him?

8. What does the night nurse do to prepare K. O. for the preoperative injections?

K. O. was transferred to the surgical area by stretcher at 7:00 a.m. At 8:45 a.m., K. O returned to the nursing unit. The nurse went into the room and prepared to take his vital signs and do the postoperative assessment. As the nurse looked under his gown for the surgical dressing, K.O. said, "Don't bother, they never did the surgery. It was canceled and I have no idea why." The nurse made K. O. comfortable and left the room to review his chart. She read the following laboratory values: CBC = normal, serum potassium = 5.0 mg/L, serum sodium = 142 mEq/L, serum chloride = 106 mEq/L, serum glucose = 108 mg/dL, serum creatinine = 1.4 mg/100 mL, BUN 26 mg/100 mL, and PT = 12 seconds.

9. What immediate care is needed for K. O. until the preoperative medications wear off?

10. Identify which laboratory values are abnormal. What is the significance of this to K. O.'s risk of having surgery? Why is it important to determine the cause of his abnormal laboratory results?

11. After 2 days of evaluation, K. O. is rescheduled for surgery. Does the surgical consent need to be resigned? Do new orders need be written for surgery?

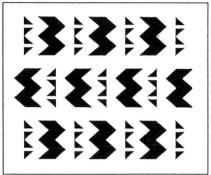

C H A P T E R 2 0

Interventions for Intraoperative Clients

LEARNING OBJECTIVES

At the end of this chapter, the student will be able to

▪ Describe the members of the surgical team

▪ Identify methods to ensure client safety during surgery

▪ Identify nursing responsibilities with anesthesia

▪ Describe the assessment of and nursing diagnoses for the client who has just entered the operating room

▪ List nursing measures to reduce the risk of impaired skin integrity and wound infection during surgery

▪ Identify the information given to the recovery room nurse as the client is being transferred from the operating room

PREREQUISITE KNOWLEDGE

Prior to beginning this chapter, the student should review

▪ The principles of sterile technique

▪ The principles of skin care

▪ The norms for vital sign measurements

▪ Normal laboratory values for hemoglobin, hematocrit, white blood cells (WBCs), red blood cells (RBCs), platelets, serum electrolytes, arterial blood gases, and urinalysis

STUDY QUESTIONS

Surgical Team and Environment

Match the following role functions (1–9) with the correct surgical team members (a–e). Answers may be used more than once.

_____ 1. sets up and hands sterile supplies and instruments to the surgeon

_____ 2. sets up room and maintains needed supplies

_____ 3. responsible for all medical acts

_____ 4. checks equipment safety and functioning

_____ 5. administers anesthetic agents (physician)

_____ 6. accounts for sponges, needles, and instruments throughout surgical procedure

_____ 7. ensures that sterile technique is maintained

_____ 8. administers anesthesia under a physician's supervision

_____ 9. coordinates activities of the operating room

a. anesthesiologist

b. circulating nurse

c. nurse anesthetist

d. scrub nurse

e. surgeon

10. List the support services to the surgical suite.

    a. _____

    b. _____

    c. _____

    d. _____

11. List the types of designated areas that ensure sterility in the operating room.

    a. _____

    b. _____

    c. _____

12. Identify examples of hygienic measures for the following sources of contamination.

    a. hair: _____

    _____

    _____

    b. skin: _____

    _____

    _____

    c. respiratory tract: _____

    _____

    _____

    d. jewelry: _____

    _____

    _____

13. Which of the following statements about the surgical scrub are true?

    a. The scrub sterilizes the hands and forearms.

    b. The effectiveness of the scrub depends on friction.

    c. The scrub is performed by the circulating nurse.

    d. Isopropyl alcohol is the preferred antimicrobial scrub solution.

    e. The scrub takes 5–6 minutes.

    f. The hands are held lower than the elbows.

    g. The hands and arms are dried with a sterile towel.

Anesthesia

14. List the purposes of anesthesia.

    a. _____

    _____

    b. _____

    _____

    c. _____

    _____

    d. _____

    _____

15. When does the administration of anesthesia begin?

    _____

    _____

16. Which of the following statements about anesthesia is correct?

    a. Most anesthetics are excreted by the lungs.

    b. Hepatic dysfunction can reduce anesthetic toxicity.

    c. Hypnosis is a commonly used form of anesthesia.

    d. Anesthesia produces multiple systemic effects.

Match the following qualities (17–24) with their associated types of anesthesia (a–c). Answers may be used more than once.

_____ 17. contraindicated in hepatic or renal disease

_____ 18. poor control once agent is administered

_____ 19. most controlled method

_____ 20. few disruptions in body functions

_____ 21. explosive

_____ 22. low incidence of postoperative nausea

_____ 23. few side effects

_____ 24. rapid induction

a. inhalation

b. intravenous (IV)

c. regional or local

25. During induction with general anesthesia, the client's

    a. hearing is most acute in stage II

    b. breathing is regular and quiet in stage III

    c. muscle tone and activity increase in stage I

    d. pulse is strong and regular in stage IV

26. Identify factors that affect the reversal of general anesthesia

    a. _____

    _____

    _____

    b. _____

    _____

    _____

    c. _____

    _____

    _____

27. During emergence, the nurse

    a. removes coverings to allow for body cooling

    b. applies protective padding to prevent injury

    c. provides suction equipment to prevent aspiration

    d. encourages deep breathing to hasten anesthesia reversal

28. Which of the following statements is correct about inhalant anesthetic agents?

    a. Urinary output is monitored carefully if isoflurane (Forane) is administered.

    b. The client is covered with warmed blankets if halothane (Fluothane) is administered.

    c. ECG changes are closely monitored if enflurane (Ethrane) is administered.

    d. Blood pressure is assessed frequently when nitrous oxide (N_2O) is administered.

29. Which of the following statements is correct about IV anesthetic agents?

    a. Barbiturates provide sustained postoperative analgesia.

    b. Opioids are used to produce unconsciousness.

    c. Neuromuscular blockers reduce postoperative nausea.

    d. Dissociative agents do not produce respiratory depression.

30. List the symptoms of malignant hyperthermia.

    a. _____

    _____

    b. _____

    _____

    c. _____

    _____

    d. _____

    _____

    e. _____

    _____

    f. _____

    _____

    g. _____

    _____

31. Briefly discuss the significance of the nurse accurately recording a client's preoperative height and weight in the record. Use a separate sheet.

32. List the four components of balanced anesthesia.

    a. _____

    _____

    _____

    b. _____

    _____

    _____

    c. _____

    _____

    _____

    d. _____

    _____

    _____

33. List the factors that affect the extent of the anesthetized field with local or regional anesthesia.

    a. _____

    _____

    b. _____

    _____

    c. _____

    _____

    d. _____

    _____

34. Identify the signs of a systemic toxic reaction related to regional anesthetic agents. Use a separate sheet.

Match the following descriptions (35–40) with their types of regional anesthesia (a–f).

____ 35. intra- or subcutaneous injection of anesthetic agent

____ 36. anesthetic applied directly to body surface

____ 37. injection of anesthetic agent through vertebral interspaces

____ 38. injection of anesthetic agent into subarachnoid spaces

____ 39. series of injections around the operative field

____ 40. nerve supplying a region is injected with an agent

a. epidural
b. field block
c. local infiltration
d. nerve block
e. spinal
f. topical

41. The *major* focus during and following regional anesthesia is

    a. administering ordered analgesics until the anesthetic wears off
    b. monitoring the position of numb body parts to protect from injury
    c. assessing the site of infiltration for signs of local tissue irritation
    d. documenting when full sensation has returned to the numbed body area

42. Nursing interventions for regional anesthesia overdose include all of the following *except*

    a. administering oxygen
    b. administering a barbiturate
    c. establishing an open airway
    d. placing in reverse Trendelenburg's position

43. Interventions for the client with a headache following spinal anesthesia include

    a. assisting the client with bathroom privileges
    b. restricting fluids to 1000 mL per day
    c. encouraging diversionary activities such as reading
    d. administering sedatives or analgesics as ordered

44. Identify what the nurse monitors in the client who is consciously sedated.

    a. _____

    b. _____

    c. _____

    d. _____

Collaborative Management

45. Identify the rationale for the following questions that the circulating nurse asks the client.

    a. "What is your name?" _____

    _____

    _____

    b. "What kind of operation are you having today?" _____

    _____

    _____

46. The record is reviewed by the circulating nurse when a client is admitted to the surgical suite. Explain the purpose for the nurse checking the following data (a–m). Use a separate sheet.

    a. history of allergies
    b. previous reaction to anesthesia
    c. previous reaction to transfusion
    d. use of blood or blood products during surgery
    e. autologous blood transfusion
    f. hemoglobin level

g. serum glucose level

h. routinely taken medications

i. history of cardiac disease

j. preoperative anticoagulant therapy

k. dentures or dental prostheses

l. osteoporosis

m. contact lenses

47. List the nursing diagnoses common to intraoperative clients.

a. _____

_____

b. _____

_____

c. _____

_____

48. Identify the factors that are considered by the nurse when positioning the client for surgery.

a. _____

b. _____

c. _____

d. _____

49. Ms. W. is having a right hip replacement. She has previously had a hip replacement on the left side. The grounding pad should be placed under her left

a. hip

b. thigh

c. arm

d. calf

50. List the purposes of the adhesive surgical drape.

a. _____

_____

b. _____

_____

51. Which of the following statements is true about the use of plastic adhesive drapes? The drape is

a. applied before the surgical scrub to protect the client from infection

b. applied immediately after the incision is made to control bleeding

c. removed quickly and all in one motion to reduce the incidence of pain

d. removed carefully in the elderly because these clients have fragile skin

52. Identify the purposes of the surgical dressing.

a. _____

_____

b. _____

_____

c. _____

_____

Match the following types of sutures (53–55) with their purposes (a–c).

_____ 53. absorbable

_____ 54. nonabsorbable

_____ 55. stay sutures

a. remain inside the body until digested by body enzymes

b. used for clients at high risk of retarded healing

c. removed from the skin

56. Identify the members of the surgical team who usually accompany the client to the postanesthesia care unit (PACU).

a. _____

b. _____

c. _____

57. List the intraoperative information on the client that the circulating nurse reports to the PACU nurse. Use a separate sheet.

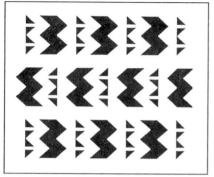

CHAPTER 21

Interventions for Postoperative Clients

LEARNING OBJECTIVES

At the end of this chapter, the student will be able to

- List the nursing assessments and interventions completed in the postanesthesia care unit (PACU)
- Describe the ongoing head-to-toe assessments of the postoperative client
- List the common nursing diagnoses for the postoperative client
- Describe common nursing interventions for the postoperative client

PREREQUISITE KNOWLEDGE

Prior to beginning this chapter, the student should review

- The assessment and care of the client having pain
- The principles of sterile technique
- Normal laboratory values for hemoglobin, hematocrit, white blood cells (WBCs), red blood cells (RBCs), platelets, serum electrolytes, arterial blood gases, and urinalysis
- The principles of fluid balance
- Normal ranges for vital sign measurements
- The principles of skin care
- The principles of teaching and learning in client care

STUDY QUESTIONS

Assessment

1. Identify factors that affect the time a client spends in the recovery area.

   a. _____

   _____

   b. _____

   _____

   c. _____

   _____

   d. _____

   _____

   _____

   e. _____

   _____

   _____

2. List the preoperative data from the client's record that the nurse reviews following report from the circulating nurse and initial client assessment.

   a. _____

   _____

   b. _____

   _____

3. List the psychosocial data relevant to the postoperative client.

   a. _____

   _____

   b. _____

   _____

   c. _____

   _____

   d. _____

   _____

   e. _____

   _____

Match the following assessment findings in the recovery area (4–32) with their correct body systems (a–g). Answers may be used more than once and more than one answer may apply to each finding.

_____ 4. eyes open on command

_____ 5. symmetrical chest wall expansion

_____ 6. Foley's catheter to straight drainage

_____ 7. absent dorsalis pedis pulsations

_____ 8. use of the accessory muscles

_____ 9. large amount of sangiunous drainage

_____ 10. negative Homans' test

_____ 11. IV infusion of D₅ Ringer's lactate

_____ 12. states name when asked

a. respiratory

b. cardiovascular

c. fluid and electrolyte balance

d. neurologic

e. renal/urinary

f. gastrointestinal

g. integumentary

_____ 13. rounded, firm abdomen

_____ 14. exhalation felt from nose or mouth

_____ 15. decreased blood pressure

_____ 16. wound edges approximated

_____ 17. dry mucous membranes

_____ 18. vomiting

_____ 19. pupils constrict equally

_____ 20. sternal retraction

_____ 21. nasogastric tube in place

_____ 22. evisceration

_____ 23. dullness over symphysis pubis

_____ 24. tenting

_____ 25. faint heart sounds

_____ 26. wound dressing dry

_____ 27. absent bowel sounds

_____ 28. bibasilar rales or crackles

_____ 29. hand grips equal

_____ 30. simultaneous apical and radial pulsations

_____ 31. dehiscence

_____ 32. snoring

33. Identify the signs that a client may exhibit when in pain.

   a. _____

   b. _____

   c. _____

   d. _____

   e. _____

   f. _____

   g. _____

   h. _____

34. Identify factors determining the frequency and type of laboratory tests that may be ordered for the postoperative client. Use a separate sheet.

35. List criteria used to determine when a postoperative client is ready for dismissal from the recovery area.

    a. _____

    b. _____

    c. _____

    d. _____

    e. _____

    f. _____

    g. _____

    h _____

    i. _____

Analysis

36. List the common nursing diagnoses for the postoperative client.

    a. _____

    b. _____

    c. _____

37. Identify preoperative factors that put the client at risk for developing postoperative respiratory complications.

    a. _____
    _____

    b. _____
    _____

    c. _____
    _____

Planning and Implementation

38. Identify the nursing interventions implemented for each of the following potential postoperative problems. Use a separate sheet.

    a. aspiration

    b. airway obstruction

    c. atelectasis

    d. pulmonary embolus

    e. thrombophlebitis

    f. urinary retention

    g. urinary tract infection

    h. wound infection

    i. wound dehiscence

    j. evisceration

39. Which of the following is correct about postoperative analgesic administration?

    a. Opioids are routinely given the first 24–48 hours after surgery to control pain.

    b. Patient-controlled analgesia (PCA) is widely used after neurologic surgery.

    c. Elderly and debilitated clients have a decreased tolerance for pain medication.

    d. Ambulatory clients usually receive IV pain medication in the recovery area.

40. Identify the rationale for early mobilization of the postoperative client. Use a separate sheet.

41. List the topics that are included in a teaching plan for the postoperative client.

    a. _____
    _____

    b. _____
    _____

    c. _____
    _____

    d. _____
    _____

    e. _____

42. Which of the following statements reflects that dismissal teaching was effective in the client returning for a postoperative check up?

    a. The client reports consuming a diet that consists of convenience foods.

    b. The client states that he has taken all of the prescribed antibiotic.

    c. The client reports persistent fatigue and wound discomfort.

    d. The client states that he has avoided activities such as walking.

CRITICAL THINKING EXERCISES

Case Study: Postoperative Care

L. P. is a 30-year-old female client who is admitted to the recovery area following a hemorrhoidectomy. She is a small woman, 5 feet 1 in. tall and weighing 103 pounds. L. P. was in surgery for 1 hour and 45 minutes and had a severe hemorrhage from the surgical site during that time. Upon admission to the postanesthesia unit, L. P.'s blood pressure is 112/62, pulse range is 84–92, and respirations are 20 and shallow. An intravenous infusion of 1000 mL of D5LR is infusing at a rate of 200 mL per hour, and 800 mL remain in the bottle. During surgery, 100 mL of D5LR and 500 mL of NS were infused. An endotracheal tube (ET) is in place.

Address the following questions:

1. What assessments should the nurse perform before removing the ET tube?

2. What complication should the nurse monitor for in L. P.? What actions should the nurse take to prevent this from occurring?

3. How often should the nurse monitor L. P.'s vital signs?

A very slight amount of sanguinous drainage is present on L. P.'s dressing. Her blood pressure has been rising slowly and is now 20 mm Hg higher than the last time recorded in surgery. She is also restless and her respirations are 24 per minute.

4. Identify the potential complications the nurse should assess for in L. P. What assessments should the nurse make?

5. The nurse contacts L. P.'s surgeon and he orders that the intravenous rate be reduced to 100 mL per hour. What is the reason for this order?

6. L. P. stablizes and is transferred to the postsurgical nursing unit. Discuss the information that the recovery room nurse should report to the unit nurse.

8. In addition to vital signs and dressing checks, what should the unit nurse monitor in L. P. for the next 24 hours? Why?

CHAPTER 22

Inflammation and the Immune Response

LEARNING OBJECTIVES

At the end of this chapter, the student will be able to

- Identify the purpose of immunity
- Describe the concept of *self* versus *nonself*
- Discuss the general organization of the immune system
- Identify the processes necessary for immunity
- Describe inflammation
- Discuss the function of neutrophils, macrophages, basophils, and eosinophils
- Discuss the seven steps of phagocytosis
- Discuss the three stages of the inflammatory response
- Describe antibody-mediated immunity (AMI) and the B-lymphocyte
- Define the seven steps of the antigen–antibody interaction
- Describe sustained immunity or memory
- Identify the categories of antibodies (immunoglobulins and gamma globulins)
- Compare and contrast the types of antibody-mediated immunity
- Discuss cell-mediated immunity (CMI)
- Describe the types of transplant rejection and immunosuppressive agents

PREREQUISITE KNOWLEDGE

Nothing is required

STUDY QUESTIONS

General Concepts

1. Which of the following statements gives the purpose of immunity?

   a. to provide protection against side effects that accompany invasion or injury from foreign organisms

   b. to prevent invasion or injury from foreign organisms from occurring in the first place

   c. to neutralize, eliminate, or destroy invading microorganisms once body defenses have been overwhelmed

   d. to mount defensive actions against infected, debilitated self cells as well as normal, healthy self cells

2. Which of the following 10 statements are true about the immune system?

   a. *Self-tolerance* is the body's ability to recognize self versus nonself.

   b. Cell membranes contain only recognition proteins that are specific for that human.

c. Antigens are substances recognized as foreign by the immune system.

d. Leukocyte antigens are present only on leukocytes.

e. Leukocyte antigens specify an individual's tissue type.

f. The total number of human leukocyte antigens is 40.

g. The number of minor human leukocyte antigens exceeds that of major antigens.

h. Identical twins have identical recognition proteins.

i. Major tissue antigens must be matched between donor and recipient for solid organ transplantation.

j. The immune system is located in the bone marrow.

3. Which of the following statements is correct about stem cells? Stem cells are

   a. highly differentiated in function

   b. undifferentiated in function

   c. composed of a variety of different blood cell types

   d. able to revert from a specific cell type to pluripotent

4. A stem cell selects a specific maturational pathway

   a. and must progress until end-state cell type is reached

   b. based on random selection and predetermined quotas

   c. based on specific body needs at a given time

   d. because erythropoietin stimulates all further commitment

5. List the defensive actions of leukocytes. Use a separate sheet.

6. Which of the following statements is correct about leukocytes?

   a. All leukocytes are capable of performing every function of WBCs.

   b. Leukocytes are the cells that protect the body from the effects of foreign microorganism invasion.

   c. Leukocytes constitute the immune system's cells along with erythrocytes and platelets.

   d. There are different categories of leukocytes based on their originating source.

Match the following types of leukocytes (7–16) with their correct descriptions (a–j).

_____ 7. cytotoxic T-cells

_____ 8. B-lympho-cytes

_____ 9. basophils

_____ 10. eosinophils

_____ 11. natural killer cells

_____ 12. memory cells

_____ 13. macro-phages

_____ 14. monocytes

_____ 15. neutrophils

_____ 16. T-lympho-cytes

a. provide sustained protection against specific invading organisms

b. most numerous type; efficient at phagocytosis

c. mature into macrophages

d. enhance cell-mediated immunity

e. competent at phagocy-tosis

f. secrete antibodies for long-lasting immunity

g. attack and destroy nonself cells selectively

h. release histamine and heparin locally

i. attack nonself cells nonselectively

j. function mostly in allergic reactions

17. List the processes necessary for immuno-competence.

   a. _____

   _____

   b. _____

   _____

   c. _____

Inflammation

18. Identify two primary ways that inflammation differs from immunity.

   a. _____

   _____

   _____

   _____

   b. _____

   _____

   _____

   _____

19. Which of the following statements is correct about inflammation?

    a. Inflammatory responses are usually not observable and are mildly uncomfortable.

    b. Inflammatory reactions are harmful but crucial to the individual.

    c. Inflammatory responses are not essential to specific immune processes.

    d. Inflammation occurs in response to both tissue injury and microorganism invasion.

Match the following examples of inflammatory response (20–27) with their correct descriptions (a–c). Answers may be used more than once.

_____ 20. allergic rhinitis

_____ 21. appendicitis

_____ 22. contact dermatitis

_____ 23. myocardial infarction

_____ 24. otitis media

_____ 25. pharyngitis

_____ 26. sprained ankle

_____ 27. surgical incision

a. inflammatory response without infection

b. inflammatory response associated with noninfectious invasion of foreign proteins

c. inflammatory response associated with invasion by pathogenic organisms

28. Briefly discuss how the inflammatory response is nonspecific. Use a separate sheet.

29. List the four types of leukocytes responsible for generating the inflammatory response.

    a. _____

    b. _____

    c. _____

    d. _____

30. Which of the following seven statements are true about neutrophils?

    a. Mature neutrophils constitute the largest portion of the WBC count.

    b. Neutrophils mature in the body's tissues where they are needed.

    c. Neutrophils take 12–18 hours to mature from time of release by the bone marrow.

    d. Maturation time can be shortened by specific chemical factors.

    e. Neutrophils are the first line of defense in blood and extracellular fluids.

f. Granules in the cytoplasm contain enzymes that degrade different components of foreign invaders.

g. Each neutrophil is capable of multiple episodes of phagocytic destruction before dying.

31. Which of the following statements is correct about neutrophils and infection?

    a. Banded neutrophils are capable of immediate effective phagocytosis of invading organisms.

    b. One's susceptibility to infection is decreased when the number of mature neutrophils is large.

    c. A left shift of neutrophils occurs during overwhelming infection and more mature cells are released.

    d. Release of immature neutrophils benefits a client because these cells mature rapidly in the blood.

32. Which of the following statements is correct about macrophages?

    a. Macrophages derive from monocytes that migrate to various tissues where they mature.

    b. Tissue macrophages have short life spans due to the amount of phagocytosis performed.

    c. Tissue macrophages are capable only of phagocytosis and do not stimulate an immune response.

    d. Each macrophage is capable of participating in only one phagocytic event during its life span.

33. Which of the following statements is correct about basophils, eosinophils, and their enzymes?

    a. Basophilic enzymes act to control or moderate the extent of inflammatory reactions.

    b. Basophilic enzymes release heparin, which constricts the smooth muscle of the respiratory tract.

    c. Kinins and serotonin released by basophils enhance the capillary permeability to plasma.

    d. Some eosinophil enzymes work to neutralize the effects associated with exposure to allergens.

34. Define phagocytosis._____

_____

_____

_____

_____

35. List the seven steps of phagocytosis.

    a. _____

    b. _____

    c. _____

    d. _____

    e. _____

    f. _____

    g. _____

36. Place the following events in proper sequence as they occur during phagocytosis.

    _____ a. vacuole forms, sealing target cell inside the phagocyte

    _____ b. recognition of nonself cell is enhanced by the presence of opsonins on the target cell wall surface

    _____ c. penetration of foreign proteins into body's internal environment

    _____ d. target cell broken into smaller molecules subject to specific enzyme actions

    _____ e. opsonization of foreign proteins by neutrophils changes cell wall surface charges

    _____ f. phagocytic cell changes shape and invaginates around target cell

    _____ g. release of chemotaxins from damaged tissue draws phagocytic cells

    _____ h. enhanced destruction of target cell by cytoplasmic granules and lytic substances

    _____ i. sequential activation of complement components increases fixation of phagocytic cells on target cell

37. List the five physical manifestations of inflammation.

    a. _____

    b. _____

    c. _____

    d. _____

    e. _____

Match the following events in the inflammatory response (38–52) with their corresponding stages (a–c). Answers may be used more than once.

_____ 38. walling off of injured site   a. stage I

_____ 39. neutrophils migrate to injured site   b. stage II

   c. stage III

_____ 40. blood flow increases to injured area

_____ 41. immediate, short-term vasoconstriction

_____ 42. revascularization

_____ 43. bone marrow production of monocytes increases

_____ 44. capillary permeability increases and plasma leaks to interstitial spaces

_____ 45. foreign matter attacked and destroyed

_____ 46. scar tissue formation

_____ 47. tissue macrophages respond to injury

_____ 48. dead tissue removed

_____ 49. bone marrow stimulated by macrophages

_____ 50. healthy tissue stimulated to replicate

_____ 51. tissue macrophages reproduce

_____ 52. swelling at injury site

Antibody-Mediated Immunity

53. List the three actions of antibody-mediated immunity.

    a. _____

    b. _____

    c. _____

54. Which of the following statements is correct about B-lymphocytes?

    a. The primary function of B-lymphocytes is to become sensitized to a variety of foreign proteins.

    b. B-lymphocytes are efficient in recognizing self versus nonself in inflammatory reactions.

    c. The entire immune system must function adequately for antibody-mediated immunity to occur.

    d. B-lymphocytes synthesize antigens, which then interact with invading foreign proteins.

55. B-lymphocytes mature in the

    a. liver

    b. kidney

    c. tonsils

    d. bone marrow

Match the following events (56–72) that occur during antigen–antibody interactions with their correct steps (a–g). Answers may be used more than once.

____ 56. antigen cell wall disrupted

____ 57. helper T-cell initiates contact of B-lymphocyte with antigen

____ 58. antigen movement through extracellular fluids slowed

____ 59. B-lymphocyte absorbs antigen

____ 60. antibody inactivates antigen

____ 61. antigen invasion overwhelms ability of inflammatory response

____ 62. memory cell forms, is sensitized but dormant

____ 63. antibody joins antigen and initiates other actions

____ 64. formation of immunoglobulins

____ 65. macrophage attaches to antigen

____ 66. B-lymphocyte becomes sensitized

____ 67. increased susceptibility of antigen–antibody complex to attack

____ 68. helper T-cell exposes antigen

____ 69. plasma cell produces antigen-specific antibody

____ 70. B-lymphocyte recognizes antigen as nonself

____ 71. complement cascade activated

____ 72. free antibodies circulate in blood

a. exposure and invasion

b. antigen recognition

c. lymphocyte sensitization

d. antibody production and release

e. antigen–antibody binding

f. antibody binding reactions

g. sustained immunity and memory

Match the following types of immune responses (73–77) with their immunoglobulins (a–e).

____ 73. responds to antigens by agglutination and precipitation

____ 74. thought to modify activity of IgM

____ 75. binds to antigens allowing phagocytosis by neutrophils and macrophages

____ 76. inhibits bacteria and viruses from adhering to skin or mucous membrane surfaces

____ 77. causes degranulation of basophils and mast cells, releasing vasoactive amines

a. IgA

b. IgG

c. IgM

d. IgE

e. IgD

78. Which of the following statements is correct about innate immunity? Innate immunity is

    a. developed by the individual

    b. a genetically determined characteristic

    c. an adaptive response to foreign protein exposure

    d. immunity acquired through vaccination or booster injections

Match the following immunity responses (79–81) with their associated immunoglobulins.

____ 79. autoimmune response

____ 80. hypersensitivity reaction

____ 81. acquired immunity

a. IgG

b. IgM

c. IgE

Match the following descriptions of acquired immunity (82–90) with their types of immunity (a–d). Answers may be used more than once and more than one answer may apply to each.

____ 82. antibodies produced in another organism, then introduced into body

____ 83. most long-lasting immunity

____ 84. deliberate introduction of antibodies produced by one organism into body

____ 85. requires booster to maintain immunity efficiency

____ 86. body makes antibodies against antigens

____ 87. antibodies transmitted via placenta, colostrum, or breast milk

____ 88. specific antigens deliberately introduced into body in small amounts

____ 89. immediate, short-term protection against specific antigens

____ 90. antigens enter body without assistance

a. natural active

b. artificial active

c. natural passive

d. artificial passive

91. Which of the following statements is correct about factors that influence antibody-mediated immunity?

    a. A client with chronic airflow limitation has a competent immune system.

    b. An individual who is malnourished can synthesize immunoglobulins effectively.

    c. The immune system of a diabetic client is as effective as that of a healthy individual.

    d. A client with a hypoactive thyroid gland may be unable to fight infections effectively.

Cell-Mediated Immunity

92. Which of the following statements is correct about cell-mediated immunity?

    a. This type of immunity is provided by leukocytes that are slow to recognize self versus nonself.

    b. The leukocytes involved respond directly by actively phagocytizing foreign proteins.

    c. Alterations in this type of immunity do not affect the other types of immunity reactions.

    d. Total immunocompetence depends on all components of the immune system.

93. Which of the following statements is correct about T-lymphocytes?

    a. They are released from the bone marrow and migrate to Peyer's patches for maturation.

    b. They have functional characteristics that are similar to those of B-lymphocytes.

    c. They differentiate into a variety of subsets, each having its own functions.

    d. They have more than one antibody on their cell membranes that interact with multiple antigens.

Match the following immunity functions (94–102) with their respective T-lymphocytes (a–c). Answers may be used more than once.

_____ 94. binding of antibody-like substance results in direct lysis of nonself cell

_____ 95. secretes substances that inhibit other cells of immune system

_____ 96. secretes lymphokines that regulate activity of other leukocytes

_____ 97. efficient at recognizing self versus nonself cells

a. helper

b. cytotoxic/cytolytic

c. suppressor

_____ 98. prevents continuous overreaction of hypersensitivity reactions from occurring

_____ 99. becomes sensitized in similar way as B-lymphocytes

_____ 100. forms antibody-like substances in response to antigens on nonself cell

_____ 101. participates indirectly in cell-mediated immunity

_____ 102. directly opposes activity of helper T-cells

103. Which of the following statements is correct about natural killer cells?

    a. They exert direct cytotoxic and cytolytic effects on nonself cells.

    b. They must first undergo sensitization before they can act against nonself cells.

    c. They must share a histocompatibility protein with the nonself cell before they can act.

    d. They depend on interactions with other leukocytes to be most effective.

104. Natural killer cells are most effective against

    a. nonself cells

    b. healthy self cells

    c. unhealthy self cells

    d. infected nonself cells

105. Describe how the actions of cell-mediated immunity are different from those of the inflammatory response.

    a. _____

    _____

    _____

    b. _____

    _____

    _____

106. Which of the following statements about cytokines is correct?

    a. Cytokine action is similar to that of other hormones.

    b. Cells that alter their activity in response to cytokines are known as initiators.

    c. Cytokines are produced in large quantity and stored in mononuclear phagocytes.

    d. Target cell membranes have multiple receptor sites where cytokines bind and initiate changes.

107. Hyperacute graft rejection is most likely to occur in someone who

   a. has had one pregnancy

   b. has never received a blood transfusion

   c. has had a previous organ transplant

   d. has an ABO blood type similar to the donor

108. Acute graft rejection is

   a. a sign that the transplanted organ has necrosed and died

   b. related to thrombolytic occlusion of the organ's blood vessels

   c. commonly seen after 6 months following organ transplantation

   d. treated with pharmacological manipulation of the host's immune responses

109. Chronic graft rejection

   a. is rare in solid organ transplants

   b. is related to fibrotic scarring of the organ

   c. occurs intermittently during acute rejection episodes

   d. is treated and cured with pharmacological manipulation

110. Which of the following pharmacological agents is used in rescue therapy during episodes of acute rejection of a transplanted organ?

   a. OKT3

   b. prednisone

   c. cyclosporine

   d. azathioprine

Match the following descriptions (111–119) with their types of tissue transplant rejection (a–c). Answers may be used more than once.

_____ 111. the most common type of rejection

_____ 112. can occur before surgery is over

_____ 113. characterized by gradual decrease in vascular supply to the organ

_____ 114. minimized by immuno-suppressive drugs

_____ 115. occurs within weeks or months of transplanta-tion

_____ 116. avoided by pretransplan-tation cross-match

_____ 117. occurs over months or years after transplanta-tion

_____ 118. managed by increasing doses of immunosup-pressive drugs

_____ 119. increased doses of immunosuppressive drugs are ineffective

   a. hyperacute

   b. acute

   c. chronic

CRITICAL THINKING EXERCISES

Case Study: Transplant Rejection

P. V. is a 35-year-old man admitted with acute rejection of a transplanted organ.

Address the following questions:

1. Explain what has happened to P. V. using concepts of the immune response, self versus nonself, the role of neutrophils and other granulocytes, and functions of the T-lymphocyte and B-lymphocyte.

2. What or who would be the best source of a donor organ for P. V.? List in order the sources of the organ least likely to be rejected and the most likely to be rejected. Explain the rationale for your answer.

3. What may have happened to P. V's self-concept during the process of transplantation and rejection? What data would indicate problems with self-concept?

(Also see Case Study: Renal Transplantation in Chapter 72.)

C H A P T E R 2 3

Interventions for Clients with Connective Tissue Disease

LEARNING OBJECTIVES

At the end of this chapter, the student will be able to

- Describe the pathophysiology, etiology, and incidence of degenerative joint disease
- Discuss assessment of the client with degenerative joint disease
- Discuss management of degenerative joint disease
- Describe management of the client having an osteotomy or a joint replacement
- Identify the pathophysiology, etiology, and incidence of rheumatoid arthritis
- Discuss assessment of the client with rheumatoid arthritis
- Describe management of the client with rheumatoid arthritis
- Describe the pathophysiology, etiology, and incidence of lupus erythematosus
- Discuss assessment of the client with lupus erythematosus
- Describe the management of clients with discoid and systemic lupus erythematosus
- Discuss progressive systemic sclerosis (PSS)
- Discuss gout
- Discuss other connective tissue diseases

PREREQUISITE KNOWLEDGE

Prior to beginning this chapter, the student should review

- The anatomy and physiology of the musculoskeletal system, joints, and connective tissue
- The concept of autoimmunity
- The inflammatory process
- The concept of body image
- The principles of pain management
- The hazards of immobility
- Joint range of motion
- Perioperative care

STUDY QUESTIONS

Degenerative Joint Disease

1. Which of the following four terms describes degenerative joint disease (DJD)?
    a. osteoanagenesis
    b. osteoarthritis
    c. osteoarthrosis
    d. osteoporosis

2. Which of the following joints is most likely to be affected by DJD?

   a. temporomandibular

   b. elbow

   c. ankle

   d. hip

3. Put the following pathological joint changes in DJD in sequence.

   _____ a. inflammatory enzymes enhance tissue destruction

   _____ b. cartilage begins to erode

   _____ c. joint deformity causes marked immobility and pain

   _____ d. bone cysts and secondary synovitis occur

   _____ e. fissures and pitting develop

   _____ f. osteophyte spur formation occurs

   _____ g. cartilage becomes soft, opaque, and yellow

   _____ h. joint space narrows

4. Which of the following is a cause of primary DJD?

   a. obesity

   b. trauma

   c. sepsis

   d. hemophilia

5. Which of the following clients is at greatest risk for developing DJD?

   a. a 40-year-old woman who works in a meat-packing plant

   b. an 18-year-old youth who is on the school swim team

   c. a 53-year-old executive with a sedentary life style

   d. a 24-year-old model in the high fashion industry

6. List the subjective client data relevant to DJD. Use a separate sheet.

7. List the objective client data relevant to DJD. Use a separate sheet.

8. The laboratory test most useful in diagnosing DJD is

   a. a complete blood count (CBC)

   b. erythrocyte sedimentation rate (ESR)

   c. antinuclear antibodies (ANA)

   d. lupus erythematosus (LE) preparation

9. Identify the common nursing diagnoses for the client with DJD.

   a. _____

   _____

   b. _____

   _____

10. Which of the following medications is usually administered to the client with DJD?

    a. auranofin (Ridaura)

    b. prednisone (Orasone)

    c. naproxen (Naprosyn)

    d. acetaminophen (Tylenol)

11. Which of the following instructions should the nurse give the client with DJD?

    a. "Place a small pillow or folded towel under your knees when you lie on your back."

    b. "Try to rest several times during the day and lie on your stomach to stretch out."

    c. "Include more dairy products in your diet to increase the amount of calcium you eat."

    d. Try applying an ice pack to your stiff joints before exercising to reduce discomfort."

12. Which of the following conditions is treated surgically with an osteotomy?

    a. rheumatoid arthritis

    b. avascular necrosis

    c. genu valgus

    d. osteoporosis

13. Briefly discuss why total joint replacement surgery is postponed if there is any infection present. Use a separate sheet.

14. An intervention to decrease the potential for infection in the client who is having a total hip replacement is

    a. beginning intravenous antibiotic therapy postoperatively

    b. using povidone-iodine (Betadine) to scrub the surgical site before surgery

    c. scheduling the operation as the last case of the day

    d. applying a large, bulky dressing to the incision

15. The preferred position following surgery for the client who has had a total hip replacement is

   a. prone with a pillow under the abdomen

   b. side-lying with a trochanter roll along the back

   c. supine with pillows between the legs

   d. sitting in a straight-backed chair with legs elevated

16. List the signs of hip dislocation:

   a. _____

     _____

   b. _____

     _____

   c. _____

     _____

17. To reduce the incidence of tape burns in the elderly client who has had total hip replacement surgery, the nurse should

   a. remove the tape from the dressing in one quick motion

   b. apply normal saline to the tape to loosen the adhesive

   c. replace the dressing's Elastoplast tape with paper tape

   d. loosen the tape on the dressing 24 hours postoperatively

18. Which of the following should the nurse report immediately to the physician when caring for a client who has had a total hip replacement?

   a. On day 2, the client requests an injectable opioid analgesic for incisional pain.

   b. Three days following surgery, the client's hematocrit is 36% and hemoglobin is 10.6 g/dL.

   c. One day postoperatively, the client is dyspneic, respiration is 40, pulse is 124, and rales are auscultated.

   d. On day 4, the wound edges are approximated and pink, and the surrounding skin is taut.

19. Which of the following is a correct intervention for the client who is using a continuous passive motion (CPM) machine?

   a. Place the control at the foot of the bed.

   b. Check that the machine is working continuously.

   c. Store the machine on the floor when not in use.

   d. Remove any dressings before beginning a CPM session.

20. All of the following joint replacement procedures may involve CPM in postoperative management *except* replacement of the

   a. wrist

   b. elbow

   c. ankle

   d. shoulder

21. All of the following are purposes of therapeutic exercises *except*

   a. restoring muscle strength

   b. increasing muscle tone

   c. improving joint range of motion

   d. achieving physical relaxation

Rheumatoid Arthritis

22. Onset of rheumatoid arthritis (RA) is characterized by

   a. pannus formation

   b. osteoporosis

   c. synovitis

   d. bony ankylosis

23. Which of the following statements is correct about RA?

   a. It is a systemic inflammatory disease.

   b. It affects weight-bearing joints primarily.

   c. It is associated with aging, obesity, and trauma.

   d. It involves antibody IgA-forming complexes.

24. List the subjective client data relevant to RA. Use a separate sheet.

25. List the objective client data relevant to RA. Use a separate sheet.

26. The diagnostic procedure that is performed on clients with suspected RA is

   a. amniocentesis

   b. arthrocentesis

   c. paracentesis

   d. thoracentesis

27. Identify five nursing diagnoses commonly affecting the client with RA.

   a. _____

     _____

   b. _____

     _____

c. _____

_____

d. _____

_____

e. _____

_____

28. Long-term maintenance drug therapy for RA includes
    a. salicylic acid (aspirin)
    b. sodium thiomalate (Myochrysine)
    c. prednisone (Deltasone)
    d. penicillamine (Cuprimine)

29. Total joint replacement for the client with RA is performed primarily to
    a. improve physical mobility
    b. restore self-esteem
    c. relieve pain
    d. increase activity tolerance

30. Which of the following products would be most manageable for the client with self-care deficit as a result of RA?
    a. a mechanically operated can opener
    b. toothpaste in a pump dispenser
    c. single-serving packets of nondairy creamer
    d. hand soap that comes in a bar

31. Interventions to reduce fatigue for the client with RA include
    a. physical therapy for muscle strengthening
    b. effective pain management
    c. delegation of responsibility to others
    d. all of the above

32. The client with an "arthritis personality" is
    a. manipulating the feelings of others
    b. demanding and difficult to please
    c. coping to the best of his or her ability
    d. avoiding the sick role by using denial

Lupus Erythematosus

33. Which of the following statements is correct about systemic lupus erythematosus (SLE)?
    a. The primary tissue affected is the skin.
    b. SLE progresses rapidly and survival time is limited.
    c. Most clients with SLE have kidney involvement.
    d. SLE is an autosomal recessive hereditary disease.

34. Which of the following clients is at greatest risk for developing lupus?
    a. a 37-year-old woman who frequents a tanning salon
    b. an 18-year-old girl who is a lifeguard at an indoor pool
    c. a 64-year-old man who plays golf twice a week
    d. a 43-year-old man who is a construction engineer

35. List the subjective client data relevant to lupus. Use a separate sheet.

36. List the objective client data relevant to lupus. Use a separate sheet.

37. The laboratory test most useful in diagnosing discoid lupus is
    a. LE prep
    b. ANA
    c. RA factor
    d. skin biopsy

38. Briefly discuss why there are numerous nursing diagnoses for the client with lupus. Use a separate sheet.

39. Which of the following is an intervention for the client with lupus who has impaired skin integrity?
    a. using a mild astringent on the face twice a day
    b. wearing sunglasses with polarizing lenses
    c. applying a sunblock with a sun protection factor (SPF) of 15
    d. moisturizing the skin with lotion several times a day

40. Which of the following blood components is removed during plasmapheresis?
    a. RA factors
    b. immune complexes
    c. LE cells
    d. erythrocytes

41. During dismissal teaching, which of the following symptoms should the client with lupus be instructed to report to the physician immediately?

  a. joint pain

  b. butterfly rash

  c. fever

  d. fatigue

Progressive Systemic Sclerosis

42. Which of the following statements is correct about progressive systemic sclerosis (PSS)?

  a. PSS has a lower mortality rate than SLE.

  b. Diagnosis is difficult until the disease progresses.

  c. PSS responds well to treatment with systemic steroids.

  d. There is a strong family link to the cause of PSS.

43. When assessing the client with PSS, the nurse will find

  a. swollen, reddened joints

  b. bilateral joint deformities

  c. edematous hands with skin fissures

  d. bibasilar rales and diffuse rhonchi

44. Briefly describe the CREST syndrome. Use a separate sheet.

45. The leading cause of death in clients with PSS is

  a. pneumonia

  b. cardiomyopathy

  c. malabsorption syndrome

  d. renal failure

46. Interventions for the client with PSS include

  a. eating three well-balanced meals per day

  b. taking salicylic acid (aspirin) 4 to 6 times per day

  c. maintaining a warm environment or wearing extra clothes

  d. scrubbing while bathing to débride dead skin cells

Gout

47. Which of the following diseases is a cause of secondary gout?

  a. myocardial infarction

  b. multiple myeloma

  c. peptic ulcer disease

  d. rheumatoid arthritis

Match the following clinical findings (48–55) with their phases of disease process in gout (a–d). Answers may be used more than once.

_____ 48. excruciating pain

_____ 49. asymptomatic following attack

_____ 50. urate kidney stone formation

_____ 51. elevated serum uric acid level

_____ 52. podagra

_____ 53. urate crystal deposits under skin

_____ 54. no overt signs of disease present

_____ 55. joints normal upon physical examination

  a. asymptomatic hyperuricemia

  b. acute

  c. intercritical

  d. chronic tophaceous

56. Which of the following clients is at greatest risk for developing primary gout?

  a. a 46-year-old woman

  b. a 38-year-old man

  c. a 85-year-old woman

  d. a 57-year-old man

57. List the subjective client data relevant to gout. Use a separate sheet.

58. List the objective client data relevant to gout. Use a separate sheet.

59. All of the following laboratory tests are done on the client with gout *except*

  a. serum uric acid measurement

  b. urine uric acid measurement

  c. serum alkaline phosphatase measurement

  d. blood urea nitrogen measurement

60. Identify the common nursing diagnoses for the client with gout

  a. _____

  _____

  b. _____

  _____

61. The action of the drug allopurinol (Zyloprim) in the management of gout is to

  a. increase uric acid excretion

  b. decrease uric acid excretion

  c. prevent uric acid crystal formation

  d. inhibit uric acid crystal deposits

62. Which of the following drugs is administered during acute gout episodes?

   a. allopurinol (Zyloprim)

   b. furosemide (Lasix)

   c. colchicine (Colsalide)

   d. probenecid (Benemid)

63. Which of the following foods should the client with gout avoid?

   a. strawberries

   b. cottage cheese

   c. cranberry juice

   d. cheeseburgers

72. Which of the following articles of clothing should a person wear in an area known to be a habitat for deer ticks?

   a. sandals

   b. shorts

   c. tank top

   d. sun hat

73. Initial drug therapy in the management of Lyme disease includes

   a. tetracycline

   b. steroids

   c. salicylic acid

   d. nonsteroidal anti-inflammatory agents

Other Connective Tissue Diseases

Match the following connective tissue diseases (64–71) to their most commonly associated body parts (a–h).

_____ 64. ankylosing spondylitis

_____ 65. fibrositis

_____ 66. polymyalgia rheumatica

_____ 67. polymyositis

_____ 68. pseudogout

_____ 69. Reiter's syndrome

_____ 70. Sjögren's syndrome

_____ 71. systemic necrotizing vasculitis

a. striated muscle

b. arterial wall

c. shoulder girdle

d. vertebral column

e. urethra

f. vagina

g. cartilage

h. face

CRITICAL THINKING EXERCISES

Case Study: Degenerative Joint Disease

S. H. is a 65-year-old woman admitted to the nursing unit following a total hip replacement. Her vital signs are stable following the operation, and she is experiencing moderate pain. Her personal health history includes hypertension for the past 10 years which has been managed with diuretics. Her admission blood pressure prior to surgery was 138/90 mmHg. S. H. has had lower back and sciatic leg pain for the past 12–18 months which the physicians have felt was referred hip pain. She is 5 feet, 1 inch tall and weighs 222 pounds. She had recently lost 10 pounds prior to the operation. She is not employed outside the home, but takes care of her 18-month-old grandson while her daughter works.

Address the following questions:

1. List the initial assessments the nurse should perform of S. H. following surgery.

2. The physician has ordered a range of 1/6 to 1/4 grain of morphine for pain management. List various considerations the nurse should evaluate before giving the first dose of the drug. Identify the dose S. H. should have now and the rationale for the choice.

3. The morphine is available in 10 mg/mL prepackaged syringes. Calculate the amount needed in milliliters based on the dose chosen in question 2.

Following the injection of morphine, S. H. is harder to arouse. In addition, her systolic blood pressure dropped 10 mmHg in 30 minutes and her pulse slowed.

4. Is S. H. having an expected response to morphine or has she been given an overdose of the drug? Explain your answer.

5. The surgeon ordered S. H.'s legs to be abducted with a pillow. Explain the rationale for this procedure.

6. S. H. is to be transferred to a bedside chair. Develop a teaching/learning plan for her to follow as she learns to transfer to the chair. Include weight bearing, placement of the chair, and hip flexion in the plan.

Three days following surgery, S. H. is found on the floor next to her bed. She was trying to reach the phone and fell. "I slid down the side of the bed," she explained. S. H. is assisted back to bed. Upon assessment, the nurse notes that S. H.'s operative leg is externally rotated and shorter than the nonoperative leg. She has severe pain in the operative leg.

7. Discuss the significance of these findings.

8. S. H. is going to be dismissed to home. Develop a teaching/learning plan for her dismissal. Include information on turning, rising from bed, use of a toilet or low chair, hip flexion, a three-point crutch walking gait, getting into and out of a car, and precautions for traveling with the prosthesis in place. In addition, consider how and when S. H. might again take care of her grandson.

Case Study: Rheumatoid Arthritis

R. P. is a 22-year-old woman who was admitted for replacement of her wrist and finger joints. She has had rheumatoid arthritis (RA) since childhood. She currently receives prednisone (Deltasone) to control her RA. Following surgery, R. P. has increased pain, redness, and swelling in her knees, ankles, and elbows. Her physician increases her dose of prednisone and prescribes a gold injection (auranofin).

Address the following questions:

1. Describe the nursing implications prior to and following the injection of gold.
2. Develop a teaching/learning plan for R. P. about the gold injection.

R. P.'s pain decreases, and the physician orders physical therapy to begin.

3. Considering the usual pattern of pain and stiffness, what time of day should the nurse schedule physical therapy appointments for R. P.?
4. Discuss additional measures that can be used by R. P. to control her pain. Consider rest, activity, exercise, the firmness of the mattress, heat, weight control, medications, and assistive devices.

Case Study: Scleroderma

C. M. is a 47-year-old man who is admitted to the general medical nursing unit for difficulty with eating. He has lost 12 pounds in the past 3 weeks due to difficulty chewing and to diarrhea alternating with constipation. C. M. has had scleroderma for the past 9 years.

Address the following questions:

1. Identify nursing assessments for C. M that should be completed upon admission.
2. Considering the pathophysiology of scleroderma, what would be typical physical assessment findings for C. M.?

The physician orders a nasogastric (NG) feeding tube for C. M., and after placement is confirmed, he is to begin on half-strength Isocal.

3. List the methods that can be used to confirm the placement of a NG tube. Which methods provide the most reliable data? What is the risk of feeding C. M. via the NG tube prior to confirming its placement?
4. What is the rationale for beginning C. M. on half-strength tube feedings?

C. M. asks the nurse if he will need to have a feeding tube the rest of his life. He states that he feels "like a freak" already because of all the changes his body has undergone since the onset of the scleroderma.

5. How should the nurse reply? What psychosocial assessments are indicated for C. M.?
6. Discuss alternatives for the N. G. feeding tube that could be used for nutritional support.

C. M. often reports that he has pain in his hands and feet; he also feels cold. He has no palpable radial or pedal pulses. His hands and feet are yellow-white in color.

7. Discuss nursing interventions that would promote C. M.'s comfort. What classification of medication might be prescribed for this problem?

CHAPTER 24

Interventions for Clients with Immunologic Disorders

LEARNING OBJECTIVES

At the end of this chapter, the student will be able to

▮ Describe the concept of immunodeficiency

▮ Discuss the pathophysiology, etiology, and incidence of acquired immunodeficiency syndrome (AIDS)

▮ Describe the assessment of the client with AIDS

▮ List the common nursing diagnoses and goals for a client with AIDS

▮ Describe collaborative management for the client with AIDS

▮ Discuss nutritional-related immunodeficiencies

▮ Discuss congenital immunodeficiencies

▮ Discuss iatrogenic, drug-induced, and radiation immunodeficiencies

▮ Describe the four types of hypersensitivities

▮ Discuss collaborative management of anaphylaxis

▮ Discuss collaborative management of atopic allergies

▮ Discuss collaborative management of hemolytic blood transfusion reactions and drug-induced hemolytic anemia

▮ Discuss autoimmunities

▮ Discuss the gammopathy multiple myeloma

PREREQUISITE KNOWLEDGE

Prior to beginning this chapter, the student should review

▮ The concepts of immune system competence

▮ The concepts of death, dying, and grieving

▮ The concepts of human sexuality

▮ The chain of infection and the transmission of disease

▮ The normal inflammatory response and the reaction of the immune system to microorganisms

▮ Normal growth and development

▮ Normal nutrition

▮ Antimicrobial therapy

▮ Intravenous therapy and blood replacement therapy

▮ Isolation procedures

▮ Universal precautions

▮ Concepts from microbiology

▮ Shock and its management

STUDY QUESTIONS

Immunodeficiencies

1. List two conditions leading to a deficient immune system response.

   a. _____

   _____

   b. _____

   _____

2. Which of the following statements is correct about immunodeficient clients?

   a. Symptoms of an immunodeficiency disease are limited to one or two body systems.

   b. Treatment for many immunodeficiency diseases is effective and results in a high cure rate.

   c. Immunodeficiencies are chronic diseases involving intermittent periods of wellness and illness.

   d. Immunodeficient clients are at reduced risk for infection from exposure to environmental factors.

3. Which one of the following statements is correct about acquired immunodeficiency syndrome (AIDS)?

   a. Only one type of HIV virus is known to exist.

   b. The causative virus underwent random mutations.

   c. AIDS affects people between the ages of 50 and 75 years.

   d. AIDS can be caused by other immunodeficiencies

4. Briefly describe a retrovirus:

   _____

   _____

   _____

5. Which of the following is a mode of transmission for human immunodeficiency virus (HIV)?

   a. kissing

   b. sharing a drinking glass

   c. sexual intercourse

   d. using the same toilet

6. The predilection of HIV for certain cells in the immune system results in

   a. more T4 lymphocytes and general lymphocytopenia

   b. fewer activated B-cells and hypogammaglobulinemia

   c. increased response in cutaneous hypersensitivity

   d. susceptibility to opportunistic infection and neoplasm

7. HIV infection can result in

   a. acute infection

   b. asymptomatic infection

   c. lymphadenopathy

   d. neurologic symptoms

   e. all of the above

8. Which of the following statements is correct about the incidence of AIDS?

   a. The overall incidence of people diagnosed with AIDS is on the decline.

   b. Most children with AIDS become infected through their mother's breast milk.

   c. Heterosexual partners of HIV-infected people are a significant source of future AIDS cases.

   d. The overall case fatality rate for AIDS is approximately 25% and steadily rising.

9. Preventive measures for AIDS include

   a. abstaining from sexual activity

   b. screening donated blood products with enzyme-linked immunosorbent assay (ELISA)

   c. using latex condoms during sexual intercourse

   d. all of the above

10. Which of the following clients is at greatest risk for developing AIDS?

    a. a 26-year-old homosexual man who practices "safe sex"

    b. an infant delivered vaginally to an HIV-infected mother

    c. a 58-year-old housewife in a monogamous relationship

    d. a 4-year-old boy who is a hemophiliac

11. List the subjective client data relevant to AIDS. Use a separate sheet.

12. List the objective client data relevant to AIDS. Use a separate sheet.

13. The ELISA test measures

    a. the presence of HIV antibody

    b. the T4 to T8 cell ratio

    c. the total lymphocyte count

    d. reverse transcriptase activity

14. Which of the following laboratory tests is used to assess delayed skin hypersensitivity?

   a. SMAC

   b. PTT

   c. VDRL

   d. PPD

15. Which of the following is the most applicable nursing diagnosis for the client with AIDS who has incontinent diarrhea?

   a. Impaired Skin Integrity

   b. High Risk for Fluid Volume Deficit

   c. Ineffective Individual Coping

   d. High Risk for Infection

16. Which of the following interventions should the nurse implement when administering pentamidine isethionate (Pentam) intravenously for *Pneumocystis carinii* pneumonia?

   a. Elevate the head of the bed 30 degrees.

   b. Assist the client to a supine position.

   c. Place the client in Trendelenburg's position.

   d. Place the client in high-Fowler's position.

17. Which of the following foods should the nurse recommend for the client with AIDS who has a nursing diagnosis of Altered Nutrition: Less Than Body Requirements?

   a. yogurt

   b. clear broth

   c. ice cream

   d. fruit juice

18. Which of the following drugs would the nurse administer to the client with diarrhea from AIDS-related complications?

   a. codeine sulfate

   b. lactulose (Cephulac)

   c. diphenoxylate with atropine (Lomotil)

   d. trimethoprim and sulfamethoxazole (Bactrim)

19. Safety measures for the client with Altered Thought Processes related to AIDS complications include

   a. pacing activities to allow independence

   b. removing sharp utensils from food trays

   c. restraining with a jacket restraint

   d. administering a mood-altering drug

20. Which of the following four interventions is recommended for the client with AIDS who has dry, itchy skin?

   a. taking daily showers or tub baths to remove dead skin

   b. using defatted soap for cleaning to decrease dryness

   c. wearing long-sleeved shirts to discourage scratching

   d. applying an emollient lotion to retain skin moisture

21. Which of the following activites should the nurse recommend to the client with AIDS?

   a. plan an outing to a movie theater

   b. join a peer support group

   c. do volunteer work at a local shelter

   d. begin a regular exercise program

22. Which of the following people should the nurse consult prior to the dismissal of a client with AIDS?

   a. dietitian

   b. social worker

   c. clergy

   d. all of the above

23. The client with selective IgA deficiency would most likely have recurrent infections of the

   a. urinary tract

   b. middle ear

   c. scalp

   d. joints

24. Which of the following may the nurse safely administer to an immunocompromised client?

   a. measles, mumps, rubella vaccine (MMR)

   b. tetanus and diphtheria toxoid (Td)

   c. hepatitis B immune globulin (HBIG)

   d. poliovirus vaccine, trivalent (OPV)

25. An iatrogenic immunodeficiency is one that

   a. results secondarily from a disease process

   b. is induced by medical therapies or procedures

   c. is congenital and present from birth

   d. results from a hereditarily defective gene

26. Corticosteroids result in immunosuppression because they

   a. are cytotoxic and interfere with cell replication

   b. interfere with the release of lymphokines and antibodies

   c. isolate T-cells in bone marrow, resulting in lymphopenia

   d. interfere with T-helper cell growth and replication

Hypersensitivities

27. Briefly describe hypersensitivity. Use a separate sheet.

Match the following examples of hypersensitivities (28–42) with their types (a–d). Answers may be used more than once.

_____ 28. allergic asthma

_____ 29. anaphylaxis

_____ 30. contact dermatitis

_____ 31. allergic rhinitis

_____ 32. eczema

_____ 33. extrinsic and intrinsic asthma

_____ 34. hay fever

_____ 35. hemolytic anemia

_____ 36. poison ivy dermatitis

_____ 37. rheumatoid arthritis

_____ 38. sarcoidosis

_____ 39. serum sickness

_____ 40. systemic lupus erythematosus

_____ 41. tissue transplant rejection

_____ 42. transfusion reaction

a. type I
b. type II
c. type III
d. type IV

43. Preventive measures for anaphylaxis include
   a. avoiding the provoking allergen if it is known
   b. wearing a Medic Alert tag or bracelet
   c. checking for allergies prior to administering a drug
   d. alerting health care workers about allergies
   e. all of the above

44. List the subjective client data relevant to anaphylaxis. Use a separate sheet.

45. List the objective client data relevant to anaphylaxis. Use a separate sheet.

46. Identify four common nursing diagnoses for the client undergoing anaphylaxis.

   a. _____

   _____

   b. _____

   _____

   c. _____

   _____

   d. _____

   _____

47. Which of the following medications should be administered immediately to the client who is in anaphylaxis?
   a. diphenhydramine (Benadryl)
   b. metaproterenol (Alupent)
   c. epinephrine injection
   d. prednisone (Orasone)

48. Intake and output should be monitored for the client who is being treated for anaphylaxis because
   a. fluid volume depletion contributes to the shock reaction
   b. shock reversal may lead to fluid volume overload
   c. water intoxication may occur and lead to renal failure
   d. severe hypertension leads to increased cerebral edema

49. Clients who are dismissed with an anaphylaxis kit for self-administration of epinephrine should be instructed to
   a. lock the kit in a secured place
   b. carry the kit with them whenever they leave home
   c. use the autoinjector when symptoms become obvious
   d. experiment in determining the nature of the allergen

50. Which of the following statements is correct about atopic allergies?
   a. They are a result of IgG sensitization and formation.
   b. They occur only in families with a history of this problem.
   c. They are caused by genetic hypersensitivity to allergens.
   d. They result when T-cells release histamine and other agents.

51. Management of urticaria includes
   a. applying emollient lotions threes times a day
   b. administering epinephrine intramuscularly
   c. wearing long-sleeved garments to discourage scratching
   d. eliminating caffeine and alcohol from the diet

52. Intrinsic asthma is precipitated by

    a. cigarette smoke

    b. animal dander

    c. pollens

    d. dust

53. Identify the three foci of treatment for asthma

    a. _____

    _____

    b. _____

    _____

    c. _____

    _____

54. Maintenance drug therapy for asthma includes

    a. epinephrine

    b. aminophylline

    c. cromolyn sodium

    d. oxygen

55. Management of hemolytic blood transfusion reactions includes

    a. decreasing the flow rate of the transfusion

    b. maintaining IV access with normal saline

    c. collecting a urine specimen for myoglobin analysis

    d. administering furosemide (Lasix) orally twice a day

56. Drug-induced hemolytic anemia is initially managed by

    a. tapering the dose of the offending drug

    b. decreasing the dose of the offending drug

    c. eliminating the offending drug

    d. changing to an alterative drug

57. Signs and symptoms of serum sickness include

    a. wheezing

    b. nonproductive cough

    c. nausea and vomiting

    d. flank pain

58. Symptoms of serum sickness usually occur how long after administering the causative agent?

    a. immediately after

    b. within 30 minutes

    c. within 24 hours

    d. within 10 days

59. Allergens that cause contact dermatitis include

    a. fertilizers

    b. pollens

    c. noxious fumes

    d. animal dander

Autoimmunities and Gammopathies

60. Which of the following statements is correct about autoimmune diseases?

    a. They result when the host develops an immune reactivity to foreign tissue components.

    b. They result in responses that are similar to normal immune responses against nonself

    c. They have a common, underlying cause that leads to a variety of clinical manifestations

    d. They are a well-defined group of diseases that are commonly agreed to be autoimmune

61. Which of the following statements is correct about gammopathies?

    a. They are disorders involving abnormal proliferation of multiple clones of immunoglobulin-secreting plasma cells.

    b. They are derived from T-lymphocytes and result in a humoral-mediated hypersensitivity response.

    c. They are the proliferation of one clone of immunoglobulin that results in a homogeneous population.

    d. They are usually not recognized until symptoms become evident and the client is severely immunocompromised.

62. Management of gammopathies such as multiple myeloma includes

    a. bed rest to prevent pathological fractures

    b. a high-protein diet to promote tissue healing

    c. calcium supplements to rebuild bone tissue

    d. hydration with IV fluids to prevent complications

CRITICAL THINKING EXERCISES

Case Study: AIDS

J. E. is a 24-year-old man admitted to the hospital with acute flu-like symptoms including chest pain, coughing, and wheezing. The physicians are trying to rule out *Pneumocystis carinii* as the cause of the respiratory problems. He is known to be HIV-positive. He also has reported fatigue, fever, night sweats, and headache for the past 2 weeks.

Address the following questions:

1. To collect data about other probable opportunistic infections, what body systems should be assessed?

2. When asking about his social history, the nurse attempts to have J. E. disclose major risks of HIV spread. Explain why it is imperative to be strictly nonjudgmental with these sensitive questions.

J. E. discloses that he has had many sexual partners in the past 5 years, both men and women. He has no idea if any of them have HIV infections. He denies use of intravenous drugs, and no track marks are noted on his arms. He has not traveled outside of the United States, but he has had on-going treatment for genital herpes for the past 2 years.

3. What nursing education does J. E. need to avoid exposing others to the HIV virus?

The physical examination reveals that J. E. is awake and alert. He has no symptoms of cranial nerve involvement. He does have open sores in the mouth, and he has had a 15-pound weight loss over the past 6 months. He is tachycardiac, rate 114, and tachypneic, rate 48. He has rhonchi and wheezing throughout his chest, and it is difficult for him to speak in full sentences. He is 3-pillow orthopneic. He has cervical lymphadenopathy. His abdominal examination is negative. He has three open and draining lesions on the penis and near the rectum.

4. What nursing interventions are required for J. E.? What precautions does the nurse need to take when caring for J. E.?

5. He is begun on antibiotics and respiratory care for his pneumonia. While in the hospital, he develops erythematous-violaceous papules on his chest. What is the probable cause of these skin lesions? What might the nurse expect the physician to prescribe for the lesions?

6. J. E. also develops diarrhea. Since this will contribute to malnutrition and fluid loss, what interventions might be used to prevent these complications?

7. While in the hospital, J. E. is diagnosed with Kaposi's sarcoma. He says to the nurse, "Well, this is it. I'm done for. There is no cure. I guess I am getting what I deserve for living the way I did." How should the nurse respond?

8. J. E. is being dismissed to home. What preparations are needed for the home? How can dishes and clothes be sanitized? What precautions are needed for safe sex? What legal procedures should be carried out (e.g., a will or a Durable Power of Attorney)?

Case Study: Anaphylaxis

C. J. is a 56-year-old woman admitted for surgery. Following surgery, she was placed on prophylactic intravenous cephalosporin, but receives a does of penicillin by mistake. She has a known allergy to penicillin.

Address the following questions:

1. With a history of allergy to penicillin, what type of hypersensitivity reaction is C. J. most likely to experience? Using the concepts of hypersensitivity, explain this process.

C. J. calls the nurse and reports difficulty breathing and itching. Upon examination, the nurse notes severe facial edema and wheezing audible at the bedside. C. J.'s entire body is red and swollen into large welts. Her systolic blood pressure has fallen 15 mmHg from the early morning reading. The secondary intravenous set with antibiotic has approximately 25 mL remaining in the bag.

2. What should the nurse's first actions be?

3. What medications might the nurse expect the physician to prescribe to treat this anaphylactic reaction? How do the medications slow the body's allergic response?

4. What symptoms must the nurse observe for in C. J. while awaiting orders? After the medications are given?

5. What precautions should be taken by health care professionals to avert this problem in the future?

6. What information should C. J. be given to prevent such a reaction from occurring in the future?

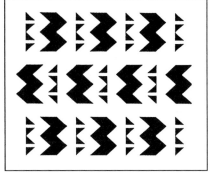

CHAPTER 25

Altered Cell Development and Growth

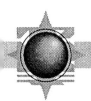

LEARNING OBJECTIVES

At the end of this chapter, the student will be able to

▮ Define *cancer* and the terminology used to describe cancer and other forms of altered cell growth

▮ Identify characteristics of normal cells

▮ Identify the process of normal cell reproduction

▮ Describe the characteristics of benign cells

▮ Describe the characteristics of malignant cells

▮ Define *carcinogenesis*

▮ Describe the TNM (tumor, nodes, and metastases) system for cancer staging and grading

▮ Compare and contrast intrinsic and extrinsic factors related to carcinogenesis

PREREQUISITE KNOWLEDGE

Prior to beginning this chapter, the student should review

▮ Normal cell reproduction from basic biology

▮ The functions and components of the immune system

STUDY QUESTIONS

Key Definitions

Match the following terms related to cancer (1–11) with their definitions (a–k).

_____ 1. anaplastic

_____ 2. benign

_____ 3. cancer

_____ 4. carcinogenesis

_____ 5. differentiation

_____ 6. dysplasia

_____ 7. hyperplasia

_____ 8. malignant

_____ 9. metastasize

_____ 10. neoplasia

_____ 11. tumor

a. large collection of cancer cells

b. abnormal cell appearance but cell function is normal

c. growth of new abnormal cells

d. large group of diseases characterized by uncontrolled growth and spread of abnormal cells

e. cells that have been transformed but are harmless

f. a swelling or lump

g. way in which cancer spreads

h. loss of shape or differentiation

i. process by which normal cells are changed into malignant cells

j. an increase in the number of cells

k. the degree of similarity of cells to their tissue of origin

Match the following descriptions of cellular reproduction (12–16) with their correct stages (a–e).

_____ 12. period in which parent cell divides into two daughter cells

_____ 13. period in which DNA is replicated

_____ 14. resting phase

_____ 15. period of time from end of mitosis to DNA synthesis

_____ 16. period of time from end of DNA synthesis to beginning of mitosis

a. gap 1
b. synthesis
c. gap 2
d. mitosis
e. gap 0

17. Which of the following statements is correct about benign cells?

a. They are always harmless.

b. They tend to metastasize early.

c. They resemble their originating tissue.

d. They are limited in the size they can attain.

18. Which of the following statement is correct about malignant cells?

a. They have a shorter life span than do their counterpart normal cells.

b. They result from the disruption in control over cellular reproduction and differentiation.

c. They develop highly specialized functions just as their normal counterpart cells do.

d. They always result in cancer and metastasize to other parts of the body.

19. Which of the following statement is correct about malignant neoplasia? These growths

a. have a structure similar to that of the original tissue

b. tend to grow slowly and progressively, then regress

c. invade and take over local surrounding normal tissue

d. are stationary and tend not to spread widely

20. List the properties of cancer cells. Use a separate sheet.

Cancer Development

21. Define the term *oncogene:* _____

_____

_____

_____

22. Which of the following statements is correct about progression and cancer?

a. Progression occurs before carcinogenesis is complete.

b. Characteristics include slowed growth rate and stability.

c. Cells change from well to poorly differentiated states.

d. Daughter cells are homogeneous to original cancer cells.

23. Put the following events of metastatic spread of cancer in sequence.

_____ a. evasion of host responses attempting to inhibit survival or growth of cancer cells

_____ b. release of tumor cells into blood

_____ c. invasion into tissues at secondary sites

_____ d. extension of primary tumor into surrounding tissues

_____ e. establishment of microenvironment conducive to continued neoplastic cell reproduction

_____ f. transport to secondary sites

_____ g. penetration of primary tumor into blood vessels

_____ h. implantation or arrest at secondary site

24. List three ways cancer cells metastasize and give an example of each.

a. _____

_____

_____

b. _____

_____

_____

c. _____

_____

_____

25. An adenoma is a neoplasia that originates from

a. connective tissue and is malignant

b. glandular tissue and is benign

c. fat tissue and is malignant

d. cartilage and is benign

26. Identify the purposes of staging and classifying specific cancers.

    a. _____

    _____

    _____

    b. _____

    _____

    _____

    c. _____

    _____

    _____

27. List the purposes for grading cancer cells.

    a. _____

    _____

    _____

    b. _____

    _____

    _____

    c. _____

    _____

    _____

28. Which of the following statements is correct about the grading of cancers?

    a. Cancers that vary histologically but come from the same organ behave similarly.

    b. The grade of a tumor is an evaluation of its potential for spreading based on cell characteristics.

    c. Low numeric grades correspond to tumors that are poorly differentiated from their original tissue.

    d. High numeric grades correspond to tumors that are well differentiated from their original tissue.

29. The basis for staging cancer is the

    a. physiological consequences of the tumor

    b. anatomical location of the tumor by body system

    c. site-specific system for size of the tumor

    d. anatomical extent of the tumor and any metastases

30. Cancers that can be staged using the TNM system include

    a. lymphomas

    b. leukemias

    c. solid tumors

    d. multiple myeloma

31. The TNM system for describing the anatomical extent of cancers includes

    a. the size of the tumor

    b. the involvement of regional lymph nodes

    c. the occurrence of distant metastases

    d. all of the above

32. In terms of doubling time, how many doublings does it take before a tumor is detectable clinically?

    a. 10

    b. 30

    c. 50

    d. 100

33. List the three primary factors that determine the development of cancer.

    a. _____

    _____

    b. _____

    _____

    c. _____

    _____

34. Which of the following statements is correct about the development of cancer?

    a. Cancer can have a short latency period.

    b. Diagnosis of cancer occurs early in the disease.

    c. Avoidance of known carcinogen exposure is primary prevention.

    d. Malignant changes make cancer treatment less complex.

35. Define *carcinogen*: _____

_____

_____

_____

36. Which of the following statements is correct about carcinogen exposure and the development of cancer?

    a. The relationship between environmental causation and cancer has been clearly defined.

    b. The time between exposure to carcinogens and cancer diagnosis is relatively brief.

    c. There is a definitive relationship between the dose of carcinogen exposure and the development of cancer.

    d. Most people who have been exposed to a carcinogen do not develop cancer.

37. Chemical carcinogens include

    a. complete carcinogens

    b. incomplete carcinogens

    c. initiating agents

    d. promoting agents

    e. all of the above

38. Which of the following statements is correct about carcinogenesis?

    a. Complete carcinogens are capable of inducing initiation and promotion.

    b. Incomplete carcinogens are capable only of inducing promotion.

    c. Initiation causes temporary, reversible alterations in a gene's DNA.

    d. Promotion-causing carcinogens can cause malignant transformation at any time.

39. Which of the following carcinogenic qualities does tobacco have?

    a. capability of inducing initiation

    b. capability of inducing promotion

    c. chemical that enhances carcinogenesis

    d. all of the above

40. Of all the risk factors involved in cigarette smoking and cancer development, which factor is the most controllable by an individual?

    a. immune function

    b. genetic predisposition

    c. deciding whether or not to smoke

    d. tar content in sidestream smoke

41. Which organ is least susceptible to the development of cancer as a result of cigarette smoking?

    a. lung

    b. skin

    c. esophagus

    d. urinary bladder

42. Which of the following statements is correct about radiation and carcinogenesis?

    a. Ionizing radiation can affect cells at all dose levels.

    b. Ultraviolet radiation produces widespread gene mutation.

    c. The risk of cancer from medical diagnostic tests is high.

    d. The incidence of radiation-related cancers is decreasing.

43. Which of the following types of tissue cells is most sensitive to the damaging effects of radiation?

    a. bone marrow

    b. muscle

    c. cardiac

    d. liver

44. Briefly discuss the role of viruses in carcinogenesis. Use a separate sheet.

45. Which of the following statements is correct about diet and carcinogenesis?

    a. The relationship between diet and carcinogenesis is clearly understood.

    b. Dietary factors are just one of many considerations in carcinogenesis.

    c. The existing evidence is overwhelming that dietary alterations can prevent cancer.

    d. Cigarette smoking and alcohol ingestion are associated with higher incidences of cancer than are dietary factors.

46. Which of the following foods is believed to be beneficial in preventing cancer?

    a. sauerkraut

    b. artificial sweeteners

    c. dill pickles

    d. strawberries

47. List the intrinsic factors that affect carcinogenesis.

    a. _____

    b. _____

    c. _____

48. Which of the following four statements is correct about immune surveillance?

    a. The part of the immune system most responsive to cancer cells is the antibody-mediated portion.

    b. Natural killer cells are the most important cells in the immune surveillance process.

    c. Cancer cells can sequester themselves in "privileged" sites such as the spleen or thymus.

    d. Cancer cells rarely outmaneuver the immune surveillance system, resulting in a low incidence rate of cancer.

49. The single most significant risk factor in the development of cancer is

    a. smoking

    b. female gender

    c. advancing age

    d. genetic predisposition

50. Identify four factors that contribute to carcinogenesis in the elderly. Use a separate sheet.

51. List four factors that are linked to genetic predisposition in carcinogenesis.

    a. _____

    _____

    b. _____

    _____

    c. _____

    _____

    d. _____

    _____

Match the following types of malignancy (52–57) with their associated carcinogenic genetic factors (a–c). Answers may be used more than once.

_____ 52. breast cancer   a. inherited cancer

_____ 53. gonadal carcinoma   b. chromosomal aberrations

_____ 54. leukemia

_____ 55. meningioma   c. familial clustering

_____ 56. retinoblastoma

_____ 57. Wilms's tumor

58. Identify the intrinsic factors other than race that should be considered as having a role in carcinogenesis.

a. _____

_____

b. _____

_____

c. _____

_____

d. _____

_____

59. Which of the following statements is correct about cancer's etiology and incidence?

    a. All cancers begin life as a single, normal cell.

    b. Causes of specific cancers are usually singular.

    c. Early diagnosis and treatment could save 80% of cancer clients.

    d. Most types of cancer have the same occurrence rate in both sexes.

60. Secondary preventive measures for cancer include

    a. performing breast self-examination yearly

    b. having a digital rectal examination yearly

    c. testing stool for occult blood every 2 years

    d. performing prostate self-examination monthly

61. Which of the following clients should be referred to a physician immediately for further evaluation of possible cancer occurrence?

    a. a 24-year-old man with a lump in one testis

    b. a 28-year-old pregnant woman with clear nipple drainage

    c. an 18-year-old youth with enlarged, nontender cervical nodes

    d. a 42-year-old woman with a lingering cough after an asthma attack

CHAPTER 26

Interventions for Clients with Cancer

LEARNING OBJECTIVES

At the end of this chapter, the student will be able to

■ Describe the effects of cancer on various body systems
■ Describe the most common treatments for cancer
■ Identify oncological emergencies

PREREQUISITE KNOWLEDGE

Prior to beginning this chapter, the student should review

■ The principles of immunology
■ The pathophysiology of cancer
■ The concept of body image
■ Normal nutrition

STUDY QUESTIONS

Consequences of Cancer and its Treatment

1. List the common changes in body systems that result from cancer development and metastasis and give an example of each.

a. _____

_____

b. _____

_____

c. _____

_____

d. _____

_____

2. Which of the following side effects occurs as a result of hematologic malignancy?

   a. diminished levels of circulating immunoglobulins

   b. cell-mediated immunity defect

   c. thrombocytopenia

   d. anemia

   e. all of the above

3. Which of the following conditions represents an effective protective barrier of the body against infection?

   a. anal fissure

   b. vaginitis (candidiasis)

   c. dry oral mucous membranes

   d. pink, moist conjunctiva

4. Altered nutrition from the effects of cancer and its treatment includes

   a. increased hunger

   b. ravenous appetite

   c. early satiety

   d. food cravings

5. Altered taste sensation related to cancer and its treatment commonly includes

   a. increased sensitivity to sweet foods

   b. decreased sensitivity to bitter foods

   c. aversion to red meats

   d. craving for fruits and vegetables

6. Hypoalbuminemia resulting from malnutrition results in

   a. ascites

   b. pleural effusion

   c. peripheral edema

   d. all of the above

7. The bone site most affected by metastasis is the

   a. skull

   b. femur

   c. radius

   d. mandible

8. Identify two purposes for cancer treatment.

   a. _____

   _____

   b. _____

   _____

9. List the types of cancer therapies.

   a. _____

   b. _____

   c. _____

   d. _____

   e. _____

10. Briefly discuss how the type and amount of cancer therapy for a client is determined. Use a separate sheet.

Match the following types of surgery for cancer treatment (11–17) with their definitions (a–g).

_____ 11. curative

_____ 12. controlling

_____ 13. diagnostic

_____ 14. palliative

_____ 15. prophylactic

_____ 16. reconstructive

_____ 17. second look

   a. removes tumor or metastases to relieve distressing symptoms

   b. restores appearances or function of body parts

   c. removes as much of tumor as possible

   d. provides a basis for deciding continuation of a specific therapy

   e. removes or destroys all gross and microscopic tumor

   f. removes at-risk tissue associated with cancer incidence

   g. provides histological proof of cancer

18. A biopsy of a cancerous tumor is necessary to

   a. establish the diagnosis of cancer

   b. remove the tumor completely

   c. check for evidence of metastasis

   d. prevent seeding of the tumor

19. Identify common nursing diagnoses associated with surgical therapy for cancer.

   a. _____

   b. _____

   c. _____

20. Identify the purpose of radiation therapy in cancer treatment. _____

_____

_____

21. Which of the following statements is correct about radiation therapy for cancer? The potential for cell injury from radiation is directly related to

    a. a slow rate of cell division

    b. the cell cycle phase

    c. an oxygenated environment

    d. homogeneous cell structure

22. List the factors that are considered in determining the type and method of radiation delivery.

    a. _____

    _____

    b. _____

    _____

    c. _____

    _____

    d. _____

    _____

    e. _____

    _____

23. Which of the following treatment modalities results in the client's body fluids being a source of external radiation "contamination"?

    a. intracavitary implantation

    b. interstitial implantation

    c. permanent implantation

    d. treatment with an unsealed isotope

24. Which of the following treatment modalities does not render the client radioactive to others?

    a. intracavitary implantation

    b. interstitial implantation

    c. external radiotherapy

    d. treatment with an unsealed isotope

25. List the three factors that affect the amount of exposure of health care workers to radiation.

    a. _____

    _____

    _____

b. _____

_____

_____

c. _____

_____

_____

26. Guidelines for health care workers who care for a client with a radioactive implant include

    a. assigning the same person to care for the client daily

    b. communicating with the client from the room's doorway

    c. wearing a lead apron to shield from radiation

    d. providing total care so as not to dislodge the implant

27. If a radium implant becomes dislodged and falls into the client's bed, the nurse should

    a. ask the client to pick up the implant and place it in the lead-lined container

    b. call the radiologist to come and retrieve the implant and prepare for its reinsertion

    c. evacuate clients from adjacent rooms and notify the radiologist what has happened

    d. place the implant in the lead-line container using tongs and notify the radiologist

28. Which of the following organs is most susceptible to acute effects from radiation therapy?

    a. heart

    b. liver

    c. ovary

    d. stomach

29. Radiation to the head and neck often results in

    a. altered taste sensation

    b. sialaporia

    c. stomatitis

    d. difficulty swallowing

    e. all of the above

30. Radiation-related nausea occurs most commonly following treatment of the

    a. femur

    b. uterus

    c. small intestine

    d. urinary bladder

31. Radiation recall phenomenon is

    a. a reaction in which skin tissue undergoes changes similar to those experienced when originally irradiated

    b. the psychological reaction of the client to the unpleasant side effects of radiation therapy

    c. a condition in which the gastrointestinal lining undergoes spontaneous sloughing and regeneration

    d. the ability of memory cells in the immune system to react to antigens following radiation therapy

32. The form of contraception recommended for the female client who is being treated for cancer with chemotherapy of radiation is

    a. birth control pills

    b. intrauterine device

    c. vaginal foams or creams

    d. condoms

33. Which of the following is needed for the client who is to receive outpatient radiation therapy following cancer staging?

    a. a source of transportation to the outpatient radiation therapy department

    b. a person or agency to assist with grocery shopping and meal preparation

    c. a support group to assist the client to cope with the diagnosis and effects of therapy

    d. all of the above

34. List the purposes for the use of chemotherapy in cancer treatment.

    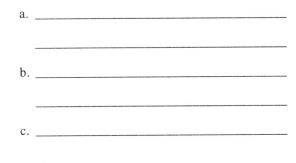

    a. _____

    _____

    b. _____

    _____

    c. _____

    _____

35. The cell cycle phase affected by most cycle-specific cancer chemotherapy agents is

    a. G_1

    b. S

    c. G_2

    d. M

    e. G_0

36. List the four factors necessary for maximal effectiveness of cancer chemotherapy agents.

    a. _____

    _____

    b. _____

    _____

    c. _____

    _____

    d. _____

    _____

37. The best preventive intervention for extravasation is

    a. assessing for blood return in the IV tubing prior to injecting a chemotherapeutic agent

    b. assessing for blood return in the IV tubing following the injection of a chemotherapeutic agent

    c. starting a new, temporary IV infusion prior to administering each dose of chemotherapy

    d. placing the IV infusion on a continuous infusion pump to administer the chemotherapy

38. Safety measures for health care workers who administer cancer chemotherapeutic agents include wearing

    a. a disposable isolation gown during preparation and administration of drugs

    b. a disposable face mask when assisting a client who is vomiting following chemotherapy

    c. surgical latex gloves when emptying a bed pan for the client who is receiving chemotherapy

    d. a disposable isolation gown when starting an IV infusion for chemotherapy

39. Which of the following statements indicates that the client has *not* resolved a problem with Body Image Disturbance related to alopecia?

    a. "I don't want to leave my room. I would feel terrible if anyone saw me looking like this."

    b. "I just took a walk to the gift shop to buy a magazine that has some interesting articles."

    c. "I have some friends coming this evening to visit and would like to put on some make-up."

    d. "I asked my hairdresser to help me choose a wig that matches my own color and style."

40. Antiemetic agents should be administered to the cancer client
    a. continuously with the administration of chemotherapy
    b. half an hour prior to administration of chemotherapy
    c. if nausea or vomiting occurs following chemotherapy administration
    d. following each session of radiation therapy

41. The response of anticipatory nausea in relation to therapy with cancer chemotherapy agents is
    a. conditioned
    b. involuntary
    c. voluntary
    d. expected

42. Clients receiving cisplatin (Platinol) should be monitored for
    a. seizures
    b. cardiac dysrhythmias
    c. decreased urinary output
    d. ineffective airway clearance

43. Interventions to improve the nutritional status of the cancer client who is experiencing nausea include
    a. marinating meats in vinegar to tenderize them
    b. rinsing mouth with a commercial mouthwash before meals
    c. arranging for half the day's calories at breakfast
    d. initiating parenteral nutrition therapy

44. Bone marrow suppression from cancer chemotherapy results in
    a. leukopenia
    b. thrombocytopenia
    c. anemia
    d. all of the above

45. The most important preventive intervention for the immunosuppressed client on chemotherapy is
    a. meticulous hand washing by all who come in contact with the client
    b. wearing a face mask if one has a cold and is caring for the client
    c. inserting an in-dwelling catheter for the client who has urinary incontinence
    d. implementing protective isolation for the client with a granulocyte count of less than 2000/mm³

46. Interventions to minimize potential injury for clients who are thrombocytopenic include
    a. shaving with a safety razor
    b. brushing teeth with a firm brush
    c. taking rectal instead of oral temperatures
    d. applying pressure to injection sites for 5 minutes

47. In addition to planned rest periods, which of the following interventions is used to assist the client with activity intolerance secondary to anemia as a result of cancer chemotherapy?
    a. platelet administration
    b. oxygen therapy
    c. low-protein diet
    d. high-impact aerobics

Match the following sites of cancer locations (48–52) with their associated routes of delivering chemotherapy (a–e).

_____ 48. blood stream   a. intraperitoneal
_____ 49. liver   b. intravenous
_____ 50. ovary   c. intrapleural
_____ 51. spinal cord   d. intra-arterial
_____ 52. thoracic cavity   e. intrathecal

53. Education about chemotherapy should include which of the following statements?
    a. There are many different types of drugs, but most have similar side effects.
    b. Most individuals can expect to react similarly to the same chemotherapeutic agents.
    c. Individuals do not react the same way to medications, and there should be no preconceived expectations.
    d. All side effects from chemotherapy can be managed to prevent their occurrence.

54. Identify the major action of biological response modifiers (BRMs) in cancer treatment. Use a separate sheet.

55. The most common side effect of interleukins is
    a. mood swings
    b. myalgias
    c. tachycardia
    d. urticaria

Oncologic Emergencies

56. Septicemia is a

    a. serious type of systemic shock reaction

    b. condition in which microorganisms invade the blood steam

    c. minor infection involving the gastrointestinal system

    d. condition involving too many circulating stem cells

57. Which of the following assessment would the nurse expect to find in the immunosuppressed client who may be going into septic shock?

    a. bradycardia

    b. cool extremities

    c. hypoventilation

    d. thready peripheral pulses

58. Intervention for disseminated intravascular coagulation includes administering

    a. cryoprecipitate

    b. antibiotics

    c. platelets

    d. heparin

    e all of the above

59. Emergency intervention for syndrome of inappropriate antidiuretic hormone (SIADH) includes

    a. restricting fluids

    b. administering D_5 0.45% saline, IV

    c. hydrating with bolus IV infusions

    d. weighing the client every other day

60. Which of the following medications should the nurse be prepared to give to the client with spinal cord compression from tumor invasion?

    a. lithium carbonate (Lithobid)

    b. demeclocycline (Declomycin)

    c. hydrocortisone (Solu-Cortef)

    d. prednisone (Deltasone)

61. The type of cancer most associated with hypercalcemia is cancer of the

    a. lung

    b. pancreas

    c. breast

    d. stomach

62. Emergency intervention for hypercalcemia includes

    a. restricting fluids

    b. administering magnesium sulfate

    c. hydrating with IV normal saline

    d. administering furosemide (Lasix) orally

63. Which of the following is an early sign of superior vena cava syndrome?

    a. eyelid edema

    b. hoarseness

    c. dyspnea with exertion

    d. distended neck veins

64. A client with leukemia who develops tumor lysis syndrome would most likely have

    a. an elevated serum acid phosphatase level

    b. a decreased serum alkaline phosphatase level

    c. an elevated serum uric acid level

    d. a decreased serum calcium level

CRITICAL THINKING EXERCISES

Case Study: Radiation Therapy

F. K. is a 54-year-old man admitted for evaluation of increasing shortness of breath. He is quickly diagnosed with lung cancer, and it is decided to treat him with radiation therapy. He will be treated as an outpatient.

Address the following questions:

1. Plan a teaching/learning process for F. K. covering the following points: the effect of radiation on cancer cells, the possible effect on normal cells, and the probable side effects F. K. will experience.

After completing the teaching, F. K. says, "Well, I am glad I'm having radiation treatments rather than those drugs. I have heard you get really sick from them."

2. How should the nurse respond?
3. Does his statement indicate that he had learned from the nurse's teaching?

Case Study: Chemotherapy

L. C. is a 63-year-old woman admitted to the hospital for a second round of chemotherapy for breast cancer. She was previously treated with chemotherapy 6 months ago and has made little progress from the treatment. Her current orders are for 5-fluorouracil 1000 mg in 500 mL of D5W over 24 hours for 5 days; ifosfamide (Ifex) 120 mg and mesna (Mesnex) 1200 mg in 1 L of D5W over 24 hours for 5 days. Both agents run simultaneously through a triple lumen subclavian line.

Address the following questions:

1. Look up the chemotherapeutic agents and list below what type of agent they are (e.g., cell cycle specific) and their major side effects.
2. How does the agent mesna differ from the other agents?
3. What specific nursing precautions are needed for handling the agents?

L. C. reports increasing pain in her legs and some pain in her back. She is more weak and requires assistance transferring to the chair. She has some tingling and numbness in her feet. Her laboratory values are Na^+ 134, K^+ 3.7, Ca 13.8, Phos 2.2, Hgb 8.5, Hct 25, RBCs 2.3, WBCs 1.8, platelets low.

4. Which values are abnormal and why?
5. Which of the altered laboratory values may explain her symptoms?
6. What should the nurse expect to be ordered to treat the problem?

CHAPTER 27

Interventions for Clients with Infection

LEARNING OBJECTIVES

At the end of this chapter, the student will be able to

- Describe the concept of infectious disease
- Define common terms used to describe the infectious disease process
- Discuss the steps within the chain of infection
- Describe host factors that influence the development of infection
- Identify techniques to prevent infection and its spread
- Identify the complications of infection
- List the pertinent and relevant data for the client with a possible infectious disease
- List possible nursing diagnoses found in the client with infection
- Describe the goals and nursing interventions for the client with Hyperthermia
- Describe the goals and nursing interventions for the client with Fatigue
- Describe the goals and nursing interventions for the client with Social Isolation
- Discuss discharge planning for the client with an infection

PREREQUISITE KNOWLEDGE

Prior to beginning this chapter, the student should review

- The concepts of immunity and inflammation
- Normal laboratory values for white blood cells
- The principles of antimicrobial therapy
- The principles of intravenous therapy
- The principles of universal precautions and isolation precautions
- The principles of stages of fever and treatment

STUDY QUESTIONS

The Infectious Process

1. An infectious disease is one that is

   a. acquired from someone or something else

   b. inherited from one's parents

   c. invasive to the surrounding tissues

   d. related to an autoimmune process

2. Which of the following four diseases is reportable to the Centers for Disease Control (CDC)?

   a. giardiasis

   b. pneumonia

   c. influenza

   d. salmonellosis

Match the following terms relating to the infectious process (3–12) with their definitions (a–j).

_____ 3. colonization

_____ 4. host

_____ 5. infection

_____ 6. invasiveness

_____ 7. normal flora

_____ 8. parasite

_____ 9. pathogen

_____ 10. pathogenicity

_____ 11. subclinical

_____ 12. virulence

a agent capable of causing disease in a human

b. degree of communicability

c. microorganisms that live at host's expense

d. presence of microorganisms in asymptomatic host

e. ability of an organism to cause disease

f. presence of infection with no obvious host reaction

g. establishment of host–parasite interaction

h. ability of an organism to spread and grow in the host

i. one's own characteristic bacteria

j. recipient of infection

13. List the factors that are necessary in the chain of infection.

a. _____

b. _____

c. _____

d. _____

e. _____

f. _____

14. Which of the following statements is correct about reservoirs of infectious agents?

a. A reservoir is usually an animate source.

b. A host's own body can harbor pathogens.

c. Someone who is incubating a pathogen is not infectious.

d. A chronic carrier is usually very ill and debilitated.

Match the following terms (15–17) with their definitions (a–c).

_____ 15. endotoxin

_____ 16. exotoxin

_____ 17. toxin

a. protein molecule released by bacteria that affects host at a distant site

b. protein molecule released from a bacterial cell wall upon its lysis

c. protein molecule produced and released by bacteria into the surrounding environment

Match the following types of pathogens (18–26) with their common disease manifestations (a–i).

_____ 18. bacteria

_____ 19. chlamydiae

_____ 20. fungi

_____ 21. helminths

_____ 22. mycoplasmas

_____ 23. prions

_____ 24. protozoa

_____ 25. rickettsiae

_____ 26. viruses

a. Creutzfeldt–Jakob disease

b. influenza

c. urethritis

d. typhus

e. psittacosis

f. osteomyelitis

g. thrush

h. malaria

i. anemia

27. Natural immunity occurs

a. following exposure to a pathogen

b. following an injection of gamma globulin

c. without previous exposure to a pathogen

d. due to maternal–fetal transfer of immunoglobulins

28. Immune system depression in the host results in increased

a. resistance to disease

b. susceptibility to infection

c. virulence of an infecting agent

d. ability to fight invading organisms

29. Which of the following clients is most susceptible to increased incidence of infectious disease?

a. a 54-year-old woman with cardiomyopathy

b. a 25-year-old pregnant woman with type I diabetes

c. an 18-year-old teenager with a fractured tibia

d. a 43-year-old woman with acute cholelithiasis

30. Which of the following drugs may suppress the immune system?

    a. azathioprine (Imuran)

    b. theophylline (Aminophylline)

    c. interferon alpha-2b (Intron A)

    d. propranolol hydrochloride (Inderal)

31. List the various ways that organisms can enter the body.

    a. _____

    b. _____

    c. _____

    d. _____

    e. _____

Match the following modes of transmission (32–38) with their descriptions (a–g).

_____ 32. airborne

_____ 33. common vehicle

_____ 34. direct contact

_____ 35. droplet spread

_____ 36. fomite

_____ 37. indirect contact

_____ 38. vector-borne

a. person-to-person transmission

b. transfer via intermediate object

c. inanimate vehicle of pathogen transfer

d. intermediary is an insect or animal between hosts

e. infected particles travel greater than 1 m

f. intermediary is contaminated food or water

g. transfer by contact with infective secretions

39. Which of the following statements is correct about portals of exit?

    a. Exit occurs from a susceptible host.

    b. Exit usually occurs from a different route than entry.

    c. Some organisms have multiple routes of exit from a host.

    d. The new susceptible host is a reservoir for infection.

Match the following host factors (40–51) with their types of defense mechanisms (a or b). Answers may be used more than once.

_____ 40. antibodies

_____ 41. cell-mediated immunity

_____ 42. ciliary action of respiratory tract

_____ 43. antibody-mediated immunity

_____ 44. inflammation

_____ 45. intact mucous membrane

_____ 46. intact skin

_____ 47. peristalsis

_____ 48. phagocytosis

_____ 49. tears

_____ 50. urine acidity

_____ 51. vaginal secretions

a. nonspecific

b. specific

52. Measures taken most often to interrupt the chain of infection are directed at the

    a. susceptible host

    b. source of an infecting organism

    c. mechanism for organism transmission to a host

    d. reservoir where an infecting organism incubates

53. The most effective mechanism for preventing the spread of infection is

    a. wearing a face mask

    b. using isolation precautions

    c. thorough hand washing

    d. wearing disposable gloves

54. Isolation precautions are recommended by the

    a. American Medical Association (AMA)

    b. Centers for Disease Control (CDC)

    c. National League for Nursing (NLN)

    d. Joint Commission on the Accreditation of Healthcare Organizations (JCAHO)

55. List the four types of guidelines used to reduce the transmission of disease.

    a. _____

    b. _____

    c. _____

    d. _____

56. Which of the following types of isolation precautions should be implemented for the client with osteomyelitis?

    a strict

    b. contact

    c. body and body fluids

    d. drainage and secretion

57. Following an injection, the nurse should

    a. cut the needle with a needle cutter prior to disposing of the syringe assembly

    b. place the syringe and needle in a puncture proof box after recapping the needle

    c. remove the needle, dispose of it in a puncture proof box, and snip the syringe adapter

    d. place the syringe and needle in a puncture proof box, intact, without recapping the needle

58. Which of the following procedures should be performed using aseptic technique in the home health care setting?

    a. preparation and administration of insulin injections

    b. intermittent bladder self-catheterization

    c. reinsertion of a nasogastric feeding tube

    d. oropharyngeal intermittent suctioning

59. List the complications that can occur from infection.

    a. _____

       _____

    b. _____

       _____

    c. _____

       _____

    d. _____

       _____

Collaborative Management

60. List the subjective client data relevant to infectious disease. Use a separate sheet.

61. List the psychosocial client data relevant to infectious disease. Use a separate sheet.

62. List the objective client data relevant to infectious disease. Use a separate sheet.

63. The most definitive laboratory test for organism identification is

    a. sensitivity testing

    b. serologic testing

    c. plasmapheresis

    d. culturing

64. In laboratory studies, the differential indicates

    a. the rate at which red blood cells fall through plasma

    b. chronic infection such as osteomyelitis

    c. the ability of the body to respond to infection

    d. the presence and location of an infection site

65. Identify the three common nursing diagnoses for the client with an infectious disease.

    a. _____

    b. _____

    c. _____

66. List the interventions that are used to control elevated body temperature.

    a. _____

       _____

    b. _____

       _____

    c. _____

       _____

    d. _____

       _____

67. The infectious organisms that are most readily treated with antimicrobial therapy are

    a. fungi

    b. yeasts

    c. viruses

    d. bacteria

68. Identify four requirements for effective antimicrobial therapy.

    a. _____

       _____

    b. _____

       _____

c. _____

_____

d. _____

_____

69. Which of the following drugs is most likely to cause an allergic reaction in the client who is allergic to penicillin?

   a. arabinoside

   b. ceftriaxone

   c. erythromycin

   d. tetracycline

70. Which of the following conditions contraindicates the use of aspirin for treatment of hyperthermia?

   a. head injury

   b. febrile seizures

   c. heart failure

   d. chickenpox

71. Which of the following interventions is indicated for the client with hyperthermia as a result of an infectious process?

   a. intragastric iced lavage

   b. body immersion in ice water

   c. tepid water sponges to the skin

   d. alcohol sponging to skin surfaces

72. Which of the following clients with hyperthermia should have fluid loss replacement therapy via IV infusions?

   a. a 22-year-old woman with chickenpox

   b. a 62-year-old man with gastroenteritis

   c. an 81-year-old man with herpes simplex

   d. a 35-year-old woman with influenza

73. Which of the following should be encouraged in the diet of a client in the early stages of an infectious process who is fatigued?

   a. custard

   b. green salad

   c. cheeseburger

   d. noodle casserole

74. Interventions for the client with activity intolerance related to an acute infectious process include

   a. prolonged bed rest

   b. sitting up at the bed side

   c. use of a tilt table for mobilization

   d. gradual increases in ambulation and self-care

75. Which of the following interventions is indicated for the client who is in isolation?

   a. discouraging family and friends from visiting

   b. limiting telephone calls to immediate relatives

   c. teaching visitors which precautions are necessary

   d. donning a mask and gown prior to ambulating the client

76. Which of the following assessments is indicated for the client who is being dismissed to home care and who will continue to have IV antimicrobial therapy?

   a. presence of cooking facilities in the home

   b. number and location of scatter rugs in the home

   c. availability of safety rails for the bathtub and toilet

   d. availability of running water and location of any sinks

77. Dismissal teaching of the client with an infectious disease includes explaining

   a. what is causing the client's illness

   b. whether the causative organism is contagious

   c. how the causative organism is spread to others

   d. the precautions necessary to prevent transmission of infection

   e. all of the above

78. Identify the information that a client who is being dismissed to home care on antimicrobial therapy needs for self-care.

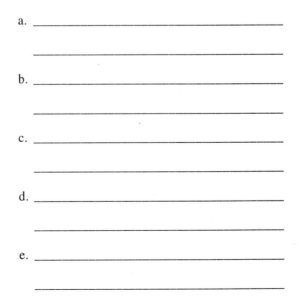

   a. _____

   _____

   b. _____

   _____

   c. _____

   _____

   d. _____

   _____

   e. _____

   _____

CRITICAL THINKING EXERCISES

Case Study: Wound Infection

P. C. is a 47-year-old type I (IDDM) diabetic who was admitted to the hospital following an exploratory laparotomy for abdominal pain. During surgery, he was found to have a ruptured appendix. Postoperative orders include triple antibiotics: Penicillin G 2 million units every 4 hours IV, gentamicin sulfate (Garamycin) 80 mg every 8 hours IV, and cefazolin sodium (Ancef) 1 g every 6 hours IV.

Address the following questions:

1. Since none of the drugs can be administered at the same time, develop a schedule for these antibiotics.

2. P. C.'s blood sugar and need for insulin has increased. Explain why this is common in these types of cases.

Three days following surgery, P. C.'s wound edges are very reddened and he develops increasing amount of seropurulent drainage.

3. What is the cause of the change in the wound? What is the probable organism causing the problem?

P. C. is treated with wound packings until his condition stabilizes. He is planning to go home and to continue the packing and IV antibiotics through a permanent infusion port in a subclavian vein.

4. Develop a teaching/learning plan for P. C. to perform his own dressing changes, wound packing, and IV antibiotic therapy.

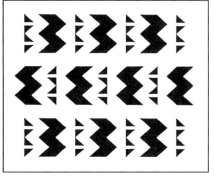

CHAPTER 28

Assessment of the Respiratory System

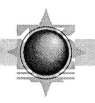

LEARNING OBJECTIVES

At the end of this chapter, the student will be able to

■ List the functions of the respiratory system

■ Describe the structure and function of the upper and lower respiratory tracts

■ Discuss the processes involved during oxygenation

■ Describe respiratory changes associated with aging

■ Obtain a history from the client with a respiratory problem

■ Complete a physical assessment of the client with a respiratory problem

■ Distinguish normal and adventitious breath sounds

■ Identify abnormal voice sounds

■ Identify diagnostic tests relevant to the care of the client with a respiratory disorder

PREREQUISITE KNOWLEDGE

Prior to beginning this chapter, the student should review

■ The anatomy and physiology of the respiratory tract

■ The process of respiration

■ The principles of diffusion, perfusion, and ventilation

■ The interpretation of blood gas measurements

STUDY QUESTIONS

Anatomy and Physiology Review

Match the following functions of the respiratory system (1–5) with their purposes (a or b). Answers may be used more than once.

_____ 1. maintain acid–base balance

_____ 2. maintain body water and heat balance

_____ 3. provide oxygen

_____ 4. remove carbon dioxide

_____ 5. aid in speech

a. primary

b. secondary

Match the following structures of the upper respiratory system (6–20) with their descriptions (a–o).

_____ 6. adenoids

_____ 7. cricoid cartilage

_____ 8. epiglottis

_____ 9. glottis

_____ 10. laryngo-pharynx

_____ 11. larynx

_____ 12. nares

_____ 13. naso-pharynx

_____ 14. nose

_____ 15. oropharynx

_____ 16. pharynx

_____ 17. septum

_____ 18. sinuses

_____ 19. tonsils

_____ 20. turbinates

a. filters, warms, humidifies air

b. throat

c. passageway for food and air

d. lymphatic tissue in oropharynx

e. contains vocal cords

f. divides nasal passages

g. provides speech resonance

h. increases nasal mucosa surface area

i. keeps food out of trachea during swallowing

j. lymphatic tissue in roof of nasopharynx

k. external openings of nasal cavities

l. contains adenoids and eustachian tubes

m. assists in coughing

n. voice box

o. gag and swallowing center

Match the following terms related to the lower respiratory system (21–31) with their descriptions (a–k).

_____ 21. alveoli

_____ 22. bronchi

_____ 23. bronchioles

_____ 24. carina

_____ 25. cilia

_____ 26. hilum

_____ 27. lungs

_____ 28. parietal pleura

_____ 29. surfactant

_____ 30. trachea

_____ 31. visceral pleura

a. point where trachea bifurcates

b. propel mucus from lower airways to trachea

c. reduces surface tension in alveoli

d. carry air to each lobe of lungs

e. elastic organs that allow for ventilation and air diffusion

f. carry air from bronchi to alveolar ducts

g. carries air from larynx to bronchi

h. lining covering lung surfaces to decrease friction

i. lines inside of thoracic cavity to decrease friction with respiration

j. basic unit where gases are exchanged

k. forms the roof of the lungs

Match the following processes of respiration (32–34) with their descriptions (a–c).

_____ 32. diffusion

_____ 33. perfusion

_____ 34. ventilation

a. movement of air in and out of lungs

b. exchange of oxygen and carbon dioxide in capillary–alveolar network

c. pumping of oxygenated blood through body and return of carbon dioxide–enriched blood to lungs

35. Identify the changes in the following parts of the respiratory system that are associated with the aging process. Use a separate sheet.

    a. chest wall

    b. alveoli

    c. lungs

    d. pharynx and larynx

    e. pulmonary artery

Subjective Assessment

36. List the subjective client data relevant to the respiratory system. Use a separate sheet.

37. Which of the following medications warrants further inquiry when collecting subjective data for the respiratory system?

    a. sulfisoxazole (Gantrisin) for chronic recurrent otitis media

    b. warfarin sodium (Coumadin) for management of thrombophlebitis of the leg

    c. lithium carbonate (Lithobid) for management of a bipolar disorder

    d. lovastatin (Mevacor) for hypercholesterolemia

38. Which of the following pathologies is significant to the respiratory system when assessing the family history?

    a. kyphoscoliosis

    b. genital herpes simplex

    c. fibrocystic breast disease

    d. rheumatoid arthritis

39. Which of the following clients has an increased risk of respiratory system problems?

    a a 45-year-old man who breeds and raises racing pigeons

    b. an 18-year-old youth who enjoys body surfing in the ocean

    c. a 68-year-old woman who does needlework for relaxation

    d. a 56-year-old man who ties flies for trout fishing

Match the following examples of dyspnea (40–50) with their classifications (a–e) and their levels of ADL performance ability (i–v). Answers may be used more than once.

____ ____ 40. no restriction in activity; dyspnea with strenuous activity

____ ____ 41. restricted to bed or chair because of dyspnea at rest

____ ____ 42. dyspnea with activities such as showering or dressing

____ ____ 43. dyspnea with minimal exertion requiring assistance with some essential activities

a. class I
b. class II
c. class III
d. class IV
e. class V

i. ADL level 4
ii. ADL level 3
iii. ADL level 2
iv. ADL level 1
v. ADL level 0

____ ____ 44. independent in ADL, but dyspnea with stair climbing, walking up incline

____ ____ 45. requires oxygen at all times

____ ____ 46. marathon runner

____ ____ 47. retired carpenter, does estimates for carpentry jobs

____ ____ 48. pauses when dressing

____ ____ 49. pauses when walking 100 yards to mailbox

____ ____ 50. cannot walk at same pace as friend the same age

51. The following is a partial client history. Discuss the significance these data have for an assessment of the respiratory system. Submit the completed exercise to the clinical instructor.

Caucasian man, 36 years old. Married, two children. History of cigarette smoking for the past 20 years, one pack per day. Works as a machinist in a factory, manufacturing metal tools and molds for tool making. In current job for 17 years. Completed vocational high school. Hobbies include making model airplanes and model railroading. Denies allergies to any medications. Suffers from seasonal allergies (rhinitis, sneezing). No difficulty with ADLs.

Objective Assessment

52. List the objective client data relevant to the respiratory system. Use a separate sheet.

53. Using the data in question 51, construct a physical assessment recording for the respiratory system. Submit the completed exercise to the clinical instructor.

54. Which of the following observations is *not* made when inspecting the lungs and thorax?

    a. symmetry of chest movement
    b. rate, rhythm, and depth of respiration
    c. color of oropharynx
    d. use of accessory muscles for breathing

55. Which of the following pieces of data is an objective sign of oxygen deprivation?

    a. complaints of shortness of breath
    b. paroxysmal nocturnal dyspnea
    c. chest pain with deep inspiration
    d. clubbing of fingernails

56. Palpation of the chest is used to assess for

    a. retractions or bulging
    b. tactile fremitus
    c. accessory muscle use
    d. friction rub

Match the following terms used in respiratory assessment (57–66) with their descriptions (a–j).

____ 57. bronchial

____ 58. bronchophony

____ 59. bronchovesicular

____ 60. egophony

____ 61. pleural friction rub

____ 62. crackles

____ 63. rhonchi

____ 64. vesicular

____ 65. wheezes

____ 66. whispered pectoriloquy

a. popping sound as air moves through moisture in small airways

b. normal sounds heard over lung periphery; sighing

c. grating, scratching sound with respiration

d. musical, squeaky sounds related to bronchospasm

e. normal sounds heard over bronchi but abnormal elsewhere

f. normal sound heard over trachea

g. rattling sounds as air moves through moisture in large airways

h. loud transmission of whispered sounds during auscultation

i. vocalized "A" is heard as "E" with stethoscope

j. loud transmission of "99" during auscultation

67. The piece of laboratory data associated with chronic airflow limitation is decreased levels of

    a. hemoglobin

    b. neutrophils

    c. eosinophils

    d. arterial oxygen

Match the following pulmonary function tests (PFTs) (68–72) with their descriptions (a–e).

_____ 68. FEV

_____ 69. FRC

_____ 70. FVC

_____ 71. RV

_____ 72. TLC

a. maximal amount of air that can be exhaled after maximal inspiration

b. amount of air in lungs at the end of maximal inhalation

c. amount of air remaining in lungs after normal exhalation

d. maximal amount of air that can be exhaled over a specific time

e. amount of air remaining in lungs at the end of full, forced exhalation

73. Pneumothorax is a serious complication that may occur following a

    a. bronchogram

    b. laryngoscopy

    c. computed tomographic scan of the lungs

    d. percutaneous lung biopsy

74. Which of the following pulse oximetry readings calls for immediate intervention?

    a. 98%

    b. 93%

    c. 89%

    d. 85%

CRITICAL THINKING EXERCISES

Case Study: Respiratory Tract Assessment

M. K. reports to the pulmonary clinic with complaints of a productive cough that "won't go away." She is a 62-year-old married housewife whose children are grown. M. K. smoked two packs of cigarettes per day for 20 years, but she has not smoked for the past 10 years. She contracted a "virus" 4 weeks ago, which "settled in her chest." Her usual remedies have not resulted in improvement in her status.

Address the following questions:

1. What additional subjective data should the nurse elicit from M. K.?

2. What physical assessments should the nurse perform on M. K.?

3. What effect does M. K.'s 10 years of not smoking have on the condition of her lungs?

4. The physician orders a chest x-ray and a sputum specimen. What should the nurse tell M. K. about these tests?

5. Following the tests, pneumonia of the right middle and lower lobes is diagnosed. What symptoms may have indicated that M. K. had pneumonia?

M. K. is placed on cefaclor (Ceclor) 500 mg every 8 hours, P.O. She is also instructed to return to the clinic in one week for a repeat chest x-ray.

6. Why is it necessary to have a follow-up x-ray and checkup?

After one week, M. K. reports no improvement and the chest x-ray results also indicate that there is no change. A bronchoscopy is scheduled to be done in the outpatient surgery unit the following day. (The physician would prefer to do an MRI, but M. K. has an inner ear implant.)

7. Prepare a teaching/learning plan for M. K. about the bronchoscopy. Consider restrictions related to breathing during the procedure.

8. When M. K. reports to the outpatient surgical unit the next morning, what assessments should the nurse make?

9. Both M. K. and her husband are very anxious. Describe interventions that the nurse should implement to assist the client and her spouse.

Thirty minutes before the procedure, M. K. is given atropine sulfate (Atropine) 0.6 mg, IM. An intravenous infusion is begun with D5/.45 NS, and diazepam (Valium) 10 mg, IV, is given.

10. Why have these medications been ordered?

11. A topical anesthetic agent is applied to the pharynx immediately before the bronchoscopy is to begin. What is the purpose of this agent?

12. What special actions must the nurse take after the procedure is completed and M. K. is taken to the PACU? What equipment should be available when she arrives? What are the reasons for this equipment?

A large mucous plug was removed during the bronchoscopy. This was thought to have contributed to the lack of improvement in M. K's condition. She will be dismissed to home care with a prescription for clindamycin hydrochloride (Cleocin) 450 mg, P.O., every 6 hours for 2 weeks.

13. What should the nurse include in the teaching/learning plan for M. K. about this antibiotic? What other information should be included in the plan?

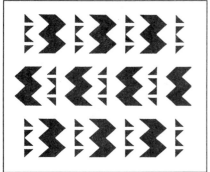

CHAPTER 29

Interventions for Clients with Upper Airway Problems

LEARNING OBJECTIVES

At the end of this chapter, the student will be able to

- Compare and contrast disorders of the nose and sinuses
- Manage care for the client with facial trauma
- Compare and contrast viral and bacterial pharyngitis
- Discuss tonsillitis
- Discuss benign laryngeal disorders
- Discuss upper airway obstruction and neck trauma
- Discuss the pathophysiology, etiology, incidence, and prevention of head and neck cancer
- Manage care for the client with head and neck cancer
- Manage care for the client undergoing a laryngectomy
- Manage care for the client with a tracheostomy

PREREQUISITE KNOWLEDGE

Prior to beginning this chapter, the student should review

- The anatomy and physiology of the upper respiratory tract
- The principles of oxygen therapy
- The principles of sterile technique
- The principles of perioperative nursing management
- The principles of human sexuality
- Grieving and loss
- The concepts of body image
- The interpretation of blood gas measurements

STUDY QUESTIONS

Disorders of the Nose and Sinuses

1. The nursing priority for the client with problems of the upper airway is to
   a. encourage fluids
   b. suction as needed
   c. ensure a patent airway
   d. promote comfort with saline gargles

2. Which of the following four statements is true about rhinitis?
    a. Allergic rhinitis and coryza are initiated by sensitivity reactions to antigens.
    b. Viral rhinitis and hay fever are initiated by sensitivity reactions to antigens.
    c. Allergic rhinitis and hay fever are initiated by sensitivity reactions to allergens.
    d. Rhinitis medicamentosa is relieved with the use of nose drops or sprays.

3. Which of the following conditions is a contraindication for drug therapy to provide symptomatic treatment of rhinitis?
    a. sleep apnea
    b. diverticulosis
    c. Meniere's disease
    d. urinary retention

4. Which of the following classes of drugs is *not* used in the treatment of viral rhinitis?
    a. antihistamines
    b. antipyretics
    c. decongestants
    d. mucolytics

5. The client with acute sinusitis experiences
    a. occipital headache
    b. nasal swelling
    c. high-grade fever
    d. copious clear nasal drainage

6. Management of sinusitis includes
    a. antiemetics
    b. rhinoplasty
    c. bronchodilators
    d. antral irrigation

7. A rhinoplasty involves
    a. straightening the nasal septum to correct sinus drainage problems
    b. cutting a "window" into the anterior portion of the inferior turbinate
    c. placing a splint on a nose that has been injured and possibly fractured
    d. reconstructing the nose surgically for cosmetic and aesthetic improvement

8. Briefly explain the term *moustache dressing:*

_____

_____

_____

9. Care of the client who has had a rhinoplasty includes
    a. applying heat to the nasal area to promote circulation
    b. applying ice to the nasal area to decrease edema
    c. encouraging coughing to prevent atelectasis
    d. giving aspirin every 4 to 6 hours for pain relief

10. Care of the client with epistaxis includes
    a. having the client lie supine
    b. placing pressure over the carotid arteries
    c. placing direct pressure over the nose
    d. having the client hyperextend the neck

11. Which of the following statements about nasal polyps is correct?
    a. They occur more often in clients with intestinal polyps.
    b. They are removed by application of liquid nitrogen.
    c. They arise more often in clients with viral rhinitis.
    d. They contribute to an increased risk of airway obstruction.

12. Hypertrophy of the turbinates is treated with steroids administered
    a. by inhalation
    b. topically
    c. orally
    d. transdermally

Facial Trauma

13. The first priority in the management of facial and neck trauma is to
    a. stop any bleeding
    b. prevent vomiting
    c. immobilize the neck
    d. maintain a patent airway

14. Management of upper airway obstruction includes
    a. repositioning the head and neck so that the head is slightly flexed
    b. using the Heimlich maneuver on the client with a partial airway obstruction
    c. performing a cricothyroidotomy and inserting a hollow tube to maintain patency
    d. intubating with an endotracheal tube to bypass any obstruction

15. Which of the following symptoms in a client with facial trauma should be reported to the physician immediately?

    a. asymmetry of the mandible

    b. bloody drainage from both nares

    c. extraocular movements not parallel

    d. pain upon palpation over the nasal bridge

16. Which of the following foods should be encouraged in the diet of a client who has an innermaxillary fixation?

    a. milk shakes

    b. cheese burgers

    c. carbonated beverages

    d. tuna noodle casserole

Disorders of the Pharynx and Tonsils

17. The most common bacterial organism to cause pharyngitis is

    a. group A beta-hemolytic *Streptococcus*

    b. *Neisseria gonorrhoeae*

    c. *Staphylococcus aureus*

    d. *Chlamydia*

18. Which of the following symptoms usually distinguishes a viral pharyngitis from a bacterial pharyngitis?

    a. degree of temperature elevation

    b. erythematous tonsils

    c. nasal discharge

    d. cervical lymphadenopathy

19. List the two most serious complications of group A streptococcal pharyngitis.

    a. _____

    b. _____

20. A quick-screening laboratory test to distinguish viral pharyngitis from group A streptococcal pharyngitis is

    a. throat culture and sensitivity

    b. latex agglutination

    c. complete blood count

    d. VDRL test

21. Management of viral pharyngitis includes

    a. oral antibiotics

    b. cool saline gargles

    c. activity as tolerated

    d. increased fluid intake

22. Antibiotic therapy for the client with bacterial pharyngitis includes

    a. oral benzathine penicillin for 10 days

    b. intramuscular tetracycline one time

    c. oral penicillin for 10 days

    d. intramuscular streptomycin one time

23. Bacterial pharyngitis is contagious

    a. if antibiotics are not given intramuscularly

    b. as long as the client's throat is red

    c. for the first 24 hours of antibiotic therapy

    d. until all the antibiotic prescribed has been taken

24. Which of the following statements is correct about acute tonsillitis?

    a. It is caused only by bacteria such as *Streptococcus.*

    b. The illness lasts from 3 to 5 days.

    c. It is transmitted by direct person-to-person contact.

    d. Tonsils are red and swollen and produce a thick exudate.

25. All of the following diagnostic studies should be done for the client with tonsillitis *except*

    a. throat culture and sensitivity

    b. monospot

    c. complete blood count

    d. VDRL test

26. Management of bacterial tonsillitis includes

    a. warm saline gargles as needed

    b. antipyretics as needed

    c. antibiotics for 7 to 10 days

    d. all of the above

27. Which of the following foods can be included in the diet of the client who has recently had a tonsillectomy?

    a. grilled cheese sandwich

    b. soft-boiled egg

    c. carrot sticks

    d. orange slices

28. Postoperative care for the client who has had a tonsillectomy should include all of the following *except*

    a. assisting the client to dangle and then ambulate progressively

    b. encouraging the client to drink cold fluids at least every hour

    c. instructing the client to cough and deep breathe

    d. positioning the client with the head at 45 degrees

29. Tonic contraction of the muscles of mastication sometimes seen in the client with peritonsillar abscess is called

    a. tenesmus

    b. trismus

    c. torticollis

    d. tic douloureux

Disorders of the Larynx

30. All of the following are associated with laryngitis *except*

    a. tobacco use

    b. alcohol ingestion

    c. overuse of the voice

    d. exposure to hot, dry air

31. List four interventions that the nurse may implement for the client with laryngitis.

    a. _____

    b. _____

    c. _____

    d. _____

32. Which of the following statements is correct about laryngeal paralysis?

    a. It results from damage to the laryngeal nerve, vagus nerve, or medulla.

    b. It is usually bilateral and results in a partial airway obstruction.

    c. It is treated with an injection of antibiotic into the affected vocal cord.

    d. It presents little risk for the client when eating or swallowing liquids.

33. Identify people who are most at risk for developing vocal cord nodules and for developing polyps. Use a separate sheet.

34. Care of the client with vocal cord nodules or polyps includes all of the following *except*

    a. restriction of warm fluids

    b. complete voice rest

    c. treatment of allergies

    d. air humidification

35. Identify alternative methods of communication for the client who is recovering from surgical removal of laryngeal polyps or nodules.

    a. _____

    b. _____

    c. _____

    d. _____

36. Symptoms of acute laryngeal edema include

    a. eupnea

    b. crackles

    c. laryngeal stridor

    d. Cheyne–Stokes respirations

37. Briefly explain why laryngeal edema can be a medical emergency: _____

    _____

    _____

38. Which of the following structures in the neck is treated with a tracheostomy if it is damaged?

    a. hyoid bone

    b. thyroid cartilage

    c. cricoid cartilage

    d. thyroid gland

39. Initial emergency management for upper airway obstruction as a result of foreign body aspiration includes

    a. several sharp blows between the scapulae

    b. cardiopulmonary resuscitation

    c. nasotracheal suctioning

    d. abdominal thrusts (Heimlich maneuver)

40. List the common causes of neck trauma.

    a. _____

    b. _____

    c. _____

Head and Neck Cancer

41. The type of tumor that most commonly affects the head and neck is

    a. adenocarcinoma

    b. basal cell carcinoma

    c. squamous cell carcinoma

    d. spongioblastoma

42. Which of the following statements is correct about head and neck carcinoma?

    a. It often metastasizes to the brain.

    b. It develops over a short period.

    c. It has no readily identifiable cause.

    d. It appears as white, patchy mucosal lesions.

43. List risk factors related to head and neck carcinoma. Use a separate sheet.

44. List at least five warning signs of head and neck cancer. Use a separate sheet.

45. Which of the following clients is most at risk for developing cancer of the larynx?

    a. a 57-year-old male alcoholic

    b. an 18-year-old marijuana smoker

    c. a 28-year-old woman addicted to diet pills

    d. a 34-year-old man who snorts cocaine

46. The most comfortable position for the client with a laryngeal tumor is

    a. Sims'

    b. contour

    c. Fowler's

    d. Trendelenburg's

47. Which of the following surgical procedures increases the client's risk of choking when eating or drinking is resumed?

    a. laryngofissure

    b. total laryngectomy

    c. transoral cordectomy

    d. supraglottic laryngectomy

48. Carotid precautions following radical neck dissection surgery include

    a. performing physical therapy exercises

    b. monitoring the flap using a doppler

    c. moving the client to an observation bed

    d. applying wet-to-dry dressings to the flap

49. List the methods for speech rehabilitation for the laryngectomy client.

    a. _____

    _____

    b. _____

    _____

    c. _____

    _____

50. Long-term maintenance of an effective airway requires a

    a. tracheostomy

    b. nasal trumpet

    c. endotracheal tube

    d. tracheotomy

51. A tracheostomy is

    a. a surgical incision into the trachea

    b. the tube inserted into an opening in the trachea

    c. the opening or stoma made during a surgical procedure

    d. necessary for the insertion of an endotracheal tube

52. List the indications for a tracheostomy being performed. Use a separate sheet.

53. List the possible complications associated with a tracheostomy. Use a separate sheet.

54. Complications of a tracheostomy that arise immediately postoperatively include

    a. septic shock

    b. neck pain

    c. leaking of foods or liquids

    d. subcutaneous emphysema

55. Hourly assessment of the intubated client includes all of the following *except*

    a. checking the tube's placement

    b. auscultating breath sounds bilaterally

    c. suctioning via a nasotracheal approach

    d. observing chest wall movement and respiratory excursion

56. To prevent accidental extubation, the

    a. client must be in four-point restraints continuously

    b. tracheostomy tube should be taped to the client securely

    c. tracheostomy tube should be flexible to permit coughing

    d. client should be instructed to steady the tube as needed

57. For a tracheostomy that is accidentally decannulated, a track that allows a patent airway forms after

    a. 2 days

    b. 4 days

    c. 7 days

    d. 14 days

58. Equipment that should be kept at the bedside of a client who has a tracheostomy includes

    a. a pair of wire cutters

    b. a thoracentesis tray

    c. gauze saturated with petroleum jelly

    d. a tracheostomy tube with obturator

Match the following terms describing tracheostomy tube equipment (59–68) with their descriptions (a–j).

_____ 59. cuff

_____ 60. double-lumen tracheostomy tube

_____ 61. face plate

_____ 62. fenestrated tracheostomy tube

_____ 63. inner cannula

_____ 64. obturator

_____ 65. outer cannula

_____ 66. single lumen

_____ 67. talking tracheostomy tube

_____ 68. tracheostomy button

a. plastic or metal tube with blunted end used during insertion of tracheostomy tube

b. one-cannula tracheostomy tube

c. maintains stoma patency while client is in transition from mechanical ventilation to spontaneous breathing

d. prevents aspiration when inflated

e. consists of inner and outer tubes and obturator

f. provides a means for communication

g. fits into outer cannula and facilitates cleaning and suctioning

h. part of outer cannula that anchors tube into trachea

i. has precut opening in outer cannula that facilitates speech

j. fits into tracheostomy and keeps airway open

69. Tracheostomy cuffs should be deflated to

    a. allow the client to speak

    b. permit suctioning more easily

    c. enable the client to eat or drink

    d. provide access for tracheostomy care

70. Prevention of obstruction of a tracheostomy by secretions includes

    a. instilling distilled water

    b. humidifying inspired air

    c. inflating the cuff to maximum pressure

    d. suctioning with a Yankauer catheter

71. Humidification and warming of air are essential for the client with an artificial airway because they

    a. prevent tracheal damage

    b. promote thick secretions

    c. dry out the airways

    d. prevent the client from chilling

72. Complications of suctioning include all of the following *except*

    a. hypoxia

    b. tissue trauma

    c. infection

    d. bronchodilation

73. Put in sequence the following steps for endotracheal or tracheal suctioning.

    _____ a. explain procedure to the client

    _____ b. pour sterile saline into sterile basin with nonsterile hand

    _____ c. preoxygenate the client

    _____ d. check suction source

    _____ e. assemble the necessary equipment

    _____ f. remove catheter wrapping keeping catheter sterile; attach to suction

    _____ g. wash hands

    _____ h. insert catheter into trachea without suctioning

    _____ i. assess need for suctioning

    _____ j. lubricate catheter tip in sterile saline solution

    _____ k. open suction kit

    _____ l. withdraw catheter while applying suction and twirling catheter

    _____ m. put on sterile gloves

    _____ n. document procedure after discarding supplies used and washing hands.

74. Briefly describe how to ensure that a tracheostomy tube is never dislodged during tracheostomy care. Use a separate sheet.

75. Put in sequence the following steps in tracheostomy care.

_____ a. remove old dressing and excess secretions

_____ b. wash hands

_____ c. suction tracheostomy tube

_____ d. put on sterile gloves

_____ e. reinsert inner cannula into outer cannula

_____ f. open tracheostomy kit and pour peroxide and saline into one sterile bowl and sterile saline into a second sterile bowl

_____ g. assemble necessary equipment

_____ h. clean stoma site and plate

_____ i. explain procedure to client

_____ j. rinse inner cannula in sterile saline

_____ k. remove inner cannula

_____ l. change tracheostomy ties if soiled

_____ m. place inner cannula in peroxide solution

_____ n. position client

_____ o. lock inner cannula to outer cannula

_____ p. place new tracheostomy dressing

_____ q. use brush and pipe cleaner to clean inner cannula

76. Interventions for the client with a tracheostomy include
   a. changing the tracheostomy ties daily
   b. suctioning continuously for 10–15 seconds
   c. providing oral hygiene with glycerine swabs
   d. cleaning the incision with hydrogen peroxide

77. Oral hygiene for the client with an artificial airway includes use of
   a. hydrogen peroxide to clean granulation tissue
   b. lemon and glycerine swabs to dry the mucosa
   c. mouthwash to alter the pH of the oral cavity
   d. toothettes dipped in water to promote healing

78. Dismissal instructions for the client with a tracheostomy include teaching about
   a. sterile suction technique
   b. tap water instillations
   c. decreasing humidity in the home
   d. wearing a medical alert bracelet

79. Which of the following will assist the client to cope with body image changes after a laryngectomy?
   a. wearing colorful scarves or jewelry
   b. obtaining a voice amplifier for the telephone
   c. purchasing a membership at a local health spa
   d. installing a hot tub or Jacuzzi for relaxation

CRITICAL THINKING EXERCISES

Case Study: Laryngeal Cancer

R. M. is a 48-year-old traveling salesman. He is divorced and has two children who are in college but live with their mother. R. M. smokes two to three packs of cigarettes per day and usually consumes several mixed drinks before dinner. He has been diagnosed with glottic carcinoma of the larynx and is now being admitted for a hemilaryngectomy and possible radical neck dissection. Prior to diagnosis, R. M. had reported being hoarse for 10 days and having some pain in the left ear.

Address the following questions:

1. Identify risk factors R. M. has for laryngeal cancer.

2. What additional data should the nurse collect from R. M. during the admission history and physical examination?

3. Based on the known data, identify the relevant nursing diagnoses for R. M.

4. Develop a perioperative teaching/learning care plan for R. M.

5. Just before surgery, R. M. states, "I guess my days as a pharmaceutical salesman are over." How should the nurse respond?

6. Will it be necessary for R. M. to learn an alternative speech pattern following surgery? Provide rationale for your answer.

The hemilaryngectomy is performed. During the procedure, it is found that two lymph nodes are positive for metastases. The surgeon also does a radical neck dissection.

7. Why is it necessary for R. M. to be transferred to the intensive care unit postoperatively?

8. What is the primary nursing priority for R. M. in the immediate postoperative period?

9. R. M. is transferred back to the surgical nursing unit the second postoperative day. Develop a care plan for him.

10. Following transfer, R. M. continues to recover uneventfully. He is scheduled for dismissal on postoperative day 10. Prepare a dismissal teaching/learning care plan for him. Include information about his job plans.

11. Will R. M. need occupational retaining? Why or why not?

12. What resources exist to assist R. M. with reentering society?

13. What information can the nurse give to R. M. to help him cope with dismissal and self-care?

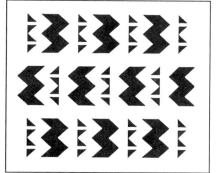

C H A P T E R 3 0

Interventions for Clients with Lower Airway Problems

LEARNING OBJECTIVES

At the end of this chapter, the student will be able to

- Compare and contrast the various types of chronic airflow limitation (CAL) diseases
- Manage care for the client with CAL
- Describe the pathophysiology, etiology, incidence, and prevention of pneumonia
- Manage care for the client with pneumonia
- Discuss the pathophysiology, etiology, incidence, and prevention of tuberculosis (TB)
- Provide care for the client with TB
- Describe lung abscess, empyema, and influenza and related treatment
- Discuss sarcoidosis
- Describe the occupational pulmonary diseases and related management

PREREQUISITE KNOWLEDGE

Prior to beginning this chapter, the student should review

- The anatomy and physiology of the lower respiratory tract
- The process of respiration
- The principles of diffusion, perfusion, and ventilation
- The principles of infection control and isolation
- The principles of perioperative nursing management
- The concepts of body image
- The principles of human sexuality
- Grieving and loss
- The interpretation of blood gas measurements
- Tracheostomy care
- The principles of suctioning

STUDY QUESTIONS

Chronic Airflow Limitation

1. All of the following diseases are commonly seen in chronic airflow limitation (CAL) *except*
   a. bronchiectasis
   b. bronchial asthma
   c. chronic bronchitis
   d. pulmonary emphysema

2. CAL is characterized by
   a. decreased airway resistance
   b. arterial blood gas imbalances
   c. reversible lung distention
   d. increased lung elastic recoil

Match the following pathophysiological changes (3–20) with their associated disease processes (a–c). Answers may be used more than once and more than one answer may apply to each.

_____ 3. affects smaller airways

_____ 4. chronic thickening of bronchial walls

_____ 5. decreased surface area of alveoli

_____ 6. destruction of alveolar walls

_____ 7. hypercapnia

_____ 8. impaired mucociliary clearance

_____ 9. increased airway resistance

_____ 10. increased eosinophils

_____ 11. increased secretions

_____ 12. increased work of breathing

_____ 13. intermittent bronchospasm

_____ 14. intermittent mucosal edema

_____ 15. intermittent periods of excess mucus production

_____ 16. loss of elastic recoil

_____ 17. mast cell destabilization

_____ 18. proteases break down elastin

_____ 19. reactive airway disease

_____ 20. respiratory acidosis

a. bronchial asthma

b. chronic bronchitis

c. pulmonary emphysema

21. Complications of CAL include all of the following *except*
    a. respiratory infections
    b. right-sided heart failure
    c. left-sided heart failure
    d. cardiac dysrhythmias

22. Status asthmaticus is potentially life threatening because
    a. it tends to intensify and progress once it begins
    b. the audible wheezing is a sign of a pneumothorax
    c. neck vein distention signals left-sided heart failure
    d. epigastric pulsations indicate an aortic aneurysm

23. All of the following are causes of CAL *except*
    a. cigarette smoking
    b. smokeless tobacco
    c. air pollution
    d. alpha-1-antitrypsin deficiency

24. If a smoker can stop smoking before serious CAL develops,
    a. lung deterioration will completely reverse itself
    b. the disease process continues but at a slower rate
    c. the rate that lung function deteriorates is unaffected
    d. medication therapy will assist in curing the disease

25. List the subjective client data relevant to CAL. Use a separate sheet.

26. The three classic symptoms of CAL are
    a. cough, dyspnea, wheezing
    b. cough, cyanosis, dyspnea
    c. cyanosis, dyspnea, wheezing
    d. cough, dyspnea, tachypnea

27. Briefly explain why smokers typically cough when they get up in the morning. Use a separate sheet.

28. The increased work of breathing causes metabolic requirements to
    a. decrease
    b. stay the same
    c. increase

29. List the objective client data relevant to CAL. Use a separate sheet.

Match the following assessment findings (30–35) with their descriptions (a–f).

_____ 30. abdominal paradox

_____ 31. asynchronous breathing

_____ 32. barrel chest

_____ 33. blue bloater

_____ 34. pink puffer

_____ 35. respiratory alternans

a. cachectic, emphysemic client

b. increased anteroposterior to lateral chest diameter

c. diaphragmatic breathing alternating with abdominal breathing

d. use of intercostal and abdominal muscles to breathe

e. cyanotic, chronic bronchitis client

f. unorganized chest motion

36. Chest radiographic findings for the client with CAL typically show

    a. hypoinflation

    b. flattened diaphragm

    c. mediastinal shift

    d. increased lung markings

37. Pulmonary function tests (PFTs) are used to

    a. help determine the oxygen liter flow rates required by the client

    b. measure arterial and venous blood gas levels before and after bronchodilators are administered

    c. evaluate the movement of oxygenated blood from the lung to the heart

    d. distinguish airway disease from restrictive lung disease

38. All of the following are major components of PFTs *except*

    a. flow volume curves

    b. diffusion capacity

    c. energy coefficient

    d. lung volumes

Match the following PFTs (39–45) with their descriptions (a–g).

_____ 39. residual volume (RV)

_____ 40. total lung capacity (TLC)

_____ 41. vital capacity (VC)

_____ 42. forced vital capacity (FVC)

_____ 43. forced expiratory volume (FEV)

_____ 44. functional residual capacity (FRC)

_____ 45. diffusion

a. total amount of gas in lungs at end of maximum inspiration

b. amount of gas remaining in lungs at end of tidal expiration

c. maximal amount of gas that can be exhaled after maximal inspiration

d. volume of gas remaining in lung after maximal expiration

e. vital capacity produced from a maximal forced expiratory effort

f. measure of carbon monoxide uptake across alveolar–capillary membrane

g. volume of air exhaled during a specified time in seconds while performing forced vital capacity

46. As CAL progresses, the FEV_1/FVC ratio

    a. decreases

    b. stays the same

    c. increases

47. List the nursing diagnoses common to most clients with CAL. Use a separate sheet.

48. High liter flows of oxygen are contraindicated in the client with CAL because

    a. the client depends on a hypercapnic drive to breathe

    b. the client depends on a hypoxic drive to breathe

    c. receiving too much oxygen over a short time results in headache

    d. response to high doses needed later will be ineffective

49. A pulse oximeter measures

    a. oxygen perfusion in the extremities

    b. carbon dioxide saturation of the blood

    c. the level of the serum pH

    d. oxygen saturation of the blood

50. Clinical indications for the use of oxygen include all of the following *except*

    a. decreased arterial PO_2 levels, as in pulmonary edema

    b. increased cardiac output, as in myocardial infarction

    c. decreased blood oxygen-carrying capacity, as in anemia

    d. increased oxygen demand, as in a sustained fever

51. Hazards of oxygen therapy include all of the following *except*

    a. increased combustion

    b. oxygen-induced hyperventilation

    c. oxygen toxicity

    d. absorption atelectasis

52. List the criteria used to determine the best type of oxygen delivery system for a client. Use a separate sheet.

Match the following systems of oxygen delivery (53–61) with their flow types (a or b). Answers may be used more than once.

_____ 53. aerosol mask

_____ 54. face tent

_____ 55. nasal cannula

_____ 56. nonrebreather mask

_____ 57. partial rebreather mask

_____ 58. simple face mask

_____ 59. T piece

_____ 60. tracheostomy collar

_____ 61. Venturi's mask

a. low-flow system

b. high-flow system

62. The purpose of diaphragmatic breathing is to

   a. increase the amount of diaphragmatic excursion

   b. promote lack of confidence and dyspnea in the client

   c. prolong exhalation and increase airway pressure

   d. maximize the amount of stagnant air in the lungs

63. All of the following are positions that a client can assume to assist in alleviating dyspnea *except*

   a. sitting on edge of chair, leaning forward with arms folded and resting on a small table

   b. leaning back in a low semireclining position with the shoulders back and several pillows under the head

   c. sitting forward in a chair with feet spread apart and elbows placed on knees

   d. leaning back against a support with feet spread apart and shoulders slumped forward

64. Which of the following statements is correct about energy conservation and usage?

   a. The biggest meal of the day is planned for when the client is the hungriest.

   b. Activities are clustered to take better advantage of the client's peak energy times.

   c. The nurse encourages the client to perform his or her own activities of daily living to avoid becoming too dependent.

   d. Light activity such as driving an automobile or vacuuming helps to improve pulmonary function.

65. Identify the main classifications of drugs that are used to manage CAL.

   a. _____

   b. _____

   c. _____

   d. _____

   e. _____

66. Identify the two types of bronchodilators that are used to manage CAL and briefly explain their actions.

   a. _____

   _____

   _____

b. _____

   _____

   _____

67. The therapeutic serum level for theophylline is

   a. 5–10 µg/mL

   b. 10–15 µg/mL

   c. 10–20 µg/mL

   d. 20–30 µg/mL

68. A factor that decreases serum theophylline levels is

   a. cigarette smoking

   b. caffeine consumption

   c. oral contraceptive use

   d. congestive heart failure

69. Briefly describe how to use an inhaler correctly. Use a separate sheet.

70. What is a major advantage of administering corticosteroids for CAL via the aerosol route?

   a. There are fewer systemic side effects.

   b. The bronchodilation effects are less.

   c. It decreases the risk of oral *Candida* infections.

   d. It is easier to manage and client compliance is better.

71. When sequencing aerosol medications for the CAL client, the

   a. steroid should be given immediately after the bronchodilator

   b. steroid should be given 5–10 minutes after the bronchodilator

   c. bronchodilator should be given immediately after the steroid

   d. bronchodilator should be given 5–10 minutes after the steroid

72. Which of the following statements is correct about the use of cromolyn sodium for the treatment of asthma?

   a. It acts by strengthening mast cell membranes to increase histamine release and decrease bronchospasm.

   b. It is useful primarily during acute episodes of asthma attacks.

   c. It is not intended for use during acute episodes of asthma attacks.

   d. It acts by weakening mast cell membranes to decrease histamine release and bronchospasm.

73. The client with CAL should perform specific coughing maneuvers to expectorate excess mucus at all the following times *except*

    a. upon arising in the morning

    b. before each meal

    c. prior to bedtime

    d. following each meal

74. Collaborative management of the client with CAL includes

    a. chest physiotherapy and postural drainage

    b. positioning and hydration

    c. coughing and deep breathing

    d. all of the above

75. Liquids to encourage in the diet of the client with CAL include

    a. fruit juices

    b. coffee, tea, or cocoa

    c. fortified milk shakes

    d. carbonated beverages

76. Interventions to reduce anxiety levels in clients with CAL include all of the following *except*

    a. hypnosis therapy

    b. physical exercise

    c. biofeedback training

    d. relaxation techniques

77. Indications for a client to be dismissed with an order for home oxygen therapy include all of the following *except*

    a. the client is clinically stable

    b. the client has severe hypoxemia

    c. the client has normal blood gas measurements on room air

    d. the client has been optimally treated

Pneumonia

78. Pneumonia results in all of the following *except*

    a. edema of interstitial lung tissue

    b. extravasation of fluid into alveoli

    c. hypoxemia and carbon dioxide retention

    d. hyperinflation of the lungs

79. Which of the following structures does pneumonia primarily affect?

    a. mainstream bronchi

    b. pharynx

    c. alveoli

    d. trachea

80. Put the following events in their correct order in the pathophysiological process of pneumonia.

    ____ a. atelectasis

    ____ b. possible septicemia

    ____ c. decreased surfactant production and compliance

    ____ d. arterial hypoxemia

    ____ e. edema formation and inflammation

    ____ f. tachypnea, tachycardia

    ____ g. migration of white blood cells (WBCs) to alveoli

    ____ h. spread of organisms to other alveoli

    ____ i. shunting of unoxygenated blood

    ____ j. thickening of alveolar wall, stiffening of lung

    ____ k. diminished capillary blood flow in alveoli

    ____ l. invasion of pulmonary tissue by pathogens

81. Decreased lung compliance in pneumonia is the result of

    a. occlusion of the bronchi and alveoli

    b. inflammatory edema and decreased surfactant production

    c. inflammatory edema and a ventilation–perfusion defect

    d. atelectasis and WBC migration to the affected area

82. Systemic effects from the release of endogenous pyrogen by phagocytes include

    a. decreased metabolic rate

    b. fever

    c. bradycardia

    d. eupnea

83. Organisms causing community-acquired pneumonias include

    a. *Legionella pneumophila*

    b. *Pseudomonas aeruginosa*

    c. *Staphylococcus aureus*

    d. *Klebsiella pneumoniae*

84. Organisms causing hospital-acquired pneumonias include

    a. *Mycoplasma pneumoniae*

    b. *Streptococcus pneumoniae*

    c. *Aspergillus*

    d. *Legionella pneumophila*

85. Which of the following is *not* a risk factor for pneumonia?

    a. smoking

    b. immunosuppression

    c. high altitude

    d. chronic illness

86. Preventive measures for pneumonia include

    a. administering vaccines to clients at risk

    b. implementing strict bed rest for debilitated clients

    c. restricting food and fluids in immunosuppressed clients

    d. decontaminating respiratory therapy equipment weekly

87. List the subjective client data relevant to pneumonia. Use a separate sheet.

88. List the objective client data relevant to pneumonia. Use a separate sheet.

89. Which of the following effects does a pneumonia infection have on blood cell components?

    a. increased erythrocyte maturation

    b. increased number of RBCs

    c. decreased number of WBCs

    d. increased number of WBCs

90. Chest radiography of a client with pneumonia will show

    a. areas of patchy consolidation

    b. pathological rib fractures

    c. tension pneumothorax

    d. stenosed pulmonary arteries

91. List the common nursing diagnoses associated with pneumonia

    a. _____

    _____

    b. _____

    _____

92. Interventions that help liquefy secretions for expectoration include

    a. performing postural drainage twice a day

    b. coughing and deep breathing every 2 hours

    c. encouraging a minimum fluid intake of 3000 mL/day

    d. administering a bronchodilator as ordered

93. Drug agents used in the management of pneumonia include

    a. cough suppressants

    b. antibiotics

    c. mucolytic agents

    d. corticosteroids

94. Which of the following medications would be given to the client with ineffective airway clearance related to nonproductive, prolonged coughing?

    a. guaifenesin (Robitussin)

    b. benzonatate (Tessalon)

    c. oxtriphylline (Brondecon)

    d. propylehexedrine (Benzedrex)

95. Which of the following instructions should be given to the client with pneumonia who is being dismissed to home care?

    a. "You may discontinue the deep breathing exercises after 2 weeks when you stop coughing."

    b. "You will continue to feel tired and fatigue easily for the next several weeks."

    c. "Try to drink 1 quart of water every day until you have finished all the antibiotics."

    d. "You should be able to return to work full time in 2 weeks when your energy returns."

Tuberculosis

96. Which of the following statements is correct about TB?

    a. It is not highly contagious to others.

    b. The causative agent of TB is transmitted via aerosolization.

    c. The tubercle bacillus travels to the alveoli via the blood stream.

    d. Exposure to TB results in active disease within 2–10 weeks.

97. According to the American Lung Association classification of TB, a "1" means

    a. no TB exposure, not infected

    b. TB infection, no disease

    c. TB exposure, no evidence of infection

    d. TB, current active disease

98. Put the following steps in the correct order in the type IV delayed hypersensitivity reaction to the infectious microbe *Mycobacterium tuberculosis*.

_____ a.   a cavity forms involving connecting bronchi

_____ b.   T-cells become sensitized to the tubercle

_____ c.   a Ghon tubercle forms

_____ d.   tubercles enter the respiratory tract

_____ e.   fibrosis and calcification of the lesion occur

_____ f.   the granuloma becomes necrotic and cheesy in appearance

_____ g.   lymphokines are released and activate macrophages

_____ h.   a multinucleated giant cell (granuloma) forms

99. Which of the following clients is at the greatest risk for developing TB?

a. a 22-year-old college woman living in a double room in a dormitory

b. a 62-year-old retired school teacher living in a house with her widowed sister

c. a 42-year-old alcoholic homeless man who occasionally stays in a shelter

d. a 53-year-old housewife who does volunteer work in a shelter for the homeless

100. List the subjective data relevant to the client with TB. Use a separate sheet.

101. Physical symptoms of TB include

a. fatigue

b. weight gain

c. high-grade fever

d. nonproductive cough

102. Diagnosis of TB is based on all of the following *except*

a. chest radiography

b. complete blood count

c. Mantoux's skin test

d. sputum culture

103. Briefly discuss why two or more pharmacological agents are used to treat TB.

_____

_____

_____

_____

104. The best time for a client to take chemotherapeutic agents for TB is

a. before breakfast

b. after breakfast

c. at midday

d. at bedtime

105. To eradicate the disease, medications for TB must be taken for

a. 7–10 days

b. 2–3 weeks

c. 3–4 months

d. 6 months or longer

Pulmonary Abscess and Empyema

106. Conditions that place a person at risk for developing a lung abscess include all of the following *except*

a. unconsciousness

b. obstruction of a bronchus

c. mononucleosis

d. immunosuppression

107. Pleuritic chest pain is usually described as

a. crushing, especially on exhalation

b. stabbing, particularly on inhalation

c. burning, especially on swallowing

d. aching, particularly with physical activity

108. An empyema often follows

a. Hansen's disease

b. chest trauma

c. viral bronchitis

d. emphysema

109. Collaborative management of the client with empyema includes antibiotics and

a. closed-chest drainage

b. bronchodilators

c. radiation therapy

d. corticosteroids

Influenza and Sarcoidosis

110. Treatment of influenza includes all of the following *except*

a. analgesics

b. antipyretics

c. antibiotics

d. bed rest

e. fluids

111. Briefly explain why the flu vaccine is given each year.

_____

_____

_____

_____

112. Which of the following should receive an annual flu vaccination?

a. people between the ages of 18 and 65 years

b. a 32-year-old client who has had a renal transplantation

c. a 54-year-old woman with degenerative joint disease

d. an 18-year-old who is inducted into the military service

113. Which of the following statements is correct about sarcoidosis?

a. It is a chronic disorder of the alveoli characterized by granuloma development.

b. It is a group of diseases also known as interstitial lung disease (ILD).

c. It is an acute disorder of the alveoli characterized by granuloma development.

d. It is caused by the sarcoid pneumonia bacterium and is highly contagious.

114. Granuloma development in sarcoidosis results from the activation of

a. B-lymphocytes

b. T-lymphocytes

c. macrophages

d. monocytes

115. Drug treatment of sarcoidosis includes

a. antibiotics

b. bronchodilators

c. corticosteroids

d. chemotherapeutic agents

Occupational Pulmonary Disease

Match the following terms related to occupational lung disease (116–122) with their definitions (a–g).

_____ 116. pneumoconiosis

_____ 117. byssinosis

_____ 118. toxic pneumonitis

_____ 119. silicosis

_____ 120. asbestosis

_____ 121. talcosis

_____ 122. berylliosis

a. interstitial lung fibrosis related to asbestos exposure

b. sarcoidosis related to exposure to highly heated or machined metals

c. pulmonary fibrosis related to long-term talc dust exposure

d. an occupational lung disease of textile workers

e. a group of chronic respiratory diseases related to occupation

f. chronic fibrosing lung disease related to silica dust inhalation

g. a group of acute respiratory diseases related to irritant gas exposure

123. The most important intervention in management of dust-related diseases is

a. using masks and adequate ventilation for prevention

b. PFTs to evaluate lung function

c. supplemental oxygen therapy to alleviate hypoxemia

d. education about bronchodilators to relieve dyspnea

CRITICAL THINKING EXERCISES

Case Study: Chronic Airflow Limitation (CAL)

C. G. is a 50-year-old man who is married, with high school and college age children. He was diagnosed with chronic obstructive lung disease at age 42. Formerly a two-pack-a-day smoker, C. G. has stopped smoking completely and has learned to minimize the effects of his disease with exercise, rest, diet, and medications. The CAL resulted in his inability to work and the need to go on disability 4 years ago. His wife supports the family through her job as a legal secretary, but finances are tight. Mrs. G. resents her husband's disease because she wanted him to stop smoking years before his diagnosis and also because the medicines and oxygen are costly. She assists her husband only minimally with his care. C. G.'s current regimen at home includes oxygen at 1 L per nasal cannula during activity and sleep. Medications include theophylline (Theo-Dur) 400 mg, bid, PO, and metaproterenol (Alupent) 20 mg, tid, via inhaler. A visiting nurse comes to the home monthly and draws a specimen for serum theophylline levels.

Address the following questions:

1. Prepare a care plan for C. G. based on the above data.

2. What does C. G. need to know about his medications? For example, consider alternating the medications times or taking them with meals.

3. Why do theophylline levels need to be monitored?

4. C. G.'s most recent theophylline level was 15 μg/mL. Is this a therapeutic level? What is the therapeutic range for this drug?

5. C. G.'s last hemoglobin was 15.6 g/mm^3 and his hematocrit was 54%. What do these laboratory values suggest? Why are the values elevated? What risk does this create for C. G.?

6. Why should be included in C. G.'s exercise program?

Recent blood gas results have shown an overall increase in C. G.'s carbon dioxide levels. The nurse discusses limiting carbohydrates in C. G.'s diet while increasing the fat content.

7. Why would this type of diet change possibly cause a decrease in C. G.'s carbon dioxide levels?

8. Does a high-fat diet provide more energy? Explain your answer.

9. What foods should the nurse encourage and discourage with a high-fat diet for C. G.?

10. Discuss whether C. G.'s order for oxygen should be reevaluated and perhaps changed.

11. C. G. comments to the visiting nurse that his wife is home less and less. He fears that she is having an extramarital affair. How should the nurse respond?

Case Study: Pneumonia

L. N., a 75-year-old married woman, reports to the outpatient clinic with her husband. She has a severe cough, says that she had left-sided chest pain, and holds her left side while coughing. L. N. appears anxious. Her face is flushed. Vital signs are temperature 102.6°F; pulse 118, apical; respirations 32, shallow; blood pressure 120/80. A diagnosis of pneumonia is suspected. A sputum specimen, chest x-ray, arterial blood gases, and CBC are ordered.

Address the following questions:

1. What should the nurse teach L. N. and her husband about the sputum collection and x-ray?
2. What will the nurse probably hear when she auscultates L. N.'s lungs? Explain your answer.

A diagnosis of pneumonia is confirmed by the chest x-ray and sputum cultures. Since L. N.'s blood gases are within normal limits, she will be managed on an outpatient basis.

3. Identify the relevant nursing diagnoses for L. N. based on the above data.

The physician orders cefaclor (Ceclor) 500 mg, P.O., every 8 hours and wants L.N. to return to the clinic in one week. If L. N.'s condition does not improve within 48 hours, or she becomes short of breath, she should call or return to the clinic.

4. Develop a teaching/learning and dismissal care plan for L. N. and her husband.

Case Study: Tuberculosis (TB)

D. H. is a 60-year-old woman who shares a three-room inner-city apartment with two of her daughters and their seven children. She comes into the neighborhood walk-in clinic complaining of extreme fatigue, a 30-pound weight loss, and a cough of 4 months' duration. A Mantoux test, sputum culture, and chest x-ray confirms a diagnosis of tuberculosis. D. H. is to begin a 12-month course of medication therapy with isoniazid (INH) 300 mg, PO, qd, and rifampin (Rifadin) 600 mg, PO, qd.

Address the following questions:

1. Discuss why two or more pharmacological agents are used to treat tuberculosis.
2. When is the best time for D. H. to take the chemotherapeutic agents to minimize the side effects?
3. Why should rifampin (Rifadin) be taken on an empty stomach?
4. What type of follow-up care should be planned for D. H.?
5. How long will D. H. be considered contagious?
6. What measures should be taken with the other family members? Explain your answer.
7. Develop a teaching/learning plan for D. H.

Three weeks after diagnosis, D. H. returns to the clinic stating that she has stopped taking her medications because they make her sick to her stomach. She is unable to eat and has continued to lose weight.

8. Identify the relevant nursing diagnoses for D. H. based on the above data.
9. Discuss what the nurse should do to assist D. H. to take her medications and eat a balanced diet.

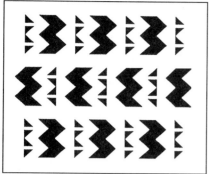

CHAPTER 31

Interventions for Critically Ill Clients with Respiratory Problems

LEARNING OBJECTIVES

At the end of this chapter, the student will be able to

- Discuss pulmonary embolism (PE) and related treatment
- Discuss the pathophysiology, etiology, incidence, and prevention of lung cancer
- Manage care for the client with lung cancer
- Describe acute respiratory failure and related treatment
- Discuss adult respiratory distress syndrome (ARDS) and related treatment
- Manage care for clients requiring mechanical ventilation
- Describe various chest traumas and related management

PREREQUISITE KNOWLEDGE

Prior to beginning this chapter, the student should review

- The anatomy and physiology of the lower respiratory tract
- The process of respiration
- The principles of diffusion, perfusion, and ventilation

- The interpretation of blood gas measurements
- The principles of oxygen therapy
- The principles of perioperative nursing management
- The concepts of body image
- The principles of human sexuality
- Grieving and loss
- Tracheostomy care
- The principles of suctioning

STUDY QUESTIONS

Pulmonary Embolism

1. The most common risk factor for a pulmonary embolism (PE) is
   a. hypercoaguability
   b. heparin therapy
   c. superficial phlebitis
   d. minor trauma

2. PEs usually originate as
   a. clots in the right side of the heart
   b. arterial microemboli
   c. fat particles in the venous system
   d. thrombi in deep veins in the legs or pelvis

3. Arterial blood gas results from early stage PE include

   a. respiratory alkalosis

   b. respiratory acidosis

   c. metabolic acidosis

   d. metabolic alkalosis

4. The test that is most diagnostic for PE is

   a. pulmonary angiography

   b. chest radiography

   c. cardiac catheterization

   d. ventilation-perfusion scan

5. Immediate intervention for PE is

   a. oral anticoagulant therapy

   b. bed rest in supine position

   c. oxygen therapy via mechanical ventilator

   d. parenteral anticoagulant therapy

6. Which of the following statements is correct about the action of heparin?

   a. It prevents platelet aggregation.

   b. It inhibits coagulation immediately.

   c. It dissolves a pulmonary embolus.

   d. It promotes deep venous thrombi absorption.

7. The antidote for heparin is

   a. prothrombin

   b. protamine sulfate

   c. fibrinogen

   d. phentolamine hydrochloride

8. The loading dose for heparin therapy is

   a. 5000 units as an IV bolus

   b. 1000 units/hour per IV infusion

   c. 10,000 units given subcutaneously (SC) stat

   d. 5000 units, SC, every 12 hours

9. Warfarin sodium (Coumadin) therapy is monitored by the

   a. PTT level

   b. PT level

   c. bleeding time

   d. sedimentation rate

Lung Cancer

10. Lung cancer survival rates are poor because

    a. chemotherapeutic agents do not cross the alveolar–capillary membrane.

    b. the ribs and sternum shield any lung tumors from radiation therapy

    c. a lung tumor can never be completely removed by surgery alone

    d. lung cancer often metastasizes before symptoms are noticed by a client

11. Which of the following statements about bronchogenic carcinoma is correct?

    a. It metastasizes primarily by direct extension to the surrounding tissue.

    b. It often metastasizes to the brain, bones, and adrenal glands.

    c. It consists of two types of tumors: small cell and large cell.

    d. It is primarily caused by air pollution and dust particle inhalation.

12. Factors that influence the development of lung cancer include all of the following *except*

    a. air pollution

    b. radon gas exposure

    c. chronic respiratory disease

    d. chewing tobacco

13. The best way to prevent the development of lung cancer is to

    a. eat four servings of green-yellow vegetables per day

    b. wear a mask when the air pollution index is high

    c. stop smoking and avoid people who are smoking

    d. avoid viral infections of the respiratory tract

14. Data indicating the possibility of lung cancer include

    a. clear, watery sputum production

    b. vague sensations of chest tightness

    c. symmetric respiratory excursion

    d. trachea midline and slightly mobile

15. List the nursing diagnoses common to the client with lung cancer.

    a. _____

       _____

    b. _____

       _____

    c. _____

       _____

16. The major complications from treatment with cisplatin is

    a. diarrhea

    b. nausea

    c. flatulence

    d. constipation

17. Immunotherapy in the management of lung cancer includes

    a. administering cytokines for neutropenia

    b. injecting an extract of live tumor cells

    c. giving a full course of hepatitis B injections

    d. administering a tetanus toxoid booster

18. The most effective intervention for pain relief due to bone metastases from lung cancer that allows for mobility is

    a. radiation therapy

    b. patient-controlled analgesia

    c. continuous morphine infusion

    d. oral meperidine hydrochloride (Demerol)

19. The nurse who is assisting with the injection of a sclerosing agent into a client's pleural cavity can expect to

    a. help position the client so that the affected lung is dependent while the drug is injected

    b. clamp the chest tube securely following the instillation of the drug

    c. instruct the client to remain very still for at least 1 hour after the drug has been injected

    d. notify the respiratory therapist to administer intermittent positive-pressure therapy and maximally inflate the lung

Match the following surgical procedures performed on the client with lung cancer (20–26) with their descriptions (a–g).

____ 20. thoracotomy

____ 21. posterolateral thoracotomy

____ 22. anterolateral thoracotomy

____ 23. median sternotomy

____ 24. pneumonectomy

____ 25. lobectomy

____ 26. wedge resection

a. incision from anterior axillary line downward

b. removal of entire lung

c. surgical opening into thoracic cavity

d. incision from submammary fold to scapular tip

e. removal of localized area of diseased lung tissue

f. straight incision from suprasternal notch to below xiphoid process

g. resection of single lobe of lung

Match the following terms related to chest tube drainage systems (27–32) with their descriptions (a–f).

____ 27. closed-chest drainage

____ 28. water seal

____ 29. suction control chamber

____ 30. drainage chamber

____ 31. sampling port

____ 32. Pleur-evac system

a. helps to regulate the amount of negative pressure applied to pleural space

b. provides access to obtain a specimen of pleural drainage

c. all-in-one piece, three-bottle system

d. keeps air from entering pleural space

e. series of connected chambers where fluid and air from the pleural space accumulates

f. drains air and blood from pleural space

33. A chest tube system to gravity drainage is functioning correctly when the water seal chamber

    a. bubbles vigorously and continuously

    b. bubbles gently and continuously

    c. fluctuates with the client's respirations

    d. fluctuates vigorously when the client coughs

34. The preferred position for the client immediately following a pneumonectomy is

    a. supine

    b. High-Fowler's

    c. lying on the operative side

    d. lying of the unaffected side

35. Interventions to promote comfort in the client with lung cancer include
    a. medicating with analgesics only when requested
    b. positioning prone with a pillow under abdomen and shins
    c. ventilating with a high tidal volume and PEEP
    d. providing supplemental oxygen via cannula or mask

36. Which side effect related to analgesics occurs infrequently in cancer clients but more frequently in clients without cancer?
    a. nausea
    b. vomiting
    c. lethargy
    d. constipation
    e. respiratory depression

37. Which of the following community resources should the nurse discuss with the client who has lung cancer and is going home?
    a. the local hospice program
    b. a home health care agency
    c. a vendor of durable medical supplies
    d. all of the above

Acute Respiratory Failure

38. Ventilatory failure usually results from
    a. ventilation-perfusion mismatching
    b. impaired respiratory muscle function
    c. impaired diffusion at the alveolar level
    d. abnormal hemoglobin that does not absorb oxygen

39. Oxygenation failure occurs when
    a. blood shunts from right to left in pulmonary vessels
    b. the client breathes air that is too concentrated with oxygen
    c. the respiratory control center in the brain malfunctions
    d. there is a mechanical abnormality of the chest wall or lungs

Match the following disorders that cause acute respiratory failure (40–58) with their classifications (a–c). Answers may be used more than once.

____ 40. lung tumors
____ 41. cerebral edema
____ 42. bronchial asthma
____ 43. near drowning
____ 44. sleep apnea
____ 45. multiple sclerosis
____ 46. pneumonia
____ 47. chronic bronchitis
____ 48. atelectasis
____ 49. gross obesity
____ 50. poliomyelitis
____ 51. smoke inhalation
____ 52. myasthenia gravis
____ 53. meningitis
____ 54. pulmonary emphysema
____ 55. carbon monoxide poisoning
____ 56. opioid overdose
____ 57. Guillian barré
____ 58. liquid aspiration

a. ventilatory failure
b. oxygenation failure
c. combination of ventilatory and oxygenation failure

59. Which of the following conditions signals impending acute respiratory failure?
    a. orthopnea
    b. tachypnea
    c. dyspnea on exertion
    d. status asthmaticus

60. Initial interventions for acute respiratory failure include all of the following *except*
    a. administration of cromolyn sodium by inhaler
    b. administration of bronchodilators
    c. energy conservation measures
    d. oxygen therapy

Adult Respiratory Distress Syndrome

61. The major site of injury in ARDS is the
    a. mainstem bronchi
    b. respiratory bronchioles
    c. alveolar–capillary membrane
    d. respiratory center in the medulla

62. Which of the following clients is at greatest risk of ARDS?

    a. a 74-year-old who aspirates a tube feeding

    b. a 34-year-old who is near drowning

    c. a 26-year-old with an electrical burn injury

    d. an 18-year-old with a fractured femur

63. Assessment findings for the client with early state ARDS include

    a. adventitious lung sounds

    b. hyperthermia and hot, dry skin

    c. intercostal and suprasternal retractions

    d. increased mental acuity and surveillance

64. Management of ARDS includes

    a. mechanical ventilation with peak inspiratory pressure (PIP)

    b. frequent, small oral feedings

    c. sedation and endotracheal suctioning

    d. antibiotics for viral superinfections

Mechanical Ventilation

65. List the goals for intubation.

    a. _____

    _____

    b. _____

    _____

    c. _____

    _____

    d. _____

    _____

Match the following parts of an endotracheal (ET) tube (66–69) with their descriptions (a–d).

_____ 66. shaft

_____ 67. cuff

_____ 68. pilot balloon

_____ 69. universal adapter

a. device to provide a seal between the trachea and tube

b. device to allow attachment of ET tube to ventilation source

c. hollow tube extending from nasaloral cavity to just above the carina

d. access site for inserting air into the cuff

70. List the equipment needed for emergency ET intubation.

    a. _____

    _____

    b. _____

    _____

    c. _____

    _____

    d. _____

    _____

71. Correct ET tube placement is conclusively verified when

    a. chest excursion is asymmetric

    b. air emerges from the ET tube

    c. breath sounds are bilaterally equal

    d. breath sounds are auscultated over the epigastrium

72. Nursing care of the client on a ventilator includes all of the following *except*

    a. monitoring the client's response to the ventilator

    b. applying soft wrist restraints as ordered

    c. suctioning every hour to prevent complications

    d. maintaining the correct placement of the ET tube

Match the following examples of ventilators (73–80) with their types (a or b). Answers may be used more than once.

_____ 73. cuirass

_____ 74. pressure cycled

_____ 75. time cycled

_____ 76. iron lung

_____ 77. volume cycled

_____ 78. poncho

_____ 79. body wrap

_____ 80. microprocessor

a. negative pressure

b. positive pressure

Match the following ventilator terms and settings (81–89) with their descriptions (a–j).

____ 81. assist-control mode (AC)

____ 82. breaths per minute (BPM)

____ 83. continuous positive airway pressure (CPAP)

____ 84. controlled ventilation

____ 85. fraction of inspired oxygen (FIO$_2$)

____ 86. peak airway inspiratory pressure (PIP)

____ 87. positive end-expiratory pressure (PEEP)

____ 88. sighs

____ 89. synchronized intermittent mandatory ventilation (SIMV)

____ 90. tidal volume (V$_T$)

a. volumes of air that are 1.5 to 2 times tidal volume

b. positive pressure throughout entire respiratory cycle to prevent alveolar collapse

c. number of ventilations delivered per minute

d. volume of air client receives each breath

e. set tidal volume and set rate delivered to client

f. positive pressure exerted during expiration to keep lungs partially inflated

g. oxygen concentration delivered to client

h. ventilator takes over the work of breathing for the client and delivers a set tidal volume

i. allows client to breathe at own rate and tidal volume but breathes for client when needed

j. pressure needed to deliver a set tidal volume

91. Identify the acid–base problems and the necessary interventions for each set of ABG data given below. Use a separate sheet.

a. pH = 7.40, PO$_2$ = 74, PCO$_2$ = 40

b. pH = 7.30, PO$_2$ = 90, PCO$_2$ = 40

c. pH = 7.30, PO$_2$ = 87, PCO$_2$ = 50

d. pH = 7.60, PO$_2$ = 94, PCO$_2$ = 21

e. pH = 7.43, PO$_2$ = 92, PCO$_2$ = 40

f. pH = 7.28, PO$_2$ = 59, PCO$_2$ = 50

Match the following complications of mechanical ventilation (92–103) with their associated body systems (a–e). Answers may be used more than once.

____ 92. pneumothorax

____ 93. stress ulcer

____ 94. muscle mass loss

____ 95. hypotension

____ 96. infection

____ 97. blood gas abnormalities

____ 98. malnutrition

____ 99. subcutaneous emphysema

____ 100. decreased strength

____ 101. fluid retention

____ 102. pneumomediastinum

____ 103. fatigue

a. cardiac
b. lung
c. gastrointestinal
d. immunologic
e. muscles

104. Which of the following situations indicates that a client is ready to wean from a ventilator? The client

a. has a respiratory infection

b. is becoming ventilator dependent

c. maintains blood gases within normal limits

d. is fatigued by the ventilator

105. Which of the following findings might delay weaning a client from a ventilator?

a. hematocrit = 42%

b. arterial PO$_2$ = 70 mmHg on a 40% FIO$_2$

c. apical heart rate = 72

d. oral temperature = 98°F

106. Which of the following clients might take the longest time to wean from a ventilator?

a. a 54-year-old man with metastatic colon cancer who has been intubated for 6 days

b. a 32-year-old woman recovering from a general anesthetic following a tubal ligation

c. a 25-year-old man intubated for 28 hours following an anaphylactic reaction

d. a 49-year-old man with a gunshot wound to the chest who was intubated for 8 hours

107. While weaning a client from the ventilator, the nurse should
   a. observe the monitoring devices regularly from a distance within the client's sight
   b. encourage family members to stay with the client and offer emotional support
   c. stay near the client's bed side as much as possible to check the ventilator
   d. leave the client alone for increasingly longer periods

108. During extubation
   a. the cuff is inflated slightly
   b. the tube is removed during expiration
   c. the client is encouraged not to cough
   d. the client is instructed to deep breathe and cough

109. An expected assessment finding in a recently extubated client is
   a. stridor
   b. dyspnea
   c. hyperpnea
   d. hoarseness

Chest Trauma

110. Which of the following is correct about pulmonary contusion?
   a. It is associated with penetrating wounds such as from a knife or gunshot.
   b. It may require mechanical ventilation with PEEP.
   c. It may result in an asymptomatic flail chest.
   d. It is treated with aggressive fluid hydration.

111. Rib fractures and flail chest are managed with
   a. potent analgesics
   b. tight bandage wraps
   c. progressive ambulation
   d. coughing and deep breathing

112. Tension pneumothorax develops when
   a. blood is lost into the thoracic cavity as a result of blunt trauma
   b. an air leak in the lung or chest wall causes the lung to collapse
   c. air accumulates in the pleural space causing a rise in intrathoracic pressure
   d. an infectious process leads to the accumulation of pus in the pleural space

113. A significant assessment finding in tension pneumothorax is
   a. tracheal deviation to the unaffected side
   b. inspiratory stridor and respiratory distress
   c. diminished breath sounds over the affected hemithorax
   d. hyperresonant percussion note over the affected hemithorax

114. During physical assessment of a client with a hemothorax, percussion of the affected side results in sounds that are
   a. hypertympanic
   b. dull
   c. hyperresonant
   d. adventitious

115. Treatment for a pneumothorax involves all of the following *except*
   a. inserting a large-bore needle into the second intercostal space at the midclavicular line, affected side
   b. placement of a chest tube into the fourth intercostal space at the midaxillary line of the affected side
   c. inserting a large-bore needle into the second intercostal space at the midclavicular line, unaffected side
   d. attaching the chest tube to a water seal drainage system until the lung is completely reinflated

CRITICAL THINKING EXERCISES

Case Study: Lung Cancer

R. C., a 54-year-old man, is married with grown children and is employed as an assistant county engineer. He reports to the pulmonary clinic with complaints of shortness of breath with activities such as working in the yard, surveying, and doing car maintenance. His history includes hypertension and hyperlipidemia, which he successfully controls with diet and, until recently, exercise. R. C. had a triple coronary artery bypass at the age of 44. An exercise treadmill test has ruled out a cardiac problem. R. C. denies smoking since his heart surgery, but there is an odor of smoke present on his breath and clothing.

Address the following questions:

1. What assessments should the nurse make?

2. What factors could be contributing to R. C.'s pulmonary problems? Consider his past diagnosis, history, and occupation.

3. Chest x-rays are completed and a hilar mass is detected. What might the nurse have detected during the assessment that would have pointed to this diagnosis?

4. What additional diagnostic studies can the nurse anticipate will be ordered for R. C.?

A mediastinoscopy and further studies indicate several brain metastatic lesions. Surgery is not an option. Radiation therapy and chemotherapy are planned on an outpatient basis.

5. Identify the relevant nursing diagnoses for R. C. based on the above data and develop a care plan for him.

Since R. C. lives 140 miles from the clinic, he plans to stay with his daughter who lives in the city. She and her husband have a new baby. Because of radiation treatments to the brain, R. C. is instructed not to drive an automobile. Mrs. C. does not drive, and R. C.'s daughter has not been medically approved to drive a car since the birth of her baby.

6. How can R. C. get to and from the clinic for his daily radiation treatments.

7. R. C.'s wife says, "I don't care if R. C. drives the car. It's his car. If he kills the two of us, at least I'll be with him." How should the nurse respond?

R. C.'s monthly chemotherapy regimen requires overnight hospitalization. He receives cisplatin (Platinol), cyclophosphamide (Cytoxan), and doxorubicin (Adriamycin).

8. What should the nurse teach R. C. to expect from these medicines? Why is a wig encouraged?

9. Which of the drugs is of most concern to R. C.'s cardiac status?

10. Discuss why complete blood counts and a 24-hour urinalysis are required before each session of chemotherapy.

11. During the chemotherapy sessions, R. C. has continuous vomiting and diarrhea. What drugs may help decrease these effects?

12. R. C. is encouraged to apply for disability insurance at the time of diagnosis. Discuss why this is so.

13. What emotional effect does R. C.'s diagnosis have on both him and his family? How can the nurse be therapeutic in this situation?

The initial weeks of radiation to the chest and head are completed and R. C. plans to return to his home. After two weeks at home, he decides to return to work and states that it helps his mental outlook. However, he does not like the way people stare at him.

14. What might the nurse suggest to help with this situation?

15. When R. C. returns for the sixth chemotherapy treatment, he complains of weakness in his legs and some problems with walking. What could be contributing to these problems?

Two months later, R. C. returns for more chemotherapy. He is weaker and thinner than before and states, "I think I've had a stroke." Further testing reveals renewed tumor growth of the metastatic brain lesions, and two additional weeks of radiation to the head are planned. R. C. states, "Just when my hair was starting to grown back, I'll lose it again!"

16. How should the nurse respond to this statement?

The radiation seems to be having no effect, and the physicians tell R. C. that there is not much more they can do besides refer him to a hospice program. R. C. responds, "I'm not ready to die. It's all happening so fast. My granddaughter will never know me."

17. How should the nurse respond?

18. Why would a hospice program be beneficial to R. C. and his family?

A month later R. C. is rehospitalized, now almost completely paralyzed and unable to walk. His wife can no longer manage him at home. R. C. has chosen his pall bearers. In two days, he develops superior vena cava syndrome and dies 12 hours later.

19. How will the hospice nurse comfort the family?

Case Study: Chest Trauma and Adult Respiratory Distress Syndrome (ARDS)

L. S., a 72-year-old widow, is brought to the hospital following a head-on car accident. She has blunt injury to the chest from hitting the steering wheel. She is having difficulty breathing and shows signs of cyanosis. Initial orders include a state chest x-ray, arterial blood gases, and oxygen at 4 L/minute per Venturi mask.

Address the following questions:

1. What other assessments should be made at this time?

2. The chest x-ray reveals a tension pneumothorax. What will an assessment reveal with this diagnosis?

A large bore needle is inserted into the pleural space on the affected side followed by the placement of a chest tube. The nurse is to attach the chest tube to a water seal drainage system.

3. At what level should the nurse set the suction?

4. What does bubbling in the water seal compartment indicate when L. S. coughs?

5. Should the nurse "strip" the chest tube? Explain your answer.

6. What should be available at L. S.'s bedside at all times in case the chest tube is accidentally pulled out?

7. Prepare a care plan for L. S.

8. Arterial blood gases are drawn. The results are PaO_2, 68 mmHg; $PaCO_2$, 32 mmHg; and pH, 7.53. What do these values suggest?

9. What interventions should be implemented based on the laboratory results?

10. L. S.'s oxygen is increased to 6 L/minute. Twenty-four hours later, L. S. develops hemoptysis, crackles, and wheezing. Discuss what may be happening to L. S. What would contribute to this condition?

11. What is the primary laboratory study used to establish the diagnosis of acute respiratory distress syndrome?

A chest x-ray and widening alveolar oxygen gradient confirm a diagnosis of ARDS. A Swan–Ganz catheter is inserted, and L. S. is intubated and placed on a respiratory with PEEP.

13. Why is PEEP necessary?

14. Explain the rationale for the use of corticosteroids, antibiotics, and colloids in the management of the client with ARDS.

15. Discuss the probability of recovery for L. S.

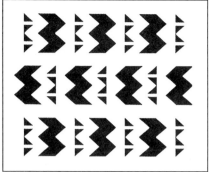

CHAPTER 32

Assessment of the Cardiovascular System

LEARNING OBJECTIVES

At the end of this chapter, the student will be able to

■ Describe the anatomy of the heart

■ Discuss the physiology of the cardiac cycle

■ Describe factors that affect cardiac performance

■ Discuss the changes in the cardiovascular system seen with aging

■ Identify the significant history findings in the client with cardiovascular disease

■ Describe the typical physical assessment findings in the client with cardiovascular disease

■ Discuss the nurse's role in diagnostic assessment of the client with cardiovascular disease

PREREQUISITE KNOWLEDGE

Prior to beginning this chapter, the student should review

■ The anatomy and physiology of the heart and peripheral vascular system, including the lymphatics

■ The effect of the nervous system on the cardiovascular system

■ The principles of normal fluid and electrolyte balance

■ The principles of acid–base balance including blood gas values

■ The physiology of muscle contraction

■ The principles of hydrostatic pressure, diffusion, osmosis, and filtration

STUDY QUESTIONS

Anatomy and Physiology Review

1. Which of the following statements about the coronary arteries of the heart is correct?

   a. There are three main coronary arteries, the left, the right, and the circumflex.

   b. In most individuals, the left coronary artery supplies both the sinoatrial (SA) and atrioventricular (AV) nodes.

   c. There is much individual variation in the branching patterns of the coronary arteries.

   d. Coronary artery blood flow to the myocardium occurs primarily during systole.

Match the following terms related to cardiac electrophysiology (2–6) with their definitions (a–e).

_____ 2. automaticity

_____ 3. conductivity

_____ 4. contractility

_____ 5. excitability

_____ 6. refractoriness

a. inability to respond to successive stimuli while contracting

b. ability to initiate an impulse spontaneously and repetitively without external influence

c. ability to respond to a stimulus by depolarizing

d. ability to transmit electrical impulses

e. ability to respond to an impulse by contracting

7. The chamber of the heart that can generate the greatest amount of blood pressure is the
    a. right atrium
    b. right ventricle
    c. left atrium
    d. left ventricle

Match the following terms related to the structure of the heart (8–22) with their descriptions (a–o).

_____ 8. aortic valve
_____ 9. atrium
_____ 10. chordae tendineae
_____ 11. coronary arteries
_____ 12. endocardium
_____ 13. epicardium
_____ 14. mitral valve
_____ 15. myocardium
_____ 16. pericardial fluid
_____ 17. pericardial space
_____ 18. pericardium
_____ 19. pulmonic valve
_____ 20. septum
_____ 21. tricuspid valve
_____ 22. ventricle

a. protective covering of heart
b. area between visceral and parietal pericardial layers
c. provides lubrication for heart's surfaces, reducing friction
d. outer layer of heart muscle
e. middle layer of heart muscle
f. inner layer of heart muscle
g. muscular wall dividing heart into halves
h. upper heart chamber
i. lower heart chamber
j. valve between right atrium and ventricle
k. valve between right ventricle and pulmonary artery
l. valve between left ventricle and aorta
m. valve between left atrium and ventricle
n. filaments that secure the atrioventricular (AV) valve leaflets
o. vessels that supply the heart with oxygenated blood

23. Which ion catalyzes a chemical interaction within the actin and myosin filaments in the myocardial muscle fibers?
    a. sodium
    b. calcium
    c. potassium
    d. magnesium

24. Put in sequence the path and the time frames of an electrical impulse along the conduction system of the heart. Include the inherent rates of the three pacemaker cell sites. Use a separate sheet.

25. Which of the following statements is correct about the cardiac cycle?
    a. Diastole is the shorter of the two phases.
    b. Systole is the longer of the two phases.
    c. S_1 results from tricuspid and mitral valve closure.
    d. S_2 results from the contraction of the ventricles.

26. Which of the following statements about the mechanical properties of the heart is correct?
    a. Blood flow to the peripheral tissues is the cardiac output.
    b. Cardiac output requirements for each person are relatively consistent.
    c. The volume of blood ejected during systole is the cardiac output.
    d. As the heart rate increases, the cardiac output proportionately decreases.

Match the following variables that affect cardiac output (27–32) with their descriptions (a–f).

_____ 27. afterload
_____ 28. compliance
_____ 29. contractility
_____ 30. heart rate
_____ 31. impedance
_____ 32. preload

a. number of times ventricles contract per minute
b. degree of myocardial fiber stretch at end-diastole
c. amount of tension ventricles develop during systole
d. pressure that ventricle must overcome to open aortic valve
e. distensibility of ventricles
f. force of contraction generated by myocardium under specified loading conditions

33. List the body systems that mediate and regulate blood pressure.

    a. _____

    _____

    _____

b. _____

_____

_____

c. _____

_____

_____

Match the following descriptions (34–40) with their type of circulatory vessel (a or b).

_____   34.   blood volume reservoir   a. artery

_____   35.   collateral circulation   b. vein

_____   36.   distribution vessels

_____   37.   high-pressure system

_____   38.   low-pressure system

_____   39.   migration depot for white blood cells

_____   40.   tissue temperature regulation

41. Which of the following statements are true about the various components of blood pressure?

    a. Systolic blood pressure is the lowest pressure during the relaxation phase of the cardiac cycle.

    b. Diastolic blood pressure is the highest pressure during contraction of the ventricles.

    c. Diastolic blood pressure is primarily determined by the amount of peripheral vasoconstriction.

    d. Pulse pressure is the difference between the systolic and diastolic pressures.

    e. Venous return to the heart is facilitated by the positive intrathoracic pressure generated during exhalation.

    f. Fluid moves from the vascular system into the interstitial spaces when the capillary endothelium is impaired.

42. Which of the following statements is correct about blood pressure regulation?

    a. Baroreceptors are stimulated when arterial walls are stretched by increased blood pressure.

    b. Chemoreceptors are sensitive primarily to hypercapnia and acidosis and secondarily to hypoxemia.

    c. Stretch receptors are sensitive to pressure and volume changes in the aortic arch.

    d. The renal system regulates cardiovascular activity by retaining sodium and water when blood pressure rises.

43. Which of the following statements is correct about the peripheral vascular system?

    a. Veins are equipped with valves that permit one-way flow of blood toward the heart.

    b. The velocity of blood flow varies directly with the diameter of the vessel lumen.

    c. Blood flow decreases and blood tends to clot as the viscosity decreases.

    d. The parasympathetic nervous system has the greatest effect on blood flow to various organs.

44. Which of the following cardiovascular assessment findings would the nurse expect to find in an elderly client?

    a. resting heart rate over 120 beats per minutes

    b. an S_3 heart sound

    c. chronic hypotension

    d. leg edema

Subjective Assessment

45. List the subjective client data relevant to a cardiovascular assessment. Use a separate sheet.

46. One of the most modifiable, controllable risk factors for cardiovascular disease is

    a. obesity

    b. diabetes mellitus

    c. ethnic background

    d. family history of cardiovascular disease

47. Calculate the number of pack-years for the client who has smoked half a pack of cigarettes per day for 2 years, one pack per day for 4 years, and two packs per day for 20 years. Discuss the significance of the number of pack-years and how those data can be used to predict a client's risk for cardiovascular or pulmonary disease. Use a separate sheet.

48. The following is a partial client history. Discuss the significance these data have for an assessment of the cardiovascular system. Submit the completed exercise to the clinical instructor.

    Caucasian male client, 45 years old. Married, three children. Works as an investment banker. Reports that he feels a lot of pressure to perform his job well. Began to have syncopal episodes 3 months ago, feeling lightheaded and sometimes dizzy. Denies loss of consciousness. States that he often skips lunch to continue working through the lunch hour. Entertains clients several times per week by taking them out to lunch or dinner. Commutes to and from work via own automobile and often gets upset and angry with traffic snarls. Tends to have late dinners with wife at home, consuming several cocktails with meals. Admits to having a "weight problem" off and on. Denies hypertension. His father has had a CVA.

Objective Assessment

49. List the objective client data relevant to a cardio-vascular assessment. Use a separate sheet.

50. Using the data in question 48, construct a physical assessment recording for the cardiovascular system. Submit the completed exercise to the clinical instructor on a separate sheet.

51. Chronic heart failure results in

    a. xanthelasma

    b. leg edema

    c. hemangioma

    d. palpitations

52. A finding of pallor is indicative of

    a. hypoxia

    b. anemia

    c. dehydration

    d. hypertension

53. The assessment technique that is infrequently performed in cardiac assessment is

    a. inspection

    b. palpation

    c. percussion

    d. auscultation

54. Which of the following assessment findings from a cardiovascular assessment is abnormal?

    a. absence of heaves, lifts, or thrills

    b. splitting of S_2, decreases with expiration

    c. jugular venous distention to level of the mandible

    d. point of maximal impulse (PMI) in fifth intercostal space at midclavicular line

55. Which of the following heart sounds is abnormal?

    a. split S_1 in an 18 year-old client

    b. S_3 in a 24-year-old client

    c. split S_2 in a 30-year-old client

    d. S_4 in a 48-year-old client

56. The laboratory test that is specific to cardiac tissue and used to assess the occurrence of myocardial infarction is

    a. aspartate aminotransferase (AST) level

    b. MB isoenzyme of creatine kinase (CK-MB) level

    c. lactate dehydrogenase, isoenzyme 2 (LDH_2) level

    d. high-density lipoprotein (HDL) level

57. All of the following laboratory tests are used to predict a client's risk of coronary artery disease *except* measurement of

    a. cholesterol level

    b. triglyceride level

    c. prothrombin time

    d. lipoprotein level

58. Preparation for electrocardiography (ECG) includes

    a. asking the client to lie on the left side

    b. applying the leads over the client's gown

    c. cleaning the client's skin with soap and water

    d. placing the leads on as flat an area as possible

59. Which of the following procedures requires informed consent from the client?

    a. ECG

    b. use of a Holter monitor

    c. stress test

    d. echocardiography

60. Which of the following assessment findings in a client who has had a cardiac catheterization should the nurse report immediately to the physician?

    a. pain at the catheter insertion site

    b. catheterized extremity dusky and cool

    c. small hematoma at the catheter insertion site

    d. intermittent nonpalpable dorsalis pedis pulse

Match the following terms relating to hemodynamic monitoring (61–63) with their descriptions (a–c).

_____ 61. central venous pressure (CVP)

_____ 62. pulmonary artery pressure (PAP)

_____ 63. pulmonary artery wedge pressure (PAWP)

    a. reflects the left atrium and left ventricle end-diastolic pressures

    b. direct measure of right atrial pressure and preload

    c. measures blood flow to lungs and the state of vascular resistance in lung tissue

64. A CVP reading of less than 3 cm H_2O indicates

    a. right-sided heart failure

    b. left-sided heart failure

    c. cardiac tamponade

    d. hypovolemia

65. Interventions for the client with a pulmonary artery catheter include

    a. continuous heparinized flush

    b. intermittent heparinized flush

    c. continuous normal saline flush

    d. heparinized flush prn

CRITICAL THINKING EXERCISES

Case Study: Assessment of the Cardiovascular System

C. K. is a 72-year-old man who had an extensive left ventricular myocardial infarction (MI) at the age of 36 years. At the time of his MI, C. K. was overweight by 50 pounds and smoked two packs of unfiltered cigarettes per day. He had smoked for 20 years. Alcohol consumption was part of his ethnic background; it was customary for C. K. to drink one or two beers per day and several mixed drinks per week. (C. K.'s father had also suffered an MI, at the age of 48, and was a chain smoker.) C. K. slowly recovered from his MI, gave up smoking, and lost weight. His weight stabilized within 15 pounds of the upper limit of his ideal weight. Mrs. K. became an active participant in C. K.'s recovery by changing her style of cooking and virtually eliminating saturated fats from their diets. C. K. no longer drank beer, but he continued to consume an average of two mixed drinks per day. C. K. began a moderate exercise program that included walking several miles a day at least three times a week. He has had stable angina for many years and has annual physical checkups and ECGs at the cardiologist's office. C. K. took up the hobby of downhill skiing at the age of 66, with his cardiologist's approval.

Over the past 6 months, C. K. has experienced infrequent periods of lightheadedness. He had "blacked out" on at least one occasion and was unable to remember any details of what happened. A second episode of loss of consciousness occurred on a clear, cold winter day while C. K. was skiing. He revived spontaneously. The next day, C. K. scheduled an appointment with his physician.

Address the following questions:

1. Identify C. K.'s risk factors for cardiovascular disease at the ages of 36 and 72 years. Which lifestyle changes decreased his risk status following his MI? Which habits increased his risk status?

2. The cardiologist performs an ECG on C. K. and orders blood work drawn for AST, CK and CK-MB, LDH and isoenzymes, and serum potassium. What is the purpose for these tests?

3. The ECG and blood work are inconclusive, but the physician is concerned about C. K.'s symptoms. Discuss why there is reason for concern.

4. C. K. is scheduled for an in-patient cardiac catheterization. The physician tells C. K. that, based on the findings at the time of the catheterization, he may go ahead and perform an angioplasty. Develop a teaching/learning plan for C. K.

The cardiac catheterization is completed, and a 95% blockage of the left anterior descending (LAD) artery is seen along with an 80% blockage of the circumflex artery. A balloon angioplasty is performed in the catheterization laboratory. Following the procedure, the LAD has a 40% blockage and the circumflex has a 25% blockage.

5. What do these findings mean? What significance does the residual blockage have for C. K.?

The physician counsels C. K. to resume activity gradually. A stress test will be scheduled in several weeks for further evaluation of C. K.'s exercise tolerance and cardiac status.

6. Develop a teaching/learning plan for C. K. to prepare him for the upcoming tests.

CHAPTER 33

Interventions for Clients with Dysrhythmias

LEARNING OBJECTIVES

At the end of this chapter, the student will be able to

- Discuss the physiology of normal electrocardiography (ECG) rhythms
- Discuss various dysrhythmias
- Describe the collaborative management of the client with dysrhythmias

PREREQUISITE KNOWLEDGE

Prior to beginning this chapter, the student should review

- The anatomy and physiology of the heart and vascular system
- The principles of fluid and electrolyte balance
- The principles of acid–base balance including blood gas values
- The principles of intravenous therapy
- The principles of perioperative nursing management
- The concepts of grief, loss, death, and dying

STUDY QUESTIONS

Electrocardiography

1. The most life-threatening consequence of cardiac dysrhythmias is

   a. hypotension

   b. bradycardia

   c. emboli

   d. sudden death

2. List in order the cardiac tissues that assume the cardiac pacemaker's role if the sinoatrial (SA) node fails to function.

   a. _____

   _____

   b. _____

   _____

   c. _____

   _____

3. ECG signal transmission is enhanced by

   a. cleaning the skin with povidone iodine solution before applying the electrodes

   b. removing excess hair from electrode sites by clipping it closely to the skin

   c. applying tincture of benzoin to the electrode sites and waiting for it to become "tacky"

   d. abrading the skin by rubbing the electrode sites briskly with sandpaper

Match the following placements (4–9) with their limb leads (a–f) for ECG monitoring.

_____ 4. right arm (+)

_____ 5. right arm (–), left arm (+)

_____ 6. left arm (–), left leg (+)

_____ 7. left leg (+)

_____ 8. left arm (+)

_____ 9. right arm (–), left leg (+)

a. lead I

b. lead II

c. lead III

d. aVR

e. aVL

f. aVF

Match the following characteristics of an ECG complex (10–15) with their descriptions (a–f).

_____ 10. P wave

_____ 11. PR interval

_____ 12. QRS complex

_____ 13. ST segment

_____ 14. T wave

_____ 15. QT interval

a. period between ventricular depolarization and beginning of ventricular repolarization

b. total time for ventricular depolarization and ventricular repolarization

c. period from atrial depolarization to just before ventricular depolarization

d. atrial depolarization

e. ventricular depolarization

f. ventricular repolarization

16. Which of the following statements is correct about ECG waves?

   a. The amplitude of the wave reflects the muscular strength of the contraction.

   b. Wave duration is measured by a series of vertical lines representing intervals of 0.04 second.

   c. Heart rate is estimated by counting the number of wave complexes in a given time if the rhythm is irregular.

   d. Assessment of rate of a rapid rhythm is best done by decreasing the recorder speed.

17. Calculate the heart rate from an ECG strip when there are 25 small blocks from one R wave to the next.

_____

18. List in sequence the eight recommended steps for analyzing ECG rhythms. Use a separate sheet.

19. Briefly differentiate between arrhythmia and dysrhythmia. Use a separate sheet.

20. Which of the following statements is correct about sinus dysrhythmias?

   a. A too-rapid heart rate lengthens diastolic filling time and leads to increased cardiac output.

   b. The body attempts to compensate for a decreased stroke volume by decreasing the heart rate.

   c. Sinus bradycardia occurs in trained athletes because the stroke volume is adequate without a higher rate.

   d. Sinus tachycardia is uncommon in the general population and causes symptoms of coronary insufficiency.

21. Which of the following statements about dysrhythmias are true?

   a. Sinus tachycardia can sustain cardiac output indefinitely.

   b. Atrial flutter is more common than atrial fibrillation.

   c. Atrial fibrillation results in incoordination of atrial contraction and decreased cardiac output.

   d. Escape beats help to maintain cardiac output when the SA node fails to regulate the rate.

   e. Atrioventricular (AV) dissociation results in the atria and the ventricles contracting independently of one another.

   f. Idioventricular rhythms are reliable for maintaining cardiac output.

   g. Most cases of ventricular tachycardia do not result in loss of consciousness.

   h. Ventricular fibrillation is the most common terminal event in sudden cardiac death.

   i. Ventricular fibrillation causes the ventricles to quiver, resulting in absence of cardiac output.

   j. Ventricular fibrillation can be initiated by a single premature ventricular contraction.

   k. Asystole results in a wavy line on the cardiac monitor.

   l. The treatment for asystole is the same as that for ventricular fibrillation.

   m. First-degree AV block is the complete blockage of impulses from the SA node.

   n. Mobitz Type II second-degree AV block does not progress to third-degree block.

   o. Third-degree AV block results in ventricular rhythms.

   p. Bundle branch blocks result in a QRS complex width that exceeds 0.12 second.

22. Identify common causes of ectopic foci for cardiac contraction. Use a separate sheet.

Collaborative Management of Dysrhythmias

23. List the subjective client data relevant to dysrhythmias. Use a separate sheet.

24. List the objective client data relevant to dysrhythmias. Use a separate sheet.

25. Identify the most common nursing diagnosis for the client with dysrhythmia.

   _____

26. Identify the factors that are considered when interventions for dysrhythmias are planned.

   a. _____

   b. _____

   c. _____

   d. _____

27. Which of the following statements is correct about antidysrhythmic agents?

   a. Class I agents slow the rate of depolarization and conduction velocity and reduce cardiac rate.

   b. Class II agents control dysrhythmias associated with too much parasympathetic stimulation.

   c. Class III agents decrease the absolute refractory time and thus help to increase cardiac rate.

   d. Class IV agents impede the flow of sodium into the cell during depolarization and slow cardiac rate.

28. Which of the following procedures should not be performed for the client who has a dysrhythmia?

   a. giving an intramuscular injection

   b. monitoring temperature rectally

   c. cleaning the mouth using a waterpick (Water Pik)

   d. assisting to a bedside commode for a bowel movement

29. Briefly discuss what *demand mode* means in cardiac pacing. Use a separate sheet.

30. List the three complications that can arise from noninvasive pacemaker therapy.

   a. _____

   b. _____

   c. _____

31. Defibrillation for cardioversion is synchronized to coincide with the client's

   a. T wave

   b. QT interval

   c. ST segment

   d. QRS complex

32. Which of the following statements is correct about cardiopulmonary resuscitation (CPR) for the client with a dysrhythmia?

   a. Respiratory arrest usually develops first, leading to cardiac arrest.

   b. CPR may not be effective in reviving the client if the underlying heart disease is extensive.

   c. Defibrillation must occur within 4 minutes of onset of a ventricular dysrhythmia to be effective.

   d. Epinephrine (adrenalin) may produce a coarse ventricular fibrillation that is unresponsive to defibrillation.

33. All clients who have a dysrhythmia should be instructed to

   a. stay at least 4 feet way from a microwave oven that is operating

   b. avoid going through any electronic metal detectors, such as at an airport

   c. learn how to take their apical pulses and have at least one houschold member also learn

   d. carry an identification card or medical alert bracelet to inform others of their disability

CRITICAL THINKING EXERCISES

Case Study: Dysrhythmia and Pacemaker

B. K. is a 75-year-old man admitted with a severe syncopal spell. He had been outside raking leaves when his wife found him lying on the ground unconscious. He was admitted to a cardiac nursing unit for monitoring through telemetry.

Address the following questions:

1. Draw a diagram showing the placement of B. K.'s leads and the expected ECG tracing from the lead placement.

2. A 12 lead ECG is ordered. Develop a teaching plan for B. K. that covers use of this diagnostic tool.

3. Using the ECG strip below, calculate the minute rate and label the rhythm. What is the nurse's responsibility for the client with this rhythm?

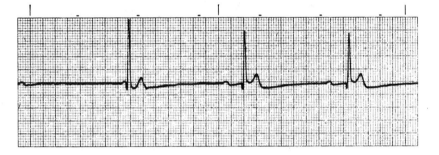

4. The physician orders an atropine drip for B. K. Discuss the rationale for the use of this medication.

5. B. K. is scheduled for insertion of a pacemaker. Develop a teaching/learning plan for the surgery.

6. Following the operation, B. K. returns to the unit and has the rhythm seen on the ECG strip below. Interpret this rhythm.

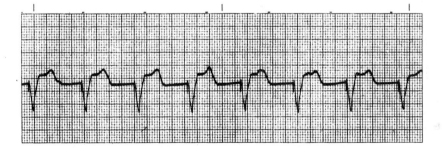

7. What assessments should the nurse perform for B. K. following the pacemaker insertion?

8. Develop a dismissal teaching/learning plan for B. K.

ECG Strip Exercise

Interpret the following ECG strips.

Strip 1: _____

_____

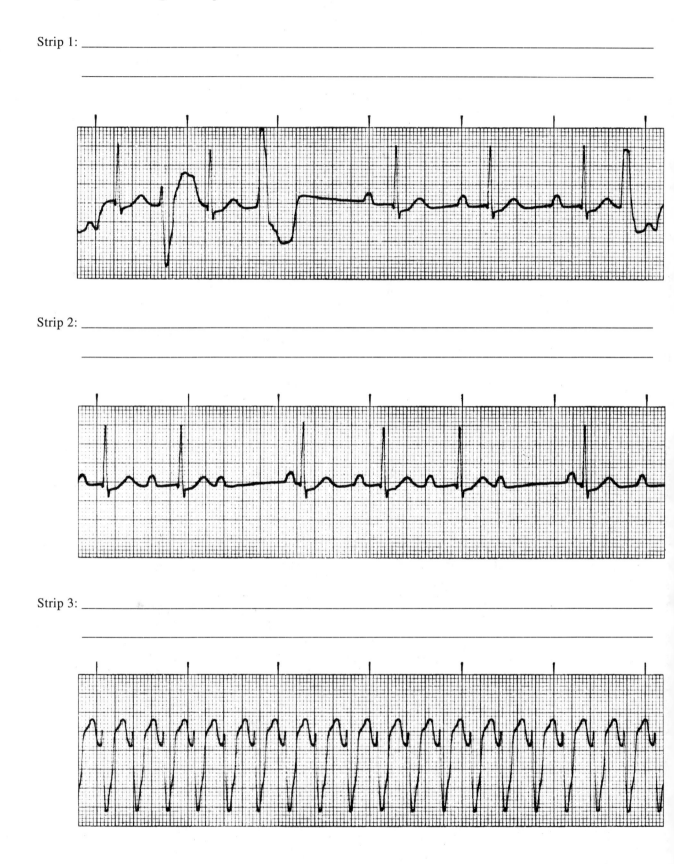

Strip 2: _____

_____

Strip 3: _____

_____

Strip 4: _____

_____

Strip 5: _____

_____

Strip 6: _____

_____

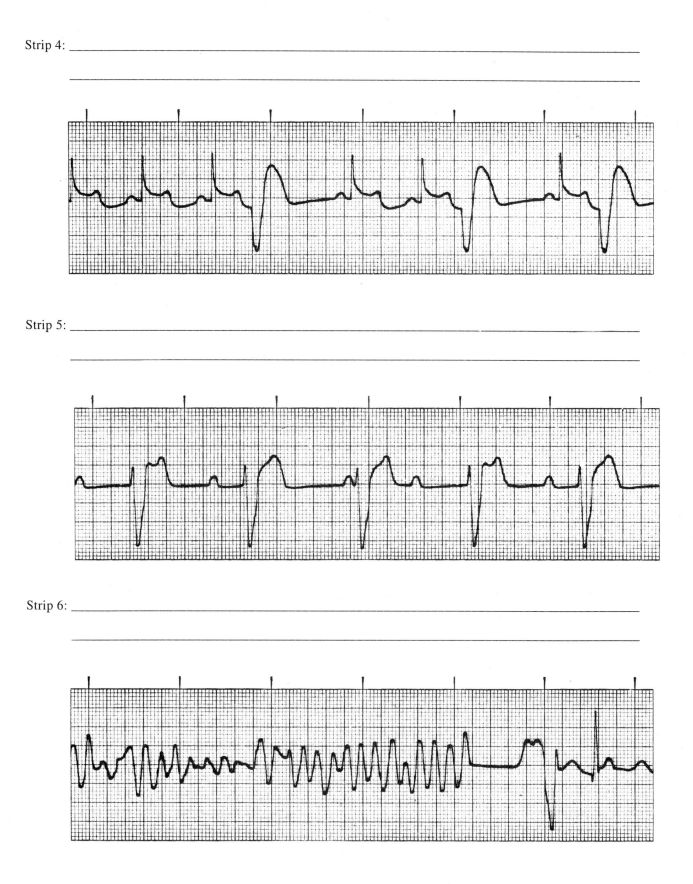

Strip 7: _____

_____

Strip 8: _____

_____

Strip 9: _____

_____

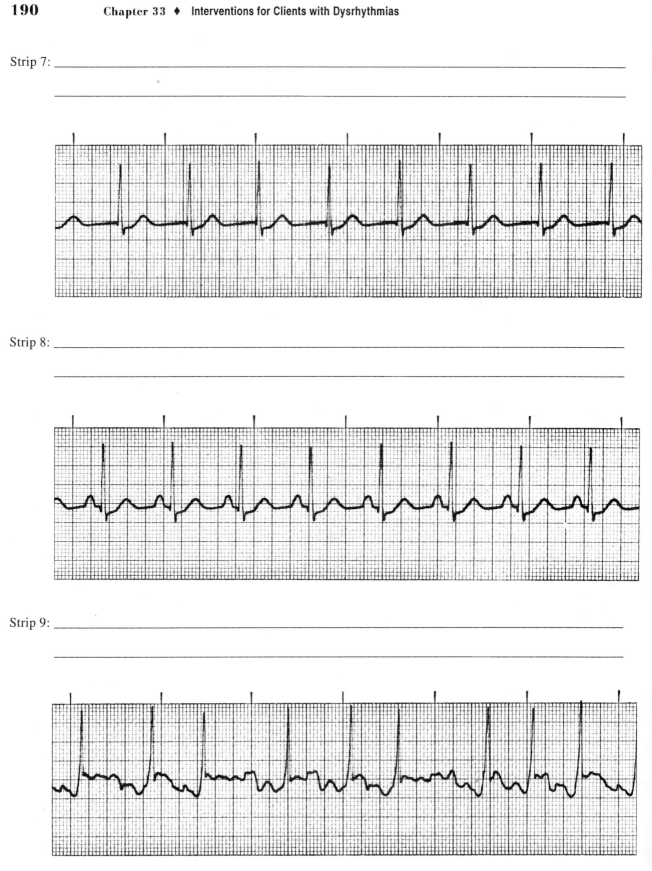

Strip 10: _____

_____

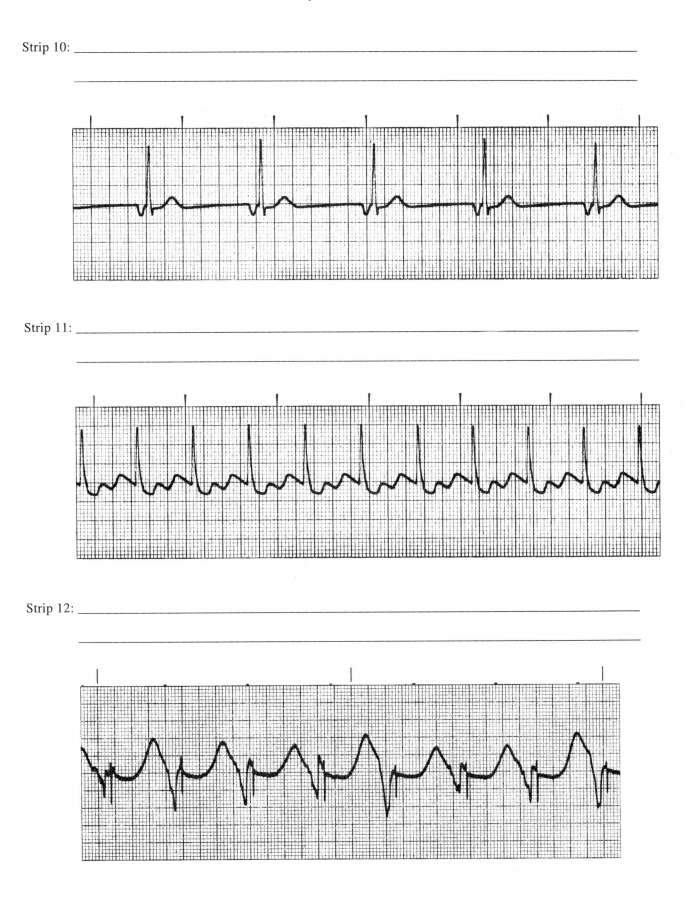

Strip 11: _____

_____

Strip 12: _____

_____

CHAPTER 34

Interventions for Clients with Cardiac Problems

LEARNING OBJECTIVES

At the end of this chapter, the student will be able to

▮ Describe the pathophysiology, classification, and etiology of heart failure

▮ Discuss collaborative management of the client with heart failure

▮ Discuss the pathophysiology, etiology, incidence, and prevention of valvular heart disease

▮ Describe the collaborative management of the client with valvular heart disease

▮ Describe the pathophysiology, etiology, incidence, and prevention of inflammatory and infectious heart disease

▮ Discuss the collaborative management of the client with inflammatory and infectious heart disease

▮ Discuss pericarditis

▮ Discuss cardiomyopathy

PREREQUISITE KNOWLEDGE

Prior to beginning this chapter, the student should review

▮ The anatomy and physiology of the pulmonary, cardiovascular, and renal systems

▮ The principles of fluid and electrolyte balance

▮ The principles of acid–base balance including blood gas values

▮ The role of the kidneys in regulating blood pressure

▮ The principles of intravenous therapy

▮ The principles of perioperative nursing management

▮ The concepts of grief, loss, death, and dying

▮ The concepts of body image and self-esteem

STUDY QUESTIONS

Heart Failure

1. Impaired cardiac function from heart failure results in
   a. low ventricular end-diastolic pressure
   b. reduced systemic diastolic blood pressure
   c. decreased pulmonary venous pressure
   d. decreased cardiac output

2. The initial compensatory mechanism of the heart that maintains cardiac output is
   a. increased parasympathetic stimulation
   b. increased sympathetic stimulation
   c. the Starling response
   d. myocardial hypertrophy

3. Which of the following statements is correct about the classification of heart failure?
   a. Forward failure is the result of the heart's inability to maintain cardiac output.
   b. Left ventricular failure is often directly related to right ventricular failure.
   c. High-output failure occurs when the body's metabolic needs are met with an increased cardiac output.
   d. Chronic heart failure develops over time and is caused by a sudden myocardial infarction (MI).

4. List the subjective client data relevant to heart failure. Use a separate sheet.

5. The client with left ventricular failure is most likely to report

   a. nocturia

   b. weight gain

   c. swollen legs

   d. nocturnal coughing

6. List the objective client data relevant to heart failure. Use a separate sheet.

7. Assessment findings of the client with left-sided heart failure are most likely to include

   a. S_2 splitting

   b. jugular venous distention

   c. splenomegaly

   d. wheezes

8. All of the following diagnostic tests are helpful in diagnosing heart failure *except*

   a. an ECG

   b. chest radiography

   c. echocardiography

   d. thallium imaging

9. Drug therapy for heart failure includes

   a. inotropic agents to increase the heart rate

   b. sympathomimetics to decrease contractility

   c. diuretics to increase the cardiac preload

   d. vasodilators to decrease systemic resistance

10. Foods that should be avoided by the client with heart failure include all of the following *except*

    a. ice cream

    b. margarine

    c. canned fruit

    d. poultry

11. Interventions for the client in acute pulmonary edema from heart failure include all of the following *except*

    a. nitroprusside (Nipride) to decrease venous return

    b. furosemide (Lasix) for diuresis

    c. dopamine (Intropin) to increase cardiac output

    d. aminophylline (Amoline) for bronchospasm

12. Identify preventive measures to delay heart failure in clients with preexisting heart disease.

    a. _____

    b. _____

    c. _____

    d. _____

    e. _____

13. Dismissal planning for the client with heart failure includes

    a. teaching the client to take diuretics at bedtime to enhance the effect on increased renal perfusion

    b. demonstrating to the client how to monitor an apical pulse and what symptoms to report to the physician

    c. determining if the client has a bathroom scale to monitor weight for a gain of more than 5 pounds

    d. providing the client with dietary exchange lists of foods allowed on a low potassium diet

Valvular Heart Disease

14. The most common site of valvular disease is in the

    a. aortic valve

    b. pulmonic valve

    c. tricuspid valve

    d. mitral valve

15. The client with paroxysmal nocturnal dyspnea usually has any one of the following valvular heart diseases *except*

    a. mitral stenosis

    b. mitral prolapse

    c. aortic stenosis

    d. aortic insufficiency

16. The most common preventable cause of valvular heart disease is

    a. congenital disease or malformation

    b. calcium deposits and thrombus formation

    c. beta-hemolytic streptococcal infection

    d. hypertension or Marfan's syndrome

17. List the subjective client data relevant to valvular heart disease. Use a separate sheet.

18. List the objective client data relevant to valvular heart disease. Use a separate sheet.

19. The diagnostic test most often performed to assess valvular heart disease is

    a. echocardiography

    b. electrocardiography

    c. exercise testing

    d. thallium scanning

20. Identify the most common nursing diagnosis for the client with valvular heart disease.

    _____

    _____

21. Long-term anticoagulant therapy for the client with valvular heart disease includes the drug

    a. heparin (Lipo-Hepin)

    b. warfarin sodium (Coumadin)

    c. tubocurarine chloride

    d. protamine sulfate

22. The most common invasive procedure that a client with valvular heart disease may have that requires prophylactic antibiotic therapy is

    a. intravenous therapy

    b. colonoscopy

    c. dental cleaning

    d. gastroscopy

23. The client undergoing heart valve surgery is instructed to

    a. continue taking oral anticoagulants until the time of admission for surgery

    b. prepare for a cardiac catheterization, at which time the defective valve will be replaced

    c. expect to have open heart surgery and be admitted to an intensive care unit postoperatively

    d. refill the prescription for oral anticoagulants because it will be resumed postoperatively

24. Home care of the client following heart valve surgery includes

    a. using an electric toothbrush for regular dental hygiene

    b. flossing of teeth daily to prevent plaque formation

    c. starting a rehabilitation regimen using weight training

    d. using clothing to camouflage the sternal incision

Inflammations and Infections

25. Which of the following clients is at greatest risk of developing infection endocarditis?

    a. an intravenous drug user

    b. a dental hygienist

    c. a radiology technician

    d. a phlebotomist

26. Which of the following procedures is the client with infective endocarditis most likely to report having had recently?

    a. teeth cleaning

    b. urinary bladder catheterization

    c. chest radiography

    d. proctoscopy

27. List the objective client data relevant to infective endocarditis. Use a separate sheet.

28. Arterial embolization to the brain resulting from infective endocarditis may cause symptoms such as

    a. dysarthria

    b. dysphagia

    c. atelectasis

    d. loquaciousness

29. Interventions for the client with infective endocarditis include

    a. administration of oral penicillin for 6 weeks

    b. hospitalization for initial intravenous antibiotics

    c. complete bed rest for the duration of the infection

    d. long-term anticoagulation therapy with heparin

30. Self-care measures for the client with infective endocarditis include

    a. taking an oral temperature reading daily for the remainder of one's life

    b. beginning a moderate exercise program to strengthen the myocardium

    c. recognizing the signs and symptoms of an infiltrated intravenous infusion

    d. weighing one's self daily to monitor for weight gain to report to the physician

31. Acute viral pericarditis commonly occurs following

    a. tuberculosis

    b. radiation therapy

    c. streptococcal pharyngitis

    d. upper respiratory infection

32. Interventions for the client with pericarditis include

    a. restricting fluids

    b. encouraging a right lateral recumbent position

    c. administering nonsteroidal anti-inflammatory agents

    d. preparing for a paracentesis if cardiac tamponade should develop

33. The clinical finding most indicative of rheumatic carditis is

    a. streptococcal infection

    b. precordial pain

    c. cardiomegaly

    d. tachycardia

34. Which of the following statements about pericarditis are correct?

   a. Tuberculosis may cause chronic constrictive pericarditis.

   b. Pericarditis pain is aggravated by holding the breath.

   c. The associated pain is relieved by lying supine.

   d. It is important to differentiate between the pain of pericarditis and that of acute MI.

   e. Atrial fibrillation is common in clients with chronic constrictive pericarditis.

   f. A complication of pericarditis is pericardial effusion.

   g. Tamponade occurs when pericardial fluid restricts atrial filling.

Cardiomyopathy

35. Which of the following statements about cardiomyopathies are correct?

   a. Cardiomyopathy always leads to heart failure with a poor prognosis.

   b. Dilated cardiomyopathy is the massive hypertrophy of the ventricles and small ventricular cavities.

   c. Dilated cardiomyopathy results in symptoms of left ventricular failure.

   d. Most clients with hypertrophic cardiomyopathy are asymptomatic until early adulthood.

   e. Sudden death may be the first manifestation of hypertrophic cardiomyopathy.

   f. Restrictive cardiomyopathy results in decreased cardiac output during exercise.

   g. Dilated cardiomyopathy and restrictive cardiomyopathy are managed the same as heart failure.

   h. Hypertrophic cardiomyopathy is managed the same as myocardial ischemia.

   i. Heart transplantation is the treatment of choice for severe hypertrophic cardiomyopathy.

36. The client with a heart transplantation will

   a. have increased risk for developing coronary artery disease

   b. respond to carotid sinus pressure and vagal stimulation

   c. experience numerous episodes of acute organ rejection

   d. report episodes of angina with increased activity

CRITICAL THINKING EXERCISES

Case Study: Heart Failure

J. W. is a 74-year-old woman who is admitted to the hospital with heart failure. She had been growing progressively weaker and had ankle edema, dyspnea on exertion, and three-pillow orthopnea. On admission, she is severely dyspneic and can only answer questions with one-word phrases. She is diaphoretic, tachycardiac (pulse 132), and hypotensive (blood pressure 96/70). She is extremely anxious.

Address the following questions:

1. Since J. W. cannot breathe or talk easily, prioritize the immediate nursing assessments upon admission.

2. Considering the process of congestive heart failure, explain the symptoms J. W. is having.

3. The physician orders the following items for
   J. W. Explain the rationale for these medications and treatments:

   • start an IV stat with D_5W TKO
   • dopamine 3 mg/kg/min IV
   • propranolol (Inderal) 80 mg PO q 6 hrs
   • verapamil (Iproveratril) 10 mg IV stat and then 60 mg PO q 6 hrs
   • furosemide (Lasix) 40 mg IV stat
   • digoxin 0.5 mg PO q 6 h × 4 doses, with ECG before doses 3 and 4
   • morphine 2 mg IV stat and then 2 mg q 1–2 hrs IV prn
   • oxygen 5 L/min per nasal prongs
   • schedule for an ejection fraction thallium scan and a signal average ECG in a.m.

4. After a few hours of treatment, J. W. is still very anxious and says to the nurse, "I'm going to die! I can't breath anymore!" How should the nurse respond?

5. J. W. is placed on a 1500-mL fluid restriction and a 2-g sodium diet while in the hospital. Discuss the nursing implications and develop a teaching/learning plan for these interventions.

6. The nurse enters J. W.'s room and finds her drinking water from the sink. How should the nurse respond to J. W.? What type of teaching reinforcement is needed?

7. J. W. has been encouraged to walk as much as she can or until she develops angina. How might she be encouraged to walk? What are the benefits of walking?

8. Over the next several days, J. W. improves and is ready to be dismissed to home. Develop a teaching/learning plan for J. W. for her diet, fluid restriction, exercise, and medications (propranolol, verapamil, furosemide, and digoxin).

Interventions for Clients with Vascular Problems

LEARNING OBJECTIVES

At the end of this chapter, the student will be able to

▪ Describe the pathophysiology, etiology, incidence, and prevention of arteriosclerosis and atherosclerosis

▪ Discuss collaborative management of the client with arteriosclerosis and atherosclerosis

▪ Describe the pathophysiology, etiology, incidence, and prevention of hypertension

▪ Discuss collaborative management of the client with hypertension

▪ Describe the pathophysiology, etiology, incidence, and prevention of chronic and acute arterial diseases

▪ Discuss collaborative management of the client with chronic and acute arterial disease

▪ Describe the pathophysiology, etiology, incidence, and prevention of aneurysms

▪ Discuss collaborative management of the client with an aneurysm

▪ Discuss other vascular disorders

▪ Describe the pathophysiology, etiology, incidence, and prevention of venous disease

▪ Discuss collaborative management of the client with venous disease

▪ Discuss vascular trauma

PREREQUISITE KNOWLEDGE

Prior to beginning this chapter, the student should review

▪ The anatomy and physiology of the cardiovascular system

▪ The role of the kidneys in regulating blood pressure

▪ The principles of fluid and electrolyte balance

▪ The principles of acid–base balance including blood gas values

▪ The principles of perioperative nursing management

▪ The principles of intravenous therapy

▪ The principles of hydrostatic pressure, diffusion, osmosis, and filtration

▪ The concepts of body image and self-esteem

▪ The concepts of grief, loss, death, and dying

STUDY QUESTIONS

Arteriosclerosis and Atherosclerosis

1. Differentiate the terms *arteriosclerosis* and *atherosclerosis*. Use a separate sheet.

2. Put in proper sequence the following events leading to atherosclerosis:

_____ a. fibrous plaque develops

_____ b. intimal layer of artery is injured

_____ c. calcification of fibrous lesion

_____ d. deposit of fatty streak on intimal layer

3. Which of the following is a primary risk factor related to atherosclerosis?

   a. obesity

   b. stress

   c. hypertension

   d. sedentary life style

4. Which of the following risk factors for atherosclerosis is modifiable?

   a. sex

   b. genetic make-up

   c. personality type

   d. hypertension

5. List the subjective client data relevant to atherosclerosis. Use a separate sheet.

6. List the objective client data relevant to atherosclerosis. Use a separate sheet.

7. Which of the following clients is at the greatest risk of atherosclerosis according to his or her total serum cholesterol level?

   a. age 27, 200 mg/dL

   b. age 38, 220 mg/dL

   c. age 43, 240 mg/dL

   d. age 62, 260 mg/dL

8. A decreased risk for atherosclerosis is associated with

   a. low high-density lipoprotein (HDL) levels

   b. high HDL levels

   c. high low-density lipoprotein (LDL) levels

   d. normal HDL levels

9. A client consumes 2100 calories per day. Which of the following represents the recommended number of grams of fat per day that this individual should consume in a step-one diet?

   a. 26

   b. 65

   c. 78

   d. 83

10. Which of the following foods is highest in water-soluble fiber?

    a. oatmeal

    b. celery

    c. white rice

    d. lettuce

11. Which of the following foods is lowest in saturated fat?

    a. egg

    b. tuna, water-packed

    c. whole milk

    d. cooked pasta

12. Which of the following is preferable as an exercise for the client with atherosclerosis?

    a. running

    b. rowing

    c. walking

    d. biking

13. Which of the following symptoms should the client with atherosclerosis be instructed to report to the physician immediately?

    a. myalgia

    b. diplopia

    c. dysarthria

    d. nocturia

Hypertension

14. Which of the following blood pressure findings should be evaluated further for hypertension?

    a. 124/62

    b. 138/78

    c. 140/96

    d. 142/88

15. List the factors that affect systemic arterial pressure.

    a. _____

    b. _____

    c. _____

16. Which of the following statements is correct about the control systems for maintaining blood pressure?

    a. The baroreceptor system counteracts a fall in arterial pressure by increasing sympathetic tone.

    b. Excess salt and water in the body cause a rise in blood pressure and cardiac output.

    c. The release of renin and angiotensin by the kidneys increases parasympathetic activity.

    d. Autoregulation responds to changes in arterial pressure by decreasing vascular resistance.

17. All of the following are target organs affected by hypertension *except*

    a. kidneys

    b. heart

    c. brain

    d. stomach

18. Factors associated with hypertension include
    a. malnutrition
    b. alcoholism
    c. vegetarianism
    d. cholelithiasis

19. List the subjective client data relevant to hypertension. Use a separate sheet.

20. List the objective client data relevant to hypertension. Use a separate sheet.

21. The initial radiographic test performed to evaluate hypertension is
    a. renal angiography
    b. intravenous pyelography
    c. computed tomographic scan of the abdomen
    d. isotope renography

22. Preventive measures for hypertension include all of the following *except*
    a. biofeedback therapy for stress management
    b. exercise to increase cardiovascular fitness
    c. switching to a low tar brand of cigarettes
    d. a diet low in salt and saturated fats.

23. Which of the following foods should the client with hypertension consume more of?
    a. fresh fruits
    b. canned soups
    c. luncheon meats
    d. organ meats

24. Initial drug therapy for a client with hypertension would include any one of the following drugs *except*
    a. chlorothiazide (Diuril)
    b. minoxidil (Loniten)
    c. propranolol (Inderal)
    d. guanethidine (Ismelin)

25. The nurse instructs the client who is to receive captopril (Capoten) for the first time to
    a. empty the bladder after the first dose
    b. continue usual activities without restriction
    c. start the drug after getting up in the morning
    d. take the drug at bedtime when in bed for the night

26. Identify reasons why a client being treated with antihypertensive medications may be noncompliant with the prescribed regimen. Use a separate sheet.

27. Which of the following items should the client with hypertension have available at home?
    a. sphygmomanometer with stethoscope
    b. exercise bicycle with odometer
    c. dietary weight scale
    d. pedometer

Peripheral Arterial Disease

28. Tissue damage in peripheral arterial disease (PAD) is related to
    a. extent of the arterial blockage
    b. chronicity of the decreased blood flow
    c. location of the arterial blockage
    d. all of the above

29. List the subjective client data relevant to PAD. Use a separate sheet.

30. How is a client with PAD, who exhibits leg pain that is severe enough to awaken him or her from sleep, classified?
    a. stage I
    b. stage II
    c. stage III
    d. stage IV

31. List the objective client data relevant to PAD. Use a separate sheet.

32. A feature of arterial ulcers that differentiates them from diabetic or venous ulcers is
    a. location over the pressure points of the feet
    b. deep, pale, even edges with little granulation tissue
    c. severe pain or discomfort at the ulcer site
    d. associated ankle discoloration and edema

33. Complications of severe PAD include
    a. gangrene
    b. septicemia
    c. amputation
    d. all of the above

34. List three noninvasive diagnostic procedures for PAD.

    a. _____

    _____

    b. _____

    _____

    c. _____

    _____

35. Exercise is contraindicated as an intervention for PAD for all of the following clients except the one with

 a. severe rest pain

 b. venous stasis ulcers

 c. gangrene of the toes

 d. intermittent claudication

36. Interventions to improve vasodilation and prevent vasoconstriction in the client with PAD include

 a. elevating the feet above the level of the heart

 b. wearing thick, soft socks and closed slippers

 c. switching to chewing tobacco from cigarettes

 d. bathing the feet in moderately hot water

37. The client with PAD may be treated initially with any of the following drugs *except*

 a. dipyridamole (Persantine)

 b. propranolol (Inderal)

 c. isoxsuprine (Vasodilan)

 d. cyclandelate (Cyclospasmol)

38. Interventions for the client who has had a percutaneous transluminal angioplasty (PTA) include

 a. maintaining bed rest for 24 hours

 b. observing for bleeding at the puncture site

 c. monitoring proximal pulses in the affected limb

 d. using crutches to assist with ambulation

39. Postoperative graft occlusion following revascularization for PAD usually occurs

 a. within the first 24 hours

 b. within the first 7 days

 c. after the first month

 d. after the first year

40. Interventions to promote graft healing in the client with PAD include

 a. passive range of motion to the affected limb

 b. early ambulation beginning the day of surgery

 c. elevation of the bed to Trendelenburg's position

 d. meticulous aseptic wound care and hand washing

41. A client who suffers an acute obstruction of a femoral graft would initially exhibit

 a. dark, dusky color in the extremity

 b. pallor of the affected extremity

 c. severe burning pain in the extremity

 d. gradual paresthesia of the extremity

42. Which of the following should the nurse do when applying a dressing to an arterial ulcer?

 a. Wrap the dressing over the limb snugly with a roll bandage.

 b. Secure the terminal ends of the roll bandage to the client's skin with paper tape.

 c. Apply fibrinolysin (Elase) to nonviable tissue to debride the ulcer.

 d. Moisten the dressing until just damp and allow it to dry before changing.

43. Identify the most common cause of peripheral arterial occlusion.

 _____

 _____

 _____

 _____

44. Complications from reperfusion in a limb following an embolectomy include

 a. rubor

 b. edema

 c. rest pain

 d. flaccidity

Aneurysms

45. The most common location for an aneurysm to develop is the

 a. abdominal aorta

 b. Circle of Willis

 c. femoral arteries

 D. popliteal arteries

46. The most common cause of aneurysms is

 a. trauma

 b. thrombus formation

 c. atherosclerosis

 d. embolization

47. List the subjective client data relevant to aneurysm. Use a separate sheet.

48. List the objective client data relevant to aneurysm. Use a separate sheet.

49. The client with a ruptured aneurysm exhibits symptoms of

 a. decreased pulse rate

 b. increased blood pressure

 c. dilated pupils

 d. diaphoretic skin

50. The first action that the nurse should take if a client has a suspected aneurysm rupture is to

    a. start an intravenous infusion with a large-bore needle

    b. take baseline measurements of blood pressure and pulse rate

    c. insert an in-dwelling urinary catheter to straight drain

    d. assess all peripheral pulses for a baseline comparison

51. The client with a repair of an abdominal aneurysm is monitored postoperatively for urinary output because

    a. the client was probably in shock preoperatively and there may be glomerular damage

    b. the client is usually in a critical care nursing unit where this is done routinely

    c. the aorta was clamped during the surgery and the kidneys may have been inadvertently damaged

    d. repair of the aneurysm improves renal perfusion and the urinary output should increase

52. Following repair of a thoracic aneurysm, the nurse monitors for and immediately reports

    a. shallow respirations and poor coughing

    b. increased drainage from the chest tubes

    c. sternal pain with coughing and deep breathing

    d. increased urinary output from the in-dwelling catheter

53. Which of the following activities is allowed after dismissal of the client who has had an aneurysm repair?

    a. playing golf

    b. washing dishes

    c. raking leaves

    d. swimming laps

Other Arterial Disorders

54. Long-term management of the client with aortic dissection includes maintaining

    a. diastolic blood pressure below 80 mm Hg

    b. diastolic blood pressure above 80 mm Hg

    c. systolic blood pressure below 140 mm Hg

    b. systolic blood pressure above 140 mm Hg

55. Which of the following is correct regarding vascular disease?

    a. Buerger's disease is often cured when the client stops smoking.

    b. Raynaud's phenomenon can be precipitated by cold or stress.

    c. Subclavian steal may develop following whiplash or clavicular fracture.

    d. Popliteal entrapment is usually a result of blunt trauma.

Match the following physical findings (56–60) with their related arterial disorders (a–e).

_____ 56. blood pressure different in each arm

_____ 57. unilateral intermittent claudication

_____ 58. blanching, then reddening, of affected extremity

_____ 59. intermittent neck and shoulder pain

_____ 60. diminished distal pulses

a. Buerger's disease

b. popliteal entrapment

c. Raynaud's phenomenon

d. subclavian steal

e. thoracic outlet syndrome

Venous Disorders

61. Thrombus formation is a result of

    a. epithelial injury

    b. venous stasis

    c. hypocoagulability

    d. interstitial edema

62. Which of the following clients is at greatest risk for developing thrombophlebitis?

    a. a 25-year-old pregnant woman

    b. an 80-year-old woman with a fractured hip

    c. a 45-year-old obese man

    d. a 52-year-old man with pneumonia

63. List the subjective client data relevant to thrombophlebitis. Use a separate sheet.

64. List the objective client data relevant to thrombophlebitis. Use a separate sheet.

65. Identify the laboratory tests that would most likely be ordered by the physician for the client with suspected thrombophlebitis.

    a. _____

    b. _____

    c. _____

66. All of the following four diagnostic tests may be ordered for the client with a deep venous thrombosis (DVT) of the calf *except*

    a. contrast venography

    b. impedance phlebography

    c. Doppler ultrasonography

    d. Allen's test

67. List the primary interventions for thrombophlebitis.

    a. _____

    b. _____

    c. _____

68. Which of the following laboratory tests is used to monitor the client receiving heparin therapy for thrombophlebitis?

    a. prothrombin time (PT)

    b. partial thromboplastin time (PTT)

    c. Lee–White clotting time

    d. bleeding time

69. Which of the following symptoms in the client with DVT who is receiving heparin therapy should the nurse report to the physician immediately?

    a. pruritus

    b. rash

    c. hematuria

    d. tinnitus

70. The therapeutic range for the PT in the client receiving warfarin (Coumadin) therapy is

    a. 1.5 to 2 times normal

    b. 2 to 2.5 times normal

    c. 2.5 to 3 times normal

    d. 3.5 to 4 times normal

71. List two surgical procedures performed for management of recurrent deep vein thrombosis or pulmonary emboli.

    a. _____

    b. _____

72. The client who is dismissed on warfarin (Coumadin) therapy should be instructed to avoid consuming

    a. fresh fruits

    b. poultry

    c. decaffeinated beverages

    d. cruciferous vegetables

73. List changes in the tissues that result from venous insufficiency.

    a. _____

    b. _____

    c. _____

74. Management protocols for treating venous stasis ulcers are

    a. well established and standardized

    b. controversial regarding the role of atmospheric oxygen

    c. dependent on the use of topical antibiotic ointments

    d. often unsuccessful, and surgery is eventually necessary

75. Health teaching for the client with chronic venous stasis includes information about

    a. elevating the legs when sitting

    b. crossing the legs only at the ankles

    c. putting on support hose immediately after arising

    d. beginning an exercise program that includes walking

76. Which of the following clients is at greatest risk for developing varicose veins?

    a. a 37-year-old mail carrier

    b. a 19-year-old retail store clerk

    c. a 40-year-old operating room scrub technician

    d. a 25-year-old woman pregnant with twins in the first trimester

77. The preferred treatment for phlebitis is

    a. dry heat

    b. ice packs

    c. warm, moist soaks

    d. compression and elevation

Vascular Trauma

78. List the common types of vascular injury.

    a. _____

    b. _____

    c. _____

79. The type of vascular injury most likely to result from blunt trauma is
    a. arteriovenous fistula
    b. aneurysm formation
    c. dissection
    d. incompetent valves

80. Which of the following clients with vascular trauma is a candidate for immediate surgery?
    a. a 54-year-old with a fractured humerus
    b. an 18-year-old with a contusion of the leg
    c. a 36-year-old with a ruptured renal artery
    d. a 67-year-old with a chronic subdural hematoma

81. List, in order of priority, the most important principles in the management of vascular trauma.

    a. _____

    b. _____

    c. _____

CRITICAL THINKING EXERCISES

Case Study: Hypertension

R. S. is a 35-year-old African-American male who is found to have hypertension (152/90) during a life insurance health assessment. He has been asymptomatic. His physician prescribes chlorothiazide (Diuril) for him as well as a reduction in dietary intake of salt.

Address the following questions:

1. Develop a teaching/learning plan for R. S. for the medication and the diet.

R. S. is seen back in the clinic one month later. His blood pressure is slightly lower (148/88). Although R. S. may require more medication to control his blood pressure, the physician asks the nurse to collect a complete history and assessment of his self-care practices.

2. What is the rationale for the physician's request?

3. What are the sequelae of poorly treated hypertension?

4. What techniques might the nurse teach R. S. to improve his compliance with the prescribed regimen?

Case Study: Thrombophlebitis and Pulmonary Embolus

C. E. is a 58-year-old woman who was dismissed from the hospital 4 days ago following lower abdominal surgery. She has been readmitted for pain and edema in her right calf. She has a tentative diagnosis of thrombophlebitis.

Address the following questions:

1. Discuss the probable etiology of C. E.'s thrombophlebitis.

2. The physician prescribes heparin sodium 1000 units per hour intravenously for C. E. Discuss the purpose of this medication, the nursing precautions, and laboratory tests to monitor its effectiveness.

3. How does heparin differ from warfarin in the treatment of thrombophlebitis?

4. C. E. is placed on strict bed rest with her legs elevated, and a warm, moist pack is to be applied. What are the purposes of these interventions?

5. The following morning C. E. complains of leg cramps and asks the nurse to massage her calf because it is "cramping." Should the nurse comply with the request? Why or why not? If not, what other things could be done for C. E. to increase her comfort?

6. The nurse removes the warm moist pack from C. E.'s leg during the bath and notices an area that does not blanche and is slightly blistered. C. E. states that the area hurts. What is the probable cause of this lesion? What should the nurse do regarding its treatment?

7. C. E.'s activated partial prothrombin time is 51 seconds and prothrombin time is 11 seconds. Discuss the significance of these test results.

8. C. E. calls the nurse and reports severe dyspnea. She had been coughing and there is blood noted in her sputum. She is unable to breathe comfortably even when sitting erect in her bed. What should the nurse do initially for C. E.?

Pulmonary embolism is suspected. The physician orders a thallium lung scan and arterial blood gases.

9. Develop a teaching/learning plan for C. E. regarding these procedures.

10. The arterial blood gas results are as follows: $PaO_2 = 82$, $PaCO_2 = 36$, pH = 7.44. Discuss the significance of these findings.

11. A pulmonary embolism is confirmed and C. E. is treated with mechanical ventilation and vasopressive agents for 48 hours until she is again stable. Develop a teaching/learning plan to reduce her risk of pulmonary emboli in the future.

Case Study: Venous Stasis Ulcers

S. T. is a 58-year-old woman who is admitted to the general medical nursing unit for the management of venous stasis ulcers. The nurse notes that S. T. has thickened, dry skin with a brownish cast. She also has 4+ edema of the legs and absent pedal pulses. The ulcer is about 5 cm in diameter, has an irregular border, and is shallow. The tissue base of the ulcer is red and bumpy, with some areas of yellow-brown adherent tissue. She has no pain in the ulcerative areas.

Address the following questions:

1. Compare and contrast the data observed from S. T.'s ulcers to those from arterial ulcers. Discuss the differences.

2. The physician orders the following medications and interventions. Discuss the rationale for them.

    • bed rest with legs elevated 30 degrees
    • elastic wraps to legs, rewrap qid
    • whirlpool for debridement bid
    • docusate sodium (Colace) po 100 mg bid
    • heparin sodium 5000 units sq bid
    • schedule for an arteriogram in 2 days

S. T.'s ulcers begin to heal, and she is to be dismissed from the hospital. The physicians feel that she can manage her own leg care and dressing changes as an outpatient. During the discussion with S. T., the nurse discovers that S. T. works as a grocery clerk during the day and then cares for her daughter's children in the evening so her daughter can work.

3. Discuss the risk of noncompliance with the prescribed regimen.

4. Consider other techniques to assist S. T.'s compliance with the dismissal instructions.

Interventions for Clients in Shock

LEARNING OBJECTIVES

At the end of this chapter, the student will be able to

▪ Define shock and its classifications

▪ Identify common clinical manifestations of all types of shock

▪ Describe the factors that influence mean arterial pressure (MAP)

▪ Describe the initial response of the body to a sustained decrease in MAP

▪ Discuss the stages of shock

▪ Describe the etiologies and specific conditions causing shock

▪ Identify emergency interventions for the client in hypovolemic (hemorrhagic) and distributive (septic) shock

▪ Explain the steps in the nursing process to provide care for the client in shock

PREREQUISITE KNOWLEDGE

Prior to beginning this chapter, the student should review

▪ The principles of fluid and electrolyte balance

▪ The principles of acid–base balance

▪ The anatomy and physiology of the pulmonary, cardiovascular, and renal systems

▪ The principles of intravenous therapy

▪ Blood administration

▪ The general adaptation syndrome (GAS) response

STUDY QUESTIONS

Anatomy and Physiology Review

1. Which of the following is the best definition of shock?

   a. a disease state involving the heart, blood vessels, or blood

   b. abnormal cellular metabolism due to inadequate delivery of oxygen

   c. a state of marked hysteria followed by syncopal episodes and prostration

   d. the physical compensatory mechanisms to counteract hypoperfusion

2. List three factors that influence MAP.

   a. _____

   b. _____

   c. _____

3. MAP is inversely related to

   a. total blood volume

   b. peripheral resistance

   c. volume of cardiac output

   d. size of the vascular bed

4. Which of the following statements about the control of blood flow is correct?

   a. The most influential factor is the regional control.

   b. The brain can independently control its own blood flow.

   c. The central nervous system is the most important factor.

   d. Blood flow is all organs is increased at the same rate.

Pathophysiology

5. Decreases in MAP are first sensed by the

   a. Golgi bodies

   b. baroreceptors

   c. chemoreceptors

   d. juxtaglomerular cells

6. Anaerobic metabolism causes all of the following *except*

   a. lactic acidosis

   b. fluid and electrolyte imbalances

   c. increased renal blood flow

   d. myocardial depression

7. Complete the following chart on the stages of shock by identifying the MAP changes and physiologic adaptations associated with each stage. Use a separate sheet.

Stage	MAP Change	Physiologic Adaptation
a. initial		
b. nonprogressive		
c. progressive		
d. refractory		

Match the following hormones (8–12) with their effects (a–c). More than one answer may apply to each hormone.

_____ 8. renin

_____ 9. antidiuretic hormone (ADH)

_____ 10. aldosterone

_____ 11. epinephrine

_____ 12. norepinephrine

a. sympathomimetic

b. conserves water

c. stimulates angiotensin

13. Complete the following chart by identifying the causes and methods of prevention for the different types of shock. Use a separate sheet.

Type of Shock	Etiology	Primary Prevention
a. hypovolemic		
b. cardiogenic		
c. distributive		
d. obstructive		

14. The most common cause of hypovolemic shock is

   a. traumatic limb amputation

   b. ruptured esophageal varices

   c. wound dehiscence and evisceration

   d. deep lacerations and blunt trauma

15. The most common cause of cardiogenic shock is

   a. heart failure

   b. myocardial infarction (MI)

   c. an intraseptal defect

   d. cardiac tamponade

16. The following clients have had MIs. The client at greatest risk for developing cardiogenic shock is the one who has

   a. a 25% infarct of the right ventricle

   b. just experienced a first infarction

   c. damage to 40% of the left ventricle

   d. an infarct of the posterior wall

17. The earliest sign of cardiogenic shock is

   a. chest pain

   b. tachycardia

   c. hypotension

   d. confusion

18. A priority for the management of cardiogenic shock is

   a. surgery to correct a mechanical heart defect once the client's condition is stable

   b. insertion of an intraortic balloon pump device to assist the right ventricle

   c. administration of thromboembolic agents to decrease the risk of embolization

   d. determining the cause of the problem and treating the shock state

19. The most common cause of distributive (septic) shock is
    a. gram-negative bacteremia
    b. gram-positive bacteremia
    c. viral sepsis
    d. yeast sepsis

20. The most common cause of anaphylaxis is
    a. poisonous snake bites
    b. poison ivy contact
    c. a drug reaction
    d. hysteria

Collaborative Management

21. List the subjective client data relevant to shock. Use a separate sheet.

22. List the objective client data relevant to the cardiovascular system in shock. Use a separate sheet.

23. An early sign of shock is
    a. cool, clammy skin
    b. decreased urinary output
    c. restlessness
    d. hypotension

24. Another common assessment finding consistent with hypovolemic shock is
    a. pulse pressure of 40 mm Hg
    b. a rapid, weak, thready pulse
    c. cyanotic, cool extremities
    d. increased muscle strength

25. List the objective client data relevant to the respiratory system in hypovolemic shock. Use a separate sheet.

26. A life-threatening pulmonary complication of shock is
    a. adult respiratory distress syndrome
    b. oxygen toxicity from free radicals
    c. status asthmaticus with bronchospasm
    d. alveolar collapse and altered perfusion

27. List the objective client data relevant to the renal system in hypovolemic shock. Use a separate sheet.

28. List the objective client data relevant to the central nervous system in hypovolemic shock. Use a separate sheet.

29. List the objective client data relevant to the musculoskeletal system in hypovolemic shock. Use a separate sheet.

30. Which of the following data indicates that a client is responding to treatment for shock?
    a. blood pH of 7.28
    b. arterial PO_2 of 65 mm Hg
    c. distended neck veins
    d. urinary output of 15 mL in 15 minutes

31. Identify three common nursing diagnoses associated with hypovolemic shock.

    a. _____

    b. _____

    c. _____

32. What size needle should be inserted into a client in hypovolemic shock?
    a. 10 gauge
    b. 12 gauge
    c. 16 gauge
    d. 22 gauge

33. Which of the following statements about colloids is correct? Colloids
    a. are less expensive than crystalloids
    b. are less readily available than crystalloids
    c. are not as similar to fluids lost as are crystalloids
    d. need to administered less often than crystalloids

34. The advantage of crystalloid solutions is that they
    a. carry oxygen to peripheral tissues
    b. substitute for blood indefinitely
    c. do not cause allergic reactions
    d. remain in the plasma for a long time

35. Which of the following statements is correct about drug therapy for hypovolemic shock?
    a. Vasoconstricting agents stimulate venous return by increasing venous pooling of blood.
    b. Beta$_2$-adrenergic agents increase the contractile response of cardiac muscle cells.
    c. Digoxin (Lanoxin) prolongs ventricular filling time and stimulates the ventricle to contract.
    d. Nitroprusside (Nitropress) dilates coronary blood vessels and causes systemic vasodilation.

36. The mental status of the client in hypovolemic shock should be assessed
    a. at the beginning of each shift rotation
    b. every hour if the client responds appropriately
    c. every half hour if the client's shock is progressing
    d. every 15 minutes to evaluate therapy effectiveness

37. Following dismissal, a common psychosocial problem faced by the client who has suffered from hypovolemic shock is
    a. anxiety about meal preparation
    b. fear of recurrence of shock or death
    c. inability to perform personal hygiene
    d. recognizing resulting limitations

38. One of the first interventions in a nonhospital setting for the client who may be in hypovolemic shock is
    a. place in Trendelenburg's position
    b. start an IV infusion
    c. apply a military anti-shock trousers (MAST) garment
    d. summon assistance

39. Which of the following statements about distributive (septic) shock is correct?
    a. The clinical manifestations in phase one are easily diagnosed.
    b. The first phase is short and rapidly progresses to the second phase.
    c. The second phase has a prolonged onset and extended downhill course.
    d. Prompt intervention during phase one has the best prognosis for the client.

40. The factor that most increases the elderly client's risk for distributive (septic) shock is
    a. reduced skin integrity
    b. diuretic therapy
    c. cardiomyopathy
    d. polycythemia

41. The clinical manifestations in the first phase of sepsis-induced distributive shock result from the body's reaction to
    a. leukocytes
    b. endotoxins
    c. hemorrhage
    d. hypovolemia

42. Disseminated intravascular coagulation (DIC) results in
    a. organ hypoxia and ischemia
    b. tachypnea and hyperventilation
    c. increased production of clotting factors
    d. adult respiratory distress syndrome

43. Which of the following assessment findings is most indicative of impending sepsis-induced distributive shock?
    a. crackles in lung bases
    b. bounding peripheral pulses
    c. cool, clammy, cyanotic skin
    d. irritability and restlessness

44. Drug therapy specific to distributive (septic) shock management includes
    a. inotropics
    b. antibiotics
    c. vasoconstrictors
    d. antidysrhythmics

45. Initial treatment for the first phase of DIC includes administration of
    a. factor XIII
    b. factor XI
    c. heparin
    d. platelets

46. Primary prevention for distributive (septic) shock includes
    a. prompt treatment of complications
    b. support of compensatory mechanisms
    c. practice of strict aseptic technique
    d. early detection of clinical manifestations

CRITICAL THINKING EXERCISES

Case Study: Hypovolemic Shock

W. R. is a 43-year-old man who was involved in a motor vehicle accident this morning. Upon admission to the Emergency Department (ED), he had multiple facial lacerations and abdominal and chest pain. Assessments of W. R. in the ED included blood pressure 102/84, pulse 128, respirations 20 and shallow, skin cool and dry, alert and oriented, in pain, and restless. An IV was started with lactated Ringer's solution, and his blood was typed and cross-matched for transfusion. W. R.'s assessments 15 minutes later are blood pressure 96/86, pulse 130, respirations 30, and skin cool, pale, and moist. W. R. is agitated, wanting to turn frequently and sit up.

Address the following questions:

1. W. R. is in hypovolemic shock. What stage of shock was he in on admission? What stage is he in now?

2. W. R. was placed in MAST trousers at the accident scene. What is the purpose of this garment?

X-rays of his chest and abdomen are taken. He is found to have three or four fractured ribs, a hemopneumothorax, and bleeding into the abdomen. It is suspected that he has a lacerated liver. A chest tube is inserted in the ED, and the operating room is notified of the need for emergency surgery to repair the liver.

3. What fluids could be given to W. R. in the ED while waiting for the blood to arrive? What type of blood could he be given?

4. What procedures should be followed to obtain a valid surgical consent for W. R.?

5. Why is a laceration of the liver dangerous?

6. W. R.'s blood pressure continues to fall and he appears to be more unstable. He is started on dopamine to maintain blood pressure of 90 mm Hg systolic. When he is awakened he complains of pain. Should he be given opioids? (Consider that severe pain can cause shock.)

7. Mrs. R. was also in the accident but sustained only minor injuries. She asks how her husband is doing. What should the nurse tell her?

Case Study: Distributive (Septic) Shock

N. M. is a 78-year-old woman admitted from a nursing home with a 3-day history of lower abdominal pain and fever. Yesterday, she developed a fever of 102.5°F with nausea and vomiting. She is presently being treated with intravenous fluids and NPO. She has a history of diverticulitis and congestive heart failure. A consultation with a general surgeon is pending. This morning N. M. is less responsive. Her blood pressure has decreased from 4 hours prior and is now 98/64.

Address the following questions:

1. What clinical problem may be occurring in N. M.? Does the problem require immediate intervention or is it sufficient to notify the physician when rounds are made?

When performing a complete assessment of N. M., the nurse notes that her extremities are cool to the touch and the skin of her legs is mottled. Her temperature has risen 1°F and her blood pressure has fallen to 92/66. Her abdomen is rigid, and she is pale in color and somewhat diaphoretic.

2. What immediate interventions are needed?

The physician arrives and orders N. M. to be transferred to the intensive care unit (ICU) for treatment of probable septic shock. There is no bed immediately available in the ICU, so the nurse must continue to care for N. M. on the nursing unit.

3. How often should vital signs be measured? In what position should the bed be placed? What other assessments and interventions are important to sustain N. M. until an ICU bed is available?

N. M. is transferred to the ICU. She is treated with vasoactive agents, a ventilator, and antibiotics.

4. Discuss the role of endotoxin/exotoxin in N. M.'s symptoms.

5. What is the probable organism causing the infection?

6. N. M. dies the following morning of overwhelming sepsis. Upon evaluation of the plan of care, what changes could have been made?

Case Study: Cardiogenic Shock

K. S. is a 44-year-old executive who was brought to the Emergency Department by ambulance from work. He was in cardiac arrest on admission and received CPR at the office and enroute. Since he was unconscious, a history was obtained from his secretary, who accompanied him. She reported that K. S. developed acute chest pain while at work. K. S. had been having pain for a few months, but he was sure it was stress or indigestion. This morning he asked her to get him a roll of antacids; when she returned, she found him slumped over his desk. She initiated CPR and he was brought to the hospital by ambulance.

On admission to the coronary care unit, K.S. is comatose. His vital signs are blood pressure 92/74, pulse 108, and ventilator-assisted respirations 22. He is in a normal sinus rhythm with occasional premature ventricular contractions (PVCs). He has an IV of 5% dextrose and water, and IV lidocaine ordered prn for PVCs over 6 per minute or multifocal in origin.

Address the following questions:

1. What other assessments should be performed on K. S.?

2. Which of the vasoactive agents would be best for K. S.'s hypotension?

Serum enzymes are drawn, and the CPK-MB and LDH are elevated. He also has an elevated white blood count. ECG findings are abnormal. K. S. is diagnosed with an anterior myocardial infarction. He does well initially with stable vital signs, a normal urine output, and low but stable cardiac output and cardiac index. The fourth day after admission, his systolic blood pressure falls to 88; his cardiac output is 2.8 L per minute (normal is 4–8 L per minute). K. S.'s cardiac index is 1.7 (normal is 2.7–3.2). (Cardiac index is calculated on body surface area based on cardiac output.) He shows increased pulmonary capillary wedge pressure at 18.5 (normal is 6–12). His systemic vascular resistance is increased to 2225 dynes/second/cm^2 (normal is 800–1200). His skin is cool and clammy and he has cyanosis of the legs and arms. An S_3 and crackles are heard on auscultation. His blood gases show hypoxemia and metabolic acidosis: pH 7.2, PaO_2 72 mm Hg, $PaCO_2$ 39 mm Hg, HCO_3 10 mEq/L, oxygen saturation 93%. He is confused and is difficult to rouse. His urine output has been 20 mL per hour for the past 2 hours.

He is diagnosed with cardiogenic shock and treated with an intraaortic balloon pump (IABP) to decrease the workload on his heart. His blood pressure is increased with inotropic agents and his fluids are carefully managed to prevent overload but maintain adequate circulation.

3. One method of calculating cardiac output (CO) is to multiply stroke volume (SV) by pulse rate (PR), or $CO = SV \times PR$. Using this equation, describe why K. S.'s cardiac output is low.

4. Explain the role of the sympathetic nervous system in the increased peripheral vascular resistance, decreased urine output, S_3, and crackles.

5. What is the etiology of his metabolic acidosis?

6. After 3 days, K. S. becomes more stable and is weaned from the ventilator, IABP, and vasoactive agents. He becomes more responsive and is transferred from the CCU to the regular nursing unit. Since K. S.'s type of MI has a 30% mortality rate, what information should be given about self-assessment upon dismissal?

CHAPTER 37

Interventions for Critically Ill Clients with Coronary Artery Disease

LEARNING OBJECTIVES

At the end of this chapter, the student will be able to

▪ Discuss the pathophysiology, etiology, incidence, and prevention of coronary artery disease

▪ Describe the collaborative management of the client with coronary artery disease

PREREQUISITE KNOWLEDGE

Prior to beginning this chapter, the student should review

▪ The anatomy and physiology of the cardiovascular system

▪ The role of the kidneys in regulating blood pressure

▪ The principles of fluid and electrolyte balance

▪ The principles of acid–base balance including blood gas measurements

▪ The principles of shock and shock management

▪ The principles of perioperative nursing management

▪ The principles of intravenous therapy

▪ The principles of hydrostatic pressure, diffusion, osmosis, and filtration

▪ The principles of rehabilitation

▪ The concepts of body image and self-esteem

▪ The concepts of grief, loss, death, and dying

▪ The concepts of human sexuality

STUDY QUESTIONS

Pathophysiology

1. The most common cause of coronary artery disease (CAD) is

   a. coronary artery spasm

   b. atherosclerosis

   c. valvular problems

   d. anemia

2. List the common causes of myocardial infarction (MI).

   a. _____

   _____

   b. _____

   _____

   c. _____

   _____

   _____

   d. _____

   _____

   _____

3. Coronary artery blood flow is unable to increase in relation to demand when the lumen is obstructed by
   a. 40%
   b. 50%
   c. 60%
   d. 70%

Match the following terms (4-7) with their descriptions (a–d).

_____ 4. myocardial infarction
_____ 5. stable angina
_____ 6. unstable angina
_____ 7. angina

   a. chest pain related to increased physical effort or stress with a familiar pattern
   b. chest pain that occurs at rest or with minimal exertion
   c. temporary imbalance between oxygen supply and demand to the myocardium
   d. formation of necrotic cardiac tissue

8. Anginal attacks should be treated promptly because
   a. the myocardium is in urgent need of oxygen
   b. accompanying dysrhythmias cause myocardial fatigue
   c. accumulated lactic acid is toxic to the myocardium
   d. the pain leads to intracellular electrolyte imbalances

9. Identify factors affecting the extent of the zone of infarction.

   a. _____

   _____

   b. _____

   _____

   c. _____

   _____

   _____

10. Which of the following statements about the heart's physiologic response to infarction is correct?
    a. The infarcted area is blue and swollen after 24 hours.
    b. Neutrophils invade the area to remove necrotic cells within 6 hours.
    c. Granulation tissue begins to form 8–10 days after infarction.
    d. Scar tissue remodeling resembles the original tissue in size and shape.

11. The location of an MI associated with the highest mortality rate is
    a. anterior
    b. lateral
    c. inferior
    d. posterior

12. Which of the following is a nonmodifiable risk factor for CAD?
    a. hypertension
    b. diabetes mellitus
    c. family history
    d. obesity

13. Which of the following clients is at greatest risk for having a fatal MI?
    a. a 36-year-old athletic man who smokes
    b. a 68-year-old woman who smokes and is obese
    c. a 24-year-old man with a family history of hypertension
    d. a 32-year-old woman with elevated serum cholesterol levels

Collaborative Management

14. List the subjective client data relevant to CAD. Use a separate sheet.

15. List the objective client data relevant to CAD. Use a separate sheet.

16. Which of the following assessments findings suggests that a client is having an MI?
    a. flushed and holding the breath
    b. diaphoretic and dyspneic
    c. talkative and restless
    d. urinary incontinence

17. The laboratory test used to confirm a diagnosis of angina is
    a. cardiac enzyme and isoenzyme levels
    b. lactate dehydrogenase level
    c. white blood cell count
    d. no specific test

18. The laboratory test used to diagnose an MI is
    a. total creatine kinase
    b. CK-MB isoenzyme
    c. LDH 1 isoenzyme
    d. LDH 2 isoenzyme

19. Which of the following electrocardiographic changes may be observed when an MI occurs but not during an anginal episode?
    a. ST elevation
    b. ST depression
    c. Q wave widened
    d. T wave inversion

20. Which of the following diagnostic tests is used to identify the client who may benefit from further invasive management after acute angina or an MI?
    a. exercise tolerance test
    b. cardiac catheterization
    c. thallium scan
    d. MUGA scan

21. All of the following are actions of nitroglycerin (NTG) *except*
    a. reduces venous return to the heart
    b. increases coronary artery blood flow
    c. reduces coronary artery spasm
    d. increases heart rate and contractility

22. Interventions for the hospitalized client who is being treated initially with antianginal agents include
    a. elevating the head of the bed to 45 degrees
    b. monitoring heart rate and rhythm by continuous ECG
    c. assisting with use of the bathroom or commode
    d. providing oxygen via intermittent positive pressure

23. Complications of thrombolytic therapy include
    a. oliguria
    b. dysarthria
    c. epistaxis
    d. diplopia

24. Which of the following assessment findings is associated with calcium channel blocker therapy?
    a. wheezes
    b. hypotension
    c. bradycardia
    d. forgetfulness

25. Activities for the client in phase 1 cardiac rehabilitation include
    a. range-of-motion exercises
    b. modified weight training
    c. warm up exercises
    d. brisk walking

26. All of the following coping mechanisms may be observed in the client who has had an MI *except*
    a. anger
    b. denial
    c. euphoria
    d. depression

27. List the indications for treating dysrhythmias.

    a. _____

    _____

    b. _____

    _____

    c. _____

    _____

28. Interventions for the client with heart failure following an MI include
    a. administering digoxin (Lanoxin), 1.0 mg, as a loading dose and then daily
    b. infusing intravenous fluids to maintain a urinary output of 60 mL per hour
    c. titrating vasoactive drugs to maintain a sufficient cardiac output
    d. observing for such complications as hypertension, flushed hot skin, and agitation

29. An intra-aortic balloon pump is regulated to inflate

    a. during diastole and deflate before systole

    b. during systole and deflate before diastole

    c. before diastole and deflate during systole

    d. before systole and deflate during diastole

30. A client with angina who is having a percutaneous transluminal angioplasty should also sign a consent for

    a. myocardial biopsy

    b. coronary artery bypass graft (CABG)

    c. carotid endarterectomy

    d. ileal–femoral bypass graft

31. During the perioperative teaching of the elderly client who is having CABG surgery, the nurse should instruct the client to

    a. report any discomfort that may occur

    b. expect to have a large abdominal incision

    c. anticipate being dismissed within the week

    d. discuss plans for a living will with the family

32. Preventive measures for CAD include

    a. consuming a diet high in saturated fats

    b. including more red meat in the diet

    c. limiting exercise to avoid inducing angina

    d. practicing stress management techniques

33. Which of the following is an appropriate activity for the client who is in a phase 3 rehabilitation program following an MI?

    a. biking in the mountains

    b. playing doubles in tennis

    c. working out with weights at a spa

    d. walking several miles three times a week

34. What information should be included in the dismissal instructions for the client who is prone to angina and is concerned about resuming sexual activity?

    a. "You will not be able to resume the same level of physical exertion as you did before."

    b. "Discuss with your partner alternative ways of achieving sexual gratification."

    c. "Try out your usual ways of intercourse to see if you can perform them without an angina attack."

    d. "Take a nitroglycerine tablet just before you engage in sexual intercourse."

35. Which of the following instructions should the nurse include in the teaching/learning plan of the client who is to take nitroglycerine tablets?

    a. "If one tablet does not relieve your angina, take two more pills within the next 5 minutes."

    b. "You can tell whether the pills are still active if they make your tongue tingle."

    c. "Keep your nitroglycerine pills with you at all times in a pill box."

    d. "The prescription should last for 6 months before you need to have it refilled."

CRITICAL THINKING EXERCISES

Case Study: Myocardial Infarction (MI) and Coronary Artery Bypass Graft (CABG)

M. C. is a 56-year-old man admitted to the hospital with severe crushing substernal chest pain. He has had the pain for 2 hours and it has not been relieved with antacids or rest. He describes the pain as being "like a vise around my chest." He admits to having had some previous chest pain with exercise, but otherwise states that he has been healthy. He is asking what can be done to relieve the pain because he wants to go home. M. C. tells the nurse that there is nothing seriously wrong to keep him in the hospital. Besides, he has an important business meeting later that day.

Address the following questions:

1. Compare and contrast the symptoms seen in M. C. to those in the textbook. Include physical and psychological findings.

2. M. C.'s ECG strip is below. Interpret the rhythm, labeling the primary rhythm and the aberrant foci.

3. What type of medication should the nurse administer for this rhythm?

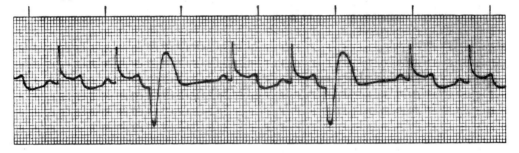

4. M. C. is scheduled for an emergency cardiac catheterization and possible percutaneous transluminal coronary angioplasty (PTCA) and intracoronary streptokinase. Develop a teaching/learning plan for these procedures.

M. C. was found to have complete occlusion (98%) of the left coronary artery, 50% occlusion of the marginal branch of the left coronary artery, and 60% occlusion of the circumflex arteries. Revascularization was achieved with the PTCA and streptokinase. The physician has ordered intravenous heparin for 12 hours and then warfarin sodium (Coumadin) to begin, as well as aspirin.

5. Discuss the rationale for these anticoagulants. Consider the timing of the drugs and their half-life.

6. M. C. also is to receive dipyridamole (Persantine) and nifedipine (Procardia). Discuss the rationale for the use of these medications for M. C.

Six days later M. C. develops severe chest pain similar to what he had on admission. His physician schedules him for an emergency coronary artery bypass graft.

7. Upon entering M. C.'s room, the nurse notices M. C. crying. She approaches him and sits near him to ask what is making him cry. M. C. screams at the nurse, "This is so stupid! Here I wasted 5 days having that procedure done. It didn't help. Now they want me to have surgery. I think all they want is my money!" What might the nurse want to consider before formulating an answer?

M. C. has the surgery and returns to the general nursing unit from intensive care 3 days later. He has had an uneventful recovery and is stable. During the night, M. C. wakes up and screams, "They are out to get me! Stop them!" He is combative and strikes out at the nurses. M. C. is unable to be calmed down despite reassurance that he is in a hospital and is safe.

8. Discuss the options available to prevent M. C. from hurting himself or others. Consider the use of physical and chemical restraints and the ethical issues surrounding their use.

9. Discuss what may have happened to M. C. to cause his confusion and paranoia.

10. M. C. is to continue with cardiac rehabilitation. Discuss the purpose of rehabilitation for cardiac clients. Include the concept of on-going exercise for M. C. after dismissal.

C H A P T E R 3 8

Assessment of the Hematologic System

LEARNING OBJECTIVES

At the end of this chapter, the student will be able to

∎ Describe the structure and function of the bone marrow

∎ Discuss the process of hemostasis

∎ Describe the hematologic changes with aging

∎ Discuss the significant history findings in the client with hematologic disease

∎ Describe typical physical assessment findings in the client with hematologic disease

PREREQUISITE KNOWLEDGE

Prior to beginning this chapter, the student should review

∎ The anatomy and physiology of the hematologic system

∎ The anatomy and physiology of the body systems, e.g., integumentary, respiratory, musculoskeletal, gastrointestinal, central nervous, and cardiovascular, including the lymphatics, renal, and immunologic functions

∎ Normal laboratory values for serum values, e.g., red blood cells (RBCs), white blood cells (WBCs), and platelets

∎ The principles of acid–base balance

∎ The role of nutrition in the formation of hematologic elements, e.g., RBCs, WBCs, and platelets

STUDY QUESTIONS

Anatomy and Physiology Review

1. As a person ages, functional blood-forming marrow is limited to the
   a. ends of long bones
   b. liver and spleen
   c sternum and pelvis
   d. ribs

2. The pluripotent stem cells give rise to
   a. RBCs
   b. WBCs
   c. platelets
   d. all of the above

3. The humoral protein required for RBC maturation is
   a. erythropoietin
   b. leukopoietin
   c. thrombopoietin
   d. immunopoietin

Match the following plasma proteins (4–6) with their descriptions (a–c).

_____ 4. albumin

_____ 5. fibrinogen

_____ 6. globulin

a. transports substances that protect against infection

b. contributes to osmotic pressure in the capillary bed

c. forms polymeric structures basic to the clotting of blood

7. Active hemoglobin synthesis occurs in which of these stages of RBC development?

   a. polychromatic erythroblast

   b. orthochromatic erythroblast

   c. reticulocyte cell

   d. mature RBC

8. Pathological conditions that cause increased oxygen release at the tissue level include all of the following *except*

   a. hypercapnia

   b. alkalosis

   c. acidosis

   d. fever

9. The minerals required for hemoglobin formation include all of the following *except*

   a. copper

   b. zinc

   c. iron

   d. nickel

10. The normal life span of an RBC is

   a. 14 days

   b. 28 days

   c. 60 days

   d. 120 days

11. The element most essential to the growth of WBCs is

   a. folic acid

   b. pyridoxine

   c. cobalt

   d. selenium

12. Platelets are stored in the

   a. liver

   b. spleen

   c. kidney

   d. pancreas

13. The normal life span of a platelet is

   a. 5 days

   b. 14 days

   c. 28 days

   d. 120 days

14. List the functions of the spleen in hematopoiesis.

   a. _____

   _____

   b. _____

   _____

   c. _____

   _____

   d. _____

   _____

15. List the roles of the liver in the hematologic system.

   a. _____

   _____

   b. _____

   _____

   c. _____

   _____

   d. _____

   _____

16. Put the following events in the correct order as they occur in the coagulation of blood.

____ a. platelets adhere to injured blood vessels and form plugs

____ b. clot retracts and pulls the edges of the blood vessel together

____ c. platelets produce phospholipids

____ d. fibrin forms a network of threads that traps cells to form a clot

____ e. vascular injury occurs

____ f. the extrinsic coagulation system is initiated

____ g. clear serum is released from the clot into the blood

____ h. blood flow decreases and tissue thromboplastin is released

____ i. the clot occludes the lumen of the blood vessel, preventing further blood loss

____ j. vessel wall constricts

17. Identify events that can activate the intrinsic coagulation cascade.

a. _____

_____

b. _____

_____

c. _____

_____

d. _____

_____

e. _____

_____

18. Dissolution of a fibrin clot involves

a. fibrinogen

b. prothrombin

c. thromboplastin

d. plasmin

19. All of the following are normal changes in the hematologic system associated with the aging process *except*

a. lymphopenia

b. decreased antibody response

c. thrombocytopenia

d. increased erythrocyte sedimentation rate

Subjective Assessment

20. List the subjective client data relevant to the hematologic system. Use a separate sheet.

21. Which of the following clients is at greatest risk for developing a hematologic disorder?

a. auto mechanic

b. house painter

c. file clerk

d. gourmet chef

22. Which of the following symptoms may be indicative of a hematologic disorder?

a. weight gain

b. bradycardia

c. constipation

d. fatigue

23. The following is a partial client history. Discuss the significance these data have for an assessment of the hematologic system. Submit the completed exercise to the clinical instructor on a separate sheet.

Quiet female client, age 27. Mother of two young children, ages 2 and 4. States she has been feeling increasingly tired the past few months; tries to get 9 hours sleep per night, but wakes up feeling tired. Usually enjoys playing with her children, but finds that she gets short of breath after just a few minutes of activity. Used to exercise (aerobics) three times per week but has stopped. Denies allergies. Takes occasional OTC drugs for headaches (Tylenol). No other medications. It's becoming difficult for her to keep up with housework and meal preparation. Concerned about whether she has an infection or something contagious. Has had a sore throat off and on for the past 2 weeks.

Objective Assessment.

24. List the objective client data relevant to the hematologic system. Use a separate sheet.

25. Using the data in the client history of question 23, construct a physical assessment recording for the hematologic system. Submit the completed exercise to the clinical instructor on a separate sheet.

26. Which of the following clinical findings is suggestive of a hematologic disorder?

    a. coffee ground drainage from a nasogastric tube 2 days after gastric resection

    b. slight oozing of serosanguinous drainage from a colostomy 1 day postoperatively

    c. continuous sanguinous oozing from multiple sites of prior and current punctures

    d. intermittent episodes of epistaxis when indoors during the winter months.

27. Which of the following assessment findings in an elderly client is significant for hematologic disorders?

    a. progressive loss of body hair

    b. dry, scaly skin on elbows

    c. capillary refill lasting more than 5 seconds

    d. pale skin on trunk and legs

28. Which of the following laboratory test results cannot occur? An elevated

    a. RBC count

    b. hemoglobin level

    c. mean corpuscular volume

    d. mean corpuscular hemoglobin concentration

29. The client with sickle cell anemia will have an elevated level of

    a. hemoglobin A_1

    b. hemoglobin C

    c. hemoglobin S

    d. hemoglobin F

30. Which of the following laboratory tests is used to determine blood compatibility between a donor and a recipient?

    a. direct Coombs

    b. capillary fragility

    c. indirect Coombs

    d. reticulocyte count

31. A laboratory finding of decreased total iron-binding capacity (TIBC) indicates

    a. pernicious anemia

    b. overwhelming sepsis

    c. sickle cell anemia

    d. chronic malnutrition

32. Which of the following statements is correct about coagulation laboratory tests?

    a. Bleeding time tests are used to evaluate platelet activity during hemostasis.

    b. The prothrombin time (PT) test is used to assess the intrinsic coagulation cascade.

    c. The partial thromboplastin time (PTT) test evaluates the extrinsic coagulation cascade.

    d. Platelet aggregation determines the ability of platelets to form a fibrin network.

33. In addition to the iliac crest, bone marrow aspiration can be taken from the

    a. ribs

    b. scapulae

    c. sternum

    d. skull

34. When preparing the client for a bone marrow aspiration test, the nurse should

    a. tell the client that the procedure will be done under general anesthesia

    b. explain that the skin over the aspiration site may be anesthetized prior to the procedure

    c. reassure the client that the procedure is relatively painless and risk free

    d. inform the client that the physician will take multiple samples for comparison

CRITICAL THINKING EXERCISES

Case Study: Hematology Assessment

L. K. is a 45-year-old woman who is married to a career military officer. Her father was a miner, leading an itinerant life as he worked in uranium mines. L. K. grew up in a western state and remembers playing with other children on slag heaps from the mines. She recalls being ill often as a child and attributes this to being chronically undernourished. The family was often cold during the winter months when there was no money to buy warm clothing or fuel for heat.

Over the past 6 months, L. K. has had episodes of epistaxis and prolonged bleeding after having her teeth cleaned by the dental hygienist. She has also noticed that she seems to bruise easily. There are multiple ecchymotic areas on her legs and arms. L. K. reported to the military hospital for a checkup and was referred to a regional civilian hospital for further evaluation. During the admission history, L. K. tells the nurse that she tires easily and often has little energy. Her husband and children are worried about her.

Address the following questions:

1. What additional data should the nurse elicit from L. K. at this time?

2. Based on the above data, formulate relevant nursing diagnoses for L. K.

As part of the diagnostic workup, L. K. is scheduled to have blood work drawn for CBC with differential, platelets, electrolytes, bleeding time, PT, PTT, iron, TIBC, total proteins, and albumin.

3. What is the purpose of these laboratory studies?

4. L. K. is scheduled to have a bone scan. Prepare a teaching/learning plan for her.

Th results of the laboratory tests and bone scan indicate that L. K. has depressed bone marrow function. The hematologist discusses plans to perform a bone marrow aspiration with her.

5. What is the purpose of this procedure?

6. Develop a teaching/learning plan for the bone marrow aspiration procedure.

7. Just before the hematologist is expected to arrive to perform the aspiration, L. K. asks the nurse if she is going to die. She says she is scared and begins to cry. How should the nurse respond?

CHAPTER 39

Interventions for Clients with Hematologic Problems

LEARNING OBJECTIVES

At the end of this chapter, the student will be able to

▪ Describe the pathophysiology, etiology, incidence, and prevention of red blood cell disorders

▪ Discuss collaborative management of the client with red blood cell disorders

▪ Discuss polycythemia vera

▪ Describe the pathophysiology, etiology, and incidence of leukemia

▪ Discuss collaborative management of the client with leukemia

▪ Discuss the malignant lymphomas Hodgkin's disease and non-Hodgkin's disease

▪ Discuss autoimmune thrombocytopenic purpura

▪ Discuss hemophilia

▪ Discuss transfusion therapy

PREREQUISITE KNOWLEDGE

Prior to beginning this chapter, the student should review

▪ The anatomy and physiology of the hematologic system

▪ The anatomy and physiology of the body systems, e.g., integumentary, respiratory, musculoskeletal, gastrointestinal, central nervous, and cardiovascular, including the lymphatics, renal, and immunological functions

▪ Normal laboratory values for serum values, e.g., red blood cells (RBCs), white blood cells (WBCs), and platelets

▪ The principles of acid–base balance

▪ The principles of intravenous therapy

▪ The principles of normal nutrition

▪ The principles of infection and the inflammatory response

▪ The concepts of loss, grief, death, and dying

▪ The concepts of body image and self-esteem

STUDY QUESTIONS

Red Blood Cell Disorders

1. Which of the following statement is correct about sickle cell anemia?

   a. Sickle cell anemia is a sex-linked, recessive hereditary disorder.

   b. The inheritance of one abnormal gene results in the sickle cell trait.

   c. Offspring have a one-in-four chance of being affected if one parent has the disorder.

   d. The disorder is treatable by genetic engineering to replace the defective gene.

2. The average life span of a sickled cell compared with that of a normal RBC is

   a. one-sixth

   b. one-fourth

   c. one-third

   d. one-half

3. Events that may precipitate a sickle cell crisis include

   a. warm weather

   b. overhydration

   c. infection

   d. gentle exercise

4. The organ affected most often by the clumping of sickled cells is the

   a. liver

   b. stomach

   c. lungs

   d. spleen

5. The most common clinical finding in clients who are in sickle cell crisis is

   a. jaundice

   b. diarrhea

   c. pain

   d. bradycardia

6. Management of sickle cell crisis includes

   a. restricting fluids to decrease sickling

   b. administering oxygen to reverse hypoxia

   c. counseling to discourage childbearing

   d. transfusing packed cells to replace defective cells

7. A deficiency in glucose 6-phosphate dehydrogenase (G6PD) results in

   a. an inability of the RBCs to produce their own glucose for energy metabolism

   b. an inability of the RBCs to carry the usual amount of oxygen to the tissues

   c. the RBCs being more susceptible to damage and early hemolysis

   d. the RBCs being deficient in an enzyme that stabilizes their cell walls

8. Assessment findings for the client with G6PD deficiency include

   a. clubbing

   b. oliguria

   c. bradypnea

   d. hypertension

9. List the interventions used in the management of G6PD deficiency.

   a. _____

   _____

   _____

   b. _____

   _____

   _____

   c. _____

   _____

   _____

10. Which of the following interventions is preventive for the client with cold antibody-type autoimmune hemolytic anemia?

    a. keeping the client well hydrated

    b. administering oxygen via mask

    c. encouraging iron-rich foods in the diet

    d. warming the car before driving in winter

11. Initial treatment for the client with autoimmune hemolytic anemia includes

    a. intensive immunosuppressive therapy

    b. high-dose corticosteroid therapy

    c. transfusion with cryoprecipitate

    d. radiation and chemotherapy

Match the following descriptions (12–19) with their associated types of anemias (a–d). Answers may be used more than once.

_____ 12. bone marrow transplantation

_____ 13. causes include increased metabolic demands

_____ 14. inhibits folate transportation

_____ 15. intrinsic factor deficiency

_____ 16. most common type of anemia

_____ 17. often seen in clients with cirrhosis

_____ 18. oral contraceptives are a contributing cause

_____ 19. pancytopenia

a. iron deficiency

b. vitamin B_{12} deficiency

c. folic acid deficiency

d. aplastic

20. List the subjective client data relevant to the client with anemia. Use a separate sheet.

21. List the objective client data relevant to the client with anemia. Use a separate sheet.

22. Typical physical assessment data for the client with sickle cell anemia includes

    a. hepatosplenomegaly

    b. acromegaly

    c. acrocyanosis

    d. phimosis

23. Which of the following clients is most at risk for developing anemia?

    a. a 26-year-old man who is a strict vegetarian

    b. a 47-year-old woman with dysfunctional uterine bleeding

    c. a 53-year-old man with chronic back pain

    d. an 80-year-old woman who has a fractured wrist

24. Interventions for the client with anemia include

    a. moderate exercise to increase aerobic capacity

    b. frequent periods for socialization during the work day

    c. short work sessions with rest periods interspersed

    d. transfusion with WBCs and platelets

25. Drug therapy for anemia includes

    a. oral vitamin supplements

    b. vitamin K injections

    c. parenteral hyperalimentation

    d. intravenous iron dextran

26. Which of the following foods provides the vitamins and iron that are lacking in the deficiency anemias?

    a. white bread

    b. egg substitutes

    c. liver

    d. green vegetables

27. A major laboratory finding in polycythemia vera is

    a. thrombocytopenia

    b. leukopenia

    c. anemia

    d. erythrocytosis

28. Clinical findings in polycythemia vera include

    a. pallor

    b. dyspnea

    c. fatigue

    d. giddiness

29. Routine management of polycythemia vera includes

    a. chordotomy

    b. lobectomy

    c. myotomy

    d. phlebotomy

White Blood Cell Disorders

30. The most common type of leukemia in adults is

    a. acute lymphocytic leukemia (ALL)

    b. acute myelogenous leukemia (AML)

    c. chronic lymphocytic leukemia (CLL)

    d. chronic myelogenous leukemia (CML)

31. List the three classic laboratory findings in WBC disorders.

    a. _____

    b. _____

    c. _____

32. Briefly discuss why leukemia leads to a deficiency in other blood components and what the consequences of these deficiencies are. Use a separate sheet.

33. A chemical that is commonly found in industrialized societies that is linked to leukemia is

    a. ammonia

    b. benzene

    c. alcohol

    d. carbon

34. List the subjective client data relevant to leukemia. Use a separate sheet.

35. The age group most susceptible to developing leukemia is

    a. children

    b. adolescents

    c. young adults

    d. elderly people

36. Which of the following hobbies is most likely to increase a person's risk for developing leukemia?

    a. model airplane building

    b. stamp collecting

    c. butterfly collecting

    d. model railroading

37. List the objective client data relevant to leukemia. Use a separate sheet.

38. Anemia associated with leukemia produces clinical findings such as

    a. rectal bleeding

    b. somnolence

    c. fever

    d. seizures

39. Thrombocytopenia associated with leukemia produces clinical findings such as

    a. oral lesions

    b. lymphadenopathy

    c. carotid bruit

    d. melena

40. Leukopenia associated with leukemia produces clinical findings such as

    a. petechiae

    b. lethargy

    c. splenomegaly

    d. tachycardia

41. List the phases of drug therapy used for AML and briefly describe them. Use a separate sheet.

42. An antifungal agent often give to leukemic clients is

    a. amikacin sulfate (Amikin)

    b. amphotericin B (Fungizone)

    c. acyclovir sodium (Zovirax)

    d. tobramycin sulfate (Nebcin)

43. The most important intervention for infection control for the leukemic client is

    a. wearing a mask

    b. aseptic technique

    c. frequent hand washing

    d. reverse isolation

44. Which of the following is contraindicated in the room of a leukemic client?

    a. framed pictures

    b. greeting cards

    c. flower bouquets

    d. stuffed animals

45. Which of the following condiments is contraindicated on the food tray of the leukemic client?

    a. refined sugar

    b. salt substitute

    c. brown sugar

    d. ground pepper

46. Which of the following assessments should the nurse perform to monitor for infection in the leukemic client?

    a. auscultate lung sounds every 4 hours

    b. insect the oral mucosa once daily

    c. percuss for costovertebral tenderness daily

    d. palpate for precordial thrills every shift

47. Interventions for the leukemic client include

    a. using a disposable razor to prepare the skin for a bone marrow aspiration

    b. taking blood pressure every 4 hours to monitor for signs of bleeding

    c. administering glycerine suppositories for management of constipation

    d. transfusing platelets rapidly through a special filter to prevent bleeding

48. The most successful bone marrow grafts are

    a. autologous

    b. bovine

    c. porcine

    d. allogenic

49. The host tissue most commonly affected in graft versus host disease (GVHD) is the

    a. kidney

    b. liver

    c. pancreas

    d. heart

50. Which of the following statements is correct about GVHD?

    a. This immune phenomenon often occurs following autologous bone marrow transplantation.

    b. The transplanted tissue contains mature T-cells, which then begin to reject the recipient's body.

    c. Symptoms of GVHD usually occur in the kidneys, lungs, and bone marrow tissues.

    d. The major cause of death in clients with GVHD is fluid and electrolyte imbalances.

51. Interventions for the leukemic client with extreme fatigue include

    a. encouraging brief sessions out of bed and sitting in a chair

    b. ordering meal trays three times a day with no snacks

    c. administering blood products as ordered by the physician

    d. scheduling physical therapy sessions prior to mealtimes

52. Following dismissal, the client with leukemia should be advised to

    a. resume a normal work schedule

    b. be vaccinated yearly with the flu vaccine

    c. relax and recuperate by taking a vacation

    d. begin a hobby such as swimming at a local spa

53. Which of the following statements is correct about malignant lymphoma?

    a. These malignancies arise from stem cell precursors.

    b. Abnormal cell proliferation occurs in the bone marrow.

    c. Lymphoid tissue proliferates in the thymus and liver.

    d. Lymphomas are solid tissue masses scattered in the body.

54. The earliest clinical manifestation of Hodgkin's disease is

    a. intermittent fever

    b. night sweats

    c. painless enlarged node

    d. general malaise

55. An irreversible effect of treatment for extensive Hodgkin's disease is

    a. alopecia

    b. diarrhea

    c. dysphagia

    d. sterility

56. Which of the following statements is correct about non-Hodgkin's lymphoma?

    a. The highest incidence is in the middle-aged population.

    b. This type of lymphoma can arise in any tissue or organ.

    c. These lymphomas have a better prognosis than Hodgkin's.

    d. Most types of this lymphoma do not require treatment.

Coagulation Disorders

57. Which of the following statements are correct about autoimmune thrombocytopenic purpura?

    a. The total number of circulating platelets is diminished.

    b. Platelet production in the bone marrow is depressed.

    c. Clients make an antibody toward their own platelets.

    d. Platelets are destroyed primarily while circulating in the blood stream.

    e. This disorder is more prevalent in clients with a preexisting autoimmune condition.

    f. This disorder has a higher occurrence rate in women between the ages of 20 and 40.

    g. Anemia may be a coexisting problem.

58. Identify the common nursing diagnosis for the client with autoimmune thrombocytopenic purpura:

    _____

59. Interventions for the client with autoimmune thrombocytopenic purpura include

    a. routine platelet transfusions

    b. girth measurement daily

    c. rectal temperature measurement

    d. gentle skin care

60. Dismissal instructions for the client with autoimmune thrombocytopenic purpura include

    a. reassuring the client that it is all right to resume use of a safety razor for shaving

    b. teaching the client to take an oral temperature daily to monitor for infection

    c. warning the client to remain on strict bed rest at home to decrease chances of injury

    d. suggesting that the client seek a diversionary hobby such as wood carving

61. Which of the following statements is correct about the incidence of hemophilia?

    a. The majority of people with hemophilia have a deficiency of factor IX.

    b. Hemophilia is a Y-linked dominant trait and predominantly a disease affecting women.

    c. The daughters of male hemophiliacs are obligatory carriers of the hemophilic trait.

    d. All sons of male hemophiliacs have the gene for hemophilia and have the disorder.

62. Laboratory test results for a true hemophiliac client include

    a. normal activated partial thromboplastin time

    b. prolonged bleeding time

    c. normal prothrombin time

    d. increased RBCs

63. List the complications that may occur with repeated transfusions for hemophilia.

a. _____

_____

b. _____

_____

c. _____

_____

64. Identify measures used to ensure that the correct blood component is delivered to the client. Use a separate sheet.

65. A needle or intravenous catheter used for a transfusion should be

a. 25 gauge

b. 22 gauge

c. 20 gauge

d. 18 gauge

66. Infusions for blood transfusions should be started with solutions of

a. dextrose in water

b. lactated Ringer's

c. dextrose in saline

d. normal saline

67. Which of the following blood products is *not* administered through a standard filter?

a. whole blood

b. packed cells

c. platelets

d. washed RBCs

68. If a severe reaction occurs from a blood transfusion, it usually happens

a. during the infusion of the first 50 mL

b. after the entire unit is infused

c. about half way through the infusion

d. during transfusion of the second unit of blood

69. Which of the following transfusions will result in a hemolytic transfusion reaction? Administering

a. Rh-negative blood to a client with Rh-negative blood

b. type B blood to a client with type AB blood

c. type AB blood to a client with type O blood

d. type O blood to a client with type A blood

70. List the types of transfusion reactions that can occur.

a. _____

b. _____

c. _____

d. _____

71. DIC, a complication of transfusion therapy, is most commonly seen in which type of transfusion reaction?

a. hemolytic

b. allergic (anaphylactic)

c. febrile

d. bacterial (septicemia)

CRITICAL THINKING EXERCISES

Case Study: Sickle Cell Anemia

D. S. is a 26-year-old African-American male admitted to the hospital with right-sided flank pain radiating to the groin. He also has sickle cell anemia, but has been asymptomatic for the past 9 years. He is married but has no children. Renal calculi are found in the right renal pelvis, and he is scheduled for immediate lithotripsy.

Address the following questions:

1. From the above data, determine if D. S. is at increased risk of sickle cell crisis. Explain your answer.

Following the lithotripsy, D. S's urine is strained and small particles of stones are found. He continues to complain of severe flank pain and receives meperidine hydrochloride (Demerol) 100 mg and hydroxyzine (Vistaril) 50 mg I.M. every 3 hours for the pain. Two days following the procedure, the flank pain continues. The physician orders an abdominal x-ray to reassess for the presence of calculi; none are found.

2. What could be contributing to D. S.'s pain?

3. The physician suspects that D. S. is in sickle cell crisis. What laboratory tests are likely to be ordered and why?

D. S. reports pain in the entire abdomen, knees, hips, and wrists. He has shaking chills, and when his temperature is taken, it is 102.2°F. His white blood cell count is 15,600/mm^3. Based on these data, sickle cell crisis is confirmed.

4. Discuss the rational for the following orders for D. S.:

   • oxygen at 4 L/minute by nasal prongs

   • bed rest

   • warm moist packs to the joints prn pain

   • increase IV rate to 125 mL/hour

   • ceftazidime (Fortaz) 1 g IV q 6 hours

   • acetaminophen (Tylenol) gr x for temp over 101°F

5. From the above data, identify three priority nursing diagnoses.

Two days later as D. S. is recovering from the crisis, he comments to his nurse that his father and an older brother have sickle cell disease. "The last two days have started me thinking about whether my wife and I should continue to try to have kids. What are the chances of my kids getting sickle cell disease? I sure wouldn't want any kid of mine to have this curse."

6. What information should the nurse consider while formulating a reply?

7. What other health care team members should be consulted to assist D. S. and his wife with this decision?

Case Study: Leukemia

K. A. is an 18-year-old woman admitted to the oncology nursing unit with acute myelogenous leukemia (AML). The following admission data are recorded in the chart: Has had difficulty completing first year of college due to recurrent upper respiratory infections, fatigue, and heavy menstrual flow (18 pads in 2 days). Pallor evident with ecchymotic areas on shins and lower arms. Unable to sit in bedside chair for 30 minutes during interview due to fatigue. Height is 5 feet, 3 inches, weight is 92 pounds. Denies bone pain. Laboratory results reveal the following: Hgb, 7.4 g/dL normochromic cells; platelets, 114,000/mm^3; white blood cells, 18.7/mm^3.

Address the following questions:

1. Compare K. A.'s signs and symptoms to those presented in the textbook in the discussion of leukemia. Discuss similarities and differences.

2. K. A.'s physician documents that she is pancytopenic. Discuss this term and its significance in leukemia.

3. A bone marrow biopsy is scheduled. Develop a teaching/learning plan for this procedure.

4. Who should sign the permit for this procedure? Discuss your answer.

The bone marrow biopsy reveals blastic WBCs, and the diagnosis of AML is confirmed. The physician plans to begin with the first phase of chemotherapy.

5. Discuss the three phases of chemotherapy and the treatment goals in each stage.

6. Does K. A. need to be on neutropenic precautions? Explain your answer.

7. K. A. has a triple-lumen subclavian catheter inserted. Discuss the nursing interventions for her with regard to this catheter. Consider the frequency of dressing changes, the need for aseptic technique, and the advantages and disadvantages of a central line for chemotherapy.

Following confirmation of the location of the catheter, chemotherapeutic agents are ordered for K. A. Her physician has ordered cytosine arabinoside (Cytarabine) and daunorubicin hydrochloride (Cerubidine).

8. What specific precautions by the nurse are required for the administration of these agents?

9. What side effects of the agents should also be monitored for?

One morning following her bath, K. A. is brushing her hair and cries out, "What's happening to my hair? It's all coming out!" The nurse notices that there are large fist-size clumps of hair in K. A.'s hairbrush and bed.

10. How should the nurse respond to K. A.?

11. What interventions could the nurse implement to assist K. A. in coping with the alopecia?

12. K. A. has several laboratory tests to be drawn. Describe the procedure for withdrawing blood from a triple-lumen line.

13. Four days after chemotherapy begins, K. A.'s hemoglobin is 7.0 g/dL, her WBC count is 1200/mm^3, and her platelets are 90,000/mm^3. Identify three priority nursing diagnoses for K. A.

14. K. A. has a slow but complete remission. Eighteen months later she is scheduled for an autologous bone marrow transplant. Develop a teaching/learning plan for her about this procedure. Include the techniques used to harvest the marrow; the typical hospital course, possible complications (e.g., graft versus host disease), and long-term management.

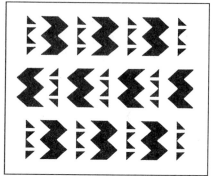

C H A P T E R 4 0

Assessment of the Nervous System

LEARNING OBJECTIVES

At the end of this chapter, the student will be able to

- Describe the anatomy and physiology of the neuron and the glial cell
- Discuss the structure and function of the peripheral nervous system (PNS)
- Discuss the structure and function of the autonomic nervous system (ANS)
- Discuss the structure and function of the central nervous system (CNS)
- Describe the neurological changes associated with aging
- Obtain a neurological history from a client
- Identify the assessment of mental status
- Describe the assessment of cranial nerves
- Discuss the assessment of sensory function
- Describe the assessment of motor function
- Identify aspects of cerebellar function
- Describe the assessment of reflex activity
- Describe the steps of a rapid neurological assessment
- Discuss various neurological diagnostic studies and client preparation

PREREQUISITE KNOWLEDGE

Prior to beginning this chapter, the student should review

- The anatomy and physiology of the neurological system (central and peripheral)
- The process of nerve conduction
- The principles of acid–base balance
- The principles of fluid and electrolytes

STUDY QUESTIONS

Anatomy and Physiology Review

Match the following terms related to the neuron (1–10) with their definitions (a–j).

_____ 1. afferent pathway

_____ 2. axon

_____ 3. dendrite

_____ 4. efferent pathway

_____ 5. gray matter

_____ 6. myelination

_____ 7. node of Ranvier

_____ 8. soma

_____ 9. synaptic knob

_____ 10. white matter

a. cell body

b. brings information to cell body

c. distal end of an axon

d. coat of lipid cells

e. axonal process

f. dendritic process

g. axons that have myelin

h. nonmyelinated axons

i. transmits impulses from cell body to other neurons

j. gap in myelin sheath

11. Which of the following statements is correct about interneurons?

    a. They are the largest neurons in the nervous system.

    b. They are located in the peripheral nervous system.

    c. They form complex circuits with other neurons.

    d. They provide support for the principal neurons.

12. Briefly discuss the all-or-nothing principle in relation to nerve conduction. Use a separate sheet.

13. The rate of speed with which a nerve impulse is conducted depends on

    a. whether the nerve dendrite is myelinated

    b. the relative diameter of the nerve fiber

    c. the type of stimulus to be transmitted

    d. the width of the synaptic cleft

Match the following factors that affect neuron transmission (14–23) with their effects (a or b). Answers may be used more than once.

_____ 14. hypoxia

_____ 15. low extracellular fluid (ECF) calcium

_____ 16. cocoa

_____ 17. high serum pH

_____ 18. high ECF magnesium

_____ 19. theophylline

_____ 20. anesthesia

_____ 21. low serum pH

_____ 22. caffeine

_____ 23. low ECF sodium

a. inhibit

b. excite

24. The function of a neuromodulator is to

    a. influence a neuron's sensitivity to a neurotransmitter

    b. act directly on the postsynaptic membrane

    c. use an enzyme process to create a membrane potential

    d. alter the speed of impulse transmission along a fiber

25. Which of the following statements is correct about glial cells?

    a. astroglia help regulate cerebrospinal fluid (CSF) composition

    b. oligodendrocytes form the myelin sheath in the cerebrum

    c. microglia provide physical support for the neurons

    d. ependymal cells have a phagocytic function in infection

26. List the components of the peripheral nervous system (PNS).

    a. _____

    _____

    b. _____

    _____

    c. _____

    _____

27. Which of the following statements is correct about spinal nerves?

    a. The posterior branches transmit motor impulses to the muscles of the body.

    b. The anterior branches carry sensory information to the spinal cord.

    c. There are specific sensory receptors throughout the body, except for pressure.

    d. Spinal nerves form plexuses that eventually branch into individual peripheral nerves.

28. Which of the following statements is correct about reflexes?

    a. They are consciously controlled body functions.

    b. They consist of multibranching circuits called *arcs.*

    c. They control input to the central nervous system (CNS).

    d. They are responsible for maintaining muscle tone.

29. List the components of the CNS.

    a. _____

    b. _____

30. Which of the following statements is correct about the cranial nerves?

    a. Eye muscle movement is controlled by cranial nerves II, III, IV, and VI.

    b. Cranial nerves with mixed sensory and motor functions include V, VII, IX, and X.

    c. Cranial nerves that stimulate parasympathetic glandular functions are III, VII, IX, and X.

    d. Tongue muscle movement is controlled by cranial nerves V, VII, IX, and XII.

31. Which of the following statements is correct about the autonomic nervous system?

    a. The sympathetic system is craniosacral.

    b. Norepinephrine is the primary transmitter of the parasympathetic system.

    c. The parasympathetic system is thoracolumbar.

    d. Cholinergic fibers secrete acetylcholine as their primary transmitter.

32. Which of the following statements is correct about the sympathetic nervous system?

    a. The sympathetic nervous system is responsible for the "feed-breed" functions of the body.

    b. Injury to the upper spinal cord results in impaired function of the sympathetic nervous system.

    c. Receptor cells at the termination of nerve endings determine the effect of transmitter substances.

    d. The adrenal medulla is an adrenergic receptor organ and is stimulated by norepinephrine.

33. Which of the following statements is correct about the parasympathetic nervous system?

    a. The parasympathetic nervous system is responsible for the fight-or-flight functions of the body.

    b. Parasympathetic inhibition of the sympathetic nervous system results in vasoconstriction.

    c. Bladder and bowel emptying are controlled by the sacral parasympathetic system.

    d. Injury to the spinal cord above the sacral level results in erectile dysfunction.

Match the following functions (34–37) with their associated spinal cord tracts (a–d).

____ 34. transmits impulses for voluntary muscle movement

____ 35. transmits pain, temperature, light touch, and pressure sensations

____ 36. transmits sensations of vibration, discrete localization, and two-point discrimination

____ 37. transmits impulses of proprioception from lower extremities

a. spinothalamic

b. spinocerebellar

c. fasciculi gracilis and cuneatus

d. corticospinal

Match the following structures of the brain stem and diencephalon (38–45) with their functions (a–h).

____ 38. epithalamus

____ 39. hypothalamus

____ 40. medulla

____ 41. mesencephalon

____ 42. pons

____ 43. reticular formation tissue

____ 44. subthalamus

____ 45. thalamus

a. responsible for arousal and other functions

b. initiates physiological changes to maintain homeostasis

c. contains the pneumotaxic center

d. contains auditory and visual reflex centers

e. serves as the major relay point for the CNS

f. regulates internal environment

g. connects to basal ganglia reciprocally

h. contains neurons responsible for sense of smell

46. List the two primary functions of the cerebellum.

    a. _____

    _____

    b. _____

    _____

Match the following structures of the cerebrum (47–57) with their functions (a–k).

____ 47. Broca's area

____ 48. eyefield

____ 49. general interpretative area

____ 50. limbic lobe

____ 51. occipital lobe

____ 52. parietal lobe

____ 53. prefrontal cortex

____ 54. premotor area

____ 55. primary motor area

____ 56. temporal lobe

____ 57. Wernicke's area

a. survival functions

b. control of muscle groups

c. voluntary eye movement

d. word formation

e. skilled muscle movement

f. sensory interpretation

g. sound interpretation

h. judgment, foresight

i. complex sound interpretation

j. sight interpretation

k. complex thought

58. If a client had an infarction of the posterior cerebral artery, he or she would exhibit the inability to
    a. perform skilled motor acts
    b. regulate body temperature
    c. perform simple calculations
    d. distinguish odors

59. The blood–brain barrier is normally impervious to
    a. alcohol
    b. bacteria
    c. oxygen
    d. water

60. Which of the following statements is correct about the cerebral spinal fluid (CSF)?
    a. It is similar in composition to plasma.
    b. It is secreted by the arachnoid villi.
    c. It circulates through the subarachnoid space.
    d. It collects in the cavernous sinus.

61. Moving outward from brain tissue itself, list the structures that protect the CNS.

    a. _____

    b. _____

    c. _____

    d. _____

    e. _____

62. Which of the following findings is abnormal in an otherwise healthy elderly client?
    a. decreased intellectual level
    b. hypoactive deep tendon reflexes
    c. decreased sense of smell
    d. wakefulness and insomnia at night

Subjective Assessment

63. List the subjective client data relevant to the nervous system. Use a separate sheet.

64. Which of the following health problems is significant in the history of the client with a neurological deficit?
    a. peptic ulcer
    b. bladder infection
    c. cholecystitis
    d. diabetes mellitus

65. Which of the following occupations increases a client's risk for developing a neurological deficit?
    a. machinist
    b. farmer
    c. courtesy clerk
    d. travel agent

66. The following is a partial client history. Discuss **CT** the significance these data have for an assessment of the neurological system. Submit the completed exercise to the clinical instructor on a separate sheet.

    Female client, 74 years old, admitted for diagnostic workup of headaches. Describes pain as "achy" and located over left temporal area; present for 4 days. Denies nausea and vomiting. Aspirin does not relieve headache. "I was walking my dog last week in the park when he began to chase a cat. The leash got tangled around my ankles and I tripped and fell on the sidewalk." Denies hitting head or any loss of consciousness. "I am having trouble concentrating and staying awake. My right hand is clumsy and sometimes I find myself unable to lift things. My right foot also gets caught on things in the way." No visual changes.

Objective Assessment

67. List the objective client data relevant to the neurological system. Use a separate sheet.

68. Using the data in question 66, construct a physical assessment recording for the neurological **CT** system. Submit the completed exercise to the clinical instructor using a separate sheet.

69. Which of the following factors may bias the nurse's assessment of a client's mental status?
    a. being elderly
    b. gross obesity
    c. foul breath odor
    d. soiled clothing
    e. all of the above

Match the following questions (70–74) with their associated parts of the mental status assessment (a–e).

_____ 70. "What is your name?"   a. attention span

_____ 71. "What brings you to the hospital?"   b. cognition

_____ 72. "How much is 5 plus 8?"   c. language skills

_____ 73. "What is the definition of the word *library*?"   d. level of consciousness

_____ 74. "What would you do if your shoe were untied?"   e. memory

Match the following eye functions (75–80) with the descriptions of how to test for them (a–f).

_____ 75. accommodation

_____ 76. central vision

_____ 77. consensual pupil reaction

_____ 78. corneal reflex

_____ 79. eye movements

_____ 80. peripheral vision

a. client reads out loud from printed material

b. client is asked when he or she sees a wiggling object at the boundary of the visual fields

c. client's eyes follow an object through the six cardinal positions of gaze

d. shine light into one eye and observe for constriction of pupil in the opposite eye

e. observe for pupil constriction and eye convergence as an object is moved toward the nose

f. move an object quickly toward the client's eye, approaching from behind and to one side

81. Which of the following tests for cranial nerve function is performed with the client's eyes closed?

a. Weber's test

b. Rinne's test

c. gag reflex

d. whisper test

Match the following sensory functions (82–87) with the equipment used to test for them (a–f).

_____ 82. light touch

_____ 83. pain

_____ 84. pressure

_____ 85. stereognosis

_____ 86. touch discrimination

_____ 87. vibration

a. small object

b. tuning fork

c. fingertip

d. sharp end of pin

e. cotton wisp

f. dull end of pin

88. Which of the following sensory function tests may be omitted if pain perception is intact?

a. light touch

b. pressure

c. temperature

d. vibration

89. The test that assesses cerebral and brain stem integrity is

a. grip strength

b. arm drift

c. muscle strength

d. equilibrium

90. All of the following are deep tendon reflexes *except*

a. Achilles' reflex

b. biceps reflex

c. patellar reflex

d. plantar reflex

91. The Glasgow Coma Scale establishes baseline data for

a. the level of consciousness

b. response to painful stimuli

c. language comprehension and speech

d. eye opening and motor and verbal response

Match the following radiographic examinations used to assess the nervous system (92–95) with their descriptions (a–d).

_____ 92. cerebral angiography

_____ 93. computed tomography

_____ 94. flat plate

_____ 95. myelography

a. visualization of the skull and spine

b. visualization of carotid, vertebral, and cerebral circulation

c. visualization of the spinal cord and lower brain stem

d. visualization of the brain or spinal cord on many planes

96. Contrast medium is always used in the following radiographic examinations of the nervous system *except*

a. cerebral angiography

b. computed tomography

c. digital subtraction method

d. myelography

97. Follow-up care of the client who has had cerebral angiography includes

a. changing the puncture site dressing every 3–4 hours

b. placing the client in a modified Fowler's position

c. monitoring pulse and blood pressure every 4 hours

d. checking the circulation of the affected extremity

98. Which of the following instructions should the nurse give to the client who is having a lumbar puncture?

    a. "Slide over to the side of the bed so your buttocks are right on the edge."

    b. "Now that the needle is in the right place, you can slowly straighten your legs."

    c. "Hold your breath and bear down like you're having a bowel movement once the needle is in."

    d. "You will be able to get up and go to the bathroom as soon as the test is over."

99. Which of the following findings from a cerebral spinal fluid specimen is abnormal?

    a. pressure = 14 mmHg

    b. color = straw

    c. protein = 45 mg/100 mL

    d. glucose = 35 mg/100 mL

100. Which of the following beverages may the client have prior to scheduled electroencephalography?

    a. coffee

    b. herbal tea

    c. cola drink

    d. hot cocoa

101. Diagnostic neurological tests that require special handling of the client's urine following the procedure include

    a. positron emission tomography

    b. magnetic resonance imaging

    c. radionuclide brain scan

    d. none of the above

CRITICAL THINKING EXERCISES

Case Study: Neurological Assessment

F. N. is a 48-year-old male client, married and the father of three children. He works as a draftsman, designing decorative iron products and other metals. He is scheduled for a neurological diagnostic workup. Over the past month, F. N. has noticed that he has had difficulty drawing figures accurately. At times, he has been unable to hold a pencil with sufficient strength to mark the drawing paper. He denies visual changes; however, at times he has difficulty walking without tripping. A lumbar puncture is scheduled following x-rays of the skull and spine.

Address the following questions:

1. What additional data should the nurse collect initially?

2. Describe the preparation of F. N. for the x-ray studies.

3. Develop a teaching/learning plan for F. N. about the lumbar puncture.

4. The hospital requires that a consent form be signed by F. N. prior to the lumbar puncture. What is the purpose of this document?

5. F. N. asks about complications from the procedure. He asks, "Will the test may my symptoms worse? I don't need anymore problems right now." What should the nurse reply?

6. The lumbar puncture is performed and five tubes of cerebrospinal fluid (CSF) are collected. The CSF pressure is 165 mmH$_2$O). What is the significance of this finding?

The physician orders that the specimens be analyzed for cells, protein, and glucose. The laboratory results are color = straw; cells = 7 lymphocytes/mm^3; RBCs = absent; protein = 60 mg/100 mL; glucose = 68 mg/100 mL.

7. Which of the laboratory findings are normal? Which are abnormal?

Following the lumbar puncture, F. N. is to be kept on bedrest for 24 hours with the head of the bed flat. A regular diet may be resumed and fluids encouraged.

8. What is the purpose of these post-procedure interventions?

9. What assessments should the nurse make following the procedure?

10. F. N. calls the nurse and says that he has a throbbing headache. What should the nurse do? What is the most likely explanation for his headache? What interventions are indicated to help make F. N. more comfortable?

CHAPTER 41

Interventions for Clients with Problems of the Central Nervous System: The Brain

LEARNING OBJECTIVES

At the end of this chapter, the student will be able to

- Describe the pathophysiology, etiology, and incidence of migraine headache
- Describe management of the client with migraine headache
- Discuss cluster headaches
- Discuss collaborative management of epilepsy
- Discuss collaborative management of central nervous system infections
- Describe the pathophysiology, etiology, and incidence of Parkinson's disease
- Discuss collaborative management of the client with Parkinson's disease
- Discuss the pathophysiology, etiology, and incidence of Alzheimer's disease
- Describe collaborative management of the client with Alzheimer's disease
- Discuss Huntington's chorea

PREREQUISITE KNOWLEDGE

Prior to beginning this chapter, the student should review

- The anatomy and physiology of the central nervous system
- The process of nerve conduction
- The principles of acid-base balance
- The principles of fluid and electrolytes
- The normal function of the musculoskeletal system, including joint range of motion (ROM)
- The process of rehabilitation and related interventions
- The concepts of body image and self-esteem
- The concept of sexuality
- The concepts of loss, death, and grieving
- The principles of perioperative nursing management
- Pain and pain management
- Coping and stress management techniques
- Isolation techniques

STUDY QUESTIONS

Headaches

1. Which of the following statements is correct about migraine headaches?

   a. Headaches occur when pain-sensitive areas of the brain parenchyma have been stimulated.

   b. Migraine headaches tend to involve the same symptoms each time in the susceptible individual.

   c. The causes and mechanisms of migraine headaches are well understood, permitting effective treatment.

   d. Migraine headaches tend to occur more frequently as an individual ages.

2. Which of the following statements is correct about the pathophysiology and etiology of migraine headaches?

   a. During the prodromal phase, a rise in the plasma serotonin level causes arterial vasodilation.

   b. Following vasodilation, cerebral vasoconstriction and spasm occur, causing the headache.

   c. The onset of migraine headaches in the premenstrual period is related to the estrogen level.

   d. Migraine headaches are precipitated by neuroses, certain personality characteristics, and too much sleep.

3. List the subjective client data relevant to the client with migraine headaches. Use a separate sheet.

4. List the objective client data relevant to the client with migraine headaches. Use a separate sheet.

5. The drug that is administered at the client's first awareness of a migraine headache attack is

   a. ergotamine tartrate (Ergomar)

   b. propranolol hydrochloride (Inderal)

   c. metoclopramide (Reglan)

   d. imipramine hydrochloride (Tofranil)

6. List the preventive measures for migraine headaches.

   a. _____

   _____

   b. _____

   _____

   c. _____

   _____

   _____

   d. _____

   _____

   _____

7. Which of the following statements indicates that a client understands how to manage migraine headache attacks?

   a. "I have started to play tennis again and will be working out every day to perfect my backhand."

   b. "I am going to have heavy shades installed in the bedroom to block out more of the light."

   c. "My job involves a lot of business entertainment. I'll switch to wine coolers instead of mixed drinks."

   d. "I've tried other birth control methods, but the pill is the one that works the best for me."

8. Which of the following statements is correct about cluster headaches?

   a. These headaches occur erratically and unpredictably.

   b. After onset, cluster headaches persist for several hours.

   c. Incidence is highest in Caucasian women, 45 to 63 years of age.

   d. Onset occurs with relaxation, napping, or rapid eye movement sleep.

9. Which of the following assessment findings would the nurse expect to find in the client experiencing a cluster headache?

   a. nausea and vomiting

   b. tachycardia

   c. restlessness and fidgeting

   d. hyperventilation

10. Which of the following instructions should the nurse give to the client with cluster headaches for whom ergotamine tartrate (Gynergen) is prescribed?

    a. Take the medicine every 4 hours around the clock.

    b. Make sure to take the pills with plenty of water.

    c. Lie down in a dark room after taking the medicine.

    d. You will feel warm and flushed after taking the medicine.

11. Preventive measures for cluster headaches include
    a. taking frequent, short rest periods such as napping
    b. avoiding food such as cheese, red meat, and mushrooms
    c. wearing sunglasses and avoiding glare from bright light
    d. engaging in regular physical activity such as running

Epilepsy

12. Which of the following statements is correct about seizure activity?
    a. The mechanisms responsible for the development of seizures are well understood.
    b. Triggering mechanisms cause sudden abnormal bursts of electrical brain activity.
    c. Seizure activity follows the all-or-none principle and the entire brain responds to a trigger.
    d. Seizures are an inherited disorder and linked to findings of below normal intelligence.

13. Which of the following symptoms would a client with a partial seizure disorder exhibit?
    a. tonic, clonic activity of the extremities
    b. periods of inattention and daydreaming
    c. sudden loss of muscle tone and falling
    d. repetitive, small muscle group activity

14. List the subjective client data relevant to seizure activity. Use a separate sheet.

15. List the objective client data relevant to seizure activity. Use a separate sheet.

16. The test that is most diagnostic for epilepsy is
    a. electrocardiography (ECG)
    b. electroencephalography (EEG)
    c. computed tomography (CT)
    d. magnetic resonance imaging (MRI)

17. All of the following medications are used in the management of epilepsy *except*
    a. diazepam (Valium)
    b. carbamazepine (Tegretol)
    c. promazine (Sparine)
    d. phenytoin (Dilantin)

18. Seizure precautions include
    a. securing a padded tongue blade at the bedside
    b. padding the client's bed rails
    c. inserting an intravenous lock
    d. posting a seizure "alert" sign on the door

19. Interventions for the client who is having a generalized seizure include
    a. turning the client to one side
    b. inserting a padded tongue blade between the teeth
    c. ventilating with room air and Ambu bag
    d. restraining the client's limbs

20. Interventions for status epilepticus include
    a. inserting an oral airway and administering oxygen
    b. monitoring cardiac status and blood pressure
    c. administering medications to stop the seizures
    d. all of the above

21. Which of the following is an appropriate self-care activity for the client with epilepsy?
    a. skipping a medication dose because it is embarrassing to be seen taking pills at work
    b. packing medication in checked-in luggage to avoid lengthy explanations if carry-on baggage is inspected
    c. volunteering to work overtime and off-shifts to convince the boss that seizures are not a problem
    d. wearing a Medic Alert tag regularly to inform others of a potentially serious health problem

Infections

22. List the routes by which infecting organisms enter the central nervous system.

    a. _____

    _____

    b. _____

    _____

    c. _____

    _____

    d. _____

    _____

    e. _____

    _____

23. Which of the following changes occurs in viral meningitis?

    a. The cerebral spinal fluid thickens.

    b. Brain cell metabolism is altered.

    c. Exudate covers the brain and cranial nerves.

    d. Cerebral vessels dilate.

24. List the subjective client data relevant to meningitis. Use a separate sheet.

25. Which of the following symptoms is associated with meningitis?

    a. feeling sleepy

    b. feeling continually out of breath

    c. perceiving an aura

    d. seeing halos around objects

26. List the objective client data relevant to meningitis. Use a separate sheet.

27. Which of the following clinical signs is associated with meningitis?

    a. nuchal rigidity

    b. persistent headache

    c. positive Kernig's sign

    d. all of the above

28. Which of the following diagnostic tests should the nurse anticipate will be performed on the client with meningitis?

    a. myelography

    b. lumbar puncture

    c. brain scan

    d. pneumoencephalography

29. Which of the following findings in the client with meningitis should the nurse report to the physician immediately?

    a. temperature = 101.8°F

    b. pulse = 126, regular

    c. inability to follow an object with the eyes

    d. pain with neck flexion

30. Which of the following medications is contraindicated in the management of meningitis?

    a. acetaminophen

    b. codeine sulfate

    c. penicillin G

    d. morphine sulfate

31. Interventions for the client with viral meningitis include

    a. suicide precautions

    b. seizure precautions

    c. strict isolation

    d. rehabilitation

32. List the structures affected in encephalitis.

    a. _____

    b. _____

    c. _____

33. Which of the following are vectors for encephalitis?

    a. mosquitos

    b. amoebae

    c. ticks

    d. all of the above

34. Which of the following questions is pertinent to the history of the client with suspected encephalitis?

    a. "Have you had any recent cold sores or fever blisters?"

    b. "Are you allergic to any foods that you know of?"

    c. "Is there any family history of mental illness?"

    d. "Do you have any difficulty falling asleep at night?"

35. Drug therapy in the management of encephalitis includes all of the following *except*

    a. cytarabine (Ara-C)

    b. adenine arabinoside (Ara-A)

    c. vidarabine (Vira-A)

    d. acyclovir (Zovirax)

36. Briefly discuss why encephalitis is managed aggressively to prevent pulmonary complications. Use a separate sheet.

Match the following treatments (37–39) with their associated CNS infections (a–c).

_____ 37. hyperimmune equine serum   a. botulism

_____ 38. symptomatic treatment   b. Creutzfeldt–Jakob disease

_____ 39. trivalent antitoxin   c. tetanus

Parkinson's Disease

40. Symptoms of Parkinson's disease are a result of

    a. decreased production of serotonin

    b. decreased availability of acetylcholine

    c. increased production of dopamine

    d. decreased production of dopamine

41. List the subjective client data relevant to the client with Parkinson's disease. Use a separate sheet.

42. Which of the following comments by a client's spouse is consistent with a diagnosis of Parkinson's disease?

    a. "His handwriting is large and embellished with lots of loops and swirls."

    b. "When we talk over the telephone, it's almost impossible to understand what he says."

    c. "Sometimes when we take our evening walk, he just lags behind and forgets where we are going."

    d. "I think he's getting deaf because he claims to never hear what I'm saying to him."

43. List the objective client data relevant to the client with Parkinson's disease. Use a separate sheet.

44. Which of the following observations is most indicative of Parkinson's disease?

    a. demonstrates regular fine tremor of both hands that persists with intentional activity

    b. has difficulty arising from chair and beginning to walk without assistance

    c. follows objects around room with eyes and often smiles to self when left alone in room

    d. weakness of right leg becoming more noticeable after a warm bath or shower

45. When instructing a client with Parkinson's disease about levodopa (Larodopa), the nurse should tell the client to

    a. increase the dose when the tremors or stiffness become worse

    b. take the medication with milk or at mealtime to decrease stomach irritation

    c. include a multivitamin in your daily routine to balance your nutrition

    d. notify your physician if your urine or perspiration turns a darker color

46. Interventions for the client with Parkinson's disease include

    a. encouraging periods of prolonged rest interspersed with activity

    b. scheduling physical therapy sessions early in the morning after breakfast

    c. arranging for frequent, short outings to the movies or shopping mall

    d. ordering a dental soft diet that consists of small, frequent meals

Alzheimer's Disease

47. List the structural changes that occur in the brain of the client with Alzheimer's disease. Use a separate sheet.

48. Which of the following statements is correct about Alzheimer's disease?

    a. There is an inherited predisposition to the disease.

    b. Alzheimer's occurs most often between the ages of 40 and 65 years.

    c. It is the leading cause of death in the elderly.

    d. There is a higher incidence in men than in women.

49. List the subjective client data relevant to Alzheimer's disease. Use a separate sheet.

50. List rationales for including the family in the history-taking process for the client with Alzheimer's disease.

    a. _____

    _____

    _____

    b. _____

    _____

    _____

    c. _____

    _____

    _____

51. List the objective client data relevant to Alzheimer's disease. Use a separate sheet.

52. Among the first signs that the client with Alzheimer's disease manifests is

    a. disorientation to time, place, and person

    b. hesitant speech and obvious memory loss

    c. forgetfulness and short attention span

    d. ritualistic, repetitive behavior and paranoia

53. The laboratory test commonly performed that confirms the diagnosis of Alzheimer's disease is a

    a. brain biopsy

    b. brain scan

    c. positron emission tomography

    d. none of the above

54. Interventions to assist the client with Alzheimer's disease having the nursing diagnosis of Altered Thought Processes include

    a. rearranging the furniture periodically for distraction

    b. establishing and following a daily routine consistently

    c. posting a monthly calendar showing the family's activities

    d. discouraging any reminiscing because it is disorienting

55. Drug therapy for the client with Alzheimer's disease includes

    a. antidepressants

    b. neuroleptics

    c. hypnotics

    d. all of the above

56. Interventions for the family of a client with Alzheimer's disease include

    a advising them to seek legal counsel about the client's competency

    b. referring them to a local Alzheimer's support group for networking

    c. encouraging them to arrange for regular respite care of their stricken family member

    d. doing all of the above because they are all important in assisting the family to cope with the disease's effects

57. When instructing the family of a client with Alzheimer's disease about home care, the nurse includes information about

    a. considering the need for long-term care in a nursing home

    b. training in defensive techniques to use when the client becomes agitated or combative

    c. arranging for a durable power of attorney to help manage the client's financial affairs

    d. all of the above

Huntington's Chorea

58. Which of the following statements is correct about Huntington's chorea?

    a. It is a hereditary disease that is autosomal recessive.

    b. It manifests with progressive changes in mental status.

    c. It can be prevented through careful genetic counseling.

    d. It is managed by replacing the neurotransmitter gamma-aminobutyric acid.

59. The most common cause of death for the client with Huntington's chorea is

    a. sepsis

    b. suicide

    c. homicide

    d. pneumonia

CRITICAL THINKING EXERCISES

Case Study: Alzheimer's Disease

K. R. is a 76-year-old widow who has lived with her son and daughter-in-law for the past 3 years. She was diagnosed with stage I Alzheimer's disease 2 years ago. Since her original diagnosis, she has become confused, especially at night. She cannot remember where she places her personal items and recently accused her grandson of stealing her purse (which was later found in the laundry hamper). Three hours ago, K. R. had a seizure and is now hospitalized for diagnostic evaluation and medication management.

Address the following questions:

1. On admission, K. R. is difficult to arouse. Develop a plan to assess K. R. Consider her cognition and physical changes due to her Alzheimer's disease and seizure.

The nurse completes a brief mental status examination. The examination proceeds as follows:

Nurse: "What year is it?"
K. R.: "1972, what do you think?"
Nurse: "What day is today?"
K. R.: "Well, how would I know?"
Nurse: "Can you tell me where you are?"
K. R.: "Quit asking me this stuff."
Nurse: "This is a pencil, a clock, and a dress. Can you repeat these names?"
K. R.: "Dress."
Nurse: "Subtract 7 from 100, what do you get for an answer?"
K. R.: "Answer."
Nurse: "What were the three items we named before?"
K. R.: "Leave me alone."
Nurse: "What are these things?" (pointing to a pencil and a watch)
K. R.: "A pencil and a watch."
Nurse: "Repeat this: 'No ifs, ands or buts.' "
K. R.: "No."
Nurse: "Take a paper in your hand, fold it in half, and put it on the floor."
K. R. takes the paper and does nothing with it.
Nurse: "Read this sign and do what it says." (It says "close your eyes.")
K. R. closes eyes.
Nurse: "Write a sentence."
K. R.: "Quit bothering me."
Nurse: "Can you copy this design?"
K.R. takes a pencil and does nothing.

2. Score the above mental status examination. What nursing diagnoses are relevant to K. R. based on these data?

3. What items might be placed in the room to assist with K. R.'s orientation ?

K. R. is given amitriptyline (Elavil) and phenytoin (Dilantin). She thinks that it is poison and refuses to take the pills.

4. What approach might be used to administer the medications? The family asks about the rationale for the medications. How should the nurse explain their purpose?

During the night, K. R. is placed in a jacket restraint and wrist restraints. She pulls at the restraints constantly and has reddened areas on her wrists.

5. What interventions could be used to reduce the risk of injury to the skin of her arms?

K. R. is to be discharged from the hospital. Her seizures appear to be controlled with anticonvulsants.

6. What data should be considered prior to her discharge about safe placement outside of the hospital?

C H A P T E R   4 2

Interventions for Clients with Problems of the Central Nervous System: The Spinal Cord

LEARNING OBJECTIVES

At the end of this chapter, the student will be able to

- Discuss back pain
- Describe the collaborative management of back pain
- Describe the pathophysiology, mechanisms of injury, etiology, incidence, and prevention of spinal cord injury (SCI)
- Describe collaborative management of the client with a spinal cord injury
- Discuss spinal cord tumors
- Describe the pathophysiology, etiology, and incidence of multiple sclerosis (MS)
- Discuss collaborative management of the client with multiple sclerosis
- Discuss amyotrophic lateral sclerosis (ALS)
- Discuss syringomyelia
- Discuss poliomyelitis and postpolio syndrome

PREREQUISITE KNOWLEDGE

Prior to beginning this chapter, the student should review

- The anatomy and physiology of the neurological nervous system (peripheral)
- The process of nerve conduction

- The normal function of the musculoskeletal system, including joint range of motion (ROM)
- The process of rehabilitation and related interventions
- The concepts of body image and self-esteem
- The concept of sexuality
- Coping and stress management techniques
- The principles of perioperative nursing management
- Pain and pain management

STUDY QUESTIONS

Back Pain

1. Identify the causes of cervical and lower back pain. Use a separate sheet.
2. Review the principles of body mechanics that are related to preventing back injuries. Use a separate sheet.
3. List the subjective client data relevant to back pain. Use a separate sheet.
4. List the objective client data relevant to back pain. Use a separate sheet.
5. List the nonsurgical interventions that may be used for the client with back pain. Use a separate sheet.

6. Which of the following assessment findings in the client who has had a lumbar laminectomy should the nurse report to the physician immediately?

   a. dorsiflexes and plantar flexes feet

   b. perceives toes being pinched

   c. clear drainage noted on dressing

   d. inability to void while flat in bed

7. Which of the following postoperative interventions is usually performed for the client who has had a spinal fusion but not for the client who has had a simple laminectomy?

   a. assisting to get out of bed while keeping the back straight

   b. applying a thoracolumbar brace before getting out of bed

   c. completing a neurological assessment, including vital signs

   d. logrolling every 2 hours until mobile

8. Which of the following statements indicates that the client understands discharge instructions after a lumbar laminectomy?

   a. "I miss my grandchildren, especially the baby who I watch during the week."

   b. "My house has a day bed and bathroom on the main floor, near the kitchen."

   c. "I plan to use my heating pad on my back overnight and when I rest."

   d. "I can't wait to get back to my own bed with its soft mattress."

Spinal Cord Injury

9. Damage to lower motor neurons results in

   a. spinal shock

   b. flaccid paralysis

   c. spastic paralysis

   d. autonomic dysreflexia

10. Autonomic hyperreflexia is a medical emergency because is may lead to

    a. bladder rupture

    b. hyperthermia

    c. cerebral vascular ischemia

    d. shock lung

Match the following causes of spinal cord injury (SCI) (11–14) with their mechanisms of injury (a–d).

_____ 11. falling backward 20 feet onto a sharp rock

_____ 12. falling onto the buttocks while roller skating

_____ 13. diving into shallow water and striking head on the bottom

_____ 14. being rear-ended in an automobile accident

a. hyperextension

b. hyperflexion

c. penetration

d. vertical compression

15. Which of the following statements is correct about incomplete lesions of the spinal cord?

    a. Anterior cord syndrome results in loss of motor function below the level of injury, while sensation is intact.

    b. Posterior cord syndrome results in loss of both motor and sensory function below the level of injury.

    c. Brown–Séquard syndrome results in loss of both motor and sensory function ipsilaterally below the level of injury.

    d. Central cord syndrome results in complete loss of motor and sensory function below the level of injury.

16. List the subjective client data relevant to SCI. Use a separate sheet.

17. Which of the following health problems should the nurse note when taking the history of a client with SCI?

    a. chronic urinary tract infections

    b. Hirschsprung's disease

    c. scoliosis

    d. all of the above

18. List the objective client data relevant to SCI. Use a separate sheet.

19. Stimuli that may result in autonomic dysreflexia in the client with SCI include

    a. constipation

    b. urinary retention

    c. draft across the legs

    d. all of the above

20. Which of the following assessment findings for the client with SCI who is in cervical traction should the nurse report to the physician immediately?

    a. dorsiflexes and plantar flexes feet upon command

    b. bilateral hand grip strength equal

    c. right pupil oval and reacts more slowly than left

    d. capillary refill to fingers and toes within 3 seconds

Match the following medications used in treating SCI (21–25) with their indications for being ordered by the physician (a–e).

_____ 21. atropine   a. hypotension

_____ 22. dantrolene   b. cord edema

_____ 23. dexamethasone   c. bradycardia

_____ 24. dextran   d. spasticity

_____ 25. dopamine   e. cord blood flow

26. List four complications related to impaired physical mobility that the client with SCI is at increased risk for developing.

    a. _____

    _____

    b. _____

    _____

    c. _____

    _____

    d. _____

    _____

27. When assisting the client with SCI to manage problems of elimination, the nurse should

    a. realize that all such clients benefit from a regular regimen

    b. consider that much of the cord damage is irreversible and retraining is a waste of time

    c. recognize that all clients can be approached in identical ways to achieve control

    d. understand that most clients will accept the necessity for help with this basic need without embarrassment

28. Identify the areas that should be included in the discharge teaching plan for the client with SCI.

    a. _____

    _____

    b. _____

    _____

    c. _____

    _____

    d. _____

    _____

    e. _____

    _____

    f. _____

    _____

Spinal Cord Tumors

29. Spinal cord tumors

    a. are usually malignant

    b. occur frequently in the elderly

    c. often develop secondarily to metastases

    d. can result in a variety of clinical manifestations

30. List the categories of physical findings that the client with a spinal cord tumor may exhibit.

    a. _____

    _____

    b. _____

    _____

    c. _____

    _____

    d. _____

    _____

    e. _____

    _____

    f. _____

    _____

31. An essential element of a bowel program for the client with a spinal cord tumor is
    a. restricting fluids to 1500 mL per day
    b. toileting at the same time every day
    c. consuming a diet low in fiber
    d. taking a daily laxative

Multiple Sclerosis

32. Multiple sclerosis (MS) is
    a. a chronic disease characterized by periods of remission and exacerbation
    b. caused by a slow-growing virus that lays dormant for many years before becoming activated
    c. known to have a strong genetic link and an increased incidence in immediate relatives of the person affected
    d. more prevalent in areas of the country that have warm, dry climates and are near large bodies of water

33. List the subjective client data relevant to MS. Use a separate sheet.

34. Early symptoms of MS include
    a. a history of abnormal scar formation.
    b. gradual onset of personality changes.
    c. increasing visual acuity over time.
    d. feeling invigorated after a warm shower.

35. List the objective client data relevant to MS. Use a separate sheet.

36. The most definitive diagnostic test for MS is
    a. CT
    b. EEG
    c. CSF white cell count
    d. none of the above

37. Which of the following self-care measures should be taught to the client who has MS?
    a. wearing dark sunglasses when outside to decrease diplopia
    b. planning all activities in advance to allow for energy conservation
    c. engaging in physical activity such as brisk walking to help improve endurance
    d. testing water temperature with the elbow to prevent possible burn injury

38. The client with MS who is being treated with adrenocorticotropic hormone (ACTH) and cyclophosphamide (Cytoxan) should be instructed to
    a. restrict daily fluid intake to 2 quarts

b. wait to purchase a wig because alopecia may not occur
c. include a banana in the daily diet
d. take aspirin for minor discomforts

Amyotrophic Lateral Sclerosis

39. Which of the following statements is correct about amyotrophic lateral sclerosis (ALS)?
    a. Mental status changes occur as a result of the disease.
    b. The disease has a strong genetic basis.
    c. Muscle weakness and atrophy result flaccid paralysis.
    d. Death is usually a result of cardiac failure.

40. Early symptoms of ALS include
    a. diplopia
    b. tinnitus
    c. dysphagia
    d. foot drop

Other Neurological Problems

41. Syringomyelia is a disease of the
    a. cervical spinal cord
    b. thoracic spinal cord
    c. lumbar spinal cord
    d. sacral spinal cord

42. The client with syringomyelia is at increased risk for
    a. falling
    b. hand injuries
    c. aspiration
    d. foot drop

43. Poliomyelitis is
    a. transmitted by direct contact
    b. more prevalent during winter and spring
    c. preventable by immunization with a vaccine
    d. a bacterial infection of the spinal cord and brain

44. Which of the following exercises is recommended for the client with postpolio syndrome (PPS)?
    a. walking a mile per day
    b. bicycling on level terrain
    c. swimming in warm water
    d. slow jogging on an indoor track

CRITICAL THINKING EXERCISES

Case Study: Herniated Disc

T. S. is a 30-year-old long-distance truck driver. He is scheduled for a CT scan of the lumbar spine to determine if he has a herniated disc. A contrast medium will be given. He is receiving analgesics every 3–4 hours and local heat therapy and is in pelvic traction.

Address the following questions:

1. What information does T. S. need to ensure his cooperation during the procedure?

2. When questioning T. S. concerning allergic reactions, about which substance should the nurse specifically inquire? Why?

3. T. S. must sign a consent form for the CT scan. When should he sign?

After the CT scan, T. S. is informed that the results were negative. He is scheduled for discharge that evening. He is given prescriptions for ibuprofen (Motrin) 400 mg qid and cyclobenzaprine hydrochloride (Flexeril) 10 mg PO, tid.

4. What information does the nurse discuss with T. S. about posture, lifting, muscle-strengthening exercises, prolonged periods of sitting, and support devices?

5. What are the common side effects of ibuprofen? Of cyclobenzaprine?

6. The pharmacy dispenses the ibuprofen in 200-mg pills. How many should T. S. be instructed to take for each dose? How many pills will he take in a 24-hour period?

7. What instruction should the nurse include about diet while T. S. is taking his medications?

8. T. S. asks whether he can resume work soon. What does the nurse tell him?

Case Study: Spinal Cord Injury

C. S. is a 26-year-old woman who suffered a C-7 quadriplegia from a motor vehicle accident 1 month ago. She has been in the critical care unit since the injury. She was ventilator dependent, with a tracheostomy, during that time. C. S. also required surgery to repair a ruptured spleen and to stabilize her cervical spine. She has been transferred to the general nursing unit for care of a 3-cm sacral pressure ulcer and is awaiting transfer to a rehabilitation unit.

Address the following questions:

1. After C. S. is transferred, a nurse from the general care unit is heard to say, "I just think it's awful to let those patients get bedsores in ICU. Those nurses only have one patient and they still can't give them good care!" What response might be offered to this comment?

The physician orders that C. S.'s wound be packed with wet-to-dry dressings qid. The nurses decide that the best way to facilitate the wound's healing is to position C. S. prone 1 hour qid.

2. What risks are likely to occur with C. S. positioned prone? For example, consider respiration, sensory stimulation, eating, and communication.

3. While turning her prone, C. S. has a strong spasm of the legs. Describe the physiological mechanisms that cause or allow the spasms.

C. S. has been lying on her stomach for about 30 minutes. She calls the nurse and tells her that she has a terrible headache and wants to turn back over.

4. After turning her over, what other assessments might the nurse perform to determine if C. S.'s headache is from autonomic dysreflexia?

Two weeks after her transfer, C. S.'s pressure ulcer is surgically repaired. After 2 weeks more to allow for healing, she is considered for transfer to a rehabilitation unit.

5. C. S. asks what will be done for her on the new unit. Develop a teaching/learning plan that discusses her functional level, bladder and bowel training program, and ability to be mobile.

Case Study: Degenerative Arthritis

R. W. is a 60-year-old male with degenerative arthritis of the lumbar spine. He has purchased a new, firm mattress for his bed, but he frequently awakens stiff, in pain, and unable to get out of bed.

Address the following questions:

1. What measures can R. W. take to improve his morning mobility?

2. What types of exercise may be beneficial for R. W. to perform upon awakening and before arising?

3. R. W. inquires about whether he will be able to continue his leisure activity of racquetball. What does the nurse tell him?

CHAPTER 43

Interventions for Clients with Problems of the Peripheral Nervous System

LEARNING OBJECTIVES

At the end of this chapter, the student will be able to

- Describe the pathophysiology, etiology, and incidence of Guillain–Barré syndrome
- Discuss collaborative management of the client with Guillain–Barré syndrome
- Describe the pathophysiology, etiology, and incidence of myasthenia gravis (MG)
- Discuss the collaborative management of the client with myasthenia gravis
- Discuss polyneuritis and polyneuropathy
- Discuss peripheral nerve trauma
- Describe diseases of the cranial nerves

PREREQUISITE KNOWLEDGE

Prior to beginning this chapter, the student should review

- The anatomy and physiology of the neurological nervous system (peripheral)
- The process of nerve conduction
- The normal function of the musculoskeletal system, including joint range of motion (ROM)
- The process of rehabilitation and related interventions
- The concepts of body image and self-esteem
- The concept of sexuality
- Coping and stress management techniques
- The principles of perioperative nursing management
- Pain and pain management

STUDY QUESTIONS

Guillain–Barré Syndrome

1. Which of the following statements is correct about Guillain–Barré syndrome (GBS)?
   a. Occurrence tends to be seasonal, with more cases reported during the winter.
   b. Demyelination of peripheral nerves interferes with the conduction across the synaptic cleft.
   c. GBS is associated with the vaccination for influenza.
   d. Clients stricken with GBS recover quickly and have few residual deficits.

2. List the subjective client data relevant to the client with GBS. Use a separate sheet.

3. Which of the following symptoms is associated with GBS?
   a. tinnitus
   b. diplopia
   c. vertigo
   d. nausea

4. List the objective client data relevant to the client with GBS. Use a separate sheet.

5. Which of the following signs would the nurse observe in the client suspected of having GBS?

   a. nystagmus

   b. vomiting

   c. tremor

   d. myalgia

6. Which of the following observations in a client with suspected GBS should the nurse report to the physician immediately?

   a. ataxia

   b. dilated pupils

   c. tachycardia

   d. cyanosis

7. Interventions for the client with GBS who has respiratory compromise include

   a. auscultating breath sounds once per 8-hour shift

   b. positioning to maintain a patent airway

   c. suctioning prn using a clean technique

   d. measuring vital capacity once per 8-hour shift

8. The procedure used in the management of GBS that reduces the length of hospitalization is

   a. electrophoresis

   b. plasmapheresis

   c. diaphoresis

   d. diapedesis

9. Discuss the rationale for the following interventions for maintaining skin integrity in the client with GBS: monitoring for incontinence, keeping bed linen taut, providing fluids, and enteral feedings. Use a separate sheet.

10. Providing the client in the acute or plateau stage of GBS with alternatives to choose from is an intervention for

    a. Powerlessness

    b. Self-Care Deficit

    c. Anticipatory Grieving

    d. Anxiety and Fear

11. Psychosocial adjustment in the client with GBS depends on the client's

    a. age and gender

    b. available support systems

    c. residual deficit

    d. coping strategies

    e. all of the above

Myasthenia Gravis

12. Which of the following neurotransmitters is deficient in myasthenia gravis (MG)?

    a. epinephrine

    b. norepinephrine

    c. acetylcholine

    d. dopamine

13. Which of the following terms describes MG?

    a. acute

    b. autoimmune

    c. curable

    d. hereditary

14. List the subjective client data relevant to MG. Use a separate sheet.

15. Which of the following comments by a client with MG should the nurse report to the physician immediately?

    a. "I feel nauseated and have stomach cramps."

    b. "My eyelid keeps twitching and it's very annoying."

    c. "My eyes are watering and it's hard to see."

    d. "It's impossible for me to take a breath and cough."

16. List the objective client data relevant to MG. Use a separate sheet.

17. Which of the following is a significant assessment finding in the client with MG?

    a. decreased deep tendon reflexes in lower extremities

    b. decreased ability to discern the colors red and green

    c. voice becomes progressively softer with conversation

    d. able to sit in chair with safety belt applied

18. Which of the following problems is associated with MG?

    a. rheumatoid arthritis

    b. myocardial infarction

    c. meningitis

    d. spina bifida

19. The drug used most often in the procedure for diagnosing MG is

    a. neostigmine bromide (Prostigmin)

    b. edrophonium chloride (Tensilon)

    c. tubocurarine chloride

    d. atropine sulfate

20. Equipment that should be kept at the bedside of the client with MG for maintaining adequate ventilation includes

    a. an emesis basin

    b. a sphygmomanometer

    c. an intubation set-up

    d. a nasogastric tube

21. Identify four principles of energy conservation that guide the planning of care for the client with MG.

    a. _____

    _____

    b. _____

    _____

    c. _____

    _____

    d. _____

    _____

22. Which of the following medications should *not* be administered to the client with MG?

    a. prednisone (Orasone)

    b. tetracycline (Panmycin)

    c. acetaminophen (Tylenol)

    d. piroxicam (Feldene)

23. Briefly discuss the rational for administering medications on time to the client with MG. Use a separate sheet.

24. For the client in myasthenic crisis, administering the Tensilon test results in

    a. temporary improvement of symptoms

    b. no improvement of symptoms

    c. worsening of symptoms

    d. cholinergic crisis

25. Immunosuppressant drugs are administered to the client with MG to

    a. supplement the action of acetylcholine

    b. reduce the number of acetylcholine receptor antibodies

    c. increase the number of acetylcholine receptors

    d. help prevent the development of cholinergic crisis

26. Interventions for the client with MG who is undergoing plasmapheresis include

    a. teaching the client to fast before the procedure

    b. weighing the client after each session

    c. checking for shunt bruit every 2–4 hours

    d. securing bulldog clamps to a necklace the client wears

27. Interventions for the client with MG who has a thymectomy include

    a. administering pyridostigmine (Mestinon) intramuscularly

    b. administering kanamycin (Kantrex) intravenously

    c. monitoring ventilatory status until remission occurs

    d. weaning from the respirator gradually

28. Interventions for the client with MG include

    a. discouraging independence in activities of daily living (ADL) to decrease fatigue

    b. providing assistance to decrease undue frustration

    c. patching each eye alternately every day for diplopia

    d. asking the client to repeat when not understood

29. Interventions for the client with MG who has inadequate nutritional status include

    a. administering anticholinesterase medications 1 hour prior to mealtime to prevent aspiration

    b. encouraging hot liquids such as tea or coffee 30 minutes before meals to prevent constipation

    c. providing small, frequent meals around the clock to increase nutritional intake

    d. administering diphenoxylate (Lomotil) as needed for diarrhea and abdominal cramping

30. Discharge instructions for the client with MG include

    a. teaching the client to self-manage minor infections with aspirin

    b. reminding the client to include recreational activities such as biking in the weekly routine

    c. counseling the client to seek outlets for relaxation such as a sauna or hot tub

    d. advising the client to arrange for a regular schedule of activities and rest periods

Polyneuritis and Polyneuropathy

31. List the hallmarks of peripheral neuropathy. Use a separate sheet.

32. Which of the following is associated with the occurrence of peripheral neuropathy?

    a. Parkinson's disease

    b. diabetes insipidus

    c. pernicious anemia

    d. hemophilia

33. Which of the following findings is abnormal for peripheral neuropathy?

    a. miosis

    b. stereognosis

    c. graphesthesia

    d. agraphia

34. Which of the following should the client with peripheral neuropathy avoid?

    a. white socks

    b. warm boots

    c. smoking

    d. carbonated beverages

Peripheral Nerve Trauma

35. Which of the following statements is correct about peripheral nerve trauma?

    a. The nerve distal to a transection injury degenerates and retracts within 48 hours.

    b. The more well aligned the transsected nerve stumps, the better the return of nerve function.

    c. Successfully realigned damaged nerves are capable of full conduction velocities.

    d. Nerve regeneration must be complete before any sensory function can return.

36. Which of the following are significant data in the assessment of the client with suspected peripheral nerve damage?

    a. shooting leg pain from buttock to popliteal area

    b. discerns a pungent, rancid odor not noted by others

    c. reports seeing halos around lights and bright objects

    d. tinnitus and vertigo occur without warning

37. List the objective client data relevant to peripheral nerve trauma. Use a separate sheet.

38. Which of the following findings in a client with trauma should the nurse report to the physician immediately?

    a. toes warm, pink, and blanche response within 3 seconds

    b. ability to move digits on request without hesitancy

    c. fasciculations noted in the left thenar eminence

    d. bilateral patellar reflexes rated 2+ on a 4+ scale

39. Following surgery to repair damage peripheral nerves, the nurse assesses the client's skin around the cast or splint frequently because

    a. sensation may be heightened and the client will report even minor discomfort more readily

    b. excessive vasodilation occurs and the area distal to the repair will be diaphoretic

    c. hypertrophy of the epidermis and underlying tissue makes the skin more resistant to injury

    d. edema from the inflammatory process causes tissues to swell, making the cast or splint too tight

40. The member of the health care team who works most closely with the client following peripheral nerve surgery is the

    a. nurse

    b. physician

    c. physical therapist

    d. social worker

Diseases of the Cranial Nerves

41. Trigeminal neuralgia is associated with a specific type of facial pain that is

    a. dull and aching

    b. sharp and shooting

    c. dull and throbbing

    d. burning and continuous

42. Which of the following treatments for trigeminal neuralgia is preferred to provide permanent relief from pain?

    a. alcohol injection

    b. glycerin injection

    c. retrogasserian rhizotomy

    d. electrocoagulation

43. Which of the following assessment findings is abnormal after a successful rhizotomy of the trigeminal nerve?

    a. blinks when a puff of air is directed at the cornea

    b. extraocular movements intact throughout all fields, conjugate gaze

    c. reports an itching sensation over cheek and forehead

    d. facial movements asymmetric during conversation

44. Which of the following findings is associated with Bell's palsy?

    a. eyes closed tightly against resistance

    b. face mask-like and sagging on one side

    c. excessive tearing from one eye

    d. oral mucous membranes dry

45. Interventions for the client with Bell's palsy include

    a. instilling prednisone eye drops qid

    b. keeping the affected eye patched continuously

    c. practicing facial exercises three or four times per day

    d. using a straw to drink liquids

CRITICAL THINKING EXERCISES

Case Study: Guillain–Barré Syndrome

S. B. is a 54-year-old retired military officer who was admitted through the Emergency Department with ascending paralysis. During the past 2 days, he had noticed leg pain and eventually was unable to walk at all.

Address the following questions:

1. Considering the pathophysiology of Guillain–Barré syndrome, prioritize the assessments and interventions for the next few hours for S. B.

2. During the shift, he becomes increasingly paralyzed and is unable to turn in bed or lift his arms. Identify the relevant nursing diagnoses and prioritize them.

S. B. is transferred to the ICU for ventilatory management and is treated with plasmapheresis. He returns to the general medical nursing unit after 4 days and is still receiving plasmapheresis. Since he is now able to speak, he asks the nurse about the treatment and specifically if he can get AIDS from it.

3. Develop a teaching/learning plan for S. B. about plasmapheresis. Consider how it works, what specific nursing interventions are needed, and what the potential complications are while a client is receiving this therapy.

4. S. B. is very weak and unable to perform any ADLs. Consider the hazards of immobility, and develop a plan of care to prevent complications while he regains his strength.

5. One morning while assisting S. B. with his bath, he comments, "I am so helpless! I used to tell hundreds of people what to do and now I can't even bathe myself." He then starts to cry. How should the nurse respond to these feelings of powerlessness?

S. B. has regained some strength and is ready to transfer to a long-term rehabilitation center for continued care. He asks many questions about his upcoming care, such as how he will regain strength since he still gets dizzy every time he raises his head, how he will learn to control his bladder and bowels, and whether he could ever get this sick again.

6. Discuss how each of these concerns could be answered by the nurse.

Case Study: Myasthenia Gravis

P. G. is a 32-year-old woman admitted for an evaluation of fatigue, muscle weakness, difficulty swallowing, and a weak voice. Her symptoms developed very suddenly. She reports that she is normally physically active, but since the birth of her last baby 1 month ago, she has been increasingly fatigued, is unable to climb stairs, and has trouble lifting objects. P. G. admitted that initially she did not pay much attention to the symptoms and thought that she was just recovering from the birth more slowly, especially since she has a second child at home, who is 3 years old. When she developed "double vision and droopy eyelids," she became worried and saw the physician.

Address the following questions:

1. What additional data should the nurse collect from P. G?

The physician plans to test P. G.'s response to edrophonium chloride (Tensilon), a cholinergic agent.

2. Discuss the purpose of this test. Consider the pathophysiology of myasthenia gravis and how the drug Tensilon works.

3. Develop a teaching/learning plan for P. G. about the Tensilon test.

4. The next morning, P. G.'s physician asks for 0.2 mg of Tensilon. It is supplied in an ampule containing 10 mg/2 mL. How much of the medication should the nurse draw into a syringe?

5. After giving the medication, what would be the expected response in P. G.?

6. The next morning there is an emergency on the unit and medications are not given to the clients at prescribed times. What problem is likely to occur in P. G. when she does not receive her medication at the correct time?

7. Construct a teaching/learning plan for P. G. about her self-care after discharge. The physician is prescribing pyridostigmine bromide (Mestinon) 60 mg tid, prednisone 60 mg every a.m., and azathioprine (Imuran) 2 mg per day. Include symptoms of overmedication, undermedication, techniques to conserve energy, and other home management concerns.

Five days after P. G. is discharged, her husband calls the nursing unit and reports that his wife is unable to breathe or clear the secretions in her throat. She had increased her dosages of the medications because she thought her symptoms were getting worse.

8. What initial care does P. G. need?

9. How can her teaching/learning plan be reviewed to prevent this problem from occurring in the future?

CHAPTER 44

Interventions for Critically Ill Clients with Neurologic Problems

LEARNING OBJECTIVES

At the end of this chapter, the student will be able to

- Discuss the pathophysiology, etiology, and incidence, of cerebrovascular accident (CVA)
- Discuss assessment of the client following a cerebrovascular accident
- Describe collaborative management of the client following a CVA
- Describe the pathophysiology, etiology, incidence, and prevention of head injury
- Describe collaborative management of the client with a head injury
- Describe the pathophysiology, complications, classification, etiology, and incidence of brain tumors
- Discuss collaborative management of the client with a brain tumor
- Discuss brain abscess and related management

PREREQUISITE KNOWLEDGE

Prior to beginning this chapter, the student should review

- The anatomy and physiology of the neurological system (central and peripheral)
- The process of nerve conduction
- The normal function of the musculoskeletal system, including joint range of motion (ROM)
- The process of rehabilitation and related interventions
- The concepts of body image and self-esteem
- The concept of sexuality
- The concepts of loss, death, and grieving
- Coping and stress management techniques
- The principles of perioperative nursing management
- Pain and pain management

STUDY QUESTIONS

Cerebrovascular Accident (CVA)

1. The circle of Willis is a
   a. network of blood vessels at the base of the brain
   b. series of channels for the circulation of cerebrospinal fluid (CSF)
   c. complex neural network between cerebral hemispheres
   d. structure of supporting connective tissue for the brain

2. Which of the following functions is the brain capable of performing in the absence of a normal blood supply?

   a. storing oxygen and glucose

   b. removing metabolic wastes

   c. anaerobic metabolism

   d. none of the above

3. The ability of the brain to maintain cerebral blood flow is called

   a. autogenesis

   b. autoregulation

   c. autonomic reflexia

   d. autosynthesis

Match the following causes of CVAs (4–8) with their types (a or b). Answers may be used more than once.

_____ 4. hypertension   a. ischemic

_____ 5. ruptured aneurysm   b. hemorrhagic

_____ 6. embolus

_____ 7. thrombus

_____ 8. arteriovenous malformation

9. Which of the following statements is correct about CVAs?

   a. Thrombotic strokes have a quick onset and resolution and few lingering effects.

   b. The anterior cerebral artery is usually the site of embolic strokes.

   c. Transient ischemic attacks (TIAs) last less than 24 hours and cause minimal damage.

   d. Reversible ischemic neurological deficits (RIND) do not damage brain tissue.

10. Which of the following statements is correct about the etiology of CVAs?

    a. The most common cause of hemorrhagic strokes is arteriovenous malformations.

    b. Aneurysms are embryonic abnormalities in cerebral blood vessels that can rupture.

    c. Vasodilation occurring after a CVA increases the extent of neurological damage.

    d. Risk factors for cerebral vascular disease are the same as those for cardiac disease.

11. Which of the following clients is at greatest risk for developing a CVA?

    a. a 52-year-old man with renal disease

    b. an 82-year-old woman who exercises regularly

    c. a 33-year-old sedentary male executive

    d. a 45-year-old female schoolteacher

12. List the subjective client data relevant to CVA. Use a separate sheet.

13. Which of the following symptoms are associated with cerebrovascular disease?

    a. intermittent muscle cramps in the legs

    b. squeezing, substernal chest pain

    c. sore, scratchy throat

    d. numbness of the face

14. List the objective client data relevant to CVA. Use a separate sheet.

15. Which of the following would the nurse expect to find in the client who has had a CVA of the left cerebral hemisphere?

    a. neglect of the left visual field

    b. loss of ability to hear varying tones

    c. quick anger and frustration

    d. euphoria and impulsiveness

16. All of the following radiographic tests are usually performed in the differential diagnosis of stroke *except*

    a. magnetic resonance imaging (MRI)

    b. computing tomography (CT) scan

    c. myelography

    d. angiography

17. Which of the following interventions does the nurse implement for a client who has had a CVA within the past 24 hours?

    a. Elevate the head of the bed to 60 degrees.

    b. Turn to the unaffected side and support with pillows.

    c. Monitor vital signs once per 8-hour shift.

    d. Assess level of consciousness every 4 hours.

18. Which of the following drugs would the nurse expect to administer to the client who has had an intracranial hemorrhage?

    a. heparin sodium (Lipo-Hepin)

    b. epsilon-aminocaproic acid (Amicar)

    c. warfarin sodium (Coumadin)

    d. dipyridamole (Persantine)

19. Cerebral vasospasms following stroke are managed with

    a. nimodipine (Nimotop)

    b. phenytoin (Dilantin)

    c. minoxidil (Loniten)

    d. belladonna (Belladenal)

20. Identify the precautions implemented by the nurse for the client with cerebral aneurysm. Use a separate sheet.

21. Care for the client who has had a stroke and has impaired mobility includes

    a. performing active ROM to affected areas tid

    b. using splints and trochanter rolls for positioning

    c. assessing for a positive Romberg's sign daily

    d. measuring the diameters of thighs and calves daily

22. Interventions for the client with a right hemisphere CVA include

    a. approaching the client from the left side of the bed

    b. teaching the client to move his or her eyes to see objects

    c. placing objects on the right side of the overbed tray

    d. encouraging the client to be independent with ADLs

23. Interventions for the client with a left hemisphere CVA include

    a. giving the client a series of instructions to follow

    b. reorienting the client frequently to the environment

    c. providing the client with simple reading material

    d. leaving the television on for distraction

24. Which of the following devices should be used to assist the client with a stroke to communicate?

    a. magnetic letters and backboard

    b. hand-held slate and chalk

    c. computerized, hand-held letter board

    d. picture story board

25. Which of the following foods is preferred for the client with a stroke who has difficulty swallowing?

    a. scrambled egg

    b. broiled fish

    c. orange juice

    d. club sandwich

26. Management of total incontinence in the client with a stroke includes

    a. inserting an in-dwelling urinary catheter

    b. ambulating the client to the bathroom every 4 hours

    c. restricting fluid intake to 1000 mL per 24 hours

    d. determining the cause of the incontinence

27. Identify areas that are included in the discharge teaching plan for the client who has had a stroke.

28. Briefly discuss respite care and its significance for the family of a client who has had a stroke and is being treated at home. Use a separate sheet.

Head Injury

29. Which of the following statements about head injury is correct?

    a. The most common cause of head trauma is falls, especially in the elderly.

    b. Preventive measures for head trauma include wearing seat belts and protective head gear.

    c. The most common sites of injury to the brain are the occipital and cerebellar lobes.

    d. Secondary responses to brain injury are inconsequential to morbidity and mortality rates.

Match the following types of head injuries (30–42) with their descriptions (a–m).

_____ 30. acceleration injury

_____ 31. basilar skull fracture

_____ 32. closed head injury

_____ 33. concussion

_____ 34. contusion

_____ 35. deceleration injury

_____ 36. depressed skull fracture

_____ 37. direct injury

_____ 38. indirect injury

_____ 39. laceration

_____ 40. linear skull fracture

_____ 41. open head injury

_____ 42. open skull fracture

a. force produced by direct blow to head

b. rebound effect from a force to a body part other than the brain

c. skull is fractured or pierced

d. result of blunt trauma leaving skull intact

e. simple, clean break in skull

f. skull presses into brain tissue

g. scalp is lacerated and brain tissue is exposed to the environment

h. usually occurs along paranasal sinus, resulting in CSF leakage

i. brief loss of consciousness

j. bruising of brain at site of impact or opposite side of impact

k. actual tearing of cortical surface vessels

l. caused by the head being in motion

m. caused when the head is suddenly stopped or hits a stationary object

43. List the causes of increased intracranial pressure (ICP).

a. _____

b. _____

c. _____

d. _____

e. _____

f. _____

g. _____

44. Briefly describe the effects of increased ICP when the brain can no longer compensate for further volume changes. Use a separate sheet.

45. List the types of cerebral edema leading to increased ICP.

a. _____

b. _____

c. _____

Match the following terms related to cerebral hemorrhage (46–48) with their descriptions (a–c).

_____ 46. epidural hematoma

_____ 47. intracranial hemorrhage

_____ 48. subdural hematoma

a. venous bleeding into the space between the dura and the arachnoid

b. arterial bleeding into the space between the dura and skull

c. accumulation of blood within brain tissue

49. Identify the process by which the blood flow to the brain remains relatively constant.

a. autolysis

b. autoregeneration

c. autoregulation

d. autohypnosis

50. Hydrocephalus is a condition of increased CSF volume as a result of dilation of the

a. ventricles

b. cerebral vessels

c. hippocampus

d. putamen

51. Briefly discuss the damage that herniation of brain tissue presents to normal functioning of an individual. Use a separate sheet.

52. List the subjective client data relevant to head trauma. Use a separate sheet.

53. Which of the following chronic diseases should the nurse specifically inquire about when assessing a client with head trauma?

a. rheumatoid arthritis

b. hypertension

c. osteoporosis

d. Graves' disease

54. List the objective client data relevant to head trauma. Use a separate sheet.
55. Identify the goals of nursing assessment for the client with head trauma.

    a. _____

    _____

    _____

    b. _____

    _____

    _____

56. The first priority in physical assessment of the client with recent head trauma is
    a. determining if spinal cord injury exists
    b. ascertaining that there is a patent airway
    c. checking for signs of increased ICP
    d. verifying that there is a carotid pulse

57. Papilledema is
    a. a normal finding in the funduscopic examination
    b. a sign that the client is about to have a seizure
    c. a sign that is always associated with increased ICP
    d. an indication that a basilar skull fracture exists

58. Assessment of the client with severe head trauma in a critical care unit usually includes
    a. monitoring vital signs every 4 hours
    b. continuous cardiac monitoring
    c. measuring arterial blood gases once a day
    d. measuring urine specific gravity twice a day

59. Drug therapy for the client with severe head trauma includes
    a. prednisone (Orasone)
    b. haloperidol (Haldol)
    c. mannitol (Osmitrol)
    d. tolbutamide (Orinase)

60. Interventions to reorient the client with head trauma who has loss of sensation include
    a. serving beverages that are warm, not hot, to prevent burns
    b. leaving side rails down so that the client can get up as desired and explore the room
    c. playing audiotapes of the client's favorite music during the day for relaxation
    d. explaining procedures to the client in detail before and after they are completed

61. Interventions to promote gas exchange in the client with head trauma include
    a. encouraging fluids at least every hour
    b. performing chest physiotherapy four times a day
    c. elevating the head of the bed to 45–60 degrees
    d. applying thigh-high antiembolic stockings

62. Which of the following are manifestations of post-trauma syndrome?
    a. euphoria and impulsive behavior
    b. lethargy and chronic fatigue
    c. restlessness and nervousness
    d. paranoia and compulsiveness

Brain Tumors

63. List structures that are the most common sites of secondary brain tumors (metastases).

    a. _____

    b. _____

    c. _____

    d. _____

    e. _____

64. Which of the following statements is correct about brain tumors?
    a. Primary brain tumors often metastasize to other distant structures in the body.
    b. Brain tumors expand irregularly and may invade, infiltrate, or compress normal brain tissue.
    c. Benign brain tumors often have a favorable prognosis and are readily treatable.
    d. Malignant brain tumors are often untreatable surgically and are managed with chemotherapy.

65. List the subjective client data relevant to brain tumors. Use a separate sheet.
66. The most common symptom reported by the client with a brain tumor is
    a. nausea
    b. diplopia
    c. headache
    d. fatigue

67. List the objective client data relevant to brain tumors. Use a separate sheet.

68. During a physical assessment of most clients who have a brain tumor, the nurse would expect to find

    a. seizure activity

    b. papilledema

    c. ataxia

    d. aphasia

69. Which of the following statements is correct about radiation therapy for brain tumors?

    a. Radiation to the head results in few side effects.

    b. Alopecia always occurs and hair does regrow.

    c. Radiation to the head produces serious increases in ICP.

    d. Increased fatigue is abnormal and should be reported.

70. The most effective route of administration for chemotherapy to the brain is

    a. intravenous

    b. intrathecal

    c. intraventricular

    d. intramuscular

71. List the factors that most influence the outcome of chemotherapy for a brain tumor.

    a. _____

    _____

    b. _____

    _____

    c. _____

    _____

    d. _____

    _____

72. Which of the following statements should be included in preoperative teaching for the client who is to have a craniotomy for resection of a brain tumor?

    a. "Your entire head will be shaved to reduce the chance of an infection."

    b. "Your family can wait in your room for your return since you will be brought back here after the surgery."

    c. "Your family will be able to see you just as soon as you are in the recovery room area."

    d. "One or both eyes will probably look swollen and black-and-blue for awhile."

73. The preferred position for the client following a craniotomy is

    a. high Fowler's

    b. turned to the operative side

    c. turned to the nonoperative side

    d. low Fowler's

74. The most common complication (after increased ICP) that can occur following a craniotomy is

    a. wound infection

    b. atelectasis

    c. meningitis

    d. syndrome of inappropriate antidiuretic hormone

75. Which of the following medications for pain management would the nurse expect to administer to the client who has had a craniotomy for a brain tumor?

    a. acetaminophen with codeine (Tylenol with codeine)

    b. acetylsalicylic acid (aspirin)

    c. levorphanol tartrate (Levo-Dromoran)

    d. morphine sulfate (Roxanol)

76. When planning for discharge of the client following a craniotomy, the nurse should assist the family to realize that

    a. most over-the-counter medications are safe to take

    b. there may be subtle changes in the client's behavior

    c. the incidence of seizures is low and of little concern

    d. complete bed rest and a quiet environment are needed

Brain Abscess

77. List the areas of the brain where abscesses may form.

    a. _____

    b. _____

    c. _____

78. Identify sources of infective organisms that cause brain abscess

a. _____

_____

b. _____

_____

c. _____

_____

d. _____

_____

_____

e. _____

_____

_____

79. Which of the following is relevant to the subjective assessment of a possible brain abscess?

    a. history of gout

    b. recent immunosuppressive therapy

    c. family history of mental illness

    d. glaucoma treated with medication

80. Which of the following assessment findings would the nurse report to the physician immediately in the client with a suspected brain abscess?

    a. lethargy and confusion

    b. generalized muscle weakness

    c. inability to hear low voices

    d. pupils respond sluggishly to light

81. Which of the following drugs would the nurse expect to give to the client with a brain abscess caused by an anaerobic organism?

    a. metronidazole (Flagyl)

    b. penicillin G (Deltapen)

    c. chloramphenicol (Chlormycetin)

    d. nafcillin (Unipen)

CRITICAL THINKING EXERCISES

Case Study: Cerebrovascular Accident (CVA)

D. M. is a 63-year-old African-American male who was brought to the Emergency Department (ED) by his wife. Mrs. M. reported that her husband "just wasn't acting right." D. M. is able to answer some questions during the history, but becomes dysphasic at times, forgetting the question or his answer in mid-sentence. He reported that he had been having headaches for the past few days, but he was under a lot of stress because his company was asking him to retire early. He also has hypertension, which has been controlled with a combination of a vasodilator and a beta-blocker (step 3 therapy). He has no motor or sensory deficits. D. M. is admitted to the nursing unit with a diagnosis of stroke in evolution.

Address the following questions:

1. Upon admission to the nursing unit, what additional information should the nurse collect?

2. What routine assessments will D. M. require (e.g., vital signs)?

On the day following admission, D. M. is found to have no sensation or movement on his right side. He is unable to speak and is somewhat drowsy. He is diagnosed with a left middle cerebral artery thrombotic CVA.

3. Compare D. M.'s presentation of this type of stroke to the description in the textbook.

4. The physician orders heparin sodium to be infused at 1000 units per hour. The pharmacy supplies the medication in a 1000 mL/solution of D_5W with 10,000 units per liter. At what rate should the infusion be administered? List the advantages of using an infusion pump with this solution.

5. List the nursing assessments needed for D. M. while he is on heparin therapy. Consider the subjective, objective, and laboratory data to be monitored.

D. M. is trying to relearn how to feed himself. He becomes very frustrated with his inability to eat and his spilled food. He cries easily and often will not eat his meals.

6. List various nursing approaches to D. M.'s problem with eating (consider the silverware and visual changes).

7. Develop a teaching/learning plan for Mrs. M. so that she will understand her husband's disease. Include probable language, memory, visual, behavioral, and auditory changes demonstrated by D. M.

Case Study: Head Injury

L. W. is a 19-year-old male brought to the ED following a motorcycle accident. He was unconscious on admission to the ED. The rescue squad reported that L. W. was alone on the motorcycle, not wearing a helmet, and hit by a driver who turned left in front of him at a traffic light. He was thrown from the motorcycle onto the pavement. He was conscious initially after the accident, but became comatose during the transport to the hospital. Oxygen was supplied to L. W. while in transport. Physical examination reveals a posterior right-sided head laceration, a reactive left pupil and nonreactive right pupil, spontaneous respirations at 22 breaths per minute, normal sinus rhythm at 92 bpm, and blood pressure of 118/62. A lateral cervical spine x-ray is negative for cervical spine injury and shows an open fracture of the right parietal skull. He responds to deep pain.

Address the following questions:

1. What type of primary and secondary head injury does L. W. have?

It is suspected that L. W. has a subdural hematoma, due in part to the sudden change in neurological status. He is taken to surgery, the hematoma is drained, and an intracranial pressure monitoring device is placed.

2. Discuss the risk of subdural hematoma on the autoregulation of the brain and the usual symptoms.

3. Following surgery, L. W. remains intubated and on a ventilator. He is being hyperventilated to control cerebral edema. Explain how hyperventilation lowers intracranial pressure. What other methods are used to reduce swelling in the brain?

L. W.'s intracranial pressure (ICP) is stable and near normal (16 mmHg) following surgery.

4. What data should the nurse assess continuously that would indicate an increasing ICP?

5. How should L.W. be positioned to reduce ICP? What activities increase ICP and therefore should be avoided?

During the first 3 hours after surgery, L. W. awakens slightly and becomes agitated, pulling at various tubes and lines.

6. List precautions that could be taken to prevent self-injury.

L. W.'s ICP rises and does not respond to therapy. He rapidly loses consciousness; his pupils become pin-point and nonreactive. He lays in a decerebrate posture. The physicians, in conjunction with his family, declare L. W. a "No Code."

7. Describe how the family might be approached about organ donation.

Case Study: Brain Tumor and Craniotomy

T. T. is a 19-year-old girl who is admitted for a craniotomy using a transsphenoidal approach to remove a pituitary adenoma. Her admitting symptoms include amenorrhea, headaches, and loss of vision in the upper gazes.

Address the following questions:

1. Describe the nursing history and assessment that would be required prior to surgery.

2. Develop a teaching/learning plan for T. T. about her surgery.

After surgery, T. T.'s vital signs are stable and she shows no signs of increased intracranial pressure. Her nose is packed open, and she has occasional anxiety about breathing through her mouth.

3. What interventions might be used to assist T. T. with mouth breathing? How often should oral care be given?

T. T. is having her intake and output recorded. Yesterday's intake was 1475 mL and her output was 1675 mL. Over the past 10 hours, she has had 500 mL intake with breakfast and 4450 mL output. She is complaining of thirst. The specific gravity of the urine is 1.002.

4. What is likely the cause of T. T.'s diuresis and what should the nurse do for T. T.?

5. Discuss the use of vasopressin (Pitressin) for T. T. What side effects should be observed for while the drug is used?

CHAPTER 45

Assessment of the Eye and Vision

LEARNING OBJECTIVES

At the end of this chapter, the student will be able to

▮ Review the anatomy and physiology of the eye

▮ Discuss the major functions of the eye

▮ Identify eye changes associated with aging

▮ Obtain a history of the client with eye problems

▮ Complete a physical assessment of a client's eyes and visual processes

▮ Identify the diagnostic tests used to aid in diagnosis of eye disorders

PREREQUISITE KNOWLEDGE

Prior to beginning this chapter, the student should review

▮ The anatomy and physiology of the eye

STUDY QUESTIONS

Anatomy and Physiology Review

1. Which of the following muscles is responsible for elevating the upper eyelid?

   a. superior oblique

   b. superior rectus

   c. levator palpebrae

   d. lateral rectus

Match the following extraocular muscles with their function. Answers may be used more than once.

_____ 2. inferior oblique	a. abducts the eye
_____ 3. inferior rectus	b. adducts the eye
_____ 4. lateral rectus	c. moves eye downward
_____ 5. medial rectus	d. moves eye upward
_____ 6. superior oblique	
_____ 7. superior rectus	

8. Which of the following statements is true about extraocular muscles?

   a. Rectus muscles exert their primary force when the eye is turned inward.

   b. Oblique muscles exert their primary force when the eye is turned outward.

   c. Extraocular muscles work in an agonistic relationship to position the eyes.

   d. Eye muscles position each eye's optic disk to receive visual images.

Match the following terms about the eyes (9–27) with their definitions (a–s).

_____ 9. aqueous humor

_____ 10. cilia

_____ 11. ciliary processes

_____ 12. cones

_____ 13. conjunctiva

_____ 14. cornea

_____ 15. fovea centralis

_____ 16. irido-corneal angle

_____ 17. iris

_____ 18. lacrimal fluid

_____ 19. lens

_____ 20. optic disk

_____ 21. orbit

_____ 22. puncta

_____ 23. pupil

_____ 24. retina

_____ 25. rods

_____ 26. sclera

_____ 27. vitreous body

a. bony cavity that protects the eye

b. responsible for peripheral vision

c. needed for acuity and color vision

d. central circular opening

e. colored portion of the eye

f. secretes aqueous humor

g. transparent layer over the anterior eye

h. white opaque layer of the eye

i. thin layer of eyeball where nerve endings are located

j. point where optic nerve enters the eyeball

k. the area of most acute vision

l. responsible for light refraction

m. fluid that fills anterior and posterior eye chambers

n. gelatinous substance giving shape to the posterior eye

o. spaces between the anterior chamber and the canal of Schlemm

p. thin mucous membrane lining the lids and the front of the eye

q. tiny hairs that protect the eye from particles

r. fluid that moistens corneal surface

s. channels at innermost eyelid margins where tears drain

Match the following cranial nerves with their functions.

_____ 28. cranial nerve II (optic)

_____ 29. cranial nerve III (oculomotor)

_____ 30. cranial nerve V (trigeminal)

_____ 31. cranial nerve VII (facial)

a. corneal reflex

b. visual acuity

c. eyelid closure

d. eye muscle movements

Match the following terms about vision problems (32–36) with their definitions (a–e).

_____ 32. astigmatism

_____ 33. emmetropia

_____ 34. hyperopia

_____ 35. myopia

_____ 36. presbyopia

a. ideal refraction of the eye

b. refraction power is too strong

c. loss of accommodation due to aging

d. refractive error due to an irregular curvature

e. insufficient refracting power

37. Identify the causes of the following 10 eye changes associated with aging.

a. visual acuity decreases: _____

_____

_____

b. eyes appear sunken: _____

_____

_____

c. inability to maintain an upward gaze: _____

_____

_____

d. arcus senilis: _____

_____

_____

e. astigmatism: _____

_____

_____

f. sclera become yellow: _____

_____

_____

g. loss of night vision: _____

_____

_____

h. color perception decreases: _____

_____

_____

i. cataracts: _____

_____

_____

j. presbyopia: _____

_____

_____

Subjective Assessment

38. List the subjective client data relevant to the eye. Use a separate sheet.

39. Briefly discuss the significance of questioning a client about sports activities when performing eye assessment. Use a separate sheet.

40. Identify ocular signs and symptoms that may be the result of a reaction to systemic medications.

a. _____

b. _____

c. _____

d. _____

e. _____

f. _____

g. _____

h. _____

41. The following is a partial client history. Select those data that are relevant to a subjective assessment and discuss their significance. Submit the completed exercise to the clinical instructor.

A 74-year-old female client wearing eyeglasses with bifocal lenses and hearing aid in left ear. Walks with a shuffling gait, using a cane for support. Wearing house slippers and housedress. States, "My other doctor says I should have my eyes looked at by an expert. It's been awhile and my eyes seem to be acting up lately—can't see so good anymore." The client states that she takes medication for "sugar" and her blood pressure and has worn glasses for years, with the last prescription change about 3 years ago. "I was a seamstress for many years and quit when I couldn't see to thread the needles anymore—just in time too. These new materials are too hard to work with!" Denies using any eye drops. Describes vision changes as difficulty seeing well at night, especially if trying to read. Uses a magnifying glass to help when reading. No eye pain or discharge, although eyes sometimes feel "dry and scratchy," with the left eye being worse than the right. Admits to rubbing eyes but without relief.

Objective Assessment

42. List the objective client data relevant to the eye. Use a separate sheet.

43. Using the client situation in question 41, discuss what the nurse should do to perform a physical assessment. Submit the completed exercise to the clinical instructor.

Match the following assessment techniques (44–49) with their related physical findings (a–f).

____ 44. cardinal gaze positions

____ 45. confrontation

____ 46. corneal light reflex

____ 47. count fingers

____ 48. cover/uncover test

____ 49. a Snellen chart

a. alignment of antero-posterior axes

b. visual acuity

c. peripheral vision

d. eye drifting

e. eye muscle strength

f. gross estimate of visual acuity

50. Which of the following pupil diameters is abnormal?

a. 1 mm

b. 3 mm

c. 4 mm

d. 5 mm

51. Which of the following findings is abnormal in the confrontation test?

    a. chalazion

    b. nystagmus

    c. scotoma

    d. strabismus

52. Which of the following findings is abnormal in an ophthalmoscopic examination?

    a. bright foveal reflection

    b. red glare from the pupil

    c. nasal margin of optic disk blurred

    d. presence of arteriole or venule nicking

53. When preparing for fluorescein angiography, the nurse should inform the client that

    a. a yellow dye will be instilled into the eye

    b. urine voided following the test will be green

    c. a local anesthetic will be instilled into the eye

    d. the ingested radioisotope is not harmful

CRITICAL THINKING EXERCISES

Case Study: Eye Examination

J. P. is a 66-year-old client who is being seen in the eye clinic. He is wearing bifocal lenses. J. P. is to have his intraocular pressure measured with applanation tonometry.

Address the following questions:

1. How does applanation tonometry differ from the other techniques used to measure intraocular pressure?

2. What should the nurse tell J. P. to prepare him for the test?

3. What specific instructions does J. P. need to assist him to be as cooperative as possible during the test?

4. The tonometer readings are O.D. = 20 mmHg and O.S. = 25 mmHg. What do these findings mean?

5. What instructions should the nurse provide to J. P. following the test?

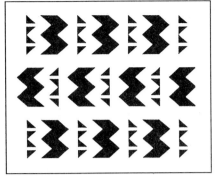

C H A P T E R 4 6

Interventions for Clients with Eye and Visual Problems

LEARNING OBJECTIVES

At the end of this chapter, the student will be able to

- Identify the various disorders of the eyelid and their related treatment
- Identify and manage care for the client with lacrimal apparatus disorders
- Identify the various conjunctival disorders and describe the related treatments
- Identify the various types of corneal disorders and related treatments
- Discuss episcleritis
- Manage care for the client with cataracts
- Manage care for the client with glaucoma
- Manage care for the client with uveitis
- Manage care for the client with retinopathy
- Manage care for the client with a retinal detachment
- Discuss the correction of refractive errors
- Identify the types of traumatic disorders to the eye

- Discuss ocular melanoma and related management
- Describe ocular manifestations of acquired immunodeficiency syndrome (AIDS)
- Discuss management of the client who is blind

PREREQUISITE KNOWLEDGE

Prior to beginning this chapter, the student should review

- The anatomy and physiology of the eye
- Care of the client with contact lenses
- How to tell a blind person the location of items in a room and on a food tray
- The procedure for instillation of eyedrops and ointments
- The concepts of body image and self-esteem
- The concepts of loss and grief
- The principles of perioperative nursing management

STUDY QUESTIONS

External Eye Disorders

Match the following eyelid disorders (1–6) with their descriptions (a–f).

_____ 1. blepharitis

_____ 2. chalazion

_____ 3. ectropion

_____ 4. entropion

_____ 5. hordeolum

_____ 6. ptosis

a. inverted lid margin

b. lid eversion

c. gland infection at lid/lash margin

d. granulomatous inflammation

e. drooping upper lid

f. eyelid margin inflammation

7. The client who is to instill an ophthalmic ointment should be instructed to

   a. rub the eyelid to distribute the ointment

   b. use a cotton swab to apply the ointment

   c. squeeze the ointment inside the lower lid

   d. refrain from blinking after instillation

8. Which of the following statements is true about keratoconjunctivitis sicca and its management?

   a. Artificial tears (Hypotears) decrease daytime dryness.

   b. Injury to the trigeminal nerve can inhibit tearing.

   c. Warm, moist compresses help restore moisture to the eye.

   d. Massaging the lacrimal glands stimulates tear production.

9. Identify interventions for the client with dry eye syndrome.

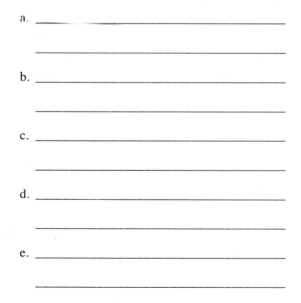

a. _____

   _____

b. _____

   _____

c. _____

   _____

d. _____

   _____

e. _____

   _____

Match the following conjunctival disorders (10–13) with their descriptions (a–d).

_____ 10. inflammatory conjunctivitis

_____ 11. bacterial conjunctivitis

_____ 12. subconjunctival hemorrhage

_____ 13. trachoma

a. has an insect vector

b. easily transmitted infection

c. often seasonal in nature

d. result of local increased pressure

14. The nurse should instruct the client with conjunctival disorders about

   a. using commercial eyedrops to reduce irritations

   b. avoiding cross-contamination from one eye to the other

   c. instillation of steroidal ophthalmic solutions

   d. wearing hypoallergenic make-up until irritation resolves

Match the following corneal disorders (15–18) with their descriptions (a–d).

_____ 15. corneal ulcer

_____ 16. dystrophy

_____ 17. keratitis

_____ 18. keratoconus

a. abnormal depositing of substances resulting in changes in corneal structure

b. degenerative thinning and forward protrusion of cornea

c. break in the corneal epithelium

d. corneal inflammation

19. Identify three common bacteria that can result in infected corneal ulcers.

a.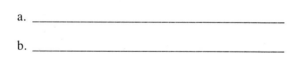

b. _____

c. _____

20. Which of the following clients are at increased risk for corneal disorders?

   a. a 15-year-old who wears contact lenses

   b. a 36-year-old using hedge trimmers wearing safety glasses

   c. a 55-year-old client who has had a renal transplantation

   d. a 19-year-old who is comatose following head trauma

   e. a 2-year-old cross-country skier wearing ski goggles

   f. an 82-year-old who has had a cerebrovascular accident

   g. a 46-year-old with Bell's palsy

21. List the subjective client data relevant to corneal disorders. Use a separate sheet.

22. List the objective client data relevant to corneal disorders. Use a separate sheet.

23. Which of the following statements is true about the administration of eye medications?

    a. Wait at least 3 minutes between instillations when instilling several medications in one eye.

    b. Both hands should be gloved when instilling any eye medications.

    c. Multidose bottles of eyedrops may be used for several clients.

    d. Hand washing is mandatory before and after administering eyedrops.

24. Postoperative care of the client following corneal transplant includes

    a. approaching the client from the operative side

    b. turning the client to the operative side

    c. setting up the client's meal trays

    d. elevating the head of the bed 15 degrees

25. Discharge instructions for the client following corneal transplant include

    a. encouraging the client to play with a pet for diversion

    b. keeping a list of emergency numbers near the telephone

    c. engaging in light exercise such as grocery shopping

    d. discontinuing use of the eyeshield 1 week postoperatively

26. Which of the following statements is correct about scleral disorders?

    a. A blue sclera is a common finding in middle-aged adults.

    b. Corticosteroids halve the duration of episcleritis.

    c. Episcleritis is associated with other systemic diseases.

    d. Episcleritis often leads to further scleral involvement.

Intraocular Disorders

27. Which of the following statements is true about cataracts?

    a. Some degree of cataract formation is expected in anyone over the age of 50 years.

    b. Any event that destroys lens capsule integrity can lead to a traumatic cataract.

    c. L-Sorbitol is responsible for cataract formation in clients with hypoparathyroidism.

    d. Lens opacification due to the aging process can be prevented with dietary management.

28. List the subjective client data relevant to cataracts. Use a separate sheet.

29. List the objective client data relevant to cataracts. Use a separate sheet.

30. Postoperative complications of cataract surgery include

    a. decreased intraocular pressure

    b. increased photophobia

    c. systemic hypertension

    d. intraocular hemorrhage

31. List activities that the client who has had cataract surgery should avoid. Use a separate sheet.

32. Briefly discuss the advantages and disadvantages of treating aphakia with eyeglasses compared with contact lenses. Use a separate sheet.

33. Which of the following statements about glaucoma is true?

    a. It is the most common cause of blindness in the United States.

    b. Increased pressure on the optic disk causes visual loss.

    c. Primary open-angle glaucoma is considered an emergency.

    d. Warning signs include gradual loss of central vision.

34. List the subjective client data relevant to glaucoma. Use a separate sheet.

35. List the objective client data relevant to glaucoma. Use a separate sheet.

36. Complete the following chart for medications used in the treatment of glaucoma. Use a separate sheet.

Medication	Purpose	Nursing Implications
a. pilocarpine hydrochloride (Pilocar)		
b. timolol (Timoptic)		
c. acetazolamide (Diamox)		
d. oral glycerin (Osmoglyn)		

37. A diabetic client with a history of glaucoma is being prepared for surgery. Which of the following medications orders should the nurse clarify with the physician?

    a. meperidine hydrochloride (Demerol) 100 mg intramuscularly preoperatively

    b. regular insulin 5 units subcutaneously the morning of surgery

    c. atropine sulfate 0.5 mg intramuscularly preoperatively

    d. diazepam (Valium) 5 mg orally the morning before surgery

38. Which of the following statements is correct about uveitis?

    a. Anterior uveitis is an inflammation of the retina.

    b. Posterior uveitis is an inflammation of the iris.

    c. Treatment is primarily symptomatic because a cure is not possible.

    d. Adhesions between the iris and the lens are complications.

39. Nursing management of the client with uveitis includes

    a. applying an occlusive eye shield to the eye

    b. keeping the room darkened

    c. encouraging light activity such as reading

    d. patching the affected eye

40. Which of the following is an appropriate nursing diagnosis for the client with uveitis?

    a. Sleep Pattern Disturbance

    b. Ineffective Individual Coping

    c. Impaired Physical Mobility

    d. Impaired Adjustment

Retinal Disorders

41. List the retinal changes that occur in hypertensive retinopathy. Use a separate sheet.

42. Which of the following statements about diabetic retinopathy is true?

    a. It is the leading cause of vision loss in the elderly.

    b. Incidence and severity increase over time in diabetics.

    c. Controlling blood sugar prevents retinopathy from occurring.

    d. Photocoagulation therapy affects both central and peripheral vision.

43. Which of the following statements about retinal detachment is true?

    a. It can be directly prevented by prompt intervention.

    b. Hyperopia is directly associated with its occurrence.

    c. High-risk activities include playing tennis or racquetball.

    d. Extracapsular cataract extraction reduces the risk of retinal detachment.

44. List the subjective client data relevant to retinal detachment. Use a separate sheet.

45. List the objective client data relevant to retinal detachment. Use a separate sheet.

46. Following a scleral buckling procedure involving a gas bubble insertion, the client should be positioned

    a. supine

    b. in high-Fowler's position

    c. in Trendelenburg's position

    d. toward the operative side

Refractive Errors

Match the following types of refractive errors (47–51) with their definitions (a–e).

_____ 47. aphakia

_____ 48. astigmatism

_____ 49. hyperopia

_____ 50. myopia

_____ 51. presbyopia

a. refractive ability is too weak

b. lens is unable to change shape

c. refractive ability is too strong

d. unequal light refraction in all directions

e. lens is absent, focus ability is lost

52. Instructions for the client who will wear contact lenses include

    a. encouraging the client to alternate hard lenses with eyeglasses until the eyes adjust

    b. teaching that soft lenses may be worn for most sports activities, including swimming

    c. reminding the client that lenses should be examined daily for nicks, scratches, and tears

    d. teaching that extended-wear lenses need to be removed once a day for cleaning and inspection

Traumatic Disorders

53. Nursing management of hyphema includes

    a. testing the client's extraocular muscle function daily

    b. instilling antibiotic eyedrops four times a day

    c. assisting the client with bathroom privileges

    d. restricting television watching and reading

54. Nursing management of contusion of the eye includes

    a. encouraging the client to lie supine quietly

    b. applying a warm compress immediately after the injury

    c. patching the eye closed until it can be examined

    d. flushing the eye with copious amounts of warm water

55. Nursing care of the client with a foreign body in the eye includes

    a. instructing the client to wear protective goggles when working with power tools

    b. assessing the client's visual acuity thoroughly after the eye is irrigated

    c. administering an intramuscular analgesic prior to irrigating the eye

    d. directing the irrigating solution across the cornea toward the inner canthus

56. Nursing care of the client with an eye laceration includes

    a. removing a penetrating object from the injured eye as carefully as possible

    b. asking the client about allergies to penicillin and sulfa drugs

    c. applying a pressure dressing and eyeshield over the injured eye at the scene

    d. reassuring the client that vision will be restored following surgery

57. Nursing care of the client with chemical burns to the eye includes

    a. determining the pH of the irritating chemical before starting to irrigate the eye

    b. using an irrigating solution that will neutralize the chemical irritant

    c. assessing the client's visual acuity following the irrigation procedure

    d. irrigating first one eye then the other if both eyes are involved

Ocular Melanoma

58. Identify which of the following descriptions about ocular melanoma are true.

    a. frequently found in uveal tract

    b. spreads easily

    c. wart-like growth on eyelid

    d. usually found on routine examination

    e. slow, painless growth

    f. treated by surgical excision

    g. diagnosed with ultrasonography

    h. treated with radioactive disks

    i. diagnosed by biopsy

    j. outpatient surgery

    k. inpatient surgery and hospitalization

59. Define *enucleation*. Use a separate sheet.

60. Postoperative nursing care of the client with an enucleation includes

    a. reporting any sign of bright red drainage on the dressing to the ophthalmologist

    b. assisting the client to achieve psychological readjustment by discharge time

    c. teaching the client exercises to increase visual acuity in the remaining eye

    d. discouraging the client from wearing glasses because it will call attention to the face

61. Develop a teaching/learning plan for the client undergoing radioactive therapy for malignant melanoma of the eye. Submit the completed exercise to the clinical instructor on a separate sheet.

Ocular Manifestations of HIV

Match the following ocular changes related to AIDS (62–70) with their disease processes (a–c). Answers may be used more than once.

_____ 62. chronic blepharitis   a. Kaposi's sarcoma

_____ 63. cotton wool exudates   b. AIDS retinopathy

     c. cytomegaloretinitis

_____ 64. discoloration on eyelid

_____ 65. optic nerve atrophy

_____ 66. papilledema

_____ 67. recurrent conjunctival hemorrhages

_____ 68. retinal hemorrhages

_____ 69. retinitis

_____ 70. keratitis

Blindness

71. Which of the following clients is classified as being legally blind? The client whose vision with correction is

    a. 20/100

    b. 20/150

    c. 20/180

    d. 20/240

72. Complete the following chart listing examples of nursing interventions that assist the blind client with orientation, ambulation, and self-care. Use a separate sheet.

Orientation	Ambulation	Self-Care
a.	a.	a.
b.	b.	b.
c.	c.	c.
d.	d.	d.
e.		e.
f.		f.
g.		
h.		

73. Describe how the nurse assists a client who has had limited vision for a long time to eat from a meal tray.

_____

_____

_____

_____

_____

_____

_____

_____

_____

_____

CRITICAL THINKING EXERCISES

Case Study: Cataract Surgery

D. K. is an 85-year-old widow who has had a cataract removed by extracapsular cataract extraction (ECCE) and an intraocular lens implanted (IOC). She is being dismissed to the care of her 80-year-old friend, who also has failing vision. The two women live together in a small apartment in a retirement complex.

Address the following questions:

1. What assessments should the nurse make concerning the home environment?

2. Plan a teaching guide for D. K.'s home care. Consider how this information can best be taught.

3. D. K. tells the nurse that she and her friend have two house cats. What information should the nurse discuss with D. K. concerning these animals?

4. The physician orders prednisolone acetate suspension (Metimyd) 0.2% eye drops, one drop qid, to the operative eye, which D. K. is to instill for one week. Discuss the procedure for instilling the eye drops with D. K. What assessments should the nurse make?

Case Study: Retinal Detachment

C. R. is a 45-year-old client who has had progressive myopia and astigmatism since age 11 years. She wears eyeglasses and has satisfactory correction. At age 37, C. R. was told by her ophthalmologist that she had retinal "latticing" (multiple fine-grade holes) in the temporal segments of each retina. C. R. has an eye examination about every 3 years.

Address the following questions:

1. At her last examination, the ophthalmologist advised C. R. to give up playing tennis and volleyball. Why did the physician say this? What are C. R.'s risk factors? How can she reduce her risk?

C. R. is working in her yard trimming hedges with an electric clipper. Despite wearing her eyeglasses, a branch whips backward and strikes C. R. in the left eye. C. R. immediately sees a bright flash of light and then a shadow when looking downward and in toward her nose.

2. What should C. R. do?

C. R. is admitted to the hospital and scheduled for an emergency scleral buckling.

3. What instructions should the nurse give to C. R. about her activity, diet, and postoperative care?

4. Postoperatively, C. R. reports being nauseated. There is an order for prochlorperazine (Compazine) 10 mg IM every 6 hours PRN. C. R. had a dose just 4 hours ago. What should the nurse do?

5. The day after surgery, the ophthalmologist removes the eye patch and examines C. R.'s eye. Later she looks in a mirror and exclaims, "My eye is all red and everything is blurred!" What should the nurse say to C. R.?

6. Four days after surgery, C. R. is discharged. Devise a discharge teaching/learning plan for her. Identify factors that should be assessed in the home environment.

7. C. R. tells the nurse that she is looking forward to going home because she wants to be able to work outside in her garden for relaxation. What should the nurse say?

CHAPTER 47

Assessment of the Ear and Hearing

LEARNING OBJECTIVES

At the end of this chapter, the student will be able to

▮ Review the anatomy and physiology of the ear

▮ Describe hearing

▮ Identify ear changes associated with aging

▮ Obtain a history of the client with a hearing disorder

▮ Complete a physical assessment of the client with a hearing disorder

▮ Identify diagnostic measures to assess hearing disorders

PREREQUISITE KNOWLEDGE

Prior to beginning this chapter, the student should review

▮ The anatomy and physiology of the ear

STUDY QUESTIONS

Anatomy and Physiology Review

Match the following structures of the ear (1–21) with their locations (a–c). Answers may be used more than once.

_____ 1. auricle

_____ 2. cochlea

_____ 3. eustachian tube

_____ 4. scala tympani

_____ 5. mastoid process

_____ 6. malleus

_____ 7. semicircular canal

_____ 8. perilymph

_____ 9. tympanic membrane

_____ 10. stapes

_____ 11. pars tensa

_____ 12. cranial nerve VIII

_____ 13. tragus

_____ 14. scala vestibuli

_____ 15. umbo

_____ 16. cerumen

_____ 17. organ of Corti

_____ 18. pars flaccida

_____ 19. incus

_____ 20. endolymph

_____ 21. helix

a. external ear

b. middle ear

c. inner ear

22. List the two functions of the ear.

    a. _____

    b. _____

23. Put in sequence the following events that lead to the sensation of hearing.

    _____ a. staples vibrates

    _____ b. sound waves strike the mastoid and tympanic membrane

    _____ c. sound wave vibrations enter the cochlea

    _____ d. sound is processed and interpreted by the brain

    _____ e. sound waves are transmitted through the air

    _____ f. eighth cranial nerve is innervated

    _____ g. malleus is set into vibration

24. Which of the following changes in the ear is related to aging?

    a. Hearing acuity for high-frequency sounds increases.

    b. The pinna becomes atrophied, shorter, and thickened.

    c. Cerumen dries, leading to impaction and hearing loss.

    d. Unsteadiness results from cochlear degeneration.

Subjective Assessment

25. List the subjective data relevant to hearing loss. Use a separate sheet.

26. During the history, a client reports taking a number of medications. Which of the client's following medications is ototoxic?

    a. digoxin (Lanoxin) 0.25 mg qd

    b. potassium chloride (K-lyte) one packet tid

    c. methyldopa (Aldomet) 500 mg tid

    d. furosemide (Lasix) 40 mg bid

27. The following is a partial client history. Select those data relevant to a subjective assessment of the ear and discuss their significance. Submit the completed exercise to the clinical instructor.

    A 68-year-old female client wearing eyeglasses. Sitting in chair, leaning forward. Maintains continuous eye contact. Occasionally asks that questions be repeated, stating she did not understand what was meant. No difficulty standing and walking to the examination table. Reports that her mother and maternal grandmother were "stone deaf" by the age of 70. Concerned about her own hearing because her family has told her that she does not always respond when they talk to her. Long-standing history of sinus problems and multiple earaches as a child, with several ruptures of each ear drum. No current ear pain or discharge. Smoked for 40 years, quitting at age 60. Uses cotton applicator to clean ears approximately every 2 weeks. Prefers tub bath, but showers daily because has difficulty getting in and out of a tub. Takes aspirin four times a day for joint stiffness. Lives alone with cat.

Objective Assessment

28. List the objective data relevant to hearing. Use a separate sheet.

29. When examining the external ear with an otoscope, the nurse should

    a. visualize the location of the incus and stapes

    b. inspect the integrity of the tympanic membrane

    c. displace the pinna downward and back in an adult

    d. position the otoscope with the nondominant hand

Match the following terms (30–33) with their definitions (a–d).

_____ 30. conductive hearing loss

_____ 31. lateralization

_____ 32. sensorineural hearing loss

_____ 33. tinnitus

a. hearing loss due to a defect in nerve conduction

b. ringing in the ears

c. hearing loss due to obstruction of sound wave transmission

d. sound heard louder in one ear

34. Which of the following statements is correct about auditory assessment?

    a. The voice test is a simple test for hearing acuity.

    b. Lateralization is indicative of a sensorineural loss.

    c. Bone conduction is twice as long as air conduction.

    d. Slight swaying is an abnormal finding on the Romberg test.

35. List two laboratory tests that may be done on ear discharge.

    a. _____

    _____

    _____

    b. _____

    _____

    _____

Match the following terms about hearing testing (36–41) with their definitions (a–f).

_____ 36. audiogram

_____ 37. audiometry

_____ 38. frequency

_____ 39. intensity

_____ 40. masking

_____ 41. threshold

a. volume of a pure tone

b. introduction of background noise to the nontested ear

c. lowest level of volume that a sound is heard

d. measurement of hearing acuity

e. high or low pitch of a pure tone

f. recording of a pure tone hearing acuity test

42. Which of the following individuals is at greatest risk for developing hearing loss? Give a rationale for your answer on a separate sheet.

    a. lead singer in a rock music band

    b. percussionist in a symphony orchestra

    c. baggage handler at an international airport

    d. logger who works for the national forest service

43. Results of an audiogram

    a. are extremely accurate for diagnostic purposes

    b. indicate the cause of the hearing loss

    c. determine the type of hearing loss by the configuration

    d. reveal that any hearing loss is often bilaterally equal

44. Briefly discuss the difference between speech reception threshold and speech discrimination. Use a separate sheet.

45. Tympanometry is a

    a. test to help determine inner ear problems such as otosclerosis

    b. subjective procedure to assess ear drum mobility

    c. procedure used to diagnose serous otitis

    d. way to assess eustachian tube patency

CRITICAL THINKING EXERCISES

Case Study: Ear Examination

J. T. is a 58-year-old man who is being seen in the ears, nose, and throat (ENT) clinic. During the history, he reports that he often has difficulty hearing what is being said to him and that this is causing problems in his job. His chief complaint today is that his ears are "plugged" and he feels as thought his head "is in a fishbowl." The nurse inspects J. T.'s ears and notes dried, brown drainage in the external meatus. Attempts to insert an otoscope are unsuccessful because dried cerumen obstructs both canals.

Address the following questions:

1. Discuss what the nurse should do next.

After J. T.'s ear canals are cleaned, otoscopic examination is again attempted. The canals appear dark pink, and white patches are noted at the ends of the canals, near the annulus and partially obstructing the tympanic membrane. The physician is consulted, and it is determined that J. T. has a fungal infection of the external ear. A prescription is written for acetic acid with hydrocortisone (VoSol HC otic solution), five drops into both ear canals tid.

2. Develop a teaching/learning plan for J. T. about the administration of the ear drops.

3. What should the nurse discuss with J. T. concerning ear hygiene?

The physician advises J. T. that his hearing should be tested once the infection is resolved. Appointments are scheduled for complete audiometry and tympanogram.

4. What information should the nurse discuss with J. T. about these tests? What must J. T. do to prepare for his appointments?

J. T. has the audiogram and tympanogram. The tympanogram is normal. Results of the pure tone audiogram indicate sensorineural loss in both ears, with the right ear being worse than the left. Speech reception threshold is 25–30 dB in the left ear and 35–40 dB in the right. Speech discrimination is 85% for the left ear and 70% for the right.

5. Discuss the meaning of these test results.

6. Formulate relevant nursing diagnoses for J. T. based on the above data.

7. What information should the nurse discuss with J. T. about self-care and learning to live with his hearing loss?

C H A P T E R 4 8

Interventions for Clients with Ear and Hearing Problems

LEARNING OBJECTIVES

At the end of this chapter, the student will be able to

- Identify conditions affecting the external ear
- Discuss external otitis
- Discuss otitis media and related management
- Discuss mastoiditis and related treatment
- Discuss otosclerosis and related management
- Discuss growths in the middle ear
- Discuss conditions of the inner ear
- Discuss Ménière's syndrome and related management
- Discuss the types of hearing loss and identify the causes of hearing loss
- Discuss interventions for the client with hearing loss

PREREQUISITE KNOWLEDGE

Prior to beginning this chapter, the student should review

- The anatomy and physiology of the ear
- The maintenance of hearing aids
- The procedure for instillation of ear drops and ear irrigations
- The concepts of body image and self-esteem
- The principles of perioperative nursing management

STUDY QUESTIONS

External Ear Conditions

1. List four conditions affecting the external ear.

   a. _____

   _____

   _____

   b. _____

   _____

   _____

   c. _____

   _____

   _____

   d. _____

   _____

   _____

2. List the subjective data relevant to otitis externa. Use a separate sheet.

3. List the objective data relevant to otitis externa. Use a separate sheet.

4. A client with otitis externa is being treated with antibiotic eardrops and has an earwick in place. After instilling the drops for the second day, the client experiences increased ear pain and calls the physician's office. The nurse should

    a. advise the client to withhold the next two doses and try again after the ear has had a chance to recover

    b. instruct the client to apply warm, moist compresses to the ear three or four times a day for 20 minutes

    c. suggest that the client switch to another analgesic and take it 45 minutes before instilling the drops

    d. instruct the client to discontinue the medication and come into the office for further evaluation

5. Preventive measures for swimmer's ear include

    a. instilling alcohol drops into the ear canals before swimming

    b. wearing snug-fitting earplugs whenever in the water

    c. drying the canals with cotton applicators after swimming

    d. swimming only in chlorinated swimming pools or hot tubs

6. Describe the characteristics of a furuncle of the external ear. Use a separate sheet.

7. Briefly discuss why water at body temperature is used to irrigate the external ear to remove excess cerumen. Use a separate sheet.

Middle Ear Conditions

Match the following characteristics (8–13) with the associated types of otitis media (a–c). Answers may be used more than once.

_____ 8. may follow repeated ear infections

_____ 9. may be a long-term complication of acute otitis

_____ 10. sterile fluid accumulates

_____ 11. sudden onset

_____ 12. associated with greater damage to middle ear structures

_____ 13. duration less than 3 weeks

    a. acute

    b. chronic

    c. serous

14. List the subjective data relevant to otitis media. Use a separate sheet.

15. List the objective data relevant to otitis media. Use a separate sheet.

16. Which of the following assessment findings are associated only with otitis media?

    a. fever and malaise

    b. itching

    c. tinnitus

    d. bulging of tympanic membrane

    e. redness of canal

17. Define *myringotomy*. Use a separate sheet.

18. Which of the following client data indicates that treatment for otitis media is ineffective?

    a. return of hearing acuity

    b. onset of vertigo and nausea

    c. reduction of fever

    d. negative Romberg's test

19. Mastoiditis is an inflammation of the

    a. bones in the middle ear

    b. temporal bone behind the ear

    c. labyrinth structure

    d. cranial nerves VI and VII

20. Postoperative management following a mastoidectomy includes

    a. elevating the head of the bed 15 degrees

    b. positioning the client on the operative side

    c. encouraging strict bed rest for 2–3 days

    d. allowing the client bathroom privileges with help

21. List the three causes of trauma to the tympanic membrane and ossicles.

22. Otosclerosis is primarily characterized by

    a. conductive hearing loss

    b. sensorineural hearing loss

    c. hearing loss of the mixed type

    d. ataxia and loss of balance

23. Otosclerosis is

    a. preventable

    b. a disease of old age

    c. more prevalent in men

    d. linked with a strong family history

24. List the subjective data relevant to otosclerosis. Use a separate sheet.

25. List the objective data relevant to otosclerosis. Use a separate sheet.

26. Which of the following statements are correct about cholesteatoma?

    a. It is a malignant growth of the middle ear.

    b. It is a cauliflower-like growth on or behind the tympanic membrane.

    c. It can invade the ossicles, mastoid, labyrinth, and facial nerve.

    d. Facial paralysis results from cranial nerve VIII involvement.

    e. Surgical removal is necessary.

Inner Ear Conditions

27. Identify five causes of tinnitus.

    a. _____

    _____

    b. _____

    _____

    c. _____

    _____

    d. _____

    _____

    e. _____

    _____

    _____

28. Differentiate between dizziness and vertigo. Use a separate sheet.

29. List the three body systems that are involved in balance and provide input to the cerebellum.

    a. _____

    _____

    b. _____

    _____

    c. _____

    _____

30. The most serious complication of labyrinthitis is

    a. nausea

    b. vertigo

    c. nystagmus

    d. meningitis

31. Which of the following statements is correct about Ménière's syndrome?

    a. Increased endolymph enhances sound wave conduction.

    b. Vertigo is a result of damage to the vestibular system.

    c. Accompanying tinnitus is a result of ossicle damage.

    d. Hearing loss is reversible even with repeated attacks.

32. List the subjective data relevant to Ménière's syndrome. Use a separate sheet.

33. List the objective data relevant to Ménière's syndrome. Use a separate sheet.

34. Management of Ménière's syndrome includes

    a. instructing the client to use short, quick head and eye movements

    b. advising the client to include foods such as organ meats in the diet

    c. counseling the client to stop smoking because of its vasoconstrictive effect

    d. teaching the client to come to the physician's office at the first sign of an attack

35. An acoustic neuroma is

    a. benign and causes relatively few problems

    b. malignant and prone to metastasizing widely

    c. benign but potentially neurologically damaging

    d. malignant but slow growing with few damaging effects

Hearing Loss

36. Compare conductive and sensorineural hearing loss by completing the following chart on a separate sheet.

	Conductive	Sensorineural
a. transmission of sound waves through ear		
b. reversibility		
c. cranial nerve conduction		
d. results of the Weber test		
e. results of the Rinne test		
f. appearance of ear canal and tympanic membrane		

37. List the causes of conductive hearing loss. Use a separate sheet.

38. List the causes of sensorineural hearing loss. Use a separate sheet.

39. The client with a conductive hearing loss will

    a. complain of constant tinnitus in both ears

    b. speak loudly and ask others to speak up also

    c. hear best when there is some background noise

    d. become dizzy on occasion and feel nauseated

40. Define *presbycusis*. _____

    _____

    _____

41. Preventive measures for hearing loss include

    a. inserting earplugs or wearing a hat on windy days

    b. wearing rigid head gear when playing contact sports

    c. cleaning ear canals weekly with cotton-tipped applicators

    d. irrigating the ears at least monthly with warm water

42. Which of the following actions demonstrates proper care of a hearing aid?

    a. using sterile alcohol to clean the earmold

    b. storing the device with the battery left in

    c. inserting the device after using hair spray

    d. clipping the battery pack to an outside pocket

43. Identify materials that may be used to replace the ossicles in a tympanoplasty.

    a. _____

    _____

    b. _____

    _____

    c. _____

    _____

    d. _____

    _____

44. Which of the following statements is appropriate to include in the discharge instructions for the client who has had a tympanoplasty?

    a. "You may resume your usual activities any time as you begin to feel better."

    b. "You may go back to work in 2 or 3 days if your temperature remains normal."

    c. "You need to drink plenty of fluids, so use a straw if it will help."

    d. "You need to keep your ear dry, so take a tub bath rather than showering."

45. The client who has had a stapedectomy should be told which of the following statements?

    a. Hearing will improve significantly immediately after the surgery.

    b. Hearing will be worse right after the surgery but will improve.

    c. Hearing loss on the affected side is rare unless there is damage to cranial nerve VIII.

    d. Vertigo, nausea, and vomiting are rare complaints and do not respond to medication.

46. Briefly discuss what the nurse should do when attempting to communicate with a hearing-impaired client in the following situations. Use a separate sheet.

    a. an 82-year-old-man with cataracts and a hearing aid who is recovering from general anesthesia

    b. a 19-year-old girl who has been deaf since she was 6 months old and attended a special school for the deaf

    c. a 26-year-old man with traumatic injury to one ear from a blow to the head

CRITICAL THINKING EXERCISES

Case Study: Ménière's Syndrome

B. R. is a 57-year-old client who has suffered from Ménière's syndrome since his 30s. He reports having attacks of vertigo about twice a year, usually in the spring and fall. The episodes have become increasingly more severe; B. R. has been hospitalized for rehydration four times in the past 5 years. B. R. tells the nurse that he can feel his left ear stuff up, and the noise in that ear gets louder about a day or so before an attack. B. R. is scheduled for a labyrinthectomy the next day.

Address the following questions:

1. Discuss assessments that the nurse should do for B. R.
2. What information should the nurse clarify with B. R. about the surgical procedure?
3. Identify safety precautions the nurse should implement for B. R.

Postoperatively, B. R. has a dressing over the left ear and an intravenous infusion.

4. What assessments should the nurse perform for B. R.? Discuss the rationale for these.

When B. R. is dismissed, he states, "I am looking forward to living a normal life again. I never knew in advance how bad an attack would be or how long it would take to recover."

5. How should the nurse respond?
6. Design a discharge teaching/learning plan for B. R.

Case Study: Otosclerosis

H. N. is a 53-year-old client who has had progressive hearing loss since her late 20s. Her ability to hear is better with her right ear, although she has been using a hearing aid for the past 5 years. After being evaluated, it is determined that H. N. has otosclerosis. H. N. discusses options with her physician and decides to have a stapedectomy of the left ear.

Address the following questions:

1. Why is H. N.'s left ear going to be operated on instead of the right ear?
2. Develop a preoperative teaching/learning plan for H. N. What should the nurse discuss about the hearing aid?
3. Discuss alternatives for H. N. to cope with her reduced hearing ability until the surgery is performed.

When H. N. is admitted to the ENT unit preoperatively, she tells the nurse, "I don't know whether I'm more excited or more worried. I realize that the surgery may not work, but I just know I'll be O.K."

4. How should the nurse respond?

Postoperatively, H. N. is nauseated and states that she is dizzy when she tries to sit up. There is a physician's order for meclizine hydrochloride (Antivert) 25 mg PO, tid, and HS and for droperidol (Inapsine) 7.5 mg IM every 6 hours as needed.

5. What side effects should the nurse monitor for in H. N. while she is receiving these medications? What interventions are implemented for client safety?

Following removal of the external dressing, H. N. becomes upset and begins to cry. She states, "I don't notice any difference; in fact, I think it's worse! Now I can't hear anything with my right ear!"

6. What is the probable cause of H. N.'s hearing loss?
7. What can the nurse say to H. N. to assist her at this time?

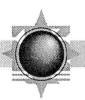

C H A P T E R 4 9

Assessment of the
Musculoskeletal System

LEARNING OBJECTIVES

At the end of this chapter, the student will be able to

- Describe the types, structure, function, growth, and metabolism of bones
- Describe the types, structure, and function of joints
- Describe the structure and function of skeletal muscles
- Identify facets in the client's history that may affect the musculoskeletal system
- Assess the musculoskeletal system
- Describe other tools to diagnose musculoskeletal disorders

PREREQUISITE KNOWLEDGE

Prior to beginning this chapter, the student should review

- The anatomy and physiology of the musculoskeletal system (muscles, bones, and joints)
- The physiology of muscle contraction
- Active and passive range-of-motion (ROM) exercises for each joint
- The effect of immobility on the musculoskeletal system
- The normal ROM for each joint

STUDY QUESTIONS

Anatomy and Physiology Review

1. Briefly describe how bone is a living tissue.

   _____

   _____

   _____

   _____

   _____

2. Which of the following hormones is primarily responsible for regulating serum calcium levels?

   a. growth hormone

   b. vitamin D

   c. parathyroid hormone

   d. calcitonin

3. Which of the following minerals is present in bone and serum in direct proportion to calcium?

   a. zinc

   b. phosphorus

   c. potassium

   d. iron

Match the following musculoskeletal terms (4–23) with their definitions (a–t).

_____ 4. atrophy

_____ 5. bursa

_____ 6. cartilage

_____ 7. cancellous

_____ 8. cortex

_____ 9. diaphysis

_____ 10. epiphysis

_____ 11. fascia

_____ 12. fasciculi

_____ 13. haversian system

_____ 14. ligament

_____ 15. osteoblast

_____ 16. osteoclast

_____ 17. osteocyte

_____ 18. periosteum

_____ 19. synovium

_____ 20. synovial fluid

_____ 21. tendon

_____ 22. trabeculae

_____ 23. Volkmann's canal

a. living bone cells

b. spongy inner layer of bone

c. membrane that secretes a lubricating fluid

d. decrease in size and number of muscle fibers

e. shaft of a long bone

f. network connecting bone marrow vessels to outer bone covering

g. sac preventing joint friction

h. band of tough, fibrous tissue attaching muscle to bone

i. bone-forming cells

j. bundles of muscle fibers

k. lubricating liquid

l. highly vascular bone covering

m. longitudinal canal network containing blood vessels

n. end of a long bone

o. band of tough, fibrous tissue attaching bone to bone

p. fibrous tissue surrounding muscle

q. bone-destroying cells

r. collagen fibers at bone ends

s. bone tissue containing marrow

t. outer layer of bone tissue

24. List the four common types of bones and give an example of each.

a. _____

_____

b. _____

_____

c. _____

_____

d. _____

_____

25. Identify the six major functions of the skeletal system.

a. _____

_____

b. _____

_____

c. _____

_____

d. _____

_____

e. _____

_____

f. _____

_____

26. List the three types of joints and give an example of each.

a. _____

_____

b. _____

_____

c. _____

_____

Match the following types of synovial joints (27–31) with their functions (a–e) and their examples (i–v).

_____ _____ 27. ball-and-socket

_____ _____ 28. biaxial

_____ _____ 29. condylar

_____ _____ 30. hinge

_____ _____ 31. pivotal

a. gliding movement

b. flex, extend only

c. rotation only

d. any direction

e. flex, extend, rotate

_____

i. knee

ii. radial/ulnar area

iii. elbow

iv. wrist

v. shoulder

32. List the three types of muscle tissue and identify their functions.

a. _____

_____

_____

b. _____

_____

_____

c. _____

_____

_____

33. Identify the changes that occur with the aging process in the following musculoskeletal system structures. Use a separate sheet.

a. bone tissue

b. muscle tissue

c. synovial joints

d. vertebral column

Subjective Assessment

34. List the subjective client data relevant to the musculoskeletal system. Use a separate sheet.

35. The following is a partial client history that is scrambled. Select the data that are pertinent and relevant to a musculoskeletal assessment. Submit the completed exercise to the clinical instructor.

African-American female, 68 years old. Fell and rolled down steep bank while fishing with grandson. Could not get up even with grandson's help because of pain in left thigh. Five feet, 3 inches tall, 240 pounds. Lying on ground over 2 hours before paramedics arrived. Retired, small pension, receives food stamps. Takes care of three grandchildren (6–14 years old) during daytime. Never hospitalized. Sees gynecologist (past 4 months) for vaginal bleeding and cardiologist (past year) for chest pain. Tires easily. Sits while ironing and preparing meals ("legs get weak"). Stays home mostly except to go to church and grocery shopping when someone is able to drive her. Fishing is favorite pastime.

Objective Assessment

36. List the objective client data relevant to the musculoskeletal system. Use a separate sheet.

37. Using the client history data from question 35, construct a physical assessment recording for the musculoskeletal system. Submit the completed exercise to the clinical instructor.

38. The instrument used to assess joint ROM is

a. an odometer

b. an ergometer

c. a goniometer

d. a spectrometer

39. Which of the following is an abnormal finding in the physical assessment of the musculoskeletal system?

a. upper extremities symmetric, equal muscle mass

b. gait balanced, stride smooth and regular

c. arms swing opposite to leg movements

d. thigh abductors and adductors rated 4 out of 5

40. Identify laboratory test results and their normal ranges that are specific to the musculoskeletal system. Use a separate sheet.

41. Identify radiographic examinations of the musculoskeletal system that require special preparation of the client.

a. _____

b. _____

c. _____

42. Which of the following diagnostic procedures involves injecting a radioactive material into the client?

a. bone biopsy

b. bone scan

c. electromyography

d. magnetic resonance imaging (MRI)

43. Which of the following assessments findings in the client who has just had a myelogram should the nurse report to the physician immediately?

a. headache unrelieved by analgesics

b. ability to dorsiflex right foot but not left

c. muscle spasms in lumbosacral area

d. intermittent nausea relieved with antiemetic

CHAPTER 50

Interventions for Clients with Musculoskeletal Problems

LEARNING OBJECTIVES

At the end of this chapter, the student will be able to

▌ Compare and contrast the pathophysiology, etiology, and incidence of various metabolic bone diseases

▌ Provide care for clients with metabolic bone diseases

▌ Discuss the pathophysiology, etiology, and management of the client with osteomyelitis

▌ Compare and contrast the types of benign bone tumors

▌ Provide care for the client with a benign bone tumor

▌ Compare and contrast the types of malignant bone tumors

▌ Provide care for the client with a malignant bone tumor

▌ Describe disorders of the hand

▌ Describe disorders of the foot

▌ Define and describe methods of treatment for scoliosis

▌ Define *osteogenesis imperfecta* and *muscular dystrophy*

PREREQUISITE KNOWLEDGE

Prior to beginning this chapter, the student should review

▌ The anatomy and physiology of the musculo-skeletal system (muscles, bones, and joints)

▌ The principles of perioperative nursing management

▌ Wound and skin isolation, contact isolation, and drainage precautions

▌ The metabolism of calcium and vitamin D

▌ The concepts of grief, loss, death, and dying

▌ The concepts of growth and development

▌ The concepts of body image and self-esteem

▌ The principles of intravenous therapy

STUDY QUESTIONS

Metabolic Bone Diseases

Match the following musculoskeletal disorders (1–3) with their pathophysiological features (a–c) and risk factors (i–iii).

____ ____ 1. osteo-
               porosis

____ ____ 2. osteo-
               malacia

____ ____ 3. Paget's
               disease

a. enlarged, weak, disorganized bone deposits

b. decreased bone density due to calcium loss

c. accumulation of poorly mineralized osteoid

i. elderly, vitamin D deficiency, insufficient exposure to sunlight

ii. possibly a result of latent viral infection

iii. female, Caucasian, menopause, immobilization, thin, lean

Match the following subjective client data (4–16) with the musculoskeletal disorders they are primarily associated with (a–c). Answers may be used more than once.

____ 4. headache

____ 5. dress hem longer in front

____ 6. muscle cramps

____ 7. smokes two packs of cigarettes per day

____ 8. back pain relieved by rest

____ 9. fatigue

____ 10. milk intolerance

____ 11. sedentary life style

____ 12. pelvic bone pain, worse at night

____ 13. drinks eight cups of coffee per day

____ 14. dizziness

____ 15. muscle weakness in legs

____ 16. loss of height

a. osteoporosis

b. osteomalacia

c. Paget's disease

Match the following objective client data (17–25) with the musculoskeletal disorders they are primarily associated with (a–c). Answers may be used more than once.

____ 17. unsteady gait

____ 18. hip flexion contractors

____ 19. flushed, warm skin

____ 20. vertebral fracture

____ 21. bone tenderness over rib cage

____ 22. kyphosis

____ 23. long bone bowing

____ 24. discomfort on vertebral palpation

____ 25. skull soft

a. osteoporosis

b. osteomalacia

c. Paget's disease

26. Identify factors that contribute to the bone pain perceived by clients with metabolic bone disease.

a. _____

_____

b. _____

_____

c. _____

_____

d. _____

_____

27. Identify the laboratory tests diagnostic for osteomalacia and Paget's disease. Use a separate sheet.

a. Osteomalacia

b. Paget's disease

c. Which of these laboratory tests requires that the client receive special instructions for managing the specimen collection?

28. List the radiographic tests commonly used to diagnose metabolic bone disease.

a. _____

_____

b. _____

_____

c. _____

_____

29. List the three common nursing diagnoses associated with osteoporosis and osteomalacia.

    a. _____

    _____

    b. _____

    _____

    c. _____

    _____

Match the following preventive measures (30–35) with the musculoskeletal disorders they are primarily associated with (a or b). Answers may be used more than once.

____ 30. exercise   a. osteoporosis

____ 31. sunlight   b. osteomalacia

____ 32. estrogen
         replacement

____ 33. vitamin D

____ 34. calcium
         supplement

____ 35. avoid alcohol, caffeine

36. Identify nursing measures used to help prevent client falls and possible resultant fractures.

    a. _____

    _____

    b. _____

    _____

    c. _____

    _____

    d. _____

    _____

37. Identify three classes of drugs commonly taken by elderly clients that may contribute to fractures.

    a. _____

    b. _____

    c. _____

38. Compare two drugs commonly used to treat osteoporosis by completing the following chart on a separate sheet. Submit the completed exercise to the clinical instructor.

	Conjugated Estrogen	Calcium Supplement
a. class		
b. pharmacodynamics		
c. side effects		
d. does range and frequency		
e. nursing implications		

39. Compile a list of foods that the osteoporotic client should consume, as well as a list of foods this client should avoid. Use a separate sheet.

40. Interventions for the client with Paget's disease include

    a. teaching the client how to apply a back brace

    b. maintaining bed rest until pain episodes subside

    c. clustering activities to provide longer rest periods

    d. discouraging naps to promote sleeping at night

Osteomyelitis

41. List the two major types of osteomyelitis and differentiate between them.

    a. _____

    _____

    b. _____

    _____

42. Define the term *sequestrum*. Use a separate sheet.

43. Briefly describe the pathophysiological process in osteomyelitis. Use a separate sheet.

44. List and define three routes of inoculation resulting in bone infection. Use a separate sheet.

45. Identify the risk factors for developing osteomyelitis in the following types of bone infections. Use a separate sheet.

    a. acute hematogenous

    b. direct inoculation

    c. contiguous spread

46. List the subjective client data relevant to bone infection. Use a separate sheet.

47. List the objective client data relevant to bone infection. Use a separate sheet.

48. Which of the following statements is correct about antibiotic therapy for the client with osteomyelitis?

   a. Single-agent therapy is the most effective treatment for acute infections.

   b. The optimal drug regimen for chronic osteomyelitis is well established.

   c. Clients usually remain hospitalized to complete the full course of antibiotic therapy.

   d. The infected wound may be irrigated with one or more types of antibiotic solutions.

49. Interventions to promote healing in the client with osteomyelitis include

   a. strengthening and ROM exercises

   b. increasing calories and protein in the diet

   c. teaching about foods high in vitamins and calcium

   d. all of the above

Bone Tumors

Match the following terms related to bone tumors (50–55) with their definitions (a–f).

_____ 50. chondrogenic

_____ 51. fibrogenic

_____ 52. osteogenic

_____ 53. primary tumor

_____ 54. sarcoma

_____ 55. secondary tumor

   a. tumor originating in bone

   b. arising from bone

   c. malignant tumor metastasizing to bone

   d. arising from cartilage

   e. arising from fibrous tissue

   f. malignant bone tumor arising from underlying tissue

Match the following types of benign tumors (56–59) with their most common locations (a–d).

_____ 56. chondroma

_____ 57. giant cell tumor

_____ 58. osteoblastoma

_____ 59. osteoid osteoma

   a. vertebra

   b. femur and tibia

   c. metastasis to lung

   d. hands and feet

Match the following types of malignant bone tumors (60–63) with their associated signs and symptoms (a–d).

_____ 60. chondrosarcoma

_____ 61. Ewing's sarcoma

_____ 62. fibrosarcoma

_____ 63. osteosarcoma

   a. local tenderness in lower extremity long bones

   b. short-term pain and swelling in distal femur

   c. long-term dull pain near proximal femur

   d. pain and swelling in lower pelvis

64. List the common sites of formation of primary tumors that metastasize to the bone.

   a. _____

   b. _____

   c. _____

   d. _____

   e. _____

65. Identify the common sites for bone tumor metastases.

   a. _____

   b. _____

   c. _____

   d. _____

66. Identify the sources of pain in clients with bone tumors.

   a. _____

     _____

     _____

   b. _____

     _____

     _____

67. List the subjective client data relevant to bone tumors. Use a separate sheet.

68. List the objective client data relevant to bone tumors. Use a separate sheet.

69. Identify the psychosocial manifestations exhibited by clients with benign and malignant bone tumors.

Benign tumors

a. _____

b. _____

c. _____

Malignant tumors

a. _____

b. _____

c. _____

d. _____

Match the following radiographic findings (70–76) with their associated types of bone tumor growths (a or b). Answers may be used more than once.

____ 70. poor margination

____ 71. intact cortices

____ 72. bone destruction

____ 73. cortical breakthrough

____ 74. smooth periosteal bone

____ 75. irregular new periosteal bone

____ 76. sharp margins

a. benign

b. malignant

77. List the interventions for pain management for the client with bone tumors.

a. _____

b. _____

c. _____

d. _____

e. _____

f. _____

78. Which of the following assessment findings in the client who has had a bone graft for a tumor should the nurse report to the physician immediately?

a. extremity distal to operative site warm and pink

b. temperature of cast over operative site cool

c. blanche response in distal digits lasting longer than 5 seconds

d. pain in operative extremity relieved by analgesics

79. Interventions to assist the client with a bone tumor who is grieving and anxious include

a. allowing the client to verbalize feelings

b. offering to call the client's clergyperson or religious leader

c. listening attentively when the client talks

d. all of the above

Disorders of the Hand

Match the following characteristics (80–90) to the hand disorders they are primarily associated with (a–c). Answers may be used more than once.

____ 80. pain worse at night

____ 81. round, cyst-like lesion

____ 82. first three digits affected

____ 83. progressive palmar flexion deformity

____ 84. joint discomfort after strain

____ 85. median nerve compression

____ 86. fourth and fifth digits affected

____ 87. swollen synovium

____ 88. familial tendency common

____ 89. Colles' fracture or hand burns

____ 90. occupational hazard

a. carpal tunnel syndrome

b. Dupuytren's contraction

c. ganglion

91. Design a discharge teaching plan for a client who has had a synovectomy. Submit the completed exercise to the clinical instructor on a separate sheet.

Disorders of the Foot

92. Identify the joint involved in hallux valgus.

_____

_____

93. Describe the changes involving the skin that occur as a hammertoe deformity progresses.

    a. _____

    _____

    b. _____

    _____

94. Differentiate between Morton's neuroma and tarsal tunnel syndrome. Use a separate sheet.

Other Musculoskeletal Disorders

Match the following spinal deformities (95–97) with their definitions (a–c).

_____ 95. kyphosis

_____ 96. lordosis

_____ 97. scoliosis

a. lateral curvature of the vertebral spine

b. increased curvature of the thoracic spine

c. increased curvature of the lumbar spine

Match the following corrective procedures for scoliosis (98–99) with their post-procedure client mobilizations (a or b).

_____ 98. insertion of Harrington's rod

_____ 99. insertion of Luque's rod

a. same day mobilization

b. several days of bed rest

Match the following characteristics and physical findings (100–105) with their associated musculoskeletal disorders (a or b). Answers may be used more than once.

_____ 100. muscle atrophy, weakness

_____ 101. fragile, deformed bones

_____ 102. cardiac involvement

_____ 103. mental retardation

_____ 104. presenile deafness

_____ 105. poor skeletal development

a. osteogenesis imperfecta

b. muscular dystrophy

106. Identify nursing diagnoses that may be applicable to an 18-year-old client with Duchenne's muscular dystrophy. Submit the completed exercise to the clinical instructor on a separate sheet.

CRITICAL THINKING EXERCISES

Case Study: Osteoporosis

A. G. is a 74-year-old female client with pathological compression fractures of T11-12 and L2-3 secondary to osteoporosis.

Address the following questions:

1. A support corset is ordered for A. G. to wear continuously when out of bed. What does the nurse do to maintain skin integrity for A. G.?

2. How should the corset be applied?

3. A. G. goes to physical therapy bid for strengthening exercises and ambulation. What does the nurse do to supplement A. G.'s scheduled therapy?

4. A. G. insists on having her bed side rails down at night. She states that she will sign a waiver to release the hospital from responsibility in case she should fall. What does the nurse tell A. G.? What does the nurse chart in A. G.'s record?

5. A. G. is scheduled for discharge to her home. She lives alone. What data does the nurse collect about A. G.'s home environment?

6. What community resources could be incorporated into the discharge plan?

Case Study: Osteomyelitis

B. D. is a 24-year-old client admitted with a diagnosis of osteomyelitis of the left tibia that resulted from a compound fracture suffered when he fell while snow skiing.

Address the following questions:

1. B. D. is scheduled for a bone scan. What does the nurse tell him in preparation for this diagnostic test?

2. Pending identification of the infecting organism, B. D. is placed on body fluid precautions. What instruction does the nurse give to B. D. about visitors?

3. B. D. is receiving intravenous antibiotics. What assessments does the nurse perform concerning the intravenous site?

4. The intravenous antibiotics are ordered as follows: oxacillin sodium (Prostaphlin) 1 g every 4 hours, cephalothin sodium (Keflin) 1 g every 6 hours, and tobramycin sulfate (Nebcin) 100 mg every 8 hours. Develop an administration schedule for these antibiotics.

5. What medication side effects should the nurse monitor for in B. D.?

6. The tobramycin sulfate (Nebcin) is mixed in 200 mL of solution. Calculate the drip rate required for the medication to infuse over 60 minutes. The administration set has a drip factor of 10 drops per mL.

7. B. D.'s wound is irrigated with an antibiotic solution tid and a new dressing applied. What observations are made at each dressing change?

B. D is to be dismissed to home care. He will continue on intermittent intravenous antibiotics and daily dressing changes. He also will need to use crutches for ambulation assistance.

8. What data does the nurse collect about B. D.'s home environment?

9. Plan discharge instructions for B. D. What should the nurse review about diet, care of the intravenous site, and dressing changes?

10. What information does B. D. need to know about his medication?

Case Study: Osteosarcoma

D. B. is a 32-year-old woman, married, and the mother of two children, ages 5 and 12 years. She recently has been diagnosed with primary osteosarcoma of the left distal femur.

Address the following questions:

1. Identify three nursing diagnoses that may apply to D. B. based on her psychosocial assessment.

2. D. B. asks the nurse if she will die soon. What does the nurse reply?

3. D. B. is scheduled for radiation therapy prior to surgery. What information does D. B. need to prepare her for this treatment?

4. After the third radiation therapy session, D. B. states that the skin on her left leg is red, dry, and itchy. She asks for some moisturizing lotion to apply to the area. What does the nurse do?

5. D. B. is scheduled to have an osteotomy and excision of the tumor. Because of the location of the tumor, the surgeon plans to insert a stabilizing implant (intramedullary rod). Design a perioperative teaching plan for D. B.

6. D. B. asks how she will be able to walk after her leg heals. What does the nurse tell D. B. to prepare her for the postoperative period?

7. What physical assessments does the nurse perform postoperatively about D. B.'s left lower extremity?

8. Prior to discharge to home, D. B. asks if she will ever be able to resume playing tennis. What does the nurse tell her?

9. Identify the stage of grief D. B. is probably experiencing. What does the nurse do to assist D. B. at this time?

CHAPTER 51

Interventions for Clients with Musculoskeletal Trauma

LEARNING OBJECTIVES

At the end of this chapter, the student will be able to

- Discuss the classifications, etiology, healing, and complications of fractures
- Provide care for the client with a fracture
- Discuss care for the client with an amputation
- Identify types of sports-related injuries to the musculoskeletal system

PREREQUISITE KNOWLEDGE

Prior to beginning this chapter, the student should review

- The anatomy and physiology of the musculoskeletal system (muscles, bones, joints)
- The principles of body mechanics
- The gaits for crutch- and cane-assisted walking and use of a walker
- The principles of perioperative nursing management
- The techniques for transferring a client from bed to wheelchair and wheelchair to bed
- The principles of hot and cold therapy
- The effect of immobility on the musculoskeletal system

- The normal ROM for each joint
- Orthopedic bed making
- The concepts of grief and loss
- The concepts of body image and self-esteem
- The principles of rehabilitation

STUDY QUESTIONS

Fractures

1. Compare and contrast the following pairs of fracture types. Use a separate sheet.

   a. complete versus incomplete

   b. open versus closed

   c. spontaneous versus fatigue

   d. greenstick versus spiral

Match the following terms related to the fracture healing process (2–5) with their definitions (a–d).

_____ 2. callus

_____ 3. granulation

_____ 4. hematoma

_____ 5. remodeling

a. mass of clotted blood at fracture site

b. process of bone building and resorption

c. outgrowth of new capillaries

d. nonbony union at fracture site

6. Identify the complications associated with fractures.

   a. _____

   b. _____

   c. _____

   d. _____

   e. _____

   f. _____

   g. _____

7. Briefly discuss why compartment syndrome is a medical emergency. Use a separate sheet.

8. List the signs and symptoms associated with compartment syndrome. Use a separate sheet.

9. Identify possible problems resulting from compartment syndrome.

   a. _____

   _____

   b. _____

   _____

   c. _____

   _____

   d. _____

   _____

10. List the sequence of complications in crush syndrome that results from involvement of multiple compartments.

   a. _____

   b. _____

   c. _____

   d. _____

   e. _____

   f. _____

   g. _____

11. Identify the type of shock that is a possible complication of fractures.

   _____

   _____

12. Identify the two sources of emboli and their mechanisms of release in fat embolism syndrome. Use a separate sheet.

13. List the types of fractures that are primarily associated with the occurrence of fat embolism.

   a. _____

   b. _____

   c. _____

14. Identify the types of clients with fractures who are at increased risk for developing deep venous thrombosis.

   a. _____

   _____

   b. _____

   _____

   c. _____

   _____

   d. _____

   _____

15. Define *avascular necrosis:* _____

   _____

   _____

Match the following fracture complications (16–18) with their definitions (a–c).

_____ 16. delayed union

_____ 17. malunion

_____ 18. nonunion

a. incorrect fracture healing

b. incomplete fracture healing

c. lack of fracture healing

19. List the subjective client data relevant to fractures. Use a separate sheet.

20. List the objective client data relevant to fractures. Use a separate sheet.

21. Identify the factors that are considered when formulating nursing diagnoses for clients with fractures.

    a. _____

    _____

    b. _____

    _____

    c. _____

    _____

    d. _____

    _____

22. Identify the emergency measures taken in an acute trauma situation to assist a client who may have suffered a fracture. Use a separate sheet.

23. List the methods used to immobilize fractures.

    a. _____

    b. _____

    c. _____

    d. _____

    e. _____

24. Describe the assessments the nurse performs of the area distal to an immobilization device. Use a separate sheet.

25. Describe nursing interventions used to preserve cast integrity, from the time of application to removal. Use a separate sheet.

26. Identify complications that may result from cast application. Use a separate sheet.

27. List the nurse's responsibilities about the maintenance of traction devices. Use a separate sheet.

28. Identify the pros and cons of performing pin care for external fixation devices. Use a separate sheet.

29. Identify nondrug interventions that may be alternatives for relieving pain in the client with a fracture.

    a. _____

    b. _____

    c. _____

    d. _____

    e. _____

f. _____

g. _____

30. List the potential complications related to impaired physical mobility in the client with a fracture.

    a. _____

    _____

    b. _____

    _____

    c. _____

    _____

    d. _____

    _____

    e. _____

    _____

    f. _____

    _____

31. Which of the following mobilization devices is usually preferred for the elderly client?

    a. crutches

    b. cane

    c. walker

    d. wheelchair

32. Describe measures within the hospital setting that the nurse may implement to prevent falls.

    a. _____

    _____

    b. _____

    _____

    c. _____

    _____

    d. _____

    _____

    e. _____

    _____

33. Interventions to prevent thromboembolism in the client who has impaired mobility as a result of fracture include

    a. applying antiembolism stockings

    b. teaching the client isometric and isotonic exercises

    c. administering anticoagulant therapy

    d. all of the above

34. Elderly clients immobilized with a fracture are prone to developing

    a. diarrhea

    b. constipation

    c. fluid volume overload

    d. increased mental alertness

35. The use of a fracture pan instead of a regular bedpan for toileting by the client following hip surgery is to prevent

    a. increased pain

    b. prosthesis dislocation

    c. wound infection

    d. decreased mobility

36. Which of the following foods should the client who is immobilized with a fracture be encouraged to eat?

    a. Cobb salad and roll

    b. fruit salad and broth

    c. hot dog and french fries

    d. cheeseburger and coleslaw

Amputations

37. Complete the following chart by comparing the open and closed methods of amputation. Use a separate sheet.

	Open	Closed
a. indication for procedure		
b. wound appearance		

38. Identify the complications that may result from an amputation.

    a. _____

    b. _____

    c. _____

    d. _____

    e. _____

    f. _____

39. List the problems that may lead to amputation.

    a. _____

    b. _____

    c. _____

    d. _____

    e. _____

    f. _____

    g. _____

40. List the subjective client data relevant to amputation. Use a separate sheet.

41. List the objective client data relevant to amputation. Use a separate sheet.

42. Identify and describe the psychosocial factors the nurse considers when assessing the client having an amputation. Use a separate sheet.

43. Identify the nursing diagnoses for a 26-year-old male client who has had an emergency above-the-knee amputation for a crushing injury. Submit the completed exercise to the clinical instructor on a separate sheet.

44. Which of the following assessment findings is abnormal in the client with an above-the-knee amputation?

    a. skin flap pink and warm

    b. femoral pulse nonpalpable

    c. reported phantom limb pain

    d. refusal to look at stump

Sports-Related Injuries

45. List the common sites of injury to the knee.

a. _____

_____

b. _____

_____

c. _____

_____

d. _____

_____

Match the following terms related to musculoskeletal injuries (46–49) with their definitions (a–d).

_____ 46. dislocation

_____ 47. sprain

_____ 48. strain

_____ 49. subluxation

a. incomplete joint surface separation

b. injury to a ligament

c. joint surfaces not approximated

d. excessive stretching of muscle or tendon

CRITICAL THINKING EXERCISES

Case Study: Fracture

P. D. is a 20-year-old client with fractures of the right tibia and fibula. He has a long leg cast that was applied 2 days ago. The nurse enters P. D.'s room to remove his lunch tray and observes him inserting a table knife under the top edge of his cast. P. D. states, "The itching is driving me crazy!"

Address the following questions:

1. What does the nurse tell P. D. about using a knife to scratch under his cast?

2. What other measures may be taken by the nurse to assist P. D. in coping with the itching?

Case Study: Fractured Femur

M. P. is a 73-year-old female client with a fractured left femur neck. She is in a Buck's boot for skin traction with 5 pounds of weight applied.

Address the following questions:

1. M. P. states that she needs to urinate. Describe how the nurse assists M. P. to use a fracture bedpan.

2. M. P. is scheduled to have a portable x-ray of her left hip. During the procedure, the traction lines catch on the bed frame. What does the nurse do when checking M. P. after the x-ray technologist leaves?

M. P. is scheduled for an open reduction and internal fixation procedure.

3. Upon return to her room from post-anesthesia recovery, describe the assessments the nurse performs for this type of surgery.

4. A wound drain to a Hemovac collective device is in place. What are the nurse's responsibilities relative to this type of drain?

5. M. P. has an order for meperidine hydrochloride (Demerol) 50–100 mg IM every 3–4 hours for analgesia. The nurse determines that M. P. is to receive 75 mg of meperidine. It is supplied in prefilled syringe cartridges. In the opioid drawer, only 50- and 100-mg/mL cartridges are in stock. Which cartridge(s) should the nurse select?

6. If meperidine hydrochloride (Demerol) is supplied in units of 50 mg/mL, how many milliliters should the nurse administer to give 75 mg?

7. M. P. has prophylactic intravenous infusion of heparin sodium 20,000 units in 500 mL of D_5W. The infusion set has a drip factor of 60 microdrops/mL and is administered via a pump. Calculate the drip rate for M. P. to receive 1000 units of heparin per hour.

Case Study: Amputation

J. M. is a 52-year-old male. He has tissue necrosis of the left foot to the level of the malleoli, related to frostbite. Amputation of the entire foot is scheduled.

Address the following questions:

1. Prepare a preoperative teaching plan.

2. J. M. is receiving 1 g cephalothin sodium (Keflin) IV every 6 hours. The medication comes already prepared in 50 mL of D_5W, which is to be administered over 30 minutes. Using an administration set with a drip factor of 10 macrodrops/mL, calculate the drip rate per minute.

3. J. M. is now postoperative. When in bed, what is the optimum position for him to prevent contractures and enhance fitting with a prosthesis?

4. J. M. enthusiastically talks about resuming his recreational hobby of alpine skiing. Is this a realistic expectation? What factors would the nurse consider when discussing J. M.'s plans?

CHAPTER 52

Assessment of the Gastrointestinal System

LEARNING OBJECTIVES

At the end of this chapter, the student will be able to

■ Describe the overall structure, function, and nerve and blood supply of the gastrointestinal (GI) tract

■ Describe the functions of the mouth, pharynx, esophagus, and stomach

■ Describe the functions of the pancreas, liver, and gallbladder

■ Describe the functions of the small and large intestines

■ Identify the physiological changes of the GI tract associated with aging

■ Complete a history and physical assessment for a client with a disorder of the digestive system

■ Identify diagnostic tools for determining GI abnormalities

PREREQUISITE KNOWLEDGE

Prior to beginning this chapter, the student should review

■ The anatomy and physiology of the gastrointestinal system

■ The effect of the central and autonomic nervous systems on the gastrointestinal organs

■ Normal nutrition, including the essential vitamins, minerals, and foods in the recommended food groups

■ Special diets for clients with gastrointestinal organ disorders, such as low salt, high or low protein, high carbohydrate, high or low fiber, low fat, bland, liquid, and puréed

■ The principles of enema administration

■ Normal fluid and electrolyte values

STUDY QUESTIONS

Anatomy and Physiology Review

Match the following terms associated with the GI system (1–21) with their definitions (a–u).

_____ 1. bile

_____ 2. chyme

_____ 3. deglutition

_____ 4. duodenum

_____ 5. elimination

_____ 6. esophagus

_____ 7. gallbladder

_____ 8. ileum

_____ 9. jejunum

_____ 10. large intestine

_____ 11. liver

_____ 12. lobule

_____ 13. mouth

_____ 14. mucosa

_____ 15. pancreas

_____ 16. plicae circularis

_____ 17. saliva

_____ 18. secretin

_____ 19. stomach

_____ 20. submucosa

_____ 21. villi

a. organ with both exocrine and endocrine functions

b. terminal portion of small intestine

c. finger-like projections into small intestine

d. oral secretion that softens food

e. thick, liquid mass of partly digested food

f. temporary reservoir for food

g. intestinal hormone that inhibits acid secretion, decreases gastric motility

h. epithelial cell layer lining GI tract

i. process of expelling feces

j. central part of small intestine

k. swallowing

l. organ where water absorption occurs

m. conduit for food from mouth to stomach

n. first 10 inches of small intestine

o. connective tissue layer of GI lumen

p. functional unit of liver

q. liver secretion essential to fat digestion

r. largest abdominal organ with numerous functions

s. organ that concentrates and stores bile

t. circular folds of mucosa projecting into GI lumen

u. beginning pathway for digestion

22. List the major functions of the GI tract and briefly describe them.

a. _____

_____

_____

b. _____

_____

_____

c. _____

_____

_____

23. Identify the layers of the GI tract and their functions

a. _____

_____

_____

b. _____

_____

_____

c. _____

_____

_____

24. Which of the following statements is correct about innervation of the GI tract?

a. Local contractile stimulation is provided by sympathetic nerve fibers.

b. Sphincter relaxation is a result of parasympathetic stimulation.

c. Sympathetic stimulation increases motor and secretory activity.

d. The myenteric and submucosal plexuses inhibit smooth muscle tone and movement.

25. Which of the following statements is correct about the blood supply to the GI tract?

    a. The blood supply originates from the aorta and branches to many arteries.

    b. The blood flow accounts for 10% of the cardiac output.

    c. Absorbed nutrients are carried away from the lumen via the hepatic vein.

    d. Blood circulates through the liver by means of the portal vein.

26. Complete the following chart by comparing the functions of the digestive organs. Use a separate sheet.

Organ	Function	Secretions and Purpose
a. mouth and pharynx		
b. esophagus		
c. stomach		
d. pancreas		
e. liver		
f. gallbladder		
g. small intestine		
h. large intestine		

27. Briefly discuss the physiological significance of the various secretions needed for digestion. Use a separate sheet.

28. Complete the following chart by givng examples of health problems illustrating the nutritional effects of the following age-related physiological changes. The first item is completed as an example. Submit the completed exercise to the clinical instructor using a separate sheet.

Change	Nutritional Effect
a. loss of teeth	*avoidance of high fiber in diet (constipation)*
b. decreased ptyalin and saliva	
c. esophageal sphincter relaxation	
d. decreased gastric HCl production	
e. decreased calcium absorption	
f. decreased vitamin B_{12} absorption	
g. decreased iron absorption	
h. loss of abdominal muscle tone	

Subjective Assessment

29. List the subjective client data relevant to the GI system. Use a separate sheet.

30. Briefly discuss the significance that psychosocial factors have for a GI assessment. Use a separate sheet.

31. The following is a partial client history. Discuss **CT** the significance these data have for a GI assessment. Submit the completed exercise to the clinical instructor using a separate sheet.

   Caucasian female, 84 years old. Lives alone in small apartment with cat for company. Admitted for observation after falling while boarding a city bus. Was on her way to grocery store to shop. States she has been unable to chew well since dentures were cracked 3 months ago when the cat knocked them off her night stand. Income consists of monthly Social Security checks. Uses food stamps. Denies problems with constipation or diarrhea.

Objective Assessment

32. List the objective client data relevant to the GI system. Use a separate sheet.

33. Using the client history data from question 31, **CT** construct a physical assessment recording for the GI system. Submit the completed exercise to the clinical instructor using a separate sheet.

34. Discuss the rationale for why the nurse should never pursue a complete abdominal assessment in the following circumstances: abdominal aneurysm, polycystic kidney disease, appendicitis, and abdominal organ transplantation. Use a separate sheet.

35. Laboratory values for the client with liver disease show

    a. decreased prothrombin time

    b. increased aspartate aminotransferase (AST) and alanine aminotransferase (ALT) levels

    c. increased amount of total protein

    d. decreased lactate dehydrogenase (LDH) level

36. List the contract media that are used in diagnostic radiographic studies of the GI tract and their routes of administration.

    a. _____

       _____

       _____

    b. _____

       _____

       _____

37. Discuss the significance of administering a laxative following barium contrast radiographic studies. What additional interventions should be implemented? Use a separate sheet.

CRITICAL THINKING EXERCISES

Case Study: Upper GI Pain

J. V. is an 87-year-old female client who is admitted to a medical nursing unit from a local nursing home. She had surgery for abdominal adhesions 4 weeks ago and is now passing blood-streaked stools. J. V. also reports that her stomach hurts, especially during the night. "It feels like someone is burning a hole inside me." J. V. states that she lives alone in a retirement apartment building. Last week, a close friend and neighbor visited J. V. at the nursing home and reported news of deaths of two residents of the apartment building who were mutual friends.

Address the following questions:

1. What additional data should the nurse collect for a thorough GI system assessment of J. V.?

2. J. V. is scheduled to have an upper GI and small bowel series the next day. What does the nurse do to prepare J. V. for these diagnostic studies? Devise a teaching/learning plan for J. V.

J. V. is unable to tolerate the barium solution, becomes nauseated, and vomits. Her physician orders that an esophagogastroduodenoscopy (EGD) be done.

3. What additional preparation is needed before this procedure can be performed on J. V.?

4. Following the EGD, J. V. is returned to her room by stretcher. The nurse assists J. V. to transfer to bed. What position should J. V. be assisted to assume? What assessments should the nurse initially perform? Why?

5. While the nurse is assessing her, J. V. asks for some water to drink because "my mouth is so dry that my tongue is sticky." What should the nurse do?

CHAPTER 53

Interventions for Clients with Oral Cavity Problems

LEARNING OBJECTIVES

At the end of this chapter, the student will be able to

- Identify the various types of stomatitis
- Discuss management of stomatitis
- Identify the types, effects, and etiology of oral cavity tumors
- Manage care for the client with an oral cavity tumor
- Identify disorders of the salivary glands and plan care for the client with these problems
- Discuss malocclusion and provide care for the client with malocclusion

PREREQUISITE KNOWLEDGE

Prior to beginning this chapter, the student should review

- The anatomy and physiology of the oral cavity
- Special diets for clients with oral cavity disorders, such as liquid, puréed, and bland
- The principles of oral hygiene
- The care of nasogastric tubes
- Normal fluid and electrolyte values
- Perioperative nursing care
- The concepts of body image and self-esteem
- The concepts of grief, loss, death, and dying

STUDY QUESTIONS

Stomatitis

1. Differentiate between primary and secondary stomatitis. Use a separate sheet.

Match the following descriptions of primary stomatitis (2–5) with their types (a–d).

_____ 2. erythema, ulceration, and necrosis of gingival margins

_____ 3. uniformly sized vesicles on tongue, palate, oral mucosa

_____ 4. circular, white, painful lesion with well-defined margins

_____ 5. circular, white lesion with undefined margins

a. aphthous
b. herpes simplex
c. Vincent's stomatitis
d. traumatic ulcer

6. List six etiological factors associated with secondary stomatitis.

   a. _____

   b. _____

   c. _____

   d. _____

   e. _____

   f. _____

Match the following descriptions of secondary stomatitis manifestations (7–11) with their types (a–c). Answers may be used more than once.

____ 7. vesicles at labial edge of mucosa

____ 8. dull, flat lesions on tongue

____ 9. white, thick patches on tongue

____ 10. symmetric with various patterns

____ 11. mouth feels as if it is burning

a. candidiasis

b. herpes simplex

c. lichen planus

12. Briefly discuss why it is difficult to prevent stomatitis. Use a separate sheet.

13. List the subjective client data relevant to assessment for stomatitis. Use a separate sheet.

14. List the objective client data relevant to oral cavity infections. Use a separate sheet.

15. List preventive measures that may be used against stomatitis.

   a. _____

   _____

   b. _____

   _____

   c. _____

   _____

   _____

   d. _____

   _____

   _____

16. Identify nursing implications for the following medications used in the treatment of stomatitis. Submit the completed exercise to the clinical instructor on a separate sheet.

   a. nystatin oral suspension

   b. gentian violet solution

   c. dyclonine HCl

17. Discharge instructions for the client with stomatitis should include

   a. frequent intake of juices such as pineapple or orange

   b. chewing aspirin gum (Aspergum) for topical analgesia

   c. frequent rinses with a commercial mouthwash solution

   d. frozen foods such as yogurt, sherbet, or ice milk

Tumors

Match the following types of oral cavity tumors (18–21) with their descriptions (a–d).

____ 18. basal cell carcinoma

____ 19. erythroplakia

____ 20. leukoplakia

____ 21. squamous cell carcinoma

a. oral cavity or neck mass

b. raised scab on lip

c. red patch on oral mucosa

d. white patch on oral mucosa

22. Identify the sites where oral cavity carcinoma may develop.

   a. _____

   b. _____

   c. _____

   d. _____

   e. _____

   f. _____

   g. _____

   _____

   h. _____

   _____

23. List the etiological factors associated with leukoplakia.

    a. _____

    b. _____

    c. _____

    d. _____

    e. _____

    f. _____

    g. _____

    h. _____

24. Identify preventive measures for oral cavity tumors.

    a. _____

    _____

    b. _____

    _____

    c. _____

    _____

    _____

    d. _____

    _____

25. List the subjective client data relevant to oral cavity tumors. Use a separate sheet.

26. List the objective client data relevant to the oral cavity. Use a separate sheet.

27. Immediate interventions following local resection of an oral tumor include

    a. performing vigorous oral hygiene every hour

    b. initiating interventions only with a physician's order

    c. suctioning oral secretions with a tonsil-tip catheter

    d. monitoring for fever by taking an oral temperature qid

28. List assessments that the nurse should make when a client resumes oral liquids following oral surgery.

    a. _____

    _____

    b. _____

    _____

    c. _____

    _____

Disorders of the Salivary Glands

29. List the common disorders of the salivary glands.

    a. _____

    b. _____

    c. _____

    d. _____

30. Which of the following statements about salivary gland disorders is true?

    a. Acute sialadenitis is often seen in young adult clients.

    b. Exposure to the mumps virus provides passive immunity.

    c. Salivary calculi within a duct can obstruct saliva flow.

    d. Xerostomia is increased salivation occurring with stimulation.

31. For a client who has had a parotidectomy, the nurse

    a. asks the client to open and close his or her eyes

    b. keeps the client turned to the operative side

    c. observes the symmetry of uvula movement

    d. avoids stimulating the gland by restricting fluids

Malocclusion

32. Differentiate between acute onset and chronic malocclusion. Use a separate sheet.

33. Identify the etiological factors for tooth and mandibular fractures.

a. _____

b. _____

c. _____

d. _____

e. _____

f. _____

g. _____

h. _____

i. _____

34. List the subjective client data relevant to malocclusion. Use a separate sheet.

35. List the objective client data relevant to malocclusion. Use a separate sheet.

36. Interventions for the client with a mandibular fracture include

a. gentle swabbing with lemon-glycerine swabs

b. use of ice packs applied to affected area

c. irrigation with a waterpick (Water Pik) on a high setting

d. providing hard candy for the client to slowly suck

37. Identify rationales for the following diet recommendations for the client with malocclusion.

a. soft or puréed foods: _____

_____

_____

b. moderate-temperature foods: _____

_____

_____

38. Postoperative care for the client having an inter-maxillary fixation (IMF) includes

a. administering oral anti-emetic medications

b. inserting a nasogastric tube to low intermittent suction

c. keeping wire cutters at the bedside continuously

d. checking presence of the gag reflex prior to feedings

39. Discharge instructions for the client with an IMF include

a. engaging in nonstrenuous activities such as fishing

b. drinking calorie-dense carbonated beverages

c. seeking professional help if the wires need to be cut

d. avoiding alcoholic beverages including wine coolers

CRITICAL THINKING EXERCISES

Case Study: Unrelenting Toothache

L. I. is a 28-year-old male client who is seen in the dental clinic following an assault during which he suffered blows to the head. Several teeth were loosened. During the oral examination, the nurse notes that L. I.'s gums are reddened and tender and bleed easily when probed with a tongue blade. The area under the left premolar is swollen, tender, and abscessed. L. I. pulls away and tells the nurse to stop because it hurts too much to touch that tooth. It had been hurting the past several weeks. When questioned, L. I. states that he brushes his teeth once a day, has never been told about flossing, and usually has several candy bars for lunch.

Address the following questions:

1. Formulate relevant nursing diagnoses for L. I. based on the above data.

2. What additional data should the nurse collect from L. I. about his oral hygiene?

3. L. I. is scheduled for a pulpectomy and incision and drainage of the abscessed tooth the next day in outpatient surgery. Design a perioperative teaching/learning plan for L. I.

4. During the follow-up clinic visit after surgery, what information should the nurse collect to evaluate L. I.'s progress in dental self care?

Case Study: Cancer of the Tongue

M. Q. is a 58-year-old client who has cancer of the tongue. He currently is receiving local radiation therapy in the form of implanted radium seeds and is in a private room. His 36-year-old wife is 3 months pregnant with their first child. M. Q. will be scheduled for tumor excision once the radiation treatment is complete.

Address the following questions:

1. When in M. Q.'s room, what are the precautions that the nursing staff should take? That Mrs. Q should take?

2. Identify actual and potential nursing diagnoses for M. Q. based on the above data.

3. What type of oral hygiene measures should M. Q. receive, if any, while the radium seeds are in place?

M. Q. is scheduled for the tumor excision, which will include part of the base of the tongue. A temporary tracheostomy and nasogastric feeding tube will be placed during surgery.

4. Design a perioperative teaching/learning plan for M. Q.

5. In addition to pain postoperatively, what other nursing diagnoses can be anticipated for M. Q.?

6. M. Q. weighs 181 pounds. Postoperatively, his estimated energy needs are 37 kcal/kg. M. Q.'s tube feedings are administered by pump at a rate of 100 mL/hour. At a calorie density of 1 calorie/mL, how many calories will M. Q. receive in 24 hours? Is this sufficient for meeting his calorie needs? His peripheral intravenous solution is D_5W, which is infusing at a rate of 125 mL/hour. How many additional calories does this provide in 24 hours?

7. M. Q. becomes frustrated with his inability to talk and express his needs. The intravenous cannula is in his dominant hand and makes using a magic slate difficult. Discuss alternatives that may be used to assist M. Q.

8. Following removal of the tracheostomy tube, M. Q. realizes that his speech is unclear and people have difficulty understanding him. He becomes upset and depressed. "How can I help coach my wife in the delivery room if I can't be understood? I won't be able to talk to the baby! I'll never be able to go back to work if no one can understand me." What can the nurse do to assist M. Q.?

9. M. Q. is allowed to begin oral fluids. What should the nurse do to prepare him for this?

CHAPTER 54

Interventions for Clients with Esophageal Problems

LEARNING OBJECTIVES

At the end of this chapter, the student will be able to
- Discuss gastroesophageal reflux disease (GERD)
- Manage care for the client with GERD
- Discuss hiatal hernia and related management
- Discuss achalasia and related management
- Discuss tumors of the esophagus
- Provide care for the client with esophageal cancer
- Discuss diverticula of the esophagus and related care
- Provide care for the client with esophageal trauma

PREREQUISITE KNOWLEDGE

Prior to beginning this chapter, the student should review
- The anatomy and physiology of the esophagus
- The care of nasogastric and nasointestinal tubes
- The care of feeding tubes and preparation of tube-feeding formulas
- The principles of total parenteral nutrition (TPN) and care of peripheral and central line catheters
- Normal fluid and electrolyte values
- Perioperative nursing care
- The concepts of grief, loss, death, and dying
- The concepts of body image and self-esteem

STUDY QUESTIONS

Gastroesophageal Reflux Disease

1. Identify two anatomical factors that support the normal function of the lower esophageal sphincter (LES).

   a. _____

   _____

   _____

   b. _____

   _____

   _____

2. List the factors that contribute to esophageal reflux.

   a. _____

   _____

   b. _____

   _____

   c. _____

   _____

   d. _____

   _____

3. The degree of esophageal inflammation is

   a. inversely related to the acid concentration of refluxed stomach contents

   b. directly dependent on the number of reflux episodes of stomach contents

   c. primarily determined by the duration of exposure to irritating material

   d. a result of increased peristaltic activity as irritants return to the stomach

4. Briefly discuss the relationship that nighttime reflux has to GERD. Use a separate sheet.

5. Complete the following chart identifying factors that affect the tone and contractility of the LES. Use a separate sheet.

Increased Tone	Decreased Tone
a.	a.
b.	b.
c.	c.
d.	d.
e.	e.
	f.

6. List the subjective client data relevant to esophageal reflux. Use a separate sheet.

7. Briefly discuss why a careful, complete nursing history is critical to GERD assessment. Use a separate sheet.

8. List the objective client data relevant to GERD. Use a separate sheet.

Match the following definitions of GERD-associated symptoms (9–14) with their terms (a–f).

____ 9. occurrence of warm fluid climbing up the throat

____ 10. painful swallowing

____ 11. excessive gas in stomach or intestines

____ 12. reflex salivary hypersecretion in response to reflux

____ 13. raising of gas from the stomach

____ 14. burning sensation in epigastric and sternal region

a. belching

b. flatulence

c. odynophagia

d. pyrosis

e. regurgitation

f. water brash

15. The most sensitive and accurate measure of reflux is

   a. the Bernstein test

   b. 24-hour pH monitoring

   c. esophageal manometry

   d. esophagoscopy

16. Dietary modifications that may decrease esophageal reflux symptoms include

   a. eating four to six small meals a day including an evening snack

   b. drinking at least 12–16 ounces of liquid with each meal

   c. restricting intake of caffeine and alcoholic beverages

   d. including carbonated beverages such as cola products

17. The lifestyle adaptation that may best reduce esophageal reflux is

   a. placing the bed in the Trendelenburg position

   b. wearing snug-fitting belts and waistbands

   c. engaging in regular exercise such as weight lifting

   d. attaining and maintaining one's ideal body weight

18. Metoclopramide hydrochloride (Reglan) may safely be given to clients with which of the following disorders?

   a. epilepsy

   b. diarrhea

   c. diabetes mellitus

   d. Parkinson's disease

Hiatal Hernia

19. Differentiate between the two types of hiatal hernias. Use a separate sheet.

20. List the subjective client data relevant to hiatal hernias. Use a separate sheet.

21. List the objective client data relevant to hiatal hernias. Use a separate sheet.

22. Interventions for the client who has had a fundoplication procedure for hiatal hernia include

    a. reinserting the NG tube if it becomes dislodged

    b. providing the client with carbonated beverages

    c. ordering small, frequent meals and snacks

    d. encouraging the supine position to promote peristalsis

Achalasia

23. Describe the possible physiological factors involved in achalasia. Use a separate sheet.

24. List the subjective client data relevant to achalasia. Use a separate sheet.

25. List the objective client data relevant to achalasia. Use a separate sheet.

26. Following esophageal dilatation, the nurse

    a. teaches the client to swallow any oral secretions that accumulate

    b. massages the client's shoulder when he or she complains of shoulder pain

    c. encourages the client to drink very cold fluids for their numbing effect

    d. palpates the neck carefully to assess for signs of esophageal perforation

27. Briefly discuss why myotomy is a more complicated surgical treatment than esophageal dilatation and requires more complex nursing management postoperatively. Use a separate sheet.

Tumors

28. Which of the following statements about esophageal tumors is true?

    a. Leiomyomas are malignant tumors and almost always fatal.

    b. Esophageal cancer is difficult to diagnose early.

    c. Other tumors commonly metastasize to the esophagus.

    d. Tumors grow quickly because of early pathological changes.

29. Complications from esophageal tumors include

    a. delayed lymph node spread because of few lymphatics

    b. iron deficiency anemia from chronic low-grade bleeding

    c. late metastasis to thoracic and mediastinal structures

    d. obstruction from tumors less than 10 cm in size

30. List the subjective client data relevant to esophageal cancer. Use a separate sheet.

31. List the objective client data relevant to esophageal tumors. Use a separate sheet.

32. Identify the common nursing diagnosis associated with cancer of the esophagus.

_____

_____

33. Prevention of esophageal tumors is

    a. simple owing to multiple identified causative factors

    b. directly related to high alcohol consumption

    c. specifically targeted to African-American males

    d. unrelated to chewing tobacco or smoking practices

34. Following esophagogastrostomy, the client is placed in

    a. high-Fowler's position

    b. supine position

    c. Sim's position

    d. Trendelenburg's position

35. Which of the following foods should be encouraged in the diet of the client who has had esophageal surgery for cancer?

    a. fresh fruit

    b. well-cooked meats

    c. enriched eggnogs

    d. raw vegetables

Esophageal Diverticula

36. Define *diverticula*. Use a separate sheet.

37. Which of the following statements is correct about esophageal diverticula?

    a. They increase the client's risk for esophageal perforation.

    b. They are a common congenital defect.

    c. They form primarily in the lower part of the esophagus.

    d. Zenker's diverticula are found more often in women.

38. List the subjective client data relevant to esophageal diverticula. Use a separate sheet.

39. List the objective client data relevant to esophageal diverticula. Use a separate sheet.

40. Nonsurgical management of esophageal diverticula includes

    a. encouraging a nap after meals

    b. including mostly liquids in the diet

    c. raising the head with a wedge pillow

    d. administering a cough suppressant for nocturnal cough

41. Postoperatively, nursing care for the client who has had an excision of a Zenker's diverticulum includes

    a. keeping the head of the bed elevated 15 degrees

    b. observing the abdominal dressing for blood drainage

    c. administering tube feedings via the gastrostomy tube

    d. offering frequent oral hygiene and analgesics

42. Instructions for the client who is dismissed to home care with a feeding tube in place for intermittent feedings include

    a. checking the tube placement once a day in the morning

    b. administering feedings while the client is sitting up in a chair

    c. scheduling feedings every 4 hours around the clock

    d. wearing a cervical collar to support the neck incision

Esophageal Trauma

43. Give examples of extrinsic causes of esophageal rupture or perforation. Use a separate sheet.

44. Give examples of intrinsic causes of esophageal rupture or perforation. Use a separate sheet.

45. Briefly discuss why an esophageal perforation is serious. Use a separate sheet.

46. List the subjective client data relevant to esophageal perforation. Use a separate sheet.

47. List the objective client data relevant to esophageal perforation. Use a separate sheet.

48. When administering steroids to the client who has suffered an esophageal perforation, the nurse

    a. monitors serum glucose levels

    b. observes for signs of hyponatremia

    c. implements reverse isolation precautions

    d. checks blood gases for metabolic acidosis

49. Which of the following statements reflects that a client has understood the discharge instructions following an esophageal repair for perforation?

    a. "I can meet my buddies at the club next week for our regular social hour."

    b. "If I have more problems with swallowing, I will contact my doctor."

    c. "I can stop all these little white pills once I get home."

    d. "I can expect to continue to lose weight while this feeding tube is in."

CRITICAL THINKING EXERCISES

Case Study: Hiatal Hernia

M. B. is a retired 82-year-old illustrator of children's books and lives with her 78-year-old sister. She is being evaluated for complaints of chest pain which have become increasingly more frequent. Yesterday, when M. B. was packing her library in preparation for a move to a retirement community, she became dyspneic and collapsed. Her sister called the ambulance, and M. B. was admitted to a medical nursing unit. This morning, M. B. had an abdominal ultrasound prior to an upper GI series. When the nurse last checked, M. B. was dozing.

Address the following question:

1. M. B.'s call light is on. As the nurse enters the room, M. B. is attempting to get out of bed. She is gasping and clutching at her chest, saying, "Please help me! I can't breathe!" What should the nurse's first action be? What are the relevant nursing diagnoses for M. B. based on the above data?

Slowly, M. B. calms and is able to breathe more easily. The physician orders a stat portable chest x-ray. The film shows a hiatal hernia in which the entire stomach is above the diaphragm. An emergency fundoplication is scheduled using a high abdominal approach.

2. What information should the nurse provide to M. B. to prepare her for surgery?
3. Following M. B.'s return to the unit postoperatively, the NG tube is attached to low intermittent suction. The nurse notes that the drainage is dark brown with heavy white streaks. Should the nurse be concerned? What measures does the nurse take to maintain tube patency? What significance does a non-functioning NG tube have for M. B.?
4. M. B. is extremely reluctant to cough and deep breathe, saying that it hurts too much and her throat is sore from the NG tube. What can the nurse do to promote M. B.'s comfort and cooperative with pulmonary hygiene?
5. M. B. has an order for 35 mg of meperidine hydrochloride (Demerol), which may be given intramuscularly every 3 hours prn. The medication comes in pre-filled syringes of 50 mg/mL. How many milliliters should the nurse give?
6. Following the removal of the NG tube, M. B. is to begin a clear liquid diet. She eagerly begins to drink the clear broth but stops, saying that she cannot swallow. What should the nurse do to assist M. B.?
7. M. B. is to be dismissed to the care of her sister. Develop a discharge teaching/learning plan.
8. M. B. asks about her planned move to the retirement community. What should the nurse tell her?

Case Study: Esophageal Cancer

C. Z. is a 71-year-old client recently diagnosed with a large esophageal tumor. He is a widower and lives with his only son and daughter-in-law. C. Z. currently is receiving hyperalimentation via a central line catheter prior to having surgery. He has completed a course of radiation therapy and is scheduled for tumor resection in 2 days.

Address the following question:

1. Formulate relevant nursing diagnoses for C. Z. based upon the above data.

2. The planned surgical procedure is a subtotal esophagectomy and anastomosis of the cervical esophageal stump to the stomach. Devise a perioperative teaching/learning plan for C. Z.

Postoperatively, C. Z. has an NG tube to low intermittent suction, a central line catheter for hyperalimentation solution, a peripheral intravenous line for antibiotic administration, and a chest tube to low continuous suction.

3. Identify additional nursing diagnoses for C. Z. using these additional data. What are the client goals and expected outcomes?

4. C. Z. is to receive 30 mL of antacid instilled into the NG tube every 2 hours. What is the purpose of this treatment? Discuss how the instillation is to be done to achieve the most beneficial effect.

5. The second postoperative day, C. Z. pulls out the NG tube. What should the nurse do?

Five days postoperatively, C. Z. begins a clear liquid diet. This is well tolerated, and supplemental oral feedings are added, which include blenderized high-protein drinks. On postoperative day seven, C. Z.'s pulse rate increases from 88 to 124 bpm, his temperature is 101.8°F, and his respiratory rate is 24 breaths per minute. A check of the chest incision dressing shows thick, brown drainage.

6. What should the nurse do initially? What further actions should the nurse take?

7. Eventually, C. Z.'s wounds begin to heal and preparations are made to discharge him to the care of his son and daughter-in-law. Discuss what factors should be considered when planning for C. Z.'s discharge.

8. C. Z.'s family inquire about hospice care. What information can the nurse give to them?

9. The night before he is to go home, the nurse finds C. Z. curled up in his bed, crying. What can the nurse do to comfort C. Z.?

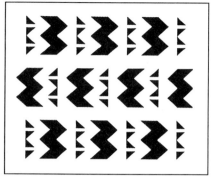

C H A P T E R 5 5

Interventions for Clients with Stomach Disorders

LEARNING OBJECTIVES

At the end of this chapter, the student will be able to

- Discuss the pathophysiology and etiology of gastritis
- Provide care for the client with gastritis
- Discuss peptic ulcer disease (PUD)
- Provide care for the client with PUD
- Discuss carcinoma of the stomach
- Provide care for the client with gastric cancer

PREREQUISITE KNOWLEDGE

Prior to beginning this chapter, the student should review

- The anatomy and physiology of the stomach
- The effect of the central and autonomic nervous systems on the stomach
- Special diets for clients with stomach disorders such as bland, liquid, and puréed
- The care of nasogastric tubes
- The care of feeding tubes and preparation of tube-feeding formulas
- The principles of total parenteral nutrition (TPN) and care of peripheral and central line catheters

- Normal fluid and electrolyte values
- Perioperative nursing care
- The concepts of grief, loss, death, and dying
- The concepts of body image and self-esteem

STUDY QUESTIONS

Gastritis

1. Identify the functions of the gastric mucosa:

_____

_____

Match the following gastric disorders (2–5) with their descriptions (a–d).

_____ 2. acute

_____ 3. atrophic

_____ 4. chronic

_____ 5. gastric atrophy

a. diffuse prolonged inflammatory process

b. complete gland loss with minimal inflammation and mucosal thinning

c. decreased number of fundal, parietal, and chief cells

d. short-lived process with complete regeneration and healing

Match the following etiological factors (6–14) with their types of gastritis (a or b). Answers may be used more than once.

_____ 6. peptic ulcer disease

_____ 7. long-term alcohol abuse

_____ 8. aspirin ingestion

_____ 9. bacterial infection

_____ 10. physiological stress

_____ 11. radiation therapy

_____ 12. emotional upset

_____ 13. pernicious anemia

_____ 14. history of smoking

a. acute

b. chronic

15. Preventive measures for gastritis include

   a. eliminating alcohol and caffeine temporarily from the diet

   b. taking H_2 antagonists (if on a chemotherapy protocol)

   c. taking nonsteroidal anti-inflammatory drugs instead of aspirin in long-term therapy

   d. including foods high in fiber and roughage in the diet

16. List the subjective client data relevant to gastritis. Use a separate sheet.

17. List the objective client data relevant to gastritis. Use a separate sheet.

18. Gastritis can often be treated successfully by

   a. encouraging the client to maintain a moderate activity level

   b. identify causative factors

   c. helping the client eliminate causative factors

   d. administering analgesics regularly

19. Collaborative management of gastritis includes

   a. devising a schedule for administering the multiple medications that are commonly ordered

   b. instructing the client to supplement the diet with iron preparations such as ferrous sulfate

   c. introducing the client to new foods to replace those that cause gastric irritation

   d. reinforcing behaviors that contribute to the client's sense of dependency

20. Which of the following statements about discharge planning is true for the client with gastritis?

   a. Family dining habits and mealtime planning will require minimal changes.

   b. Over-the-counter medications containing acetaminophen should be avoided.

   c. Life style modifications are temporary and former patterns may eventually be resumed.

   d. Family counseling will educate members to potential sources of stress.

Peptic Ulcer Disease

21. Define _peptic ulcer disease_ (PUD): _____

   _____

   _____

22. List the locations where peptic ulcers are commonly found and their frequency of occurrence in these locations.

   a. _____

   _____

   b. _____

   _____

   c. _____

   _____

23. Briefly discuss why it is important to specify the anatomical region when referring to PUD. Use a separate sheet.

24. Complete the following chart by comparing the characteristics of gastric and duodenal ulcers. Use a separate sheet.

Characteristic	Gastric Ulcer	Duodenal Ulcer
a. age of occurrence		
b. sex		
c. blood group		
d. nutritional status		
e. gastric acid production		
f. location of ulcer		
g. pain pattern		
h. response to H_2 receptor blockers		
i. type of bleeding		
j. perforation		
k. appearance of surrounding mucosa		

25. Describe the process of ulcer perforation and its associated signs and symptoms. Use a separate sheet.

26. Define *intractability* and its relationship to PUD. Use a separate sheet.

27. Preventive measures for initial PUD and recurrent disease include

    a. drinking a glass of milk with every meal

    b. including cereal grains and legumes in the diet

    c. developing stress management techniques

    d. substituting ibuprofen for aspirin

28. List the subjective client data relevant to PUD. Use a separate sheet.

29. List the objective client data relevant to PUD. Use a separate sheet.

30. Identify the nonsurgical interventions for PUD.

    a. _____

    _____

    b. _____

    _____

    c. _____

    _____

    d. _____

    _____

    e. _____

    _____

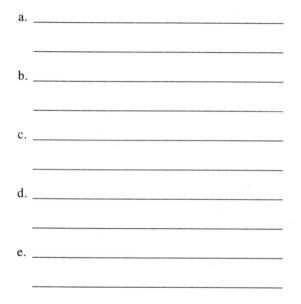 31. Complete the following chart by providing the rationale for administering these drugs in PUD management. Submit the completed exercise to the clinical instructor on a separate sheet.

Drug	Rationale
a. histamine antagonists	
b. antacids	
c. mucosal barrier fortifiers	
d. anticholinergics	
e. antisecratory agents	
f. prostaglandin analogs	

32. Which of the following antacids should preferably be taken by the diabetic client who has PUD?

    a. magnesium hydroxide (Gelusil) tablets

    b. magaldrate (Riopan)

    c. magnesium hydroxide with dried aluminum hydroxide and simethicone (Maalox Plus) tablets

    d. aluminum hydroxide (Amphojel)

33. Briefly discuss the rationale for administering the liquid form of an antacid instead of the tablet form. If a client persists in taking a tablet form of antacid, what instructions are indicated? Use a separate sheet.

34. Which of the following drugs should preferably be taken by the hypertensive client who has PUD?

    a. magnesium hydroxide with aluminum hydroxide, simethicone, and sodium (Mylanta liquid)

    b. sodium bicarbonate

    c. famotidine (Pepcid)

    d. aluminum hydroxide (Amphojel)

35. A client who has PUD has the following medications ordered: magnesium hydroxide with aluminum hydroxide (Maalox) 5 mL PO 1 hour and 3 hours after meals and at bedtime; sucralfate (Carafate) 1 g PO 1 hour before meals and at bedtime; famotidine 40 mg PO at bed time. Meal times are generally at 8 a.m., 12:15 p.m., and 5:30 p.m. An evening snack is also to be given and is delivered from the diet kitchen at 8 p.m. Devise an administration schedule that will be the most therapeutic and acceptable to the client. Consider whether the delivery of meal trays will need to be altered accommodate the schedule. Use a separate sheet.

36. Initial interventions for the client following rupture of a peptic ulcer include

    a. bed rest with bathroom privileges

    b. administration of opioid analgesics

    c. irrigation of the NG tube with normal saline

    d. administration of anticholinergics

37. Signs and symptoms of dumping syndrome include

    a. pain

    b. bradycardia

    c. profuse vomiting

    d. abdominal cramping

38. Which of the following foods should be included in the diet of the client who has dumping syndrome?

 a. scrambled eggs

 b. ice cream

 c. thin broths

 d. raw cauliflower

39. Which of the following statements is correct about Zollinger–Ellison syndrome?

 a. Lack of symptoms is a reliable guide in determining whether excess acid secretion is controlled.

 b. Diarrhea is the most common symptom and is present in over half of these clients.

 c. Required doses of H_2 receptor blockers are similar to those used for ordinary duodenal ulcers.

 d. Gastric acid hypersecretion results from the trophic effect of pancreas-related gastrin.

Carcinoma of the Stomach

40. Briefly describe the methods of gastric carcinoma extension. Use a separate sheet.

41. Which of the following statements is correct about the etiology of gastric carcinoma?

 a. Consuming cured and pickled foods reduces the risk of gastric cancer.

 b. Vitamin C is known to block nitrosamine formation and protect the stomach.

 c. Pernicious anemia is not a known risk factor for this tumor.

 d. Self-medicating for recurrent stomach pain effectively reduces its occurrence.

42. Which of the following statements is correct about gastric cancer?

 a. Treatment results for advanced stages have improved considerably over the past 15 years.

 b. The 5-year survival rate for stage IV carcinoma has improved to 20%.

 c. Most clients in the United States for whom stomach cancer is diagnosed have stage I or II.

 d. Prognosis and treatment depend on the disease stage and general health status of the client.

43. List the subjective client data relevant to carcinoma of the stomach. Use a separate sheet.

44. List the objective client data relevant to stomach cancer. Use a separate sheet.

45. Briefly discuss why there are few physical findings specifically associated with early gastric cancer. Use a separate sheet.

46. Which of the following statements is correct about the management of gastric cancer?

 a. Combination chemotherapy for advanced disease is less effective than single-agent therapy.

 b. The response to combination chemotherapy is unaffected by radiation therapy.

 c. Combining chemotherapy and radiotherapy after surgery has proved to be effective and is preferred.

 d. High-dose radiation therapy is the recommended adjuvant therapy to surgical treatment.

47. Which of the following statements about surgical interventions for gastric cancer is true?

 a. Surgery has the lowest cure rate for early gastric cancer because of tumor size.

 b. Neoplasm location in the stomach determines the type of surgical procedure.

 c. Palliative resection can help the cure rate for clients with advanced disease.

 d. Curative surgical procedures involve little resection and are associated with a low mortality rate.

48. Interventions for the client with an NG tube include

 a. turning off the suction periodically to decrease trauma to the gastric mucosa

 b. irrigating with tap water periodically to decrease gastric secretion viscosity

 c. securing the tube to the bedding with a pin to prevent accidental dislodgment

 d. observing for the return of instilled fluid to determine if the tube is obstructed

49. The nurse monitors the client with an NG tube for

 a. hyponatremia

 b. hyperkalemia

 c. fluid volume excess

 d. metabolic acidosis

50. Which of the following types of NG tube drainages should the nurse report immediately?

 a. greenish yellow

 b. dark green

 c. flecks of red

 d. bright red

51. List the specific complications that may follow gastric surgery.

    a. _____

    b. _____

    c. _____

    d. _____

    e. _____

    f. _____

    g. _____

52. Identify factors that may contribute to inadequate nutrient intake in the client who has had gastric surgery.

    a. _____

    b. _____

    c. _____

    d. _____

53. Briefly discuss the indications for placing a client on total parenteral nutrition (TPN) following gastric surgery. Use a separate sheet.

CRITICAL THINKING EXERCISES

Case Study: Peptic Ulcer Disease

J. A. is a 46-year-old male client who is being evaluated for intractable PUD. He has a history of recurrent duodenal ulcers. Last night, J. A. awakened at 2:00 a.m. and requested his antacid. This morning after breakfast, he passed a large, dark, liquid stool that tested positive for occult blood. Just prior to the 11:00 a.m. dose of antacid, J. A. turned on his call light. When the nurse enters the room, J. A. is lying on his side with his knees drawn up, moaning, and holding his pillow against his abdomen. He is diaphoretic, pale, and breathing rapidly and shallowly. J. A. states, "I was just about to take some more of my Maalox and all of a sudden I felt a burning pain in my belly. It's never hurt like this before." (J. A. point to his abdomen just above his umbilicus and to the right of the midsternal line.) "I feel like I've been stabbed and the knife is going clear through to my back."

Address the following questions:

1. What should the nurse's first actions be?

2. Based on the above description, what has probably happened to J. A.? What interventions should the nurse anticipate being ordered for him? How can the nurse prepare for these interventions and treatments?

3. Formulate relevant nursing diagnoses for J. A. based on the above data.

The physician orders J. A. to be prepared for immediate surgery and asks for a surgical consent form to be signed by J. A. The operative permit reads, "Exploratory laparotomy: hemigastrectomy and gastrojejunostomy."

4. What type of surgical procedure is this? What types of nutritional problems may be anticipated for J. A. postoperatively and long term?

5. Identify the assessments the nurse should make while awaiting J. A.'s transfer to the operating room. What laboratory values are significant to monitor in J. A.? Why?

6. Postoperatively, what are the data used to determine when the NG tube will be discontinued? When the intravenous catheter and fluids will be discontinued? How is this information communicated to J. A.?

7. On the fourth postoperative day, J. A. states that he is having more pain around his incision. His temperature is 102.4°F, his pulse is 128 bpm, and respirations are 24 breaths per minute. Inspection of the abdominal wound shows a reddened, tense area around the incision. The dressing has some green-tinged serosanguineous drainage. What should the nurse do?

The physician order cefoperazone sodium (Cefobid) 1 g every 6 hours intravenously and gentamicin sulfate (Garamycin) 80 mg every 8 hours intravenously. Nephrotoxicity is an effect common to both these drugs.

8. What assessments should the nurse make for this potential problem? What data would the nurse report immediately to the physician if adverse effects occurred?

9. Eventually, J. A. recovers from the effects of the surgery and complications and is permitted to begin an oral diet. What instruction should J. A. be given concerning his diet? What foods should he try to avoid?

10. J. A. is to be discharged. What should the nurse discuss with him prior to discharge? What adjustments will J. A. and his family need to make to enhance the success of his maintenance therapy?

Case Study: Post-Gastric Surgery

L. O. is a 52-year-old client who had a subtotal gastrectomy for stage III stomach carcinoma 10 weeks ago and has had difficulty maintaining his body weight. His usual weight is 192 pounds and he currently weighs 164 pounds.

Address the following questions:

1. Is L. O. at nutritional risk? If so, discuss the reasons.
2. Calculate his percentage of weight loss.
3. The physician orders TPN therapy to begin once a Hickman catheter is placed. What does the nurse do to prepare L. O. for this procedure?
4. What type of information does L. O. need to manage his TPN therapy successfully at home once he is discharged?
5. What type of diet should L. O. follow at home? Discuss foods he should include and avoid.
6. Identify resources that L. O. may need to assist him with his home management. What are these people's roles with respect to L. O.?

Mrs. L. O. calls the nursing unit a week after L. O. has gone home. She reports that her husband is depressed, won't eat, and sleeps all day in his chair. She states, "I don't know what to do anymore! I think he just wants to die." She then starts crying.

7. What should the nurse say to Mrs. L. O.?
8. Whom should the nurse contact to assist the family?

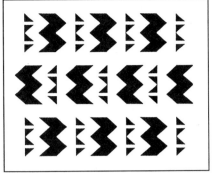

CHAPTER 56

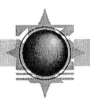

Interventions for Clients with Noninflammatory Intestinal Disorders

LEARNING OBJECTIVES

At the end of this chapter, the student will be able to

- Discuss irritable bowel syndrome (IBS) and related management
- Discuss hernias and related management
- Discuss the pathophysiology, etiology, and incidence of cancer of the intestine
- Provide care for the client with cancer of the colon
- Discuss the pathophysiology, etiology, and incidence of intestinal obstruction
- Manage care for the client with intestinal obstruction
- Discuss abdominal trauma
- Discuss management of the client with polyps
- Discuss management of the client with hemorrhoids
- Discuss malabsorption syndrome

PREREQUISITE KNOWLEDGE

Prior to beginning this chapter, the student should review

- The anatomy and physiology of the small bowel and large intestine, including the rectum and anus
- The effect of the central and autonomic nervous systems on the gastrointestinal organs
- Normal nutrition, including the essential vitamins, minerals, and foods in the recommended food groups
- Special diets for client with gastrointestinal organ disorders, such as low protein, high carbohydrate, bland, low fiber, liquid, and puréed
- The principles of oral hygiene
- The care of nasogastric and intestinal tubes
- The care of feeding tubes and the preparation of tube-feeding formulas
- The principles of total parental nutrition (TPN) and care of peripheral and central line catheters
- The principles of enema administration
- Normal fluid and electrolyte values
- Perioperative nursing care
- The concepts of grief, loss, death, and dying
- The concepts of body image and self-esteem

STUDY QUESTIONS

Irritable Bowel Syndrome

1. Briefly discuss why irritable bowel syndrome (IBS) is not a true colitis.

   _____

   _____

   _____

2. List the possible stimuli that lead to changes to GI motility.

   a. _____

   b. _____

   c. _____

   d. _____

   e. _____

   f. _____

   g. _____

3. IBS is commonly characterized by

   a. chronic diarrhea

   b. chronic constipation

   c. alternating diarrhea and constipation

4. Which of the following statements is true about IBS?

   a. IBS occurs infrequently in the Western world.

   b. Lactose intolerance may be a contributing factor.

   c. Individual life style is relatively unaffected.

   d. The disorder is reportable to the Centers for Disease Control.

5. List the subjective client data relevant to IBS. Use a separate sheet.

6. List the objective client data relevant to IBS. Use a separate sheet.

7. Which of the following interventions is implemented for the client with IBS?

   a. increasing liquids to at least 800 mL/day

   b. establishing a time for regular bowel elimination

   c. collecting multiple stool specimens for culture

   d. teaching about long-term therapy with anti-diarrheals

8. Preventive measures for IBS include

   a. consuming carbonated beverages with meals

   b. engaging in social conversation at mealtimes

   c. limiting activity unless it is in the home

   d. reducing stress levels and managing stressors

9. Which of the following statements indicates that the client with IBS understands his or her home maintenance regimen?

   a. "I enjoy having a glass or two of wine with my dinner."

   b. "A cigarette after meals helps me to relax."

   c. "It's awkward to take mediation at the office."

   d. "I take a walk after lunch before going back to work."

Herniation

10. Identify causes of increased intra-abdominal pressure leading to a hernia.

    a. _____

    b. _____

    c. _____

    d. _____

Match the following types of hernias (11–17) with their descriptions (a–g).

_____ 11. femoral

_____ 12. incarcerated

_____ 13. indirect inguinal

_____ 14. reducible

_____ 15. strangulated

_____ 16. umbilical

_____ 17. ventral

a. contents of the sac can be replaced into the abdominal cavity

b. occurring when muscle ring enlarges, allowing peritoneum through

c. occurring in the region of the navel

d. tissue follows the spermatic cord descending into the scrotum

e. cannot be replaced back into the abdominal cavity

f. blood supply to the herniated bowel segment is cut off

g. occurring at the site of a prior surgical incision

18. Which of the following statements is correct about hernias?

    a. Direct hernias are the most common type.

    b. Umbilical hernias are more common in the elderly.

    c. Indirect hernias occur most often in men.

    d. Incisional hernias are common in obese people.

19. List the subjective client data relevant to hernias. Use a separate sheet.

20. List the objective client data relevant to hernias. Use a separate sheet.

21. Briefly discuss why the nurse or the client should not attempt to reduce an incarcerated hernia.

    _____

    _____

    _____

    _____

    _____

22. Interventions for the client who uses a truss for a hernia include

    a. using a surgical binder to hold the truss in place

    b. inspecting the skin under the truss several times a week

    c. applying the truss while sitting on the edge of the bed

    d. applying powder to the skin under the truss daily

23. Postoperative measures for the male client who has had an inguinal herniorrhaphy include

    a. applying a warm pack to the scrotum

    b. elevating the scrotum on a sling

    c. encouraging aggressive coughing and deep breathing

    d. encouraging use of a urinal to void

24. Preventive measures for hernias include

    a. using proper lifting techniques

    b. being slightly underweight

    c. refraining from physical activity

    d. eating a high-fiber diet

Colorectal Cancer

25. Put in sequence the following steps describing the growth and spread of an intestinal tumor.

    _____ a. enlargement into the bowel lumen

    _____ b. presence of a polyp in the bowel

    _____ c. malignant cells found in the liver

    _____ d. malignant cells line the bowel wall

    _____ e. local invasion into layers of the bowel wall

    _____ f. spread via the lymphatics or circulatory system

26. Identify the sites where intestinal tumors metastasize.

    a. _____

    b. _____

    c. _____

    d. _____

    e. _____

    f. _____

    g. _____

27. Define *tumor seeding*. Use a separate sheet.

28. List the complications related to a growing intestinal tumor.

    a. _____

    _____

    b. _____

    _____

    c. _____

    _____

    d. _____

    _____

    e. _____

    _____

    f. _____

    _____

29. Which of the following statements is correct about the etiology of intestinal cancer?

    a. The exact cause of colorectal cancer is unknown.

    b. Decreased transit time is linked to tumor formation.

    c. Refined carbohydrates decrease transit time.

    d. Chemical mutagens are substances known to prevent cancer.

30. The primary risk factor for colorectal cancer is

    a. Crohn's disease

    b. familial polyposis

    c. ulcerative colitis

    d. ureterosigmoidostomy

31. Preventive measures for intestinal cancers include

    a. maintaining body weight slightly below the ideal

    b. consuming fewer cruciferous vegetables

    c. having an annual sigmoidoscopy beginning at age 40 years

    d. checking one's own stool for guaiac with a home test kit

32. List the subjective client data relevant to intestinal cancer. Use a separate sheet.

33. List the objective client data relevant to intestinal cancer. Use a separate sheet.

34. Discuss the psychosocial implications for the client with intestinal cancer. Use a separate sheet.

CT 35. Design a teaching/learning plan for a client who is to have stool guaiac tests done. Submit the completed exercise to the clinical instructor on a separate sheet.

36. Which of the following statements is correct about cancer of the intestine?

    a. Symptoms occur early in the disease process.

    b. Screening tests detect the disease in early stages.

    c. Deterioration is rapid once metastases have occurred.

    d. Treatment even in the early stages is not very effective.

37. Following colostomy surgery, the nurse

    a. covers the stoma with a dry, sterile dressing

    b. applies a pouch system as soon as possible

    c. makes a pinhole in the pouch for gas to escape

    d. watches for the colostomy to function by day one

38. Which of the following should the client who has a perineal wound and cavity be instructed to report to the physician immediately?

    a. serosanguinous drainage from the wound

    b. sensations of having a bowel movement

    c. constant perineal odor and pain

    d. occasional perineal pain and itching

39. A food that the client with a colostomy should avoid is

    a. cheese

    b. poultry

    c. hard candy

    d. sherbet

Intestinal Obstruction

Match the following terms related to intestinal obstruction (40–47) with their definitions (a–h).

_____ 40. adhesions

_____ 41. adynamic ileus

_____ 42. complete obstruction

_____ 43. incarcerated obstruction

_____ 44. mechanical obstruction

_____ 45. nonmechanical obstruction

_____ 46. partial obstruction

_____ 47. strangulated obstruction

a. blockage of the bowel lumen due to internal or external factors

b. incomplete blockage of intestine

c. blockage of bowel lumen due to decreased muscular activity

d. total blockage of intestinal lumen

e. blockage with compromised blood flow

f. blockage with decreased blood flow and tissue necrosis

g. decreased intestinal activity

h. bands of scar tissue encircling intestine and constricting lumen

48. Describe adynamic ileus and its progression to hypovolemic shock. Use a separate sheet.

49. Discuss how septic shock may result from a strangulated or incarcerated obstruction. Use a separate sheet.

Match the following metabolic disturbances (50–52) with their levels of bowel obstruction (a–c).

_____ 50. insignificant imbalance

_____ 51. metabolic acidosis

_____ 52. metabolic alkalosis

a. high in the small intestine

b. below the duodenum and above the large bowel

c. below the terminal ileum

53. Identify the common causes of mechanical obstructions of the small intestine and large bowel.

Small intestine:

a. _____

b. _____

Large bowel:

a. _____

b. _____

c. _____

54. Draw a diagram of a volvulus and an intussusception. Use a separate sheet.

55. Identify preventive measures for intestinal obstruction. Use a separate sheet.

56. List the subjective client data relevant to intestinal obstruction. Use a separate sheet.

57. List the objective client data relevant to intestinal obstruction. Use a separate sheet.

58. Mechanical obstruction above the ileum usually

a. causes late, profuse vomiting

b. produces emesis containing fecal contents

c. results in thick, foul-smelling vomitus

d. results in emesis of partly digested food

59. Nursing care of the client with a newly inserted nasointestinal tube includes

a. anchoring the tube firmly to the client's cheek

b. irrigating with 30 mL of sterile saline prn

c. changing the client's position every 2 hours

d. setting the tube to low continuous suction

60. Assessments for the client with a nasointestinal tube include

a. measuring drainage output every 8 hours

b. asking the client to report passing flatus

c. auscultating bowel sounds every 8 hours

d. measuring abdominal girth every other day

61. Interventions for the client with Fluid Volume Deficit related to an intestinal obstruction include

a. frequent mouth care with lemon-glycerine swabs

b. assessing for sacral and pretibial edema

c. providing ice chips prn for the client to suck

d. monitoring for bradycardia and hypertension

62. Which of the following observations should the nurse report immediately for the client with an intestinal obstruction?

a. a urinary output of 1000 mL in an 8-hour period

b. jugular venous distention halfway up the neck when sitting

c. abdominal pain changing from colicky to constant discomfort

d. the client's repeated requests for something to drink

63. Discharge instructions for the client who has had an intestinal obstruction due to fecal impaction include

a. encouragement to report episodes of diarrhea

b. information about analgesics such as oxycodone (Percodan)

c. reminding the client to limit activity

d. providing a written description of a low-fiber diet

Abdominal Trauma

64. List the two major categories of abdominal injury and identify examples of each.

a. _____

_____

_____

_____

b. _____

_____

_____

_____

65. Identify reasons for increased client mortality risk following abdominal trauma.

    a. _____

    _____

    b. _____

    _____

    c. _____

    _____

    d. _____

    _____

66. To assess the abdomen for possible trauma, the nurse

    a. exposes the abdomen and flanks from the xiphysis process to the symphysis pubis

    b. inspects for symmetry, abrasions, lacerations, ecchymosis, and penetrating wounds

    c. carefully removes pneumatic antishock trousers and splints any fractures

    d. palpates deeply over the abdominal wall for masses and areas of tenderness

67. Briefly discuss why at least two large-bore intravenous catheters are inserted in the client with abdominal trauma. Use a separate sheet.

68. Discuss why serial hemoglobin and hematocrit levels are assessed. Use a separate sheet.

69. Complete the following chart by identifying rationales for these interventions implemented for the client with abdominal trauma. Submit the completed exercise to the clinical instructor on a separate sheet.

Intervention	Rationale
a. placing on a cardiac monitor	
b. inserting an indwelling urinary catheter	
c. measuring urine specific gravity hourly	
d. inserting an NG tube	
e. assessing blood gases	
f. preparing for peritoneal aspiration and lavage	
g. preparing the client for emergency surgery	

70. Discuss why all clients who have suffered abdominal trauma are taught which signs and symptoms to report regardless of whether they have had surgery. Use a separate sheet.

Polyps

71. Which of the following statements are true about intestinal polyps?

    a. Most polyps are premalignant.

    b. Polyps of certain tissue types are more likely to be malignant.

    c. Most intestinal polyps are in the distal colon.

    d. Tubular adenomas are rare and usually malignant.

    e. Villous adenomas tend to be benign.

    f. Pedunculated polyps have stalks.

    g. Villous adenomas tend to be sessile.

    h. Familial polyposis is characterized by multiple colorectal polyps.

    i. Polyps frequently cause pain and rectal bleeding.

    j. A polypectomy can be done during a colonoscopy.

72. Care of the client who has had a colorectal polypectomy includes

    a. administering oral codeine to promote constipation

    b. examining all stools for blood or mucopurulent drainage

    c. providing a clear liquid diet for the first week

    d. reassuring the client that recurrence is unlikely

Hemorrhoids

73. Differentiate between internal and external hemorrhoids. Use a separate sheet.

74. List the common causes of hemorrhoids.

    a. _____

    b. _____

    c. _____

75. Which of the following interventions is contraindicated in the nonsurgical management of hemorrhoids?

a. encouraging a diet high in fiber and fluids

b. administering a stool softener such as docusate sodium

c. assisting with stiz baths three or four times a day

d. administering an opioid analgesic prior to defecation

76. Identify three potential postoperative problems that may occur following a hemorrhoidectomy.

a. _____

b. _____

c. _____

Malabsorption Syndrome

77. List the types of disorders that may result in malabsorption, and give an example of which nutrients are not absorbed for each.

a. _____

_____

b. _____

_____

c. _____

_____

d. _____

_____

e. _____

_____

f. _____

_____

78. List data relevant to malabsorption. Use a separate sheet.

79. Identify the changes in serum values that occur related to the following seven clinical problems.

a. iron deficiency anemia:

_____

_____

b. vitamin B_{12} and folic acid deficiency:

_____

_____

c. insufficient gastric acid:

_____

_____

d. decreased fat digestion and absorption:

_____

_____

e. vitamin D malabsorption:

_____

_____

f. bile salt deficiency:

_____

_____

g. loss of protein stores:

_____

_____

80. Which of the following statements is correct about dietary management of malabsorption syndrome?

a. A low-fat diet may improve absorption in cystic fibrosis.

b. Lactose-free diets are recommended for non-tropical sprue.

c. Gluten-free diets are advisable for gallbladder disease.

d. Low-protein diets are best after a gastrectomy.

81. Which of the following statements is correct about the pharmacological treatment of various malabsorption syndromes?

a. Belladonna taken prior to meal enhances gastric motility.

b. H_2 receptor antagonists decrease pancreatic enzyme supplies.

c. Steroids are used to control diarrhea and steatorrhea.

d. Pancreatic enzyme replacement improves fat absorption.

CRITICAL THINKING EXERCISES

Case Study: Cancer of the Intestine

C. L. is a 59-year-old married client who is admitted with intestinal bleeding. He has had a weight loss of 10 pounds over the past 5 weeks. Upon admission, C. L. is pale and moves slowly. During the nursing interview, C. L. excuses himself to go to the bathroom. He passes a large, soft, dark stool with a fetid odor. The toilet tissue is pink stained. C. L. states that the bloody stools began 2 days ago. He did not see his physician until this morning because "I just know that I have cancer in my gut. My mother had this very same thing and she died a horrible death. I finally couldn't put it off anymore, I'm so weak."

Address the following questions:

1. Formulate relevant actual and potential nursing diagnoses for C. L. based on the above data.

Radiological tests show that C. L. has a large mass in the ascending colon, near the hepatic flexure. He is to be prepared for surgery, which is scheduled for the next day. Preoperatively, C. L. is to be on clear liquids and have an intravenous infusion started for administration of blood replacement. Oral antibiotics are ordered for a bowel prep and include neomycin sulfate (Neobiotic) 1 g and erythromycin (E-Mycin) 1 g to be given PO at 1:00 p.m., 2:00 p.m., and 11:00 p.m. The physician orders two units of packed cells to be given as soon as they are available.

2. Discuss the purpose for administering these antibiotics to C. L., their dose, and the route of administration.

3. What should the nurse do prior to adding the units of blood to the infusion? What assessments should be made before and during the blood transfusions? What symptoms does the nurse observe for while the blood is transfusing that may indicate a transfusion reaction?

C. L. has a right hemicolectomy and end-to-end anastomosis of the bowel. A cecostomy tube is placed postoperatively until the anastomosis heals and will remain in place until post-surgical radiation therapy is completed. Chemotherapy is also planned.

4. Identify additional nursing diagnoses for C. L. based on the above data.

5. Design a discharge teaching/learning plan for C. L. and his wife. Include care of the cecostomy tube and drainage apparatus, skin care, diet instruction, activity restrictions, and adjustments for sexual activity.

6. What community resources should the nurse recommend to C. L. and his family to assist them in coping with home management?

7. The radiation and chemotherapy will begin 1 week post-discharge. What information should the nurse discuss with C. L. and his family concerning the therapy and its effects?

8. Once the radiation and chemotherapy begin, what instructions will C. L. and his family need about diet, hydration, and bowel and skin care?

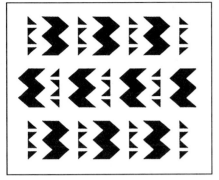

CHAPTER 57

Interventions for Clients with Inflammatory Intestinal Disorders

LEARNING OBJECTIVES

At the end of this chapter, the student will be able to

▋ Discuss the pathophysiology, etiology, and incidence of appendicitis

▋ Provide care for the client with appendicitis

▋ Discuss the pathophysiology and etiology of peritonitis

▋ Provide care for the client with peritonitis

▋ Discuss the pathophysiology, etiology, and incidence of gastroenteritis

▋ Provide care for the client with gastroenteritis

▋ Discuss the pathophysiology, etiology, and incidence of ulcerative colitis

▋ Provide care for the client with ulcerative colitis

▋ Discuss the pathophysiology, etiology, and incidence of Crohn's disease

▋ Provide care for the client with Crohn's disease

▋ Discuss the pathophysiology, etiology, and incidence of diverticular disease

▋ Provide care for the client with diverticular disease

▋ Identify problems of the anal area

▋ Discuss parasitic infections of the gastrointestinal tract

▋ Discuss food poisoning

PREREQUISITE KNOWLEDGE

Prior to beginning this chapter, the student should review

▋ The anatomy and physiology of the small bowel and large intestine, including the rectum and anus

▋ The effect of the central and autonomic nervous systems on the gastrointestinal organs

▋ Normal nutrition, including the essential vitamins, minerals and foods in the recommended food groups

▋ Special diets for client with gastrointestinal disorders, such as high protein, high carbohydrate, bland, low fiber, liquid, and puréed

▋ The principles of oral hygiene

▋ The care of nasogastric and intestinal tubes

▋ The care of feeding tubes and preparation of tube-feeding formulas

▋ The principles of total parenteral nutrition (TPN) and care of peripheral and central line catheters

▋ The principles of enema administration

▋ Normal fluid and electrolyte values

▋ Perioperative nursing care

▋ The concepts of grief, loss, death, and dying

▋ The concepts of body image and self-esteem

▋ The principles of infection control

▋ Universal or body substance precautions

STUDY QUESTIONS

Appendicitis

1. Describe the function of the appendix.

   _____

   _____

2. Put the following events related to appendicitis in chronological order.

   ____ a. hypoxia from deprived blood flow

   ____ b. peritonitis

   ____ c. intestinal mucosa secretes fluid

   ____ d. gangrene from hypoxia or perforation

   ____ e. appendix lumen is obstructed

   ____ f. intraluminal pressure exceeds venous pressure

   ____ g. bacteria invade wall of the appendix

   ____ h. further reduction of blood flow to the mucosa

   ____ i. increased swelling from infection

3. Define *fecalith* and describe the relationship of a fecalith to appendiceal obstruction:

   _____

   _____

   _____

4. Which of the following statements is correct about appendicitis?

   a. The peak incidence is between the ages of 20 and 30 years.

   b. Perforation is relatively common in middle-aged adults.

   c. Elderly people are more sensitive to normal pain signals.

   d. Diagnosis and treatment occur rapidly in the elderly.

5. Preventive measures for appendicitis include

   a. decreasing fiber in the diet

   b. treating intestinal parasites

   c. taking laxatives regularly

   d. restricting fluids to 1000 mL per day

6. List the subjective client data relevant to appendicitis. Use a separate sheet.

7. List the objective client data relevant to appendicitis. Use a separate sheet.

8. Identify the three complications of appendicitis that may result from altered tissue perfusion.

   a. _____

   b. _____

   c. _____

9. Nonsurgical management of suspected appendicitis includes

   a. administering analgesics for comfort

   b. monitoring intravenous fluids and electrolytes

   c. administering cleansing enemas

   d. applying a warm pack over McBurney's point

10. Postoperative nursing care for the client who has a wound drain following an appendectomy includes

    a. changing the dressing at least four times a day

    b. attaching the drain to low intermittent suction

    c. observing for and reporting bleeding immediately

    d. advancing the drain 1 inch every day for 4 days

11. Which of the following activities is preferable for a client following an appendectomy?

    a. gardening

    b biking

    c. tennis

    d. walking

Peritonitis

12. The fluid shift that occurs in peritonitis results in

    a. intracellular fluid moving into the peritoneal cavity

    b. a significant increase in circulatory volume

    c. eventual renal failure and electrolyte imbalance

    d. increased bowel motility due to increased fluid volume

13. The respiratory problems that may accompany peritonitis are a result of

    a. associated pain interfering with ventilation

    b. decreased pressure against the diaphragm

    c. increased oxygen demands from skeletal muscles

    d. fluid shifts to the thoracic cavity

14. Differentiate between primary and secondary peritonitis. Use a separate sheet.

15. List the preventive measures for peritonitis. Use a separate sheet.

16. List the subjective client data relevant to peritonitis. Use a separate sheet.

17. List the objective client data relevant to peritonitis. Use a separate sheet.

18. In the early stages of peritonitis, the client usually reports

    a. diffuse, vague, intermittent pain

    b. localized, continuous right lower quadrant (RLQ) pain

    c. localized, intermittent, severe RLQ pain

    d. widespread, continuous, severe abdominal pain

19. Assessment findings in the client who has generalized peritonitis include

    a. bradycardia

    b. rebound tenderness

    c. restlessness

    d. oliguria

20. Interventions following abdominal surgery for peritonitis include

    a. monitoring vital signs every 2 hours

    b. positioning the client in high Fowler's

    c. evaluating for absence of abdominal distention

    d. ambulating the client beginning day one

21. Data indicating that the client with peritonitis has a normal fluid balance include

    a. tenting of the skin over the forearm

    b. pulse rate of 84 beats per minute, regular and strong

    c. urinary output of 25 mL per hour

    d. bilateral pretibial edema rated 2+

Gastroenteritis

22. Define *gastroenteritis:*

    _____

    _____

    _____

    _____

23. Identify the two types of organisms responsible for gastroenteritis.

    a. _____

    b. _____

24. Briefly describe the symptoms commonly occurring in gastroenteritis regardless of the causative organism or specific pathophysiology.

    _____

    _____

    _____

    _____

25. List three circumstances in which invading organisms can infect a person and result in gastroenteritis and give an example of each. Use a separate sheet.

26. Discuss the primary route of transmission for invading organisms causing gastroenteritis. Use a separate sheet.

27. Identify the two age groups that are most susceptible to shigellosis and briefly discuss why.

    _____

    _____

    _____

    _____

28. Identify four ways to avoid contamination and prevent the spread of gastroenteritis. Use a separate sheet.

29. List the subjective client data relevant to gastroenteritis. Use a separate sheet.

30. List the objective client data relevant to gastroenteritis. Use a separate sheet.

31. List the two common laboratory tests used to identify pathogens that cause gastroenteritis.

    a. _____

    _____

    b. _____

    _____

32. Briefly discuss the significance of obtaining daily weights for the client with gastroenteritis. Use a separate sheet.

33. Briefly discuss the rationale for using hypotonic intravenous fluids for replacement therapy in gastroenteritis. Use a separate sheet.

34. Describe the sequence of the dietary progression for clients with gastroenteritis.

_____

_____

_____

35. Which of the following statements is correct about the treatment of gastroenteritis?

    a. Anticholinergics are routinely administered to decrease stool frequency.

    b. Antiemetics help to reduce the nausea and vomiting clients experience.

    c. Diarrhea that continues more than 10 days requires thorough investigation.

    d. Bacteriological validation of organisms is necessary in short-term diarrhea.

36. Which of the following statement indicates that a client with gastroenteritis is ready for discharge?

    a. "I can start helping my wife with the grocery shopping and cooking again."

    b. "The doctor said that I need to take these pills until the bottle is empty."

    c. "I can expect my diarrhea to continue for another 2 weeks at home."

    d. "I can't wait to start drinking my glass of milk at breakfast and lunch."

Ulcerative Colitis

37. Briefly discuss the significance of the loss of surface epithelium in the bowel lumen in ulcerative colitis. Use a separate sheet.

38. List the complications associated with ulcerative colitis. Use a separate sheet.

39. Which of the following statements is correct about ulcerative colitis?

    a. The cause of ulcerative colitis is an autoimmune dysfunction.

    b. Psychological factors contribute to the severity of attacks.

    c. There is a higher incidence of the disease in African-American people.

    d. Maintenance drug therapy helps prevent exacerbation episodes.

40. Prevention of ulcerative colitis includes

    a. no particular method of intervention

    b. following a lactose-free diet

    c. engaging in family counseling

    d. successful stress management

41. List the subjective client data relevant to ulcerative colitis. Use a separate sheet.

42. List the objective client data relevant to ulcerative colitis. Use a separate sheet.

43. Identify other disease processes that may be confused with ulcerative colitis and for which the nurse is responsible for collecting stool specimens for analysis.

    a. _____

    _____

    b. _____

    _____

44. Nonsurgical management of ulcerative colitis includes

    a. a high-roughage diet

    b. regular, moderate exercise

    c. antidiarrheal agents

    d. fluid restrictions

45. Which of the following drainage systems is the client who has had a Kock ileostomy procedure most likely to have postoperatively?

    a. gastrostomy tube set to low intermittent suction

    b. rectal tube set to low continuous suction

    c. pouch catheter set to continuous Y irrigation

    d. indwelling urinary catheter set to gravity drainage

46. Discharge instructions for the client with an ileostomy include

    a. suggesting that client empty the pouch after each meal when it is full

    b. reminding the client to include bran in the diet to increase stool bulk

    c. instructing the client to change the entire pouch system only when it becomes loose

    d. advising the client to monitor stoma output and report changes in volume to the physician

Crohn's Disease

47. Crohn's disease is similar to ulcerative colitis in that
    a. lesions extend through all bowel layers
    b. fistula formation is an early complication
    c. the underlying cause is unknown
    d. changes occur throughout the GI tract

48. Crohn's disease is different from ulcerative colitis in that
    a. the stools may show evidence of blood
    b. complications include anemia and dehydration
    c. there are associated systemic manifestations
    d. there is a higher incidence of cancer of the colon

49. Which of the following statements is correct about Crohn's disease?
    a. The highest incidence is in the 20- to 40-year age group.
    b. No known familial link correlates with its incidence.
    c. There is a decreased incidence in the Jewish population.
    d. Emotional factors can cause the disease.

50. List the subjective client data relevant to Crohn's disease. Use a separate sheet.

51. List the objective client data relevant to Crohn's disease. Use a separate sheet.

52. Identify the nursing diagnosis related to a serious, life-threatening complication seen in Crohn's disease that does not occur in ulcerative colitis.

    _____

    _____

    _____

53. Discuss the implications that an enteric fistula has for the client with Crohn's disease. Use a separate sheet.

54. Which of the following health care professionals is the best resource for skin care for the client who has an enteric fistula?
    a. physical therapist
    b. enterostomal therapist
    c. occupational therapist
    d. dermatologist

Diverticular Disease

55. Draw a diagram of a diverticulum. Use a separate sheet.

56. Which of the following statements is correct about diverticular disease?
    a. Most diverticula occur in the descending colon.
    b. Diverticula are uncomfortable even when not inflamed.
    c. High-fiber diets contribute to diverticula occurrence.
    d. Diverticula form where intestinal wall muscles are weak.

57. Preventive measures for diverticular disease include
    a. excluding whole-grain breads and cereal from the diet
    b. avoiding lettuce, spinach, and fresh pears
    c. using bulk agents such as psyllium hydrophilic mucilloid
    d. taking routine anticholinergics to reduce bowel spasm

58. List the subjective client data relevant to diverticular disease. Use a separate sheet.

59. List the objective client data relevant to diverticular disease. Use a separate sheet.

60. Briefly discuss why invasive radiographs or diagnostic tests are not done for the client with acute diverticulitis. Use a separate sheet.

61. Nonsurgical home management of diverticulitis includes
    a. following a full liquid diet
    b. engaging in light exercise such as walking
    c. applying a heating pad to the left lower quadrant (LLQ)
    d. refraining from lifting, straining, coughing, and bending

62. Nursing interventions for the client with acute diverticulitis include
    a. encouraging intake of a low-fiber diet
    b. administering laxatives or enemas daily
    c. monitoring intravenous fluids and antibiotics
    d. preparing the client for a permanent colostomy

63. Identify the complications indicating that a client with acute diverticulitis will need surgery.

    a. _____

    b. _____

    c. _____

    d. _____

    e. _____

    f. _____

    g. _____

    _____

64. Which of the following types of stomas will the client with diverticulitis have postoperatively?

    a. ileostomy

    b. Kock's pouch

    c. colostomy

    d. cecostomy

Anorectal Problems

Match the following anorectal problems (65–67) with their descriptions (a–c).

____ 65. anal fissure

____ 66. anal fistula

____ 67. anorectal abscess

a. duct obstruction and infection

b. perianal laceration

c. communicating tract

68. Discuss the significance of warm sitz baths as an intervention in managing anorectal problems. Use a separate sheet.

Parasitic Infection

69. Identify the most common route of transmission of parasitic and helminthic infections.

    _____

    _____

    _____

Match the following descriptions (70–81) with their associated parasitic infections (a–f). Answers may be used more than once.

____ 70. associated respiratory involvement

____ 71. transmitted via undercooked pork

____ 72. nocturnal perianal pruritus

____ 73. can cause liver abscess

____ 74. most prevalent parasitic infection in United States

____ 75. transmitted via raw fish

____ 76. muscular invasion occurs

____ 77. reinfection commonly occurs

____ 78. primarily invades small intestine

____ 79. generally causes few symptoms

____ 80. characteristic remission and recurrence of symptoms

____ 81. enters body through skin

a. amebiasis

b. enterobiasis

c. giardiasis

d. hookworms

e. tapeworms

f. trichinosis

82. Discuss precautions the nurse should take when collecting stool specimens from a client with suspected parasitic infection. Use a separate sheet.

83. Briefly discuss why other household members and sexual partners of the infected clients should also be examined for parasites. Use a separate sheet.

Food Poisoning

84. Complete the following chart by comparing and contrasting food poisoning and gastroenteritis. Use a separate sheet.

		Food Poisoning	Gastroenteritis
a.	communicability		
b.	incubation period		
c.	immunity status after recovery		
d.	diarrhea		
e.	nausea and vomiting		

85. Which types of food poisoning are routinely reported to local health departments?

_____

_____

86. Which type of food poisoning is the most life-threatening and why?

_____

_____

_____

CRITICAL THINKING EXERCISES

Case Study: Peritonitis

S. R. is a 75-year-old client who has had vague abdominal pain for several days. This morning she awoke at 6:15 a.m. with sharp periumbilical pain that did not respond to aspirin. She began to feel nauseated and clammy. At 8:30 a.m., S. R. phoned her daughter, saying that she was feeling weak and shaky and that the pain was getting worse. She had tried to have bowel movement but was unsuccessful. S. R. asked her daughter to contact her doctor and make an appointment for her. After talking to her daughter, S. R.'s physician arranged for immediate transportation for S. R. to the hospital. Upon arrival in the ED, S. R. had blood drawn and a portable abdominal flat plate and chest x-ray done. S. R.'s physician suspected a perforated appendix and ordered immediate preparations for surgery.

Address the following questions:

1. What laboratory work is significant to monitor in S. R. as she is being prepared for surgery? Why?

2. S. R. has been hospitalized only once before, for childbirth. Based on the above data, formulate relevant nursing diagnoses for S. R.

3. S. R. is to have an NG tube and a peripheral intravenous line inserted prior to surgery. Oxygen is ordered at 4 L per minute via nasal prongs. What does the nurse do to prepare S. R. for these treatments?

S. R. has an appendectomy and peritoneal lavage. The abdominal wound is packed and left open with three retention sutures and a Penrose drain in place. A dry sterile dressing covers the incision. There is an additional drain attached to closed bulb suction. Intravenous fluids are ordered at 100 mL per hour plus replacement for the hourly NG output. Oxygen continues to be administered at 4 L per minute. Cefamandole nafate (Mandol) 1 g every 4 hours intravenously is ordered. It is diluted in 50 mL of D_5W and administered over 20–30 minutes.

4. Discuss complications the nurse should monitor for in S. R. and give supporting rationale.

5. What additional nursing diagnoses are indicated for S. R. based on the above data?

6. Design a flow record for S. R.'s intake and output. Indicate which factors are to be monitored and recorded for a 24-hour period. If S. R.'s urinary output is 950 mL in 24 hours, is there cause for concern? Why or why not? What assessments should the nurse perform to determine if S. R.'s fluid balance is adequate?

7. Eventually S. R. recovers and is to be discharged to the care of her daughter. S. R. will go home with a wound that requires irrigation once a day with sterile normal saline and repacking with sterile gauze. Design a discharge teaching/learning plan for S. R.'s wound care.

Case Study: Ulcerative Colitis

R. B. is a 22-year-old female client diagnosed with ulcerative colitis. She has a history of exacerbations and remissions since the age of 15 years. Currently, R. B. is on a medical nursing unit being evaluated prior to surgery. Her husband is continuously at her bedside and is anxious to participate in R. B.'s physical care. R. B. was married at the age of 18 years and is a secretary. There are no children, and both sets of inlaws live out of state. R. B. is on a low-fiber diet with a peripheral intravenous line for antibiotic administration. One tablet of diphenoxylate hydrochloride and atropine (Lomotil) is to be given after each loose stool. Sulfasalazine (Azulfidine) 1 mg PO, qid, and prednisone 5 mg PO, bid, are also ordered.

Address the following questions:

1. Describe the kinds of foods R. B. may eat and those she should avoid.
2. Formulate relevant actual and potential nursing diagnoses for R. B. based on the above data.

The evaluation indicates that R. B. is a candidate for an ileostomy with a total procto-colectomy and abdominal-perineal resection. Surgery is scheduled in 3 days. R. B. is NPO except for her medications, and a subclavian catheter is inserted for TPN administration.

3. What assessments does the nurse make related to the TPN administration? Give the rationale for these.
4. Design a perioperative teaching/learning plan for R. B.

After surgery, R. B. has a stoma covered by a temporary drainable appliance, a large abdominal incision covered with a sterile dressing, and a perineal wound with a Penrose drain and sterile dressing. A Salem sump is connected to low continuous suction, and the central line has lactated Ringer's solution infusing. There are orders to resume the TPN once the solution is available from the pharmacy.

5. Describe the assessments the nurse should make relative to the stoma, any drainage from it, and the drainage appliance. What assessments are indicated for the sump drain? For the central line?
6. R. B.'s husband insists on being actively involved with the irrigations to the perineal wound, dressing changes, and stoma care. Discuss whether this is to R. B.'s benefit or not and support your answer with a rationale.

R. B.'s postoperative recovery is uneventful. She will be dismissed in 3 or 4 days. R. B. has begun empty the drainable appliance several times a day but has yet to change the appliance completely, relying on her husband to help with this. To the nurse's knowledge, neither R. B. nor her husband have discussed plans for going home. R. B. states that he is looking forward to going home; she is planning to rest and sunbathe on the beach (she lives in an ocean-side community). The discharge orders include instructions for a low-fiber diet, continued perineal wound irrigations and dressings, sitz baths three times a day, sulfasalazine (Azulfidine) 500 mg qid, and prednisone 5 mg qd.

7. Formulate relevant actual and potential nursing diagnoses for R. B. based on the above data.
8. What specific instructions are indicated for R. B. about her home medications, perineal wound care, diet, and planned activities?

R. B. comments that she is relieved to have had the surgery, stating that the pain and cramping are minimal now. She further states that she is eager to resume a "normal" life once she is fully recovered from the effects of the surgery. The nurse needs to explore R. B.'s concept of a "normal" life.

9. What information should the nurse discuss with R. B. about her recovery from ulcerative colitis? Her sexual activity? Her future childbearing plans?

Case Study: Crohn's Disease

M. W. is a 28-year-old client who has had Crohn's disease since the age of 19 years. She is 5 feet 5 inches tall and weighed 108 pounds on admission. Her usual weigh is 125 pounds. M. W. has an enterocutaneous fistula that drains 350–600 mL per 8-hour shift. Radiological study shows that the fistula's origin is in the terminal ileum. M. W. is NPO and has a central line infusion for TPN and antibiotic administration. The TPN solution has a calorie density of 1 calorie/mL.

Address the following questions:

1. Discuss the nutritional risk factors for M. W.

2. M. W.'s usual calorie needs are 1700 calories per day; she needs an additional 3000 calories to promote fistula healing. Calculate how much TPN solution must be infused in 24 hours to meet the total calorie demand. How many milliliters of TPN solution should be given in 1 hour?

Eventually, M. W.'s fistula drainage decreases and she is told that she will be able to go home. M. W. will be dismissed with the fistula, which still drains 50–100 mL per day, and will be on an oral enteric diet supplement.

3. Design a discharge teaching/learning plan for M. W. that addresses her skin care and nutritional needs.

4. What support systems may M. W. need once she is home?

Case Study: Diverticulitis

S. D. is a 66-year-old client who is admitted with left lower quadrant abdominal pain. She is known to have diverticula, and the pain has become increasingly uncomfortable for the past 3 days. A simple bowel resection and anastomosis are planned. Admission orders include placing S. D. on NPO, inserting an NG tube to low intermittent suction, intravenous fluids and clindamycin (Cleocin), and bed rest. A flat plate of the abdomen is also taken. Results show an abscess in the sigmoid area. Surgery is scheduled for the next day. The surgeon requests that the operative permit should read "exploratory laparotomy with sigmoid resection and possible temporary descending colostomy."

Address the following questions:

1. Discuss what the nurse does to prepare S. D. for the emergency surgery. What information should the nurse elicit from S. D. to proceed with the preoperative care?

2. Formulate actual and potential relevant nursing diagnoses for S. D.

S. D. returns to the nursing unit postoperatively with a temporary descending colostomy and mucous fistula. There is a temporary drainage appliance over the stoma, a small dressing over the mucous fistula, and a large abdominal wound with a dressing and Penrose drain. The next day, S. D. looks at her abdomen and asks what the dressings are for. When told about the mucous fistula, S. D. becomes upset. "My doctor didn't say anything about having two holes in my stomach! I wasn't supposed to have any holes and now I'm stuck with two of them!"

3. What should the nurse say to S. D.?

4. What does the nurse do to assist S. D. to adjust to her present circumstances?

5. Formulate additional nursing diagnoses for S. D. based on the above data.

S. D.'s postoperative recovery occurs without complication. Discharge is scheduled. Surgery to reanastomose the bowel will be scheduled at a later date. S. D. will not need to learn how to irrigate the colostomy, but she will need to be able to empty and clean the appliance, as well as change the appliance when necessary.

6. Plan a discharge teaching/learning plan for S. D. for care of her colostomy and fistula. Include diet instructions.

7. What community support system might be useful to S. D. as she continues her recovery at home?

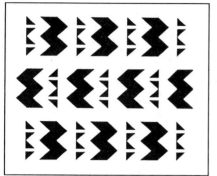

CHAPTER 58

Interventions for Clients with Liver Problems

LEARNING OBJECTIVES

At the end of this chapter, the student will be able to

■ Discuss the pathophysiology and etiology of cirrhosis

■ Provide care for the client with cirrhosis

■ Discuss the pathophysiology, etiology, and incidence of hepatitis

■ Provide care for the client with hepatitis

■ Identify other disorders of the liver and related treatment

■ Discuss indications for liver transplantation and care for the client undergoing liver transplantation

PREREQUISITE KNOWLEDGE

Prior to beginning this chapter, the student should review

■ The anatomy and physiology of the liver

■ Normal nutrition, including the essential vitamins, minerals, and foods in the recommended food groups

■ Special diets for client with disorders of the liver, such as low fat, low protein, high protein, high carbohydrate, and liquid

■ The principles of oral hygiene

■ The care of nasogastric and intestinal tubes

■ The care of feeding tubes and preparation of tube-feeding formulas

■ The principles of total parenteral nutrition (TPN) and care of peripheral and central line catheters

■ Normal fluid and electrolyte values

■ The principles of enema administration

■ Perioperative nursing care

■ The concepts of grief, loss, death, and dying

■ The concepts of body image and self-esteem

■ The principles of infection control

■ Universal or body substance precautions

STUDY QUESTIONS

Cirrhosis

Match the following descriptions (1–12) with their types of liver cirrhosis (a–d). Answers may be used more than once.

_____ 1. viral induced

_____ 2. vascular congestion

_____ 3. hobnailed capsule

_____ 4. associated with bile stasis

_____ 5. fatty infiltration of hepatocytes

_____ 6. chemical hepatotoxin induced

_____ 7. alcohol induced

_____ 8. liver anoxia

_____ 9. massive hepatocyte death

_____ 10. severe obstructive jaundice

_____ 11. increased hepatic volume

_____ 12. diffuse hepatic fibrosis

a. Laennec's

b. postnecrotic

c. biliary

d. cardiac

Match the following descriptions of pathophysiology (13–19) with their associated complications of liver cirrhosis (a–g).

_____ 13. bilirubin not excreted

_____ 14. vitamin K deficiency

_____ 15. backflow of blood to liver and spleen

_____ 16. impaired ammonia metabolism

_____ 17. plasma leaking into peritoneal cavity

_____ 18. kidneys unable to excrete solutes

_____ 19. thin-walled distended veins

a. portal hypertension

b. ascites

c. bleeding

d. esophageal varices

e. jaundice

f. encephalopathy

g. hepatorenal syndrome

20. Identify the most common form of cirrhosis in the United States. How can it be prevented?

_____

_____

_____

21. List the subjective client data relevant to cirrhosis of the liver. Use a separate sheet.

22. List the objective client data relevant to cirrhosis of the liver. Use a separate sheet.

Match the following abnormal laboratory findings in the cirrhotic client (23–32) with their causes (a–e). Answers may be used more than once.

_____ 23. serum aspartate aminotransferase elevates

_____ 24. globulins elevate

_____ 25. total proteins decrease

_____ 26. ammonia increases

_____ 27. serum alanine aminotransferase elevates

_____ 28. prothrombin time prolongs

_____ 29. direct bilirubin increases

_____ 30. albumin decreases

_____ 31. lactate dehydrogenase elevates

_____ 32. alkaline phosphatase elevates

a. hepatocyte death

b. biliary obstruction

c. decreased liver synthesis

d. increased immune response

e. decreased conversion

33. Identify rationales for the following interventions implemented for the cirrhotic client with ascites. Use a separate sheet.

a. low-sodium diet

b. fluid restriction

c. vitamin supplements

d. diuretic therapy

e. intake and output measurement

f. daily weight measurement

g. abdominal girth measurement

h. monitor electrolyte balance

i. potassium supplements

j. low-sodium antacid therapy

k. head of bed elevated

34. Which of the following antacids is preferred for the client with cirrhosis of the liver?

    a. magnesium hydroxide (Gelusil)

    b. magnesium hydroxide with aluminum hydroxide (Maalox)

    c. magaldrate (Riopan)

    d. sodium bicarbonate

35. Which of the following should the nurse do when assisting the physician with a paracentesis for a client with Laennec's cirrhosis?

    a. Ask the client to void or empty the urinary drainage bag before beginning to minimize bladder trauma.

    b. Assist the client to a left lateral recumbent position to reduce possible organ laceration.

    c. Weigh the client immediately after the procedure for comparison with the baseline weight.

    d. Discard the collected fluid carefully in the toilet to minimize cross-contamination.

36. Discuss why the cirrhotic client with medically unmanageable ascites is a poor surgical risk for a shunting procedure. Use s separate sheet.

37. Identify the purpose of a peritoneovenous shunt. Use a separate sheet.

38. Discuss the rationale for administering fresh frozen plasma, vitamin K, and packed red cells preoperatively to the client who is to have a peritoneovenous shunt procedure. Use a separate sheet.

39. Postoperatively, the client who has had a peritoneovenous shunting procedure is carefully monitored for

    a. decreased blood pressure

    b. increased blood pressure

    c. decreased central venous pressure

    d. increased urinary output

40. Nursing responsibilities related to esophagogastric balloon tamponade include

    a. identifying and labeling each lumen after the tamponade tube is inserted

    b. setting the esophageal and gastric drainage lumens to low continuous suction

    c. ensuring that balloon pressures are kept at levels needed to control bleeding

    d. repositioning the tube it if migrates upward and causes airway obstruction

41. Identify the types of intravenous products that the nurse may need to administer in cases of massive esophageal hemorrhage.

    a. _____

    _____

    b. _____

    _____

    c. _____

    _____

    d. _____

    _____

42. Vasopressin (Pitressin) therapy results in

    a. improved blood flow in the portal system

    b. relaxation of vascular bed smooth muscle

    c. effective long-term control of variceal bleeding

    d. decreased blood flow to the abdominal organs

43. Nursing management of the client have endoscopic injection sclerotherapy includes

    a. obtaining baseline vital signs after sedating the client

    b. medicating the client for acute changes in chest discomfort

    c. assessing lung sounds for hyperinflation and air trapping

    d. monitoring closely for acute hemorrhagic episodes

44. Portosystemic decompression shunting procedures

    a. are a last-resort intervention for portal hypertension

    b. improve the client's survival time significantly

    c. have few associated life-threatening complications

    d. divert portal vein blood flow to the superior vena cava

45. Following a portosystemic decompression shunting procedure, the nurse should immediately report

    a. increased urinary output

    b. decreased pulmonary artery pressure

    c. increased abdominal girth measurements

    d. decreased central venous pressure

46. Which of the following diets is indicated in early cirrhosis but contraindicated in portal systemic encephalopathy?

    a. high carbohydrate, low fat, low protein

    b. low carbohydrate, low fat, high protein

    c. high carbohydrate, moderate fat, high protein

    d. low carbohydrate, moderate fate, low protein

47. Which of the following drugs is usually contraindicated for the client with portal systemic encephalopathy?

    a. levodopa (Dopar)

    b. diazepam (Valium)

    c. lactulose (Cephulac)

    d. neomycin sulfate (Neobiotic)

48. List the stages of portal-systemic encephalopathy and discuss assessments the nurse makes relative to each stage. Use a separate sheet. Submit the completed exercise to the clinical instructor.

Hepatitis

49. Put in sequence the following steps describing the pathological changes that occur in hepatitis.

    _____ a. intrahepatic jaundice results from edema of bile channels

    _____ b. liver enlargement and congestion due to inflammatory cells, edema, and lymphocytes

    _____ c. portal circulation impaired due to distorted lobular pattern

    _____ d. eventual complete regeneration of liver cells

    _____ e. widespread inflammation, necrosis, and hepatocellular regeneration

    _____ f. exposure to causative agent occurs

    _____ g. active phagocytosis and enzyme activity remove damaged cells

50. List the types of viral hepatitis.

    a. _____

    b. _____

    c. _____

    d. _____

    e. _____

51. Identify the type of viral hepatitis that is of most concern to health care workers.

_____

Match the following descriptions (52–63) with their types of hepatitis (a–e). Answers may be used more than once.

_____ 52. occurs only in presence of hepatitis B virus

_____ 53. common cause of post-transfusion hepatitis

_____ 54. rarely life threatening

_____ 55. percutaneous route of transmission

_____ 56. does not lead to chronic infection

_____ 57. often goes unrecognized

_____ 58. spreads via close personal contact

_____ 59. major source of nosocomial infection

_____ 60. household spreading is common

_____ 61. no carrier state

_____ 62. no established preventive measures

_____ 63. vaccinations are available

a. hepatitis A

b. hepatitis B

c. hepatitis C

d. delta hepatitis

e. hepatitis E

64. Describe additional causes of hepatitis.

    a. _____

    _____

    _____

    b. _____

    _____

    _____

Match the following complications of viral hepatitis (65–67) with their descriptions (a–c).

____ 65. chronic-active hepatitis

____ 66. chronic-persistent hepatitis

____ 67. fulminant hepatitis

a. nonprogressive liver damage

b. progressive liver damage with necrosis, inflammation, and fibrosis

c. severe, frequently fatal failure of liver cells to regenerate

68. List the subjective client data relevant to hepatitis. Use a separate sheet.

69. List the objective client data relevant to hepatitis. Use a separate sheet.

70. Which of the following serum laboratory findings is detected only very briefly in delta hepatitis?

a. immunoglobulin M

b. circulating hepatitis D antigen

c. immunoglobulin G

d. immunoglobulin A

71. Interventions for the client with viral hepatitis include

a. strict bed rest

b. physical therapy

c. universal precautions

d. special diets

72. Which of the following drugs is contraindicated for managing nausea in the client with viral hepatitis?

a. trimethobenzamide hydrochloride (Tigan)

b. prochlorperazine maleate (Compazine)

c. dimenhydrinate (Dramamine)

d. benzquinamide hydrochloride (Emete-Con)

73. Discharge instructions for the client with viral hepatitis include

a. advising the client to use aspirin for relief of headache or minor pain

b. encouraging the client to begin an exercise program at a local health spa

c. telling the client that it is permissible to help with family meal preparations

d. cautioning the client to avoid sharing bathroom towels with family members

Other Liver Problems

Match the following descriptions (74–84) with their liver disorders (a–c). Answers may be used more than once.

____ 74. bacterial invasion

____ 75. result of faulty metabolism

____ 76. penetrating or blunt injury

____ 77. sudden onset of symptoms

____ 78. hemorrhagic shock

____ 79. confirmed by liver biopsy

____ 80. hepatomegaly

____ 81. right shoulder pain

____ 82. associated with chronic alcoholism

____ 83. anorexia, weight loss

____ 84. multiple blood products

a. fatty liver

b. hepatic abscess

c. liver trauma

85. Identify the sources of carcinoma metastases to the liver.

_____

_____

_____

86. Identify and briefly describe the primary type of hepatic carcinoma.

_____

_____

_____

87. List the associated causes of liver cancer.

a. _____

b. _____

c. _____

d. _____

e. _____

f. _____

Liver Transplantation

88. Briefly describe the types of clients who are and are not candidates for liver transplantation. Use a separate sheet.

89. Identify when organ rejection is most likely to occur following liver transplantation.

_____

_____

90. List the major complications that may occur following liver transplantation. Use a separate sheet.

91. Identify the assessments the nurse performs to monitor for tissue rejection following liver transplantation.

a. _____

_____

b. _____

_____

c. _____

_____

d. _____

_____

92. Identify drug therapy used to prevent tissue rejection following liver transplantation.

a. _____

_____

_____

b. _____

_____

_____

c. _____

_____

_____

CRITICAL THINKING EXERCISES

Case Study: Cirrhosis of the Liver

M. N. is a 54-year-old client admitted to a medical nursing unit with a diagnosis of prehepatic coma secondary to Laennec's cirrhosis. Admission assessment shows that he has a grossly distended abdomen, bilateral 4+ ankle edema, jaundiced sclerae and skin, and multiple bruises. M. N. has difficulty answering the nurse's questions, easily becoming distracted and preoccupied with scratching his arms and legs vigorously. Several times, he closes his eyes and dozes briefly, awakening with a start and asking where he is.

Address the following questions:

1. Identify the data that support the clinical diagnosis of prehepatic coma.

2. Discuss why M. N. has ascites and peripheral edema.

3. Based on the above data, formulate relevant nursing diagnoses for M. N.

Laboratory data for M. N. show increased serum bilirubin, decreased total proteins and serum albumin, prolonged prothrombin time, hypokalemia, and increased serum ammonia levels. The physician orders a 500 mg sodium/15 g protein diet; neomycin sulfate (Neobiotic) 20 g PO, qid; spironolactone (Aldactone) 50 mg PO, bid; furosemide (Lasix) 20 mg PO, bid; diphenhydramine (Benadryl) 50 mg PO, hs, prn; vitamin K (AquaMEPHYTON) 2 mg IM, three times per week; potassium chloride (Kaochlor) 20 mEq, PO, tid; daily tap water enema; and one unit of salt-poor albumin to be infused daily for 3 days.

4. Why was spironolactone (Aldactone) ordered? Neomycin sulfate (Neobiotic)? Vitamin K (AquaMEPHYTON)?

5. What is the purpose of also administering furosemide (Lasix)? Potassium chloride (Kaochlor)?

6. Discuss the rationale for administering salt-poor albumin to M. N.

7. What is the purpose of the daily enemas?

8. Discuss why diphenhydramine (Benadryl) is the preferred sedative for M. N.

9. What should the nurse do to assess M. N's mental status? What purpose does his diet have in treating the hepatic encephalopathy? Identify the stage of portal-systemic encephalopathy M. N. is experiencing.

10. M. N. is on a fluid restriction of 1500 mL per day. This includes the parenteral volume of fluids for administering the salt-poor albumin as well as the albumin itself, which is 250 mL. Devise a schedule for M. N.'s fluid intake that includes all his medications.

11. What does the nurse monitor for in M. N. to determine if his therapeutic regimen is achieving the desired outcomes?

Case Study: Hepatitis

D. R. is a 28-year-old female client who is admitted to a medical nursing unit. Admission assessment data include that D. R. works as a charge nurse on the same unit. She returned 3 weeks ago from her honeymoon at a resort area in a Central American country. Prior to leaving on vacation, D. R. had been caring for several oncology clients who were receiving intravenous chemotherapy and blood transfusions. D. R. has lost 10 pounds since returning from vacation and states she is always tired and has no energy. D. R. denies any jaundice, but laughs and says, "I really tanned easily!" Her appetite, which is usually good, is depressed, and she finds it difficult to eat without feeling full and becoming nauseated. Frequent headaches have become a problem, and her husband says that she is moody and becomes easily upset. Laboratory results indicate that D. R. has hepatitis A, although hepatitis B has not been completely ruled out.

Address the following questions:

1. Formulate relevant nursing diagnoses for D. R. based on the above data.

2. What precautions should the nurse take when caring for D. R.? What instructions should be given to D. R. and her husband?

3. D. R. continues to have difficulty eating. Plan a diet for her that will help to boost her oral nutrition.

4. What medications may be helpful to D. R. in improving her appetite? Which classes of drugs are contraindicated for this client? Why?

5. D. R. begins to improve and is scheduled for discharge. Design a teaching/learning plan for her concerning diet, activity, hygiene, family cooking arrangements, and sexual activity. Include specific information about transmission of hepatitis A to family members and friends.

CHAPTER 59

Interventions for Clients with Problems of the Gallbladder and Pancreas

LEARNING OBJECTIVES

At the end of this chapter, the student will be able to

▪ Describe the pathophysiology and etiology of biliary disorders

▪ Provide care for the client with cholecystitis or cholelithiasis

▪ Discuss the pathophysiology and etiology of acute pancreatitis and related management

▪ Discuss the pathophysiology and etiology of chronic pancreatitis and related management

▪ Discuss the pathophysiology and etiology of carcinoma of the pancreas and related management

PREREQUISITE KNOWLEDGE

Prior to beginning this chapter, the student should review

▪ The anatomy and physiology of the gallbladder and pancreas

▪ Normal nutrition, including the essential vitamins, minerals, and foods in the recommended food groups

▪ Special diets for clients with disorders of the gallbladder and pancreas, such as low fat, low protein, high protein, high carbohydrate, and liquid

▪ The principles of oral hygiene

▪ The care of nasogastric and nasointestinal tubes

▪ The care of feeding tubes and preparation of tube-feeding formulas

▪ The principles of total parenteral nutrition (TPN) and care of peripheral and central line catheters

▪ Normal fluid and electrolyte values

▪ The principles of enema administration

▪ Perioperative nursing care

▪ The concepts of grief, loss, death, and dying

▪ The concepts of body image and self-esteem

▪ Universal or body substance precautions

STUDY QUESTIONS

Biliary Disorders

1. Differentiate between acute and chronic cholecystitis. Use a separate sheet.

2. Which of the following statements is correct about clients with acute cholecystitis?

   a. These clients are more prone to developing biliary tract carcinoma.

   b. Intrahepatic obstructive jaundice is commonly seen in these clients.

   c. Extrahepatic obstructive jaundice is commonly seen in these clients.

   d. The gallbladder become fibrotic, contracted, and filled with debris.

3. Obstructive jaundice results in

   a. melena

   b. pallor

   c. amber urine

   d. clay-colored stools

4. Identify the common underlying factor that contributes to the etiology of acute cholecystitis.

   _____

   _____

   _____

5. A high incidence of biliary tract disease is associated with

   a. leading an active life style

   b. having a familial tendency

   c. being slightly underweight

   d. non–insulin-dependent diabetes

6. Preventive measures for biliary disease include

   a. following a high-protein diet

   b. burning fewer calories

   c. eating cruciferous vegetables

   d. having small, frequent meals

7. List the subjective client data relevant to biliary disorders. Use a separate sheet.

8. List the objective client data relevant to biliary disorders. Use a separate sheet.

9. Identify laboratory tests that are specific to biliary disease.

   _____

   _____

10. Which of the following drugs is indicated for pain management in gallbladder disease?

    a. morphine

    b. meperidine

    c. apomorphine

    d. codeine

11. Nonsurgical management for biliary colic includes

    a. encouraging a high-protein diet

    b. replacing the B vitamins

    c. administering cholestyramine

    d. giving antispasmodic medications

12. Management of a T-tube in a client who has had gallbladder surgery includes

    a. irrigating the tube with 20 mL of normal saline every 4 hours

    b. securing the collection bag to the sheet with a safety pin

    c. keeping the client in low Fowler's position when in bed

    d. administering bile output to the client via the NG tube

13. Following removal of the gallbladder, the client's dietary intake of fat should be

    a. eliminated completely

    b. limited to less than 20% of the diet

    c. adjusted according to individual tolerance

    d. resumed according to the client's preoperative preference

Match the following terms (14–17) with their definitions (a–d).

_____ 14. ascending cholangitis

_____ 15. cholangitis

_____ 16. choledocho-lithiasis

_____ 17. cholelithiasis

a. common bile duct stones

b. gallbladder stones

c. inflammation of bile ducts

d. inflammation of biliary tree

18. Identify the substances that are normally found in gallstones.

   _____

   _____

   _____

19. Pruritus resulting from obstructive jaundice is treated with

    a. ursodiol

    b. meperidine

    c. dicyclomine

    d. cholestyramine

Match the following invasive procedures (20–23) with their definitions (a–d).

_____ 20. cholecystectomy

_____ 21. cholecystotomy

_____ 22. choledocho-lithotomy

_____ 23. choledochoscopy

a. incision into common bile duct for stone removal

b. removal of gallbladder

c. direct visualization of biliary tract

d. incision into gallbladder

Acute Pancreatitis

24. Define *autodigestion*.

_____

_____

_____

25. Identify and briefly describe the four major pathophysiological processes that occur in acute pancreatitis. Use a separate sheet.

26. List the theories that attempt to explain the triggering mechanisms leading to enzyme activation in acute pancreatitis.

a. _____

_____

b. _____

_____

c. _____

_____

d. _____

_____

Match the following complications of pancreatitis (27–32) with their pathophysiologies (a–f).

_____ 27. peritoneal irritation

_____ 28. jaundice

_____ 29. hyperglycemia

_____ 30. pleural effusion

_____ 31. adult respiratory distress syndrome

_____ 32. disseminated intravascular coagulation (DIC)

a. disruption of alveolar-capillary membrane results in edema

b. release of glucagon and damaged islet cells

c. consumption of clotting factors and microthrombi formation

d. head of pancreas swells and restricts bile flow through common bile duct

e. seepage of digested proteins and lipids into mesentery

f. pancreatic exudate migrates via transdiaphragmatic lymphatics

33. Identify the two most common factors that cause injury to the pancreas.

a. _____

_____

b. _____

_____

34. Pancreatitis can develop as a complication of a perforated duodenal ulcer when

a. serum lipase levels are very high

b. the perforation extends via peritonitis

c. the client's alcohol consumption is excessive

d. the pancreatic duct is obstructed with debris

35. List the subjective client data relevant to acute pancreatitis. Use a separate sheet.

36. List the objective client data relevant to acute pancreatitis. Use a separate sheet.

37. Identify serum studies that are important in the diagnosis of pancreatitis.

a. _____

_____

_____

b. _____

_____

_____

38. Nonsurgical management of the client with acute pancreatitis includes

a. encouraging clear liquids to modify the effect of the enzymes' digestive action

b. inserting an NG tube to reduce the effect of gastric digestive juice on the pancreas

c. administering morphine sulfate by continuous intravenous infusion to control pain

d. giving anticholinergics to increase vagal stimulation and bicarbonate volume

39. The diet for a client with acute pancreatitis should be

a. high carbohydrate, high protein, low fat

b. low carbohydrate, high protein, high fat

c. high carbohydrate, low protein, low fat

d. low carbohydrate, low protein, high fat

Chronic Pancreatitis

40. Differentiate between chronic calcifying pancreatitis and chronic obstructive pancreatitis. Use a separate sheet.

Match the following complications of chronic pancreatitis (41–45) with their related causes (a or b). Answers may be used more than once.

____   41. steatorrhea

____   42. decrease in muscle mass

____   43. ketoacidosis

____   44. peripheral edema

____   45. hyperglycemia

a. loss of endocrine function

b. loss of exocrine function

46. Which of the following should the client with chronic pancreatitis avoid?

    a. taking a cough syrup such as guaifenesin (Robitussin)

    b. eating a high-protein, low-fat diet in small meals

    c. drinking beverages such as decaffeinated tea and coffee

    d. taking antacids prior to meals and snacks and at bedtime

47. List the subjective client data relevant to chronic pancreatitis. Use a separate sheet.

48. List the objective client data relevant to chronic pancreatitis. Use a separate sheet.

49. Identify the significant serum laboratory findings most commonly associated with chronic pancreatitis.

    a. _____

    _____

    b. _____

    _____

    c. _____

    _____

    d. _____

    _____

50. Discuss problems the nurse may encounter with pain management for the client with chronic pancreatitis. Use a separate sheet.

51. Nursing interventions related to administration of pancreatic enzymes include

    a. giving the drugs immediately following a meal or snack

    b. mixing the powdered forms of the drug in pudding

    c. wiping the client's lips with a tissue afterward

    d. recording the number and consistency of stools daily

52. Hospitalized clients with chronic pancreatitis often require

    a. monitoring for hyperglycemia as a result of the extra insulin given during TPN therapy

    b. replacement therapy with large doses of intramuscular vitamin C on a weekly basis

    c. careful cleaning of perianal skin after thorough inspection once a day

    d. application of a protective skin barrier such as zinc oxide or vitamin A and D cream (Sween cream)

53. Discharge planning for the client with chronic pancreatitis includes

    a. renting a commode for bedside use

    b. arranging transfer to a psychiatric care facility

    c. gradually tapering the dosage of the pancreatic enzymes

    d. asking a member of Alcoholics Anonymous to visit

54. Discuss interventions that the nurse can use to promote compliance in the client with chronic pancreatitis. Submit the completed exercise to the clinical instructor on a separate sheet.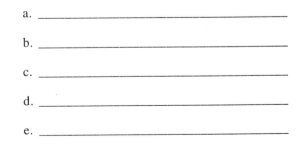

Pancreatic Carcinoma

55. Briefly discuss why cancer of the pancreas has a poor prognosis. Use a separate sheet.

56. List the primary sources of tumors that metastasize to the pancreas.

    a. _____

    b. _____

    c. _____

    d. _____

    e. _____

57. List the sites where pancreatic cancer commonly metastasizes.

  a. _____

  b. _____

  c. _____

  d. _____

  e. _____

58. Tumors in the head of the pancreas

  a. are usually large and invade the entire organ

  b. frequently cause jaundice and gallbladder dilation

  c. spread more extensively than tumors in the tail

  d. are the least common of the pancreatic cancers

59. A common complication of pancreatic carcinoma is

  a. seizures

  b. pneumonia

  c. thrombophlebitis

  d. uncontrolled bleeding

60. Identify the etiological factors that have been linked to cancer of the pancreas.

  a. _____

  b. _____

  c. _____

61. List the subjective client data relevant to cancer of the pancreas. Use a separate sheet.

62. List the objective client data relevant to cancer of the pancreas. Use a separate sheet.

63. List five serum laboratory values that are usually elevated in a client with cancer of the pancreas.

  a. _____

  b. _____

  c. _____

  d. _____

  e. _____

64. Identify the test that is most diagnostic for cancer of the pancreas.

  _____

  _____

65. Nonsurgical management of the client with cancer of the pancreas includes

  a. medicating with opioid analgesics without inducing drug dependency

  b. intense radiation therapy to improve the chance of survival

  c. keeping the client's fingernails clipped to decrease injury from scratching

  d. bathing daily using soap to remove dead skin and body wastes from the skin

66. Identify the rationales for the following interventions that the nurse performs after a client has had a Whipple procedure. Use a separate sheet.

  a. monitoring of wound drainage and drainage tubes

  b. maintaining patency of NG tube

  c. protecting the skin from wound drainage

  d. positioning in semi-Fowler's

  e. monitoring vital signs

  f. administering ordered intravenous fluids

  g. measuring hourly urinary output

  h. checking serum glucose levels

  i. changing the central venous line dressing

67. Discuss why a feeding jejunostomy tube is preferred for enteral feedings in the late stages of pancreatic carcinoma. Use a separate sheet.

68. Develop a discharge plan for a client with end-stage pancreatic cancer. Focus on the psychosocial preparation and include the family. Submit the completed exercise to the clinical instructor on a separate sheet.

CRITICAL THINKING EXERCISES

Case Study: Cholelithiasis

K. M. is a 43-year-old client admitted with a diagnosis of cholelithiasis. She is married and has four children ranging in age from 3 to 20 years. K. M. tells the nurse that she has had right upper quadrant abdominal pain for several weeks and nausea for the last 2 days. Since yesterday, K. M. has noticed that her urine is dark brown and frothy and her stool is pale yellow. With some embarrassment, K. M. admits to having trouble with "gas." She also says that she has been bothered with itching and tries not to scratch because her "skin is getting rubbed raw." K. M. states that she gains weight easily and has always had difficult losing weight after having a baby. She is currently 25 pounds overweight. The nurse notes that K. M.'s skin and sclerae have a yellow cast. There are several superficial scratches on her arms and bruises on her legs and left arm. All laboratory studies are within normal limits except for serum potassium, which is 3.2 mEq/L, and the prothrombin time, which is 22 seconds.

Address the following questions:

1. Identify the data that support the clinical diagnosis of cholelithiasis.

2. The nurse needs to assess the pain episodes more thoroughly. What additional data should be collected?

3. Why does K. M. have changes in her urine and stool, itching, jaundice, and bruising?

K. M.'s ultrasound of the gallbladder is positive for gallstones. Further tests show that there is no sign of a tumor obstructing the biliary tract. K. M. is scheduled for a cholecystectomy and exploration of the common bile duct the next morning. The physician orders a low-fat diet. Medications include meperidine hydrochloride (Demerol) 75–100 mg IM for pain every 3–4 hours; cholestyramine (Questran) 6 g PO, qid; diphenhydramine (Benadryl) 50 mg PO every 3–4 hours prn; phytonadione (AquaMEPHYTON) 10 mg IM stat; and potassium chloride (Kaochlor) 20 mEq PO, pc and HS.

4. What are the purposes for these specific orders? What side effects should the nurses monitor for in K. M.?

5. What information should the nurse reinforce with K. M. about the upcoming surgery?

K. M. returns from surgery with the intravenous infusion, an NG tube to low intermittent suction, an abdominal dressing covering the incision, which has a Penrose drain, and a T-tube connected to a closed, drainable collection bag. The postoperative orders include D_5W with 20 mEq potassium chloride at 125 mL per hour; meperidine 75–100 mg IM every 4 hours prn for pain; and prochlorperazine (Compazine) 10 mg IM every 4 hours prn for nausea.

6. What observations does the nurse make relative to the T-tube? The abdominal dressing?

7. That evening, K. M. becomes nauseated and vomits. What should the nurse do prior to administering any prochlorperazine?

There is also an order to empty and measure the T-tube drainage every 4 hours. Beginning the first postoperative day, the drainage is to be instilled via the NG tube and the tube clamped for 30 minutes.

8. What is the rationale for this intervention?

9. K. M. continues to recover. She is to be discharged with the T-tube in place. Develop a discharge teaching/learning plan for home care management of the T-tube.

10. What instruction does K. M. need about her diet?

Case Study: Acute Pancreatitis

B. V. is a 39-year-old client admitted through the ED with severe epigastric pain radiating to the back. He is jaundiced, his abdomen is full and tense, and guarding is evident upon palpation. B. V.'s former records show that he was recently treated for acute pancreatitis and discharged to home management 2 weeks ago. A stat ultrasound examination indicates a large mass near the head of the pancreas. Immediate surgery is scheduled.

Address the following questions:

1. Formulate relevant nursing diagnoses for B. V. based on the above data.
2. What does the nurse do to prepare B. V. for the surgery?

B. V. has a laparotomy, incision and drainage of a large pancreatic pseudocyst, and cysto-duodenostomy. Postoperatively, he has an intravenous infusion, an NG tube to low intermittent suction, an abdominal dressing, two sump drains into the pancreas connected to low continuous suction, and an indwelling urinary catheter.

3. Discuss what the nurse should do to manage the care of the sump drains and abdominal incision.
4. What is the purpose of the NG tube?
5. B. V.'s skin around one of the sump drains begins to show signs of redness and excoriation the first postoperative day. What should the nurse do?

Slowly, B. V. recovers and advances to oral feedings. A high-carbohydrate, high-protein, low-fat diet is ordered.

6. What foods should be included in this type of diet? What foods should be avoided?
7. How can B. V. be assisted to consume sufficient calories to meet his nutritional needs?
8. B. V. is scheduled for discharge. Construct a discharge teaching/learning plan for him about diet and disease management.

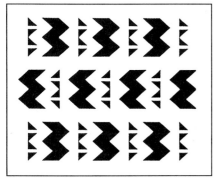

CHAPTER 60

Interventions for Clients with Anorexia Nervosa and Bulimia Nervosa

LEARNING OBJECTIVES

At the end of this chapter, the student will be able to

- Discuss the pathophysiology, etiology, and incidence of anorexia nervosa
- Identify history, physical, and psychosocial assessment findings seen in the anorexia nervosa client
- Provide care for the client with anorexia nervosa
- Discuss the pathophysiology, etiology, and incidence of bulimia nervosa
- Identify history, psychosocial, and physical assessment factors to be identified with the bulimia nervosa client
- Provide care for the bulimia nervosa client

PREREQUISITE KNOWLEDGE

Prior to beginning this chapter, the student should review

- Normal nutrition, including the essential vitamins, minerals, and foods in the recommended food groups

- The principles of oral hygiene
- The principles of total parenteral nutrition (TPN) and care of peripheral and central line catheters
- Normal fluid and electrolyte values
- The concepts of body image and self-esteem

STUDY QUESTIONS

Anorexia Nervosa

1. Which of the following statements are true about anorexia nervosa?
   a. It is a clinical syndrome of self-induced starvation.
   b. Anorexia nervosa occurs primarily in men.
   c. Onset most often occurs early in the 20s.
   d. Medical problems are the result of the illness.
   e. The anorexic ignores feelings of hunger.
   f. Anorexia nervosa is a medical illness.
   g. Many anorexics are well educated in nutrition.
   h. The anorexic client feels fat even when emaciated.

2. List the diagnostic criteria for anorexia nervosa as outlined by the American Psychological Association (*Diagnostic and Statistical Manual of Mental Disorders III-R*).

   a. _____

   _____

   b. _____

   _____

   c. _____

   _____

   d. _____

   _____

3. Briefly discuss why clinical manifestations such as amenorrhea, lowered body temperature, and bradycardia develop in the anorexic client. Use a separate sheet.

4. Identify the type of person who is at risk of developing anorexia nervosa. Use a separate sheet.

5. Which of the following statements is correct about the prevention of anorexia nervosa?

   a. Parents should discuss weight concerns with their children.

   b. Family eating patterns have little influence on prevention.

   c. Parental behavior toward food intake is influential.

   d. Perpetual dieting has little effect on the family.

6. Which of the following statements is correct about the anorexic client?

   a. Self-esteem is usually quite high in these individuals.

   b. Maintaining thinness is a way to avoid self-control.

   c. A slim person is seen as a failure and unhappy.

   d. Regulating food intake is a way of exerting control.

7. List the subjective client data relevant to anorexia nervosa. Use a separate sheet.

8. List the objective client data relevant to anorexia nervosa. Use a separate sheet.

9. List the psychosocial client data relevant to anorexia nervosa. Use a separate sheet.

10. Discuss why a thin, healthy weight is the initial goal for an anorexic client. Use a separate sheet.

11. Discuss the rationale for not permitting parents, spouses, or friends of an anorexic client to be present at mealtimes. Use a separate sheet.

12. Rationales for allowing the anorexic client to have no more than three food dislikes for menu selections include

   a. the client will try to choose more food than can be safely consumed

   b. the client will become distraught at having to choose more foods to eat

   c. the opportunity to refuse foods provides the client with some control in the situation

   d. there should be no limit on the number of times that the client changes the dislikes

13. Rationales for weighing the anorexic client three times a week include

   a. fewer weighing sessions will increase the client's anxiety level

   b. accurate weight measurements are essential to decision making about treatment

   c. the client will determine when the weighings are done to promote control

   d. periodic unannounced spot weights are avoided to promote client trust

14. Drug therapy for the anorexic client routinely includes

   a. appetite stimulants

   b. anticholinergics

   c. nonopioid analgesics

   d antidepressants

15. Rationales for reintroducing milk and milk products gradually into the diet for the anorexic client include

   a. the liquid volume provided by milk is needed to supplement fluids required for rehydration

   b. the client will retain a sense of control by taking oral fluids instead of intravenous fluids

   c. the lactose in large quantities of milk products causes indigestion and abdominal discomfort

   d. small quantities facilitate regeneration of the enzymes needed to digest the lactose

16. Refeeding edema in the anorexic client can be avoided by

   a. restricting fluid intake to 800 mL per day

   b. limiting sodium in the diet to 2 g per day or less

   c. administering a diuretic ordered by the physician

   d. increasing the calorie allowance to 2100 calories per day

17. An anorexic client states that her stomach is "fat" and that all the food she is being forced to eat is making her obese. The nurse's best reply is

    a. "Your body is starting to work normally again and is getting stronger and healthier."

    b. "You have a bloated stomach because there is too much salt in your food."

    c. "No, it's not, you look much better now than when you were first admitted."

    d. "Maybe we have been feeding you too much and you're gaining weight too fast."

18. Which of the following health care professionals should be consulted to assist the family of an anorexic client to adjust to the client's discharge?

    a. physician

    b. occupational therapist

    c. social worker

    d. public health nurse

Bulimia Nervosa

19. Which of the following statements are true about bulimia nervosa?

    a. The bulimic has an intense fear of fatness.

    b. Binge eating usually results in mood elevation.

    c. Binge eating involves ingestion of large amounts of food over a short period of time.

    d. Purging behavior eliminates the calories ingested.

    e. Purging behavior represents a loss of control.

    f. Bulimia nervosa has a possible physiological etiology.

    g. Bulimics are usually women in their 20s.

20. List the criteria used to diagnose bulimia nervosa. Use a separate sheet.

21. Which of the following statements is correct about the bulimic client?

    a. Most bulimics report that they eat because of hunger.

    b. Many bulimics report weight gain on very few calories.

    c. Bulimics view dietary restrictions as offering control.

    d. Binges engender feelings of mastery and accomplishment.

22. Which of the following statements is correct about bulimic clients?

    a. They may experience difficulty with other types of impulse control as well.

    b. They suffer from euphoria and must be considered at risk for bipolar disorders.

    c. They know that they can control their eating once they have begun by just stopping.

    d. They experience satisfaction and enhanced self-esteem following purge episodes.

23. Complete the following chart by comparing anorexia nervosa and bulimia nervosa. Use a separate sheet.

	Anorexia Nervosa	Bulimia Nervosa
a. presence of vomiting		
b. amount of weight loss		
c. age at diagnosis		
d. personality type		
e. reaction to hunger		
f. attitude toward eating		
g. sexual activity		
h. presence of associated psychological features		
i. cause of mortality		
j. menstrual pattern		
k. prognosis		
l. associated behavior abnormalities		

24. List the subjective client data relevant to bulimia nervosa. Use a separate sheet.

25. List the objective client data relevant to bulimia nervosa. Use a separate sheet.

26. List the psychosocial client data relevant to bulimia nervosa. Use a separate sheet.

27. Discuss why a psychiatric consultation is important if a bulimic client is depressed and expressing suicidal thoughts. Use a separate sheet.

28. Drug therapy for the bulimic client routinely includes

    a. calcium supplements

    b. antidepressants

    c. laxatives

    d. antiemetics

29. Discuss the rationale for encouraging regular exercise by the bulimic client. Use a separate sheet.

30. Bulimic clients who binge and purge are most at risk for developing

    a. hyponatremia

    b. hypocalcemia

    c. hypokalemia

    d. hypochloremia

31. Interventions to promote self-esteem in the bulimic client include

    a. reinforcing socially acceptable behaviors with a favorite treat such as a special dessert

    b. assisting the client to role play new coping skills and critiquing them for ways to improve

    c. teaching the client new problem-solving techniques, including confrontation and aggression

    d. helping the client to identify activities that are enjoyable and do not involve food

CRITICAL THINKING EXERCISES

Case Study: Anorexia Nervosa

S. C. is a 19-year-old Caucasian female who is a freshman in college away from home. She is 5 feet 1 inch tall. S. C. has been steadily losing weight, although she participates in the campus meal plan and takes her meals in the dormitory cafeteria. S. C. was active in sports in high school but has not gone out for any team sports in college. Most freshmen have been discussing the upcoming Thanksgiving holiday break and making plans for going home over the long weekend. The dorm counselor has noticed that S. C. has not voiced similar plans and seems to avoid any discussion about her family or home. A week before Thanksgiving, S. C. is found unconscious on the floor in the dormitory communal bathroom. An ambulance is called and S. C. is admitted to the community hospital. Her college admission physical health record states that she weighed 98 pounds in June and had no known medical problems.

Address the following questions:

1. Identify physical assessment date that should be collected upon S. C.'s admission to the hospital.

2. S. C. weighs 80 pounds on admission. Calculate her percentage of weight loss since June. Is S. C. at any nutritional risk? If so, provide supporting rationale for the answer.

The next day, S. C. asks the nurse how long she will be in the hospital. The nurse tells S. C. that test results are pending and that the physician will be in during the morning to talk to her. Discharge depends on what the laboratory tests find. The nurse also tells S. C. that her parents have been called and that they are driving to town and will arrive later in the day. S. C. becomes upset, saying that there was no reason to notify her parents. S. C.'s parents go to her room as soon as they arrive. Mrs. C. becomes visibly upset at her daughter's appearance and says, "You haven't been eating again, have you? I knew that we shouldn't have let you leave home to go to school! You're coming home with us as soon as you can leave here."

3. What should the nurse do to intervene at this point?

4. Formulate relevant nursing diagnoses for S. C. based on the above data.

5. What additional data does the nurse need to collect about S. C.'s weight loss?

S. C. is on a 1200 calorie diet with a fluid goal of 1000 mL per day. She has difficulty eating the food on her trays. Mrs. C. offers to stay with S. C. during mealtime to help her eat.

6. Should Mrs. C. be permitted to stay in S. C.'s room during mealtime? Why or why not?

7. Discuss interventions the nurse can implement to assist S. C. in increasing her food intake. The textbook states that the nurse should stay with the client while the client eats. Discuss whether this intervention is feasible on a busy adult medical-surgical unit. Consider other alternatives.

8. For which complications should the nurse monitor as S. C. begins to eat more?

9. What foods should be included on S. C.'s trays? Devise a day's sample menu for S. C., indicating types of foods, quantities, and when they should be consumed.

10. Discharge is planned for S. C. Discuss what factors must be considered in preparing S. C. and her family for discharge.

Case Study: Bulimia Nervosa

K. H. is a 26-year-old client admitted to the ED following a suspected suicide attempt. She lives with her parents, who found her in bed and could not arouse her. There was an empty medicine bottle, a bottle of gin, and a partially filled glass of gin on her bedside tray. K. H. was resuscitated and admitted. The next day, the nurse entered K.H.'s room with a breakfast tray. K. H. looked at the tray and commented that there wasn't enough foods on it to fill her up. "I'm able to eat more than that when I'm in the mood." Another tray is ordered and brought to K. H. After breakfast, the nurse begins to interview K. H. for a nursing history.

Address the following questions:

1. What subjective data should the nurse collect from K. H.?

2. What objective data should the nurse collect initially?

Later in the morning, K. H.'s parents come to visit their daughter. The nurse notices them going to her room and observes that both parents are grossly overweight. When the nurse enters the room, K. H. is lying on her side facing the window and turned away from her parents. The parents comment that they are relieved to see their daughter looking better. Mrs. H. notices that the lunch trays are being delivered and suggests that she and Mr. H. leave to get some lunch in the cafeteria while K. H. has her tray. After they leave, K. H. says, "Just look at them. All they ever talk about is where their next meal is coming from! No wonder I look like this."

3. What should the nurse reply to K. H.?

4. Formulate actual and potential nursing diagnoses for K. H. based on the above data.

5. Which health care professionals should the nurse consult to assist in planning care for K. H.?

6. Part of K. H.'s treatment includes the drug nortriptyline hydrochloride (Aventyl) 25 mg PO, qid. What information should the nurse discuss with K. H. about this medication? Which specific side effects of the drug could precipitate or aggravate potential complications of bulimia nervosa?

7. What resources are available to K. H. and her parents when discharge is planned and K. H. returns home to the care of her parents?

CHAPTER 61

Interventions for Clients with Other Nutritional Problems

LEARNING OBJECTIVES

At the end of this chapter, the student will be able to

- Identify various dietary standards
- Complete an initial nutritional assessment
- Discuss protein–calorie malnutrition (PCM)
- Complete a history and physical assessment of a client with PCM
- Provide care for the PCM client
- Discuss obesity
- Provide care for the obese client

PREREQUISITE KNOWLEDGE

Prior to beginning this chapter, the student should review

- The anatomy and physiology of the gastrointestinal system
- The effect of the central and autonomic nervous systems on the gastrointestinal organs
- Normal nutrition, including the essential vitamins, minerals, and foods in the recommended food groups
- The care of nasogastric tubes
- The care of feeding tubes and preparation of tube-feeding formulas

- The principles of total parenteral nutrition (TPN) and care of peripheral and central line catheters
- Normal fluid and electrolyte values
- Perioperative nursing care
- The concepts of body image and self-esteem

STUDY QUESTIONS

Nutrition

1. Identify the factors that define nutritional health. Use a separate sheet.
2. Recommended Dietary Allowances (RDA) are
   a. a standard for determining malnutrition
   b. a guide for selecting daily food choices
   c. a guide for estimating nutrient intake over time
   d. a standard for evaluating nutritional adequacy of dietary intake
3. The Dietary Guidelines for Americans recommend
   a. consuming a variety of foods
   b. limiting the daily intake of caffeine
   c. adjusting activity level to control weight
   d. decreasing consumption of complex carbohydrates

4. Identify factors that influence nutrient requirements.

   a. _____

   b. _____

   c. _____

5. Identify factors that influence nutrient intake.

   a. _____

   b. _____

   c. _____

   d. _____

   e. _____

   f. _____

6. List the components of nutritional status assessment. Use a separate sheet.

7. Initial nutritional screening includes

   a. the client's stated height and weight

   b. visual inspection of body shape and type

   c. anthropometric measurements for body fat

   d. a detailed 24-hour dietary intake recall

8. Significant involuntary weight loss affecting nutritional status is defined as

   a. 2%

   b. 5%

   c. 7%

   d. 10%

Malnutrition

9. Identify factors that contribute to protein–calorie malnutrition (PCM). Use a separate sheet.

10. Which of the following statements is correct about malnutrition and the immune system?

   a. Malnutrition can impair any aspect of the immune system.

   b. Excess nutrients have little effect on the immune system.

   c. Nutritional problems are limited to one deficiency.

   d. Immune system impairment relates indirectly to nutrition.

11. Preventive measures for PCM include

   a. limiting the amount of fat in the diet

   b. providing the client with favorite foods

   c. increasing the amount of free liquid consumed

   d. supplementing IV fluids with nutrients

12. List the subjective client data relevant to malnutrition. Use a separate sheet.

13. List the objective client data relevant to malnutrition. Use a separate sheet.

Match the following laboratory tests (14–19) with their indications of nutritional status (a–f).

____ 14. hemoglobin	a. sepsis
____ 15. hematocrit	b. anemia
____ 16. serum cholesterol	c. protein depletion
____ 17. serum transferrin	d. hemorrhage
	e. iron-binding capacity
____ 18. total lympho-cyte count	f. immune function
____ 19. thyroxine-binding prealbumin	

20. The preferred diet for the client who is without teeth is

   a. clear liquid

   b. full liquids

   c. mechanical soft

   d. regular

21. Complete the following chart by comparing enteral and parenteral nutrition. Use a separate sheet.

	Enteral	Parenteral
a. route of administration		
b. candidates for therapy		
c. methods of administration		
d. complications		

22. Which of the following clients would *not* be a candidate for tube feeding? The client who

   a. is unconscious

   b. has severe arthritis of the hands

   c. has massive full thickness burns

   d. has extensive jaw and mouth surgery

23. Which of the following complications may result from the administration of hypertonic tube feeding solutions?

    a. paralytic ileus

    b. venous thrombosis

    c. pulmonary edema

    d. fluid volume excess

24. The nurse is caring for a client who is to begin total parenteral nutrition (TPN) therapy. The client currently has a peripheral IV line and asks why it cannot be used for the TPN administration. Which of the following is the best response for the nurse?

    a. "Everybody who gets TPN must have an IV line in the neck or chest."

    b. "The IV line in your arm is not large enough to handle the amount of solution."

    c. "The new IV site will allow the nurses to regulate the flow rate better."

    d. "The IV line in your chest will reduce your chances of getting an infection."

 25. Develop a plan of care for the client receiving TPN. Include necessary assessments and interventions. Submit the completed exercise to the clinical instructor.

Obesity

Match the following terms related to obesity with their definitions.

_____ 26. obesity

_____ 27. overweight

_____ 28. morbid obesity

    a. weight that negatively affects health status

    b. excessive amount of body fat

    c. increase in body weight for height as compared to a standard

29. Which of the following people is at the greatest risk for obesity?

    a. a 42-year-old woman who has a body mass index of 26

    b. a 24-year-old male athlete who takes anabolic steroids

    c. a 50-year-old woman who has a waist-to-hip ratio of 0.92

    d. a 28-year-old diabetic man who is 120% of ideal body weight

30. List the subjective client data relevant to obesity. Use a separate sheet.

31. List the objective client data relevant to obesity. Use a separate sheet.

32. List the criteria used to determine a client's eligibility for obesity-reducing surgery. Use a separate sheet.

33. Which of the following diets promotes safe weight loss?

    a. low-energy diet

    b. liquid formula diet

    c. the grapefruit diet

    d. short-term fasting

34. List the major side effects of drugs used to treat obesity.

    a. _____

    b. _____

    c. _____

    d. _____

    e. _____

    f. _____

35. Identify surgical procedures that may be performed to reduce the food intake of an obese client.

    a. _____

    b. _____

    c. _____

    d. _____

36. Briefly discuss why obese clients are at a higher risk for developing postoperative wound infections and dehiscence. Use a separate sheet.

37. Which of the following exercises is recommended for the obese client who is beginning a weight loss program?

    a. bicycling

    b. walking

    c. jogging

    d. swimming

CHAPTER 62

Assessment of the Endocrine System

LEARNING OBJECTIVES

At the end of this chapter, the student will be able to

▋ Describe the function of the endocrine system

▋ Discuss the structure and function of the hypothalamus and pituitary gland

▋ Discuss the function of the gonads

▋ Discuss the structure and function of the adrenal glands

▋ Discuss the structure and function of the thyroid gland

▋ Discuss the structure and function of the parathyroid glands

▋ Discuss the structure and function of the pancreas

▋ List changes in the endocrine system associated with aging

▋ Obtain a history from the client with endocrine dysfunction

▋ Complete a physical and psychosocial assessment for the client with suspected endocrine abnormalities

▋ Identify laboratory tests that aid in the diagnosis of endocrine dysfunction

PREREQUISITE KNOWLEDGE

Prior to beginning this chapter, the student should review

▋ The anatomy and physiology of the endocrine system and the kidney

▋ The functions of the various hormones in the body

▋ Normal growth and development and the effects of the endocrine system on these processes

STUDY QUESTIONS

Anatomy and Physiology Review

Match the following terms (1–26) with their correct definitions (a–z).

_____ 1. adrenal glands

_____ 2. adrenocorticotropic hormone

_____ 3. aldosterone

_____ 4. baroreceptors

_____ 5. calcitonin

_____ 6. catecholamines

_____ 7. cortisol

_____ 8. endocrine gland

_____ 9. glucagon

_____ 10. growth hormone

_____ 11. hormone

_____ 12. hypothalamus

_____ 13. insulin

_____ 14. islets of Langerhans

_____ 15. osmoreceptors

_____ 16. oxytocin

_____ 17. parathyroid hormone

_____ 18. parathyroid glands

_____ 19. pituitary gland

_____ 20. prolactin

_____ 21. target tissue

_____ 22. thyroid gland

_____ 23. thyroid-stimulating hormone

_____ 24. T_3

_____ 25. T_4

_____ 26. vasopressin (antidiuretic hormone)

a. tissue affected by a hormone

b. hormone affecting growth and metabolism

c. hormone affecting permeability of kidney tubules

d. hormone secreting tissue

e. hormone precipitating milk letdown

f. triiodothyronine

g. gland releasing several tropic hormones that affect other glands

h. hormone affecting breast tissue development and lactation

i. adrenal hormone regulating sodium reabsorption

j. control center for central nervous system (CNS) and endocrine system to maintain homeostasis

k. glands located on each kidney

l. chemical substance with widespread effect in the body

m. blood pressure–sensitive sensors located in the aorta and carotid arteries

n. respond to changes in plasma osmolality

o. hormone weakly stimulating aldosterone secretion

p. two hormones produced by the adrenal medulla

q. hormone produced by pancreatic beta cells

r. pituitary hormone regulating thyroid hormone secretion

s. thyroxine

t. adrenal cortex hormone affecting metabolism and stress response

u. hormone regulating calcium and phosphorus metabolism

v. produces hormones affecting cell activity and metabolism

w. hormone lowering serum calcium levels

x. four small glands

y. pancreatic endocrine cells

z. hormone produced by pancreatic alpha cells promoting glycogenolysis

27. List the hormones produced by the following endocrine glands. Use a separate sheet.

    a. anterior pituitary

    b. posterior pituitary

    c. thyroid

    d. parathyroid

    e. adrenals

    f. islet cells of pancreas

    g. gonads

28. Explain the endocrine feedback control system. Use a separate sheet.

29. The hypothalamus

    a. exerts only endocrine functions

    b. consists of two distinct lobes

    c. is connected to the CNS by afferent and efferent fibers

    d. produces hormones affecting the posterior pituitary

30. Which of the following statements is correct about the pituitary gland?

    a. The posterior pituitary gland secretes tropic hormones, which stimulate the thyroid, adrenal cortex, and gonads.

    b. The anterior pituitary gland secretes oxytocin and vasopressin.

    c. The posterior pituitary gland secretes prolactin and luteinizing hormone.

    d. The anterior pituitary gland secretes growth hormone and prolactin.

31. Which of the following statements about pituitary hormones is true?

    a. Adrenocorticotropic hormone (ACTH) acts on the adrenal medulla.

    b. Follicle-stimulating hormone stimulates sperm production in men.

    c. Growth hormone promotes protein catabolism.

    d. Vasopressin decreases systolic blood pressure.

32. Which of the following statements is correct about the gonads?

    a. Ovaries and testes develop from the same embryonic tissue.

    b. Differentiation into male or female gonads is precipitated by maternal human chorionic gonadotropin secretion.

    c. The placenta secretes testosterone for the development of male external genitalia.

    d. External genitalia maturation is stimulated by gonadotropins in late adolescence.

33. Which of the following statements is correct about the adrenal glands?

    a. The cortex secretes androgens in women.

    b. Catecholamines are secreted from the cortex.

    c. Glucocorticoids are secreted from the medulla.

    d. The medulla secretes hormones essential for life.

Match the following adrenal hormones (34–40) with their origins (a or b). Answers may be used more than once.

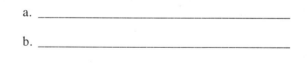

____	34. ACTH	a. adrenal cortex
____	35. androgen	b. adrenal medulla
____	36. epinephrine	
____	37. estrogen	
____	38. norepinephrine	
____	39. cortisol	
____	40. aldosterone	

41. Which of the following statements is correct about the thyroid gland and its hormones?

    a. The gland is located posteriorly in the neck directly below the cricoid cartilage.

    b. Thyroid hormone production depends on sufficient iodine and protein intake.

    c. The gland has four distinct lobes joined by a thin isthmus.

    d. All body tissues increase oxygen consumption in response to triiodothyronine (T_3) and thyroxine (T_4).

42. Identify the target organs of parathyroid hormone in the regulation of calcium and phosphorus.

    a. _____

    b. _____

    c. _____

43. Which of the following statements is correct about the pancreas?

    a. Endocrine functions of the pancreas include secretion of digestive enzymes.

    b. Exocrine functions of the pancreas include secretion of glucagon and insulin.

    c. The islets of Langerhans are the only source of somatostatin secretion.

    d. Somatostatin inhibits pancreatic secretion of glucagon and insulin.

44. Which of the following statements is correct about glucagon secretion?

    a. It is stimulated by an increase in blood glucose levels.

    b. It is stimulated by a decrease in amino acid levels.

    c. It exerts its primary effect on the pancreas.

    d. It acts to increase blood glucose levels.

45. Which of the following statements is correct about insulin secretion?

    a. It drops sharply following the ingestion of a meal.

    b. It is stimulated primarily by fat ingestion.

    c. It occurs continuously at a basal rate.

    d. It promotes glycogenolysis and gluconeogenesis.

46. The blood steam delivers the fuel glucose to the cells for energy production. The hormone that controls the cells' use of glucose is

    a. T_4

    b. growth hormone

    c. adrenal steroids

    d. insulin

47. Which of the following diseases involves a disorder of the islets of Langerhans?

    a. diabetes insipidus

    b. diabetes mellitus

    c. Addison's disease

    d. Cushing's syndrome

48. For each of the following structures, identify a physiological change in the endocrine system associated with aging and the cause of each change.

    a. gonad: _____

    _____

    _____

    b. pancreas: _____

    _____

    _____

    c. posterior pituitary gland: _____

    _____

    _____

    _____

    d. thyroid: _____

    _____

    _____

Subjective Assessment

49. List the subjective data relevant to the endocrine system. Use a separate sheet.

50. The following is a partial client history. Discuss **CT** the significance these data have for an endocrine assessment. Submit the completed exercise to the clinical instructor on a separate sheet.

    African-American, 55 years old. Lives with his wife, daughter, and his daughter's three children. Has been sleeping longer (10–12 hours per night), is unable to get through the day without a nap, has no appetite, and has lost 15 pounds in the past month. For the past 3 months, he has been unable to have sex with his wife because he has been too tired and because "nothing happens down there, it just hangs." Also states that his beard is thinner and his pubic hair is falling out. Past medical history includes gout and left ear deafness from childhood ear infections.

Objective Assessment

51. List the objective client data relevant to the endocrine system. Use a separate sheet.

52. Using the data from question 50, construct a **CT** physical assessment recording for the endocrine system. Submit the completed exercise to the clinical instructor.

53. Which of the following statements is correct about thyroid gland assessment?

    a. The thyroid gland is easily palpated in all clients.

    b. The client is instructed to swallow to aid palpation.

    c. The anterior approach is preferred for thyroid palpation.

    d. The thumbs are used to palpate the thyroid lobes.

54. Briefly discuss the rationale for suppression and stimulation testing of hormonal levels. Use a separate sheet.

55. If a routine urine specimen cannot be sent immediately to the laboratory, the nurse should

    a. take no special action

    b. discard and collect a new specimen later

    c. refrigerate the specimen until it can be transported

    d. store the specimen on the "dirty" side of the utility room

56. Which of the following nursing interventions is most appropriate when collecting a 24-hour urine specimen?

    a. Recording the client's intake and output for the duration.

    b. Checking whether any preservatives are needed in the container.

    c. Placing the collection container on ice for the 24 hours.

    d. Weighing the client before beginning the collection.

57. Identify the purposes of the following tests for the function of the islet cells of Langerhans. Use a separate sheet.

    a. fasting blood sugar

    b. 2-hour postprandial blood sugar

    c. 3-hour glucose tolerance

    d. 5-hour glucose tolerance

58. List the types of radiographic tests that may be performed on the endocrine system.

    a. _____

    _____

    b. _____

    _____

    c. _____

    _____

    d. _____

    _____

    e. _____

    _____

CRITICAL THINKING EXERCISES

Case Study: Endocrine Assessment

P. F. is a 48-year-old male client who is being evaluated for endocrine dysfunction. He is to have a series of laboratory tests, including a fasting blood sugar, a 5-hour glucose tolerance test, a 2-hour postprandial blood sugar, a routine urinalysis, a 24-hour urine test for catecholamines, and a 24-hour urine test for 17-ketosteroids.

Address the following questions:

1. Which of these tests require that P. F. be fasting?

2. Which of these specimens may be collected without regard for the time of day?

3. Devise a schedule for P. F. to complete the collection of these specimens in the most time efficient and comfortable manner.

4. Develop a teaching/learning plan for P. F. about the specimen collections.

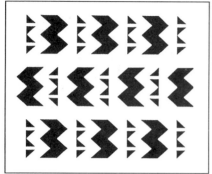

CHAPTER 63

Interventions for Clients with Pituitary and Adrenal Gland Problems

LEARNING OBJECTIVES

At the end of this chapter, the student will be able to

- Describe the pathophysiology and etiology of hypopituitarism
- Manage care for the client with hypopituitarism
- Describe the pathophysiology and etiology of hyperpituitarism
- Manage care for the client with hyperpituitarism
- Describe the pathophysiology and etiology of diabetes insipidus (DI)
- Provide care for the client with diabetes insipidus
- Discuss the pathophysiology and etiology of the syndrome of inappropriate antidiuretic hormone (SIADH), or Schwartz–Bartter syndrome
- Provide care for the client with SIADH
- Discuss the pathophysiology and etiology of hypofunction of the adrenal gland
- Describe treatment for acute adrenal insufficiency, or Addisonian crisis
- Provide care for the client with adrenal hypofunction
- Discuss the pathophysiology and etiology of hypercortisolism, or Cushing's syndrome
- Manage care for the client with hypercortisolism, or Cushing's syndrome
- Discuss the pathophysiology and etiology of hyperaldosteronism

- Manage care of the client with hyperaldosteronism
- Discuss the pathophysiology and etiology of pheochromocytoma
- Provide care for the client with pheochromocytoma

PREREQUISITE KNOWLEDGE

Prior to beginning this chapter, the student should review

- The anatomy and physiology of the hypothalamus, pituitary gland, and adrenal glands
- The functions of hormones of the pituitary gland and the adrenal glands
- Normal growth and development and the effects of the pituitary and adrenal gland hormones on these processes
- Normal laboratory values for serum and urine potassium and sodium levels and for urine specific gravity
- The principles of fluid and electrolyte balance and acid–base balance
- The technique for subcutaneous and intramuscular injections
- The concepts of body image and self-esteem
- The concepts of loss and grief
- The concept of human sexuality
- Perioperative nursing care

STUDY QUESTIONS

Disorders of the Anterior Pituitary Gland

1. Differentiate between primary and secondary pituitary dysfunction.

    a. Primary: _____

    _____

    _____

    b. Secondary: _____

    _____

    _____

2. Define *panhypopituitarism.* _____

    _____

    _____

    _____

3. Which of the following statements about hypopituitarism is true?

    a. Adrenocorticotropic hormone (ACTH) and thyroid-stimulating hormone (TSH) deficiencies are not life threatening.

    b. Luteinizing hormone (LH) and follicle-stimulating hormone (FSH) deficiencies are the most common problems.

    c. Growth hormone (GH) deficiency is the most common pituitary problem.

    d. GH deficiency is diagnosed by suppression tests.

4. Which of the following statements is correct about the etiology of hypopituitarism?

    a. Secondary dysfunction can result from radiation treatment to the pituitary gland.

    b. Primary dysfunction can result from infection or a congenital defect.

    c. Postpartum hemorrhage is the most common cause of pituitary trauma.

    d. Severe malnutrition and body fat depletion can depress pituitary gland function.

5. Which of the following statements is correct about the incidence and prevention of hypopituitarism?

    a. Hypopituitarism and panhypopituitarism are common diseases.

    b. Wearing protective head gear during contact sports is advisable.

    c. Genetic counseling is not recommended for clients with GH deficiency.

    d. Wearing seat belts has little effect on the incidence of head injury.

6. List the subjective client data relevant to hypopituitarism. Use a separate sheet.

7. List the objective client data relevant to hypopituitarism. Use a separate sheet.

8. Identify hormone assays that can be done to determine basal levels of target organ hormones.

    a. _____

    b. _____

    c. _____

    d. _____

    Match the following stimulation tests (9–11) with their pituitary hormones (a–f). Answers may be used more than once and there may be more than one answer for each.

    ____ 9. insulin tolerance test   a. ACTH

    ____ 10. metyrapone   b. FSH

    ____ 11. thyrotropin-releasing hormone   c. GH

         d. LH

    ____ 12. gonadotropin-releasing hormone   e. Prolactin

         f. TSH

13. Identify the common nursing diagnoses for the client with hypopituitarism.

    a. _____

    _____

    b. _____

    _____

    c. _____

    _____

14. Interventions for the client with hypopituitarism include

    a. relating to the client according to physical appearance

    b. encouraging the client to express feelings and concerns

    c. suggesting the client purchase an elevated toilet seat

    d. recommending clothing stores that stock adolescent sizes

15. Which of the following statements is correct about hormone therapy for hypopituitarism?

    a. Somatropin (Humatrope) is given after closure of the epiphyses.

    b. Therapy usually corrects physiological and psychological problems.

    c. Testosterone replacement therapy does not promote male fertility.

    d. Clomiphene citrate (Clomid) is used to suppress ovulation in women.

16. Female clients receiving hormone replacement therapy should be instructed to

    a. report any recurrence of symptoms between injections such as decreased libido

    b. monitor blood pressure at least weekly for potential hypotension

    c. treat leg pain, especially in the calves, with gentle muscle stretching

    d. scheduling periodic gynecological and breast examinations with the physician

17. List the types of cells that are used to classify hyperpituitarism.

    a. _____

    _____

    b. _____

    _____

    c. _____

    _____

18. Identify the hormone whose oversecretion produces gigantism and acromegaly.

    _____

19. Compare *gigantism* and *acromegaly*. Use a separate sheet.

20. Identify the most common and least common pituitary tumors.

    Most common: _____

    _____

    Least common: _____

    _____

21. List the subjective client data relevant to hyperpituitarism. Use a separate sheet.

22. List the subjective client data relevant to hyperpituitarism. Use a separate sheet.

23. Identify the common nursing diagnoses for the client with hyperpituitarism.

    a. _____

    _____

    b. _____

    _____

24. Interventions for the drug bromocriptine mesylate (Parlodel) include

    a. advising the client to get up slowly from a lying position

    b. instructing the client to take the medication half an hour before meals

    c. telling the client to resume usual activities including mild exercise

    d. teaching the client to begin with a maintenance level dose

25. Following hypophysectomy, the nurse should observe the client for

    a. urinary retention

    b. respiratory distress

    c. bleeding at suture site

    d. increased intracranial pressure

26. Postoperative care for the client who has had a trassphenoidal hypophysectomy includes

    a. encouraging coughing and deep breathing to decrease pulmonary complications

    b. testing nasal drainage for glucose to determine if it contains cerebrospinal fluid

    c. keeping the bed flat to decrease central cerebrospinal fluid leakage

    d. assisting the client with tooth brushing to decrease halitosis

27. Which of the following statements is *incorrect* about postoperative instructions for the diabetic client who has had a hypophysectomy? For the remainder of his or her lifetime, the client will

    a. be unable to have any children

    b. have to take cortisol replacement medication

    c. have to take thyroxine replacement medication

    d. require a larger does of insulin than preoperatively

Disorders of the Posterior Pituitary Gland

28. Antidiuretic hormone (ADH) influences normal kidney function by stimulating the

    a. glomerulus to control the filtration rate

    b. proximal nephron tubules to reabsorb water

    c. distal nephron tubules to reabsorb water

    d. glomerulus to prevent loss of protein in urine

29. Briefly compare diabetes insipidus (DI) with syndrome of inappropriate antidiuretic hormone (SIADH). Use a separate sheet.

30. Which of the following statements is correct about diabetes insipidus?

    a. The level of injury to the hypophyseal tract determines the extent of ADH deficiency.

    b. Nephrogenic diabetes insipidus is an acquired defect resulting from nephrotoxicity.

    c. Psychogenic polydipsia is an inherited defect resulting in ADH deficiency.

    d. Following hypophysectomy, polyuria is transient and normal urinary output returns.

31. Identify etiological factors associated with secondary diabetes insipidus. Use a separate sheet.

32. List the subjective client data relevant to diabetes insipidus. Use a separate sheet.

33. List the objective client data relevant to diabetes insipidus. Use a separate sheet.

34. Laboratory findings in diabetes insipidus include

    a. urinary output of more than 30 L per 24 hours

    b. urine specific gravity is 1.010 and osmolality is 250 mOsm

    c. serum osmolality within normal limits if taking fluids

    d. serum potassium level decreased owing to renal tubular excretion

35. All of the following drugs are used in the management of diabetes insipidus *except*

    a. chlorpropamide (Diabinese)

    b. clofibrate (Atromid S)

    c. regular insulin

    d. Lypressin (Diapid)

36. Clients with permanent diabetes insipidus must be instructed to

    a. continue vasopressin therapy until symptoms disappear

    b. monitor for recurrence of polydipsia and polyuria

    c. monitor and record their weight twice a week

    d. check urine specific gravity three times per week

37. Which of the following statements is correct about the pathophysiology of SIADH?

    a. ADH secretion is inhibited in the presence of low plasma osmolality.

    b. Water retention results in dilutional hyponatremia and expanded extracellular fluid (ECF) volume.

    c. The glomerulus is unable to increase its filtration rate to reduce the excess plasma volume.

    d. Renin and aldosterone are released and help to decrease the loss of urinary sodium.

38. Usually as the amount of ADH increases in the blood

    a. urine concentration tends to decrease

    b. glomerular filtration tends to decrease

    c. tubular reabsorption of sodium and water increases

    d. tubular reabsorption of potassium and water increases

39. Which of the following statements about the etiology and incidence of SIADH is correct?

    a. Malignant cells act on the posterior pituitary to decrease ADH release.

    b. Clofibrate (Atromid S) can potentiate the action of vasopressin.

    c. Ectopic ADH production can result from benign gastrointestinal polyps.

    d. SIADH results from vasopressin overdose in diabetes insipidus is irreversible.

40. List the subjective client data relevant to SIADH. Use a separate sheet.

41. List the objective client data relevant to SIADH. Use a separate sheet.

42. An early sign of SIADH is

    a. seizure activity

    b. excess thirst

    c. peripheral edema

    d. lethargy

43. Which of the following laboratory findings is consistent with the diagnosis of SIADH?

    a. elevated urine sodium level and increased urine specific gravity

    b. elevated serum sodium level and increased circulating fluid volume

    c. decreased urine specific gravity and decreased plasma osmolality.

    d. decreased serum sodium level and decreased circulating fluid volume

44. Identify the two common nursing diagnoses associated with SIADH.

    a. _____

    _____

    b. _____

    _____

45. A therapeutic fluid restriction level for the client with SIADH is

    a. 300–400 mL per 24 hours

    b. 500–700 mL per 24 hours

    c. 1200–1800 mL per 24 hours

    d. 2500–3000 mL per 24 hours

46. Interventions for the client with SIADH with neurological involvement include

    a. assigning the client to a quiet room away from the nurses' station

    b. assessing the client's neurological status as often as every hour if indicated

    c. restraining the client in bed with jacket and hand restraints

    d. administering hypotonic saline solutions to induce diuresis

Adrenal Gland Hypofunction

47. Identify the causes of decreased production of adrenocortical steroids.

    a. _____

    _____

    _____

    b. _____

    _____

    _____

    c. _____

    _____

    _____

48. Briefly compare the significance of adrenal cortex function loss to that of adrenal medulla function loss. Use a separate sheet.

49. Identify the functions of the following adrenal hormones and their effects on laboratory values. Use a separate sheet.

    a. cortisol

    b. aldosterone

    c. androgens

50. Briefly discuss Addisonian crisis. Use a separate sheet.

51. Preventive measures for adrenocortical insufficiency include

    a. maintaining the client on long-term, high-dose glucocorticoid therapy

    b. vaccinating clients at increased risk for contracting tuberculosis and acquired immunodeficiency syndrome (AIDS)

    c. tapering glucocorticoid doses quickly and discontinuing the drug as soon as possible

    d. decreasing glucocorticoid doses gradually, permitting pituitary and adrenal function to return

52. Which of the following statements is correct about emergency care in acute adrenal crisis?

    a. Intravenous hydrocortisone is administered to stabilize the client prior to drawing blood specimens.

    b. The initial dose of hydrocortisone is 100 mg per hour to provide a loading dose and stabilize the client.

    c. Intramuscular hydrocortisone is administered along with intravenous doses to provide a constant supply.

    d. Oral glucocorticoids and mineralocorticoids may be discontinued following crisis resolution.

53. List the subjective client data relevant to adrenal insufficiency. Use a separate sheet.

54. List the objective client data relevant to adrenal insufficiency. Use a separate sheet.

55. Briefly discuss why definitive stimulatory studies are required to confirm a diagnosis of adrenal hypofunction rather than relying on basal cortisol and ACTH levels. Use a separate sheet.

56. A client with the diagnosis of chronic adrenal insufficiency is admitted to a nursing unit. Which of the following room assignments is contraindicated?

    a. a double room with an elderly client who has had a cerebrovascular accident

    b. a double room with a middle-aged client who has bacterial pneumonia

    c. a private room that is away from the nurses' station but within view

    d. a double room next to a teenager who has a fractured leg and is in traction

57. A client with adrenal hypofunction reports weakness and dizziness on arising in the morning. The nurse explains to the client that this is most likely related to

    a. postural hypertension

    b. a potassium deficiency

    c. a hypoglycemic reaction

    d. salt and fluid retention

58. A client's laboratory results indicate that the client has Addison's disease. The nurse plans to discuss with the client the need for

    a. a special low-salt diet

    b. using an alcohol-based skin cleaner

    c. physical activity restrictions

    d. lifelong hormone replacement therapy

59. In teaching the client with adrenal hypofunction about diet, the nurse should advise the client to

    a. add a little extra salt to food at the table

    b. limit the daily intake of fluids to 1500 mL

    c. restrict the daily intake of calories to 1200

    d. decrease protein intake to 20–30 g per day

60. The client on prolonged cortisone therapy should be instructed to observe for and report signs of

    a. anuria and hypoglycemia

    b. weight gain and moon face

    c. anorexia and muscle twitches

    d. hypotension and fluid loss

61. A female client with Addison's disease has been on cortisone therapy for several months and expresses concern that she is beginning to look more masculine. The nurse should tell the client

    a. that the changes are a sign of the disease's progression

    b. not to worry because the changes are only temporary

    c. that the changes are related to the cortisone therapy

    d. that the changes are a minor inconvenience compared to dying

62. When observing the client for cortisone overdose, the nurse should be alert for

    a. behavioral changes

    b. severe anorexia

    c. hypoglycemia

    d. macular rash

Adrenal Gland Hyperfunction

63. The most common cause of hypercortisolism or Cushing's syndrome is

    a. pituitary hypoplasia

    b. insufficient ACTH production

    c. adrenocortical hormone deficiency

    d. hyperplasia of the adrenal cortex

64. List the subjective client data relevant to Cushing's syndrome. Use a separate sheet.

65. List the objective client data relevant to Cushing's syndrome. Use a separate sheet.

66. When assessing the client with Cushing's syndrome, the nurse would expect to find

    a. dehydration

    b. pitting edema

    c. hypertension

    d. muscle atrophy

67. Explain why samples for plasma cortisol levels should always be taken at the same time of day.

    _____

    _____

    _____

68. Complete the following chart by comparing the clinical findings in Addison's disease with those in Cushing's syndrome. Use a separate sheet.

Finding	Addison's Disease	Cushing's Syndrome
a. serum sodium level		
b. serum potassium level		
c. ECF volume		
d. blood pressure		
e. serum glucose level		
f. serum calcium		
g. blood urea nitrogen level		
h. cortisol		
i. eosinophil count		
j. leukocyte count		

69. List the common nursing diagnoses associated with Cushing's syndrome.

    a. _____

       _____

    b. _____

       _____

    c. _____

       _____

    d. _____

       _____

    e. _____

       _____

Match the following drugs (70-73) with their clinical uses for hypercortisolism (a–d).

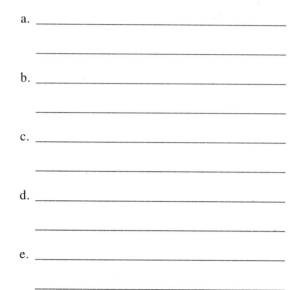

_____ 70. mitotane (Lysodren)

_____ 71. amino-glutethimide (Cytadren)

_____ 72. metyrapone (Metopirone)

_____ 73. cypro-heptadine (Periactin)

a. adrenal enzyme inhibitor used in combination with other antiadrenal agents

b. adrenal cytotoxic agent used for inoper-able adrenal tumors

c. used to treat adrenal hyperfunction resulting from pituitary disease

d. adrenal enzyme inhibitor that decreases cortisol production

74. Which of the following drugs should the nurse be prepared to administer preoperatively to the client scheduled for a bilateral adrenalectomy?

    a. ACTH

    b. regular insulin

    c. vasopressin

    d. hydrocortisone succinate

75. A client is scheduled for bilateral adrenalectomy. Prior to surgery, steroids are ordered to be given. The reason for administering this medication is to

    a. promote glycogen storage by the liver for body energy reserves

    b. compensate for sudden lack of adrenal hormones following surgery

    c. increase the body's inflammatory response to promote scar formation

    d. enhance urinary excretion of salt and water following surgery

76. Following a bilateral adrenalectomy and before having regulatory steroid replacement therapy, the client may have symptoms of

    a. hypotension

    b. hypertension

    c. hypernatremia

    d. hypokalemia

77. A client who has had a bilateral adrenalectomy is upset and crying following visiting hours because of news of a death in the family. The nurse helps to comfort the client and then notifies the physician because the client

    a. will require a sedative to promote restful sleep and reduce energy demands on the body

    b. should have the steroid medication dosage reduced in order to cope with the additional stress

    c. has decreased ability to cope with stress even with steroid replacement therapy

    d. will have feelings of exhaustion and lethargy as a result of the demands of the stressful episode

78. Discharge teaching about medications for the client following bilateral adrenalectomy includes emphasizing that

    a. the dosage of steroid replacement medications will remain the same throughout the client's lifetime

    b. the steroid medications should be taken in the evening so as not to interfere with sleep

    c. dietary salt intake may need to be restricted while the client is taking the steroid medications

    d. the steroid replacement therapy will be given in conjunction with insulin therapy

79. Discuss the significance of a medical alert (Medic Alert) tag for the client who has had a bilateral adrenalectomy. Use a separate sheet.

80. Which of the following statements is correct about hyperaldosteronism?

    a. Peripheral edema due to hypernatremia is common.

    b. It occurs more often in men than in women.

    c. It is a common cause of hypertension in the population.

    d. Fluid and electrolyte disturbances are resulting effects.

81. List the subjective client data relevant to hyperaldosteronism. Use a separate sheet.

82. List the objective client data relevant to hyperaldosteronism. Use a separate sheet.

83. Identify two special laboratory tests that may be ordered for a client with hyperaldosteronism for diagnostic purposes.

    a. _____

    _____

    b. _____

    _____

84. Which of the following statements is correct about the client with hyperaldosteronism following a successful unilateral adrenalectomy?

    a. The low-sodium diet must be continued postoperatively.

    b. Glucocorticoid replacement therapy is temporary.

    c. Spironolactone (Aldactone) must be taken for life.

    d. Additional measures are needed to control hypertension.

Pheochromocytoma

85. Which of the following statements is correct about pheochromocytoma?

    a. It is most often malignant.

    b. It is a catecholamine-producing tumor.

    c. It is found only in the adrenal medulla.

    d. It is manifested by hypotension.

86. Alpha-receptor stimulation by pheochromocytoma-produced epinephrine and norepinephrine results in

    a. diarrhea and weakness

    b. chilling and feeling cold

    c. euphoria and elation

    d. diaphoresis and flushing

87. Beta-receptor stimulation by pheochromocytoma-produced epinephrine and norepinephrine results in

    a. bradycardia

    b. hypotension

    c. bronchospasm

    d. heat intolerance

88. List the subjective client data relevant to pheochromocytoma. Use a separate sheet.

89. List the objective client data relevant to pheochromocytoma. Use a separate sheet.

90. List the laboratory specimens for which the nurse is responsible to collect for use in diagnosing pheochromocytoma.

    a. _____

    _____

    b. _____

    _____

    c. _____

    _____

91. Interventions for the client with pheochromocytoma include

    a. assisting the client to sit in a chair for blood pressure monitoring

    b. instructing the client to get up slowly from a sitting or lying position

    c. encouraging the client to maintain an active exercise schedule such as running

    d. advising the client that there are no special dietary restrictions to follow

92. Identify the medications commonly used to treat hypertension resulting from pheochromocytoma.

    a. _____

    _____

    b. _____

    _____

    c. _____

    _____

93. Following surgery for pheochromocytoma, the client should be monitored for

    a. hypertensive episodes

    b. overwhelming anxiety

    c. hemorrhage and shock

    d. diuresis and hypernatremia

CRITICAL THINKING EXERCISES

Case Study: Diabetes Insipidus

M. L. is a 22-year-old male client who was hospitalized following a motorcycle accident. He sustained multiple abrasions, a fractured right femur, and a head injury despite wearing a helmet. On day 3 of his hospitalization, M. L. was diagnosed as having diabetes insipidus.

Address the following questions:

1. Identify physical and laboratory findings that would be present in M. L.

2. Discuss whether M. L. is a candidate to undergo the fluid deprivation and hypertonic saline test to confirm the diagnosis of diabetes insipidus. Why or why not?

3. Identify the nursing diagnoses for M. L. based on the above data.

4. Identify nursing measures that would assist M. L. to maintain an adequate fluid balance. State the rationale for these measures.

5. The physician initially orders aqueous vasopressin (synthetic Pitressin) 10 units IM every 3–4 hours as indicated for M. L. How does the nurse determine when to give the medication?

M. L. recovers sufficiently to be dismissed to home care. He is to continue the vasopressin (Pitressin) via nasal spray.

6. Develop a teaching/learning plan for M. L. for self-administration of the Pitressin.

7. M. L. asks why the medication cannot be taken orally. What does the nurse tell him?

8. M. L. tells the nurse that taking the medication by nasal spray is going to be a nuisance and he questions whether it is necessary. What should the nurse reply? What alternative routes of administering the medication are available? Considering M. L.'s expressed concern about taking the medication, which route of administration is least disruptive to a daily schedule?

9. Formulate discharge teaching/learning plan for M. L.

Case Study: SIADH

M. H. is a 43-year-old female client who has metastatic carcinoma of the lung. She also has been diagnosed as having SIADH. In recent weeks, she has retained fluid and reports a loss of appetite, lethargy, headaches, and weight gain. Her pulse is 120, her temperature is 97.0°F, and her serum sodium level is 120 mEq/L. M. H. is admitted for therapy to stabilize her condition.

Address the following questions:

1. What additional data should the nurse collect?

2. Identify the relevant nursing diagnoses for M. H. and develop a care plan for these.

3. M. H. is placed on a fluid restriction of 600 mL per 24 hours. Discuss the interventions that will increase her comfort level. What should the nurse do to monitor M. H.'s compliance with the restrictions?

4. M. H. states that she has been taking aspirin at home for her headaches. What should the nurse discuss with M. H. about this drug?

5. M. H. slowly stabilizes, and her serum sodium level returns to normal limits. She is to be discharged to home care. Develop a discharge teaching/learning care plan for M. H. for the SIADH.

Interventions for Clients with Problems of the Thyroid and Parathyroid Glands

LEARNING OBJECTIVES

At the end of this chapter, the student will be able to

▌ Discuss the pathophysiology, etiology, and incidence of hyperthyroidism

▌ Provide care for the client in a thyroid storm or crisis

▌ Provide care for the client with hyperthyroidism

▌ Discuss the pathophysiology, etiology, and incidence of hypothyroidism

▌ Provide emergency care for the client in a myxedema coma

▌ Manage care of the client with hypothyroidism

▌ Identify other conditions of the thyroid gland

▌ Discuss the pathophysiology and etiology of hyperparathyroidism

▌ Manage care for the client with of hyperparathyroidism

▌ Discuss the pathophysiology, etiology, and incidence of hypoparathyroidism

▌ Provide care for the client with hypoparathyroidism

PREREQUISITE KNOWLEDGE

Prior to beginning this chapter, the student should review

▌ The anatomy and physiology of the thyroid and parathyroid glands

▌ The functions of the hormones of the thyroid and parathyroid glands

▌ Normal growth and development and the effects of the thyroid and parathyroid glands on these processes

▌ Normal laboratory values for serum and urine sodium, calcium, and phosphorus

▌ The principles of fluid and electrolyte balance and acid–base balance

▌ The principles of airway management

▌ The concepts of body image and self-esteem

▌ The concepts of loss and grief

▌ The concept of human sexuality

▌ Perioperative nursing care

STUDY QUESTIONS

Hyperthyroidism

1. Increased thyroid hormone production is known as
   a. thyrotoxicosis
   b. euthyroid function
   c. Graves' disease
   d. hypermetabolism

2. Management of the client with hyperthyroidism focuses on
   a. blocking the effects of excessive thyroid secretion
   b. treating the signs and symptoms the client experiences
   c. establishing euthyroid function
   d. all of the above

3. Excess thyroid hormone production increases
   a. glucose tolerance and insulin production
   b. protein synthesis and degradation
   c. peripheral resistance to blood flow
   d. cardiac alpha-adrenergic receptor sites

4. Identify the effects hyperthyroidism has on the following nutrients. Use a separate sheet.
   a. proteins
   b. carbohydrates
   c. lipids

5. The most common cause of hyperthyroidism is
   a. radiation
   b. Graves' disease
   c. thyroid carcinoma
   d. hyperpituitarism

6. Briefly define *thyroid storm* (or *crisis*) and discuss why this condition is an emergency. Who is likely to have a thyroid storm? Use a separate sheet.

7. Identify emergency concerns for the client in a thyroid storm.
   a. _____
   _____
   b. _____
   _____
   c. _____
   _____

8. List the signs and symptoms of the client in a thyroid storm. Use a separate sheet.

9. Which of the following medications would the nurse administer to the client who is in a thyroid storm?
   a. acetylsalicylic acid (aspirin) 10 g orally (PO)
   b. propylthiouracil (PTU) 50 mg PO qd
   c. propranolol hydrochloride (Inderal) 2 mg IV stat
   d. phentolamine mesylate (Regitine) 20 mg IV stat

Match the following medications (10–13) with their purposes in treating the client having a thyroid storm (a–d).

____ 10. methimazole (Tapazole)

____ 11. prednisone (Orasone)

____ 12. propranolol hydrochloride (Inderal)

____ 13. potassium iodide (SSKI) or Lugol's solution

a. prevent release of thyroid hormone from gland

b. stop release of thyroid hormone already in gland

c. block synthesis, secretion, and peripheral effects of thyroid hormone

d. decrease excess sympathetic stimulation in presence of dysrhythmias

14. List the subjective client data relevant to hyperthyroidism. Use a separate sheet.

15. Which of the following symptoms will the client with hyperthyroidism report?
   a. heat intolerance
   b. weight gain
   c. fainting
   d. constipation

16. List the objective client data relevant to hyperthyroidism. Use a separate sheet.

17. Assessment findings for the client with hyperthyroidism include
   a. bradycardia
   b. exophthalmos
   c. dysuria
   d. edema

18. Which of the following laboratory results in consistent with hyperthyroidism?
   a. decreased serum triiodothyronine (T_3) and thyroxine T_4) levels
   b. elevated serum thyrotropin-releasing hormone (TRH) level
   c. decreased radioactive iodine uptake
   d. increased free T_3 and T_4

19. List the common nursing diagnoses for hyper-thyroidism.

    a. _____

    _____

    b. _____

    _____

    c. _____

    _____

20. Instructions for the client who is to receive radioactive iodine therapy for hyperthyroidism include

    a. assuring the client that relief of symptoms will occur within the first week following treatment

    b. instructing the client to plan on hospitalization for 2 to 3 days following treatment

    c. teaching the client about radiation precautions for saliva, urine, and stool

    d. discussing with the client the need for supplemental medication until hyperthyroid symptoms are relieved

21. Preoperative instruction for the client who is to have a thyroidectomy includes

    a. instructing the client to avoid coughing postoperatively so as not to disrupt the sutures

    b. demonstrating to the client how the head should be supported when coughing or moving

    c. explaining that hoarseness after surgery is common due to permanent laryngeal nerve damage

    d. telling the client that tingling around the mouth is a temporary, minor discomfort

22. List the complications that may arise from thyroid surgery.

    a. _____

    _____

    b. _____

    _____

    c. _____

    _____

    d. _____

    _____

23. Discharge preparations for the client who has had a thyroidectomy include

    a. referring the client to the dietitian for help in planning a daily diet of 1200 calorie and 20 g of protein

    b. evaluating the client's home environment about the availability of air conditioning or a fan

    c. discussing with the client's family that the client will be calmer and less moody upon return to the home

    d. reassuring the client that energy levels and activity tolerance will quickly return

Hypothyroidism

24. Untreated hypothyroidism in infants results in

    a. goiter

    b. myxedema

    c. cretinism

    d. gigantism

25. Briefly define *goiter*. _____

    _____

    _____

    _____

26. List the causes of simple goiter.

    a. _____

    _____

    _____

    b. _____

    _____

    _____

    c. _____

    _____

    _____

    d. _____

    _____

27. Describe the effects that low thyroid hormone levels have on the following. Use a separate sheet.

    a. stomach

    b. intestines

    c. heart rate

    d. body temperature

    e. arteries

    f. interstitial fluid

    g. erythropoiesis

Match the following types of hypothyroidism (28–31) with their causes (a–d).

_____ 28. decreased TRH production

_____ 29. pathological changes within the thyroid gland

_____ 30. failure of thyroid gland to develop

_____ 31. inadequate pituitary production of thyroid-stimulating hormone

   a. congenital

   b. primary

   c. secondary

   d. tertiary

32. List the subjective client data relevant to hypothyroidism. Use a separate sheet.

33. List the objective client data relevant to hypothyroidism. Use a separate sheet.

34. Identify the three common nursing diagnoses for the client with hypothyroidism and briefly discuss their priorities for intervention. Use a separate sheet.

35. Identify rationales for administering the following medications intravenously to the client in myxedema coma.

    a. levothyroxine

    b. glucose

    c. corticosteroids

36. Interventions for the client with hypothyroidism include

    a. teaching the client about the need for lifelong drug replacement therapy

    b. sedating the client to help with relaxation and relieve chest pain

    c. referring the client and family for intensive psychotherapy and counseling

    d. instructing the client to restrict fluid intake to help control diarrhea

37. Which of the following types of thyroiditis requires thyroid hormone replacement?

    a. acute suppurative

    b. subacute granulomatous

    c. chronic (Hashimoto's)

38. Which of the following thyroid carcinomas is the most common?

    a. anaplastic

    b. follicular

    c. medullary

    d. papillary

Hyperparathyroidism

39. The parathyroid glands regulate homeostasis of

    a. calcium and chloride

    b. phosphorus and sodium

    c. calcium and phosphorus

    d. sodium and chloride

40. Describe the effects of hyperparathyroidism on the following physiological processes. Use a separate sheet.

    a. renal tubular reabsorption of calcium

    b. renal tubular excretion of phosphate

    c. serum pH balance

    d. serum potassium levels

    e. serum bicarbonate levels

    f. osteoblast activity

    g. osteoclast activity

    h. nerve transmission

    i. muscle contractility

    j. blood pressure

    k. cardiac muscle contractility

Match the following causes (41–46) with their types of hyperparathyroidism (a–d). Answers may be used more than once.

_____ 41. chronic renal disease

_____ 42. autonomously functioning hyperplastic glands

_____ 43. carcinoma of lung, kidney, or GI tract producing PTH-like substance

_____ 44. benign autonomous adenoma in one gland

_____ 45. vitamin D deficiency

_____ 46. radiation to the neck

   a. primary

   b. secondary

   c. tertiary

   d. ectopic

47. List the subjective client data relevant to hyperparathyroidism. Use a separate sheet.

48. List the objective client data relevant to hyperparathyroidism. Use a separate sheet.

49. Identify the most common nursing diagnosis for the client with hyperparathyroidism.

_____

_____

50. Identify rationales for administering the following medications to the client with hyperparathyroidism. Use a separate sheet.

    a. furosemide (Lasix)

    b. IV saline

    c. oral phosphates

    d. calcitonin

    e. mithramycin (Mithracin)

51. Preoperative instruction of the client who is to have removal of the parathyroid glands includes teaching the client

    a. that hoarseness commonly occurs

    b. that the bed will remain flat

    c. to report any tingling in the hands

    d. that dressings will be changed every 2 hours

52. Postoperative care for the client who has had removal of the parathyroid glands includes

    a. monitoring the serum calcium levels daily

    b. observing for signs of respiratory stridor

    c. keeping a tracheostomy tray in the supply room

    d. assessing the client for Phalen's sign every shift

Hypoparathyroidism

53. The most common cause of hypoparathyroidism is

    a. idiopathic and related to an autoimmune process

    b. related to hypomagnesemia from chronic alcohol abuse

    c. a hereditary disorder causing resistance to PTH

    d. iatrogenic, related to removal of the thyroid gland

54. List the subjective client data relevant to hypoparathyroidism. Use a separate sheet.

55. List the objective client data relevant to hypoparathyroidism. Use a separate sheet.

56. List the medications used to treat hypoparathyroidism.

    a. _____

    _____

    b. _____

    _____

    c. _____

    _____

    d. _____

    _____

57. Discharge planning for the client who has chronic hypoparathyroidism should include

    a. reinforcing that the prescribed medications must be taken for the client's entire life

    b. teaching the client to avoid taking vitamin D supplements and sunbathing

    c. advising the client's family that the client should be fully independent in self-care activities

    d. reinforcing instructions about including foods such as milk products and cheese in the diet

CRITICAL THINKING EXERCISES

Case Study: Hyperthyroidism

L. T. is a 38-year-old female client who is admitted to a surgical nursing unit for a thyroidectomy following a radioactive thyroid scan. It is 20°F outside, and L. T. has on a light cotton dress with short sleeves, sandals, and no hosiery. She is carrying a sweater. L. T. is thin and pale; there are dark circles under both eyes. Admission assessment indicates that there are no other major health problems.

Address the following questions:

1. Discuss the type of room accommodation L. T. should have. Consider her exposure to the radioactive iodine.

2. Based on the above data, formulate relevant nursing diagnoses for L. T.

3. Develop a perioperative teaching/learning care plan for L. T.

4. L. T. has a total thyroidectomy. Discuss the assessments that the nurse should make during the immediate postoperative period. What equipment should be available in L. T.'s room following her return from the postanesthesia recovery area? Explain your answer.

5. The day after surgery, L. T.'s diet has been advanced from full liquids to soft. L. T. reports that she is having difficulty talking, her voice is hoarse, and her throat is sore. Discuss what the nurse should do to assist L. T.

6. The surgeon removes the sutures on the fourth postoperative day. Later that morning, L. T. comments, "My neck is sore and it looks so ugly! Will I always have such an obvious scar?" What should the nurse reply to L. T.?

7. L. T. is scheduled for discharge. Develop a discharge teaching/learning care plan for her. Include instructions that the nurse should discuss her immediate family members.

Case Study: Myxedema

G. S. is a 56-year-old woman who is admitted in myxedema coma. Assessment findings include BP = 68/30; apical pulse = 42, irregular; respirations = 8, shallow; serum sodium = 132 mEq/L; serum glucose = 46 mg/100 mL; inability to arouse except with painful stimuli.

Address the following questions:

1. Based on the above data, identify the relevant nursing diagnoses for G. S.

2. What interventions should the nurse initiate immediately?

3. What medications should the nurse be prepared to administer?

4. G. S.'s condition begins to stabilize. What assessments should the nurse make to monitor G. S.'s progress?

5. The physician orders Synthroid (levothyroxine sodium) 0.1 mg PO, qd, for G. S. prior to her discharge. Formulate a discharge teaching/learning care plan for G. S. What factors should the nurse consider when talking to her?

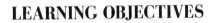

CHAPTER 65

Interventions for Clients with Diabetes Mellitus

LEARNING OBJECTIVES

At the end of this chapter, the student will be able to

- Discuss the types of diabetes mellitus
- Identify the complications, etiology, and incidence of diabetes mellitus
- Assess the client who has diabetes mellitus
- Provide care for the client with diabetes mellitus

PREREQUISITE KNOWLEDGE

Prior to beginning this chapter, the student should review

- The anatomy and physiology of the pancreas and kidney
- The function of insulin in the body
- Normal growth and development and the effects of insulin on these processes
- Normal laboratory values for serum and urine glucose levels, osmolarity, and electrolyte levels
- The principles of fluid and electrolyte balance and acid–base balance
- The principles of intravenous therapy
- The technique for subcutaneous injections
- The concepts of body image and self-esteem
- The concepts of loss and grief
- The concept of human sexuality
- Perioperative nursing care

STUDY QUESTIONS

Pathophysiology Review

1. Briefly describe the syndrome of diabetes mellitus. Use a separate sheet.

2. Identify the common types of diabetes mellitus.

   a. _____
   _____

   b. _____
   _____

   c. _____
   _____

3. Which of the following statements is correct about insulin?

   a. It is secreted by alpha cells in the islets of Langerhans.

   b. It is a catabolic hormone that builds up glucagon reserves.

   c. It is necessary for glucose transport across cell membranes.

   d. It is stored in muscles and converted to fat for storage.

4. Glucose is vital to the body's cells because it

   a. is used to build cell membranes

   b. is used by cells to extract energy

   c. affects the process of protein metabolism

   d. provides nutrients for genetic material

5. List the counter-regulatory hormones released during episodes of hyperglycemia.

   a. _____

   b. _____

   c. _____

   d. _____

   e. _____

Match the following terms (6–8) with their correct definitions (a–c).

____ 6. polydipsia   a. frequent urination

____ 7. polyphagia   b. frequent fluid intake

____ 8. polyuria   c. frequent eating

9. Untreated hyperglycemia results in

   a. respiratory acidosis

   b. metabolic alkalosis

   c. respiratory alkalosis

   d. metabolic acidosis

10. The respiratory pattern of the client with untreated hyperglycemia is

    a. rapid and shallow (tachypnea)

    b. deep and labored (Cheyne-Stokes)

    c. rapid and deep (Kussmaul's)

    d. shallow and labored (Biot's)

11. The electrolyte most affected by hyperglycemia is

    a. sodium

    b. chloride

    c. potassium

    d. magnesium

12. The primary difference between diabetic ketoacidosis (DKA) and hyperglycemic hyperosmolar nonketotic coma (HHNC) is the

    a. level of hyperglycemia

    b. amount of ketones produced

    c. level of hyperosmolarity

    d. amount of volume depletion

13. Both insulin-dependent diabetes mellitus (IDDM) and non–insulin-dependent diabetes mellitus (NIDDM) are associated with

    a. disruption of the glycolytic pathway

    b. deficiencies in the amount of insulin produced

    c. problems with the use of insulin inside the cell

    d. malfunctioning receptor sites on the cell membrane

Match the following types of glucose intolerance (14–17) with their descriptions (a–d).

____ 14. impaired

____ 15. previous abnormality

____ 16. potential abnormality

____ 17. gestational

a. at risk for developing diabetes mellitus

b. develops during pregnancy

c. currently normal with a history of abnormal blood glucose results

d. having a normal fasting blood sugar but reactive hypoglycemia

Match the following diabetic complications (18–25) with their pathophysiologies (a–c). Answers may be used more than once.

____ 18. neovascularization

____ 19. end-stage renal disease

____ 20. muscle atrophy

____ 21. proteinuria

____ 22. hemorrhage into vitreous cavity

____ 23. pain or numbness

____ 24. hard exudates on fundus

____ 25. permanent blindness

a. nephropathy

b. neuropathy

c. retinopathy

26. List lower extremity complications that may result from compromised circulation in the diabetic client.

   a. _____

   _____

   b. _____

   _____

   c. _____

   _____

Match the following etiological factors (27–33) with their types of diabetes mellitus (a or b). Answers may be used more than once.

_____ 27. aging process

_____ 28. autoimmune process

_____ 29. remission period

_____ 30. obesity

_____ 31. heredity

_____ 32. viral infection

_____ 33. decreased physical activity

a. IDDM

b. NIDDM

34. Which of the following individuals is at greatest risk for developing diabetes mellitus?

a. African-American woman, age 25 years

b. African-American man, age 64 years

c. Hispanic woman, age 56 years

d. Hispanic man, age 42 years

35. Preventive measures for diabetes mellitus include

a. controlling hypertension

b. maintaining ideal body weight

c. working in a high-stress environment

d. prenatal care beginning the third trimester of pregnancy

36. List the three emergencies in diabetes mellitus and their causes.

a. _____

_____

_____

_____

b. _____

_____

_____

_____

c. _____

_____

_____

_____

37. Complete the following chart comparing the characteristics of DKA and HHNC. Use a separate sheet.

Characteristic	DKA	HHNC
a. temperature		
b. respirations		
c. pulse		
d. level of consciousness		
e. urinary output		
f. serum glucose level		
g. serum acetone level		
h. arterial pH		
i. serum sodium level		
j. serum potassium level		
k. serum bicarbonate level		
l. anion gap		
m. blood urea nitrogen (BUN) level		

38. The type of insulin used in the emergency treatment of DKA and HHNC is

a. NPH

b. lente

c. regular

d. protamine zinc

39. Early treatment of DKA and HHNC includes intravenous

a. glucagon

b. potassium

c. bicarbonate

d. normal saline

40. A client is admitted with a blood glucose level of 900 mg/dL. Intravenous fluids and insulin are administered. Two hours after treatment is initiated the blood glucose level is 400 mg/dL. Which of the following complications is the client most at risk for developing?

a. hypoglycemia

b. cerebral edema

c. renal shutdown

d. pulmonary edema

41. In determining whether a client is hypoglycemic or hyperglycemic, a characteristic to consider is

a. skin moisture

b. irritability

c. rapid pulse

d. nausea

42. The client recovering from DKA will need
    a. assistance in identifying the cause of the episode to prevent a recurrence
    b. instruction in self-administration of glucagon to prevent further episodes
    c. intensive teaching to promote compliance with self-administration of insulin
    d. assistance in gaining a clear understanding of the nature of diabetes and its management

43. Which of the following types of cells is capable of using glucose in the absence of insulin?
    a. cardiac
    b. brain
    c. kidney
    d. pancreas

44. Glucagon is used primarily to treat the client with
    a. DKA
    b. idiosyncratic reaction to insulin
    c. insulin-induced hypoglycemia
    d. HHNC

45. Glucagon is given in a dextrose solution because dextrose
    a. promotes more storage of glucose in the liver
    b. stimulates the pancreas to produce more insulin
    c. increases blood sugar levels at a controlled rate
    d. inhibits glycogenesis, gluconeogenesis, and lipolysis

46. When glucagon is administered, it
    a. competes for insulin at the receptor sites
    b. frees glucose from hepatic stores of glycogen
    c. supplies glycogen directly to the vital tissues
    d. provides a glucose substitute for rapid replacement

Collaborative Management

47. List the subjective client data relevant to diabetes mellitus. Use a separate sheet.

48. List the objective client data relevant to diabetes mellitus. Use a separate sheet.

49. Which of the following four laboratory findings is most diagnostic of diabetes mellitus?
    a. fasting blood sugar = 80 mg/dL
    b. 2-hour postprandial blood sugar = 120 mg/dL

    c. 1-hour glucose tolerance blood sugar = 110 mg/dL
    d. 2-hour glucose tolerance blood sugar = 140 mg/dL

50. A diabetic client is scheduled to have a blood glucose test the next morning. Which of the following should the nurse tell the client to do before coming in for the test?
    a. Eat the usual diet but have nothing after midnight.
    b. Take the usual oral hypoglycemic tablet in the morning.
    c. Eat a clear liquid breakfast in the morning.
    d. Follow the usual diet and medication regimen.

51. Briefly discuss the rational for determining BUN and creatine levels in the diabetic client. Use a separate sheet.

52. The frequency with which a client should monitor capillary blood glucose levels depends on levels of
    a. urine glucose
    b. serum ketones
    c. serum glucose
    d. urine ketones

53. Discuss the concept of *renal threshold* and its significance for using measurement of urine glucose levels to manage diabetes mellitus. Use a separate sheet.

54. List the problems of using urine tests for monitoring glucose levels. Use a separate sheet.

55. The nurse should instruct the client who is taking oral hypoglycemic agents that
    a. dietary restrictions can be relaxed while taking the medication
    b. the exercise program should be changed to include more intensive aerobics
    c. there are no particular restrictions for taking over-the-counter medications
    d. drinking alcoholic beverages will cause nausea and a hot-flash feeling

56. Which of the following oral hypoglycemic agents is safe to give to the diabetic client with renal impairment?
    a. acetohexamide (Dymelor)
    b. chlorpropamide (Diabinese)
    c. glyburide (Micronase)
    d. tolbutamide (Orinase)

57. Which of the following statements is correct about insulin?

   a. Exogenous insulin is necessary for management of all cases of type II diabetes.

   b. Insulin action effectiveness depends on the individual client's absorption of the drug.

   c. Insulin doses should be regulated according to self-monitoring urine glucose levels.

   d. Insulin administered in multiple doses per day decreases a client's life style flexibility.

58. Which of the following statements is correct about insulin administration?

   a. Insulin may be given either orally, intravenously, or subcutaneously.

   b. Insulin injections should be spaced no closer than one-half inch apart.

   c. Rotating injection sites improves absorption and prevents lipodystrophy.

   d. In a mixed-dose protocol, the longer acting insulin should be withdrawn first.

59. A diabetic client is on a mixed-dose insulin protocol of 8 units regular insulin and 12 units NPH insulin at 7 a.m. At 10:30 a.m., the client reports feeling uneasy and shaky. Which of the following is the probable explanation for this?

   a. The NPH insulin's action is peaking, and there is an insufficient blood glucose level.

   b. The regular insulin's action is peaking, and there is an insufficient blood glucose level.

   c. The client consumed too many calories at breakfast, and now has an elevated blood glucose level.

   d. The symptoms are unrelated to the insulin or diet, and the client is at risk of a cardiovascular emergency.

60. A client has order for 40 units insulin zinc suspension (Lente insulin) and 10 units regular insulin every morning. Explain how these drugs should be prepared for administration. What should the client be told about the actions and side effects of these medications? Submit the completed exercise to the clinical instructor on a separate sheet.

61. Describe the three problems with blood glucose levels that may occur during the night if a client is on insulin therapy.

   a. _____

   _____

   _____

   b. _____

   _____

   _____

   _____

   c. _____

   _____

   _____

62. The client who is to use an external insulin pump should be told that

   a. self-monitoring of blood glucose levels can be done only once a day

   b. the insulin supply must be replaced every 2–4 weeks

   c. the pump's battery should be checked on a regular weekly schedule

   d. the needle site must be changed every 1–3 days

63. A client with type II diabetes mellitus, usually controlled with a sulfonylurea, develops a urinary tract infection. Due to the stress of the infection, she must be treated with insulin. She should be instructed that

   a. the sulfonylurea must be discontinued and insulin taken until the infection clears

   b. insulin will now be necessary to control the client's diabetes for life

   c. the sulfonylurea dose must be reduced until the infection clears

   d. the insulin is necessary to supplement the sulfonylurea until the infection clears

64. Identify the factors that should be considered when developing an individualized meal plan for the diabetic client.

   a. _____

   _____

   b. _____

   _____

   c. _____

   _____

   d. _____

   _____

65. Basic principles of meal planning for the diabetic client include

    a. five small meals per day plus a bedtime snack

    b. providing a favorite sweet dessert once a day

    c. high-protein, low-carbohydrate, and low-fiber foods

    d. considering the action time of the client's insulin

66. List the food groups in the exchange system of diabetic meal planning.

    a. _____

    b. _____

    c. _____

    d. _____

    e. _____

    f. _____

67. Which of the following food exchange examples is not equivalent?

    a. 1 teaspoon butter = 1 strip bacon

    b. 1 tablespoon peanut butter = 1 ounce ground beef

    c. 1 cup milk = 1 cup yogurt

    d. 1/2 cup carrots = 1/2 cup broccoli

68. Which of the following statements is correct about the diet a diabetic client should follow?

    a. Alcoholic beverage consumption is unrestricted.

    b. Dietetic foods may contain more fat than regular foods.

    c. Sweeteners should be avoided because of the side effects.

    d. Both soluble and insoluble fiber foods should be limited.

69. The recommended protocol for most diabetic clients to lose weight is to

    a. participate in an aerobic program twice a week for 20 minutes each session

    b. reduce calorie intake and walk briskly for 30 minutes daily

    c. slowly increase insulin dosage until mild hypoglycemia occurs

    d. reduce daily calorie intake to 1200 calories and monitor for ketones

70. The recommended calorie reduction for the diabetic client who must lose weight is

    a. 500 calories per week

    b. 1500 calories per week

    c. 2500 calories per week

    d. 3500 calories per week

71. List the eating disorders that the diabetic client may develop if food becomes an unhealthy focus of attention.

    a. _____

    b. _____

72. The diabetic client who swims for exercise should be advised to administer insulin prior to exercising in the

    a. abdomen

    b. thighs

    c. arms

    d. hips

73. Discuss the purpose for the diabetic client's having a supply of simple sugar available when exercising. Use a separate sheet.

74. Diabetic foot care includes

    a. using rubbing alcohol to toughen the skin on the soles of the feet

    b. wearing open-toed shoes or sandals in warm weather to prevent perspiration

    c. applying lotion to moisturize the skin and keep it smooth and supple

    d. using cool water for bathing feet to prevent inadvertent thermal injury

75. A 25-year-old female client with diabetic nephropathy tells the nurse, "I have two kidneys and I'm still young. I expect to be around for a long time, so why should I worry about it?" The best reply for the nurse to make is

    a. "You have little to worry about as long as your kidneys keep making urine."

    b. "You should discuss this with your physician because you are being unrealistic."

    c. "You would be correct if your diabetes could be managed with insulin."

    d. "The damage being done affects both kidneys, even with insulin management."

76. Which of the following statements is correct about education for diabetic clients?

    a. General education promotes a sense of well-being because it helps the client feel he or she has control over the disease.

    b. Survival education includes assisting the client to adapt self-care practices to meet his or her needs.

    c. Home management education includes information about when to call the physician.

    d. Life style improvement education includes emphasis on daily care such as hygiene.

77. Which of the following statements about sexual intercourse for diabetic clients is correct?

    a. The incidence of sexual dysfunction is lower in men than in women.

    b. Retrograde ejaculation does not interfere with male fertility.

    c. Impotence is often associated with diabetes mellitus in male clients.

    d. Sexual dysfunction in female clients results in inability to attain orgasm.

78. List the fears that are most common in diabetic clients.

    a. _____

    _____

    b. _____

    _____

    c. _____

    _____

    d. _____

    _____

79. An insulin-dependent diabetic client is planning to travel by air and asks the nurse about preparations for the trip. The nurse should tell the client to

    a. pack insulin and syringes in a labeled, crush-proof kit in the checked luggage

    b. carry all necessary diabetic supplies in a clearly identified pack aboard the plane

    c. ask the stewardess to put the insulin in the galley refrigerator once aboard

    d. take only minimal supplies and get the prescription filled at his or her destination

80. Which of the following statements reflects that the diabetic client understands the principles of self-care?

    a. "I don't like the idea of sticking myself so often to measure my sugar."

    b. "I plan to measure the sugar in my urine at least four times a day."

    c. "I plan to get my spouse to exercise with me to keep me company."

    d. "If I get a cold, I can take my regular cough medicine until I feel better."

CRITICAL THINKING EXERCISES

Case Study: Diabetes Mellitus

J. R. is a 48-year-old woman who is admitted to the emergency department. She is unconscious. She has a known history of insulin-dependent diabetes mellitus. J. R.'s daughter accompanies her and tells the staff that J. R. has had the "flu" and has been unable to eat or drink very much. The daughter is uncertain whether J. R. has taken her insulin in the past 24 hours. J. R.'s vital signs are temperature = 101.8°F; pulse = 120, weak and irregular; respirations = 22, deep with a fruity odor; and blood pressure = 64/42. Blood specimens and arterial blood gases are drawn and an intravenous infusion begun.

Address the following questions:

1. Based on J. R.'s history, give the probable changes in laboratory results for serum glucose, serum osmolarity, serum acetone, BUN, arterial pH, and arterial pCO_2. What medical emergency do these data indicate?

2. What type of intravenous solutions should the nurse be prepared to administer to J. R.? What drugs should the nurse be prepared to give? Explain your answers.

3. Identify the relevant nursing diagnoses for J. R. based on the above assessments.

4. A large-bore intravenous needle is inserted, and J. R. is placed on continuous cardiac monitoring. What is the rationale for these interventions?

5. During the first 24 hours, what complications should the nurse monitor for in J. R.? Why?

6. J. R. eventually becomes normoglycemic, regains consciousness, and begins a 1500-calorie diabetic diet. Develop a teaching/learning plan for her about this diet.

7. Prior to this emergency, J. R. had been monitoring urine glucose and ketones for self-care and insulin administration. Her physician prescribes blood glucose monitoring instead of urine testing. What is the rationale for this change?

8. Which aspect of diabetic self-care should the nurse discuss with J. R. prior to her discharge?

9. J. R. is to be discharged on a mixed-dose protocol for insulin. She is to receive 10 units regular insulin and 18 units NPH insulin before breakfast and another 5 units regular insulin and 12 units NPH at dinner time. Develop a teaching/learning plan for these medications.

10. What should the nurse discuss with J. R. about diabetes, insulin, and illness? What can J. R. do to prevent future emergency episodes? Consider "Instructions for Sick Days" rules.

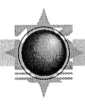

C H A P T E R 6 6

Assessment of the Skin, Hair, and Nails

LEARNING OBJECTIVES

At the end of this chapter, the student will be able to

■ Describe the structure and function of the skin

■ Describe the structure and function of the skin appendages

■ Describe the changes in the skin that occur with aging

■ Discuss the assessment of the client with a possible skin disorder

■ Discuss forms of diagnostic assessment for skin lesions

PREREQUISITE KNOWLEDGE

Prior to beginning this chapter, the student should review

■ The anatomy and physiology of the skin and its appendages

■ The principles of fluid and electrolyte balance

■ The principles of infection control

■ The concepts of body image and self-esteem

STUDY QUESTIONS

Anatomy and Physiology Review

1. List four factors that may alter the appearance and function of the skin.

a. _____

_____

b. _____

_____

c. _____

_____

d. _____

_____

Match the following terms and functions associated with the skin (2–15) with their layers of skin (a–c). Answers may be used more than once.

_____ 2. basement membrane

_____ 3. collagen, dermoblasts, elastin

_____ 4. fat formation and storage

_____ 5. ground substance

_____ 6. horny layer

_____ 7. innermost layer

_____ 8. insulating layer

_____ 9. keratin and myelin

_____ 10. Langerhans' cells

_____ 11. middle layer

_____ 12. oxygen and heat transfer

_____ 13. pads against mechanical injury

_____ 14. protective interface with environment

_____ 15. rich in sensory nerves

a. adipose tissue

b. dermis

c. epidermis

16. Which of the following statements is correct about the skin appendages?
   a. Hair growth is continuous and resistant to stressors.
   b. Nail growth and appearance are often altered in illness.
   c. Sebum secretion helps to regulate body temperature.
   d. The secretions of the apocrine glands are odorless and colorless.

17. The most important factor that contributes to the degeneration of the skin is
   a. genetic predetermination
   b. hormonal changes with aging
   c. chronic exposure to the sun
   d. presence of internal disease

18. Skin changes in elderly people leave them more susceptible to
   a. heat exhaustion and stroke
   b. acne and comedone formation
   c. hirsutism and heat retention
   d. seborrhea and scalp scaliness

Subjective Assessment

19. List the subjective client data relevant to assessment of the skin. Use a separate sheet.

20. Which of the following data are relevant to the subjective assessment of the client with a skin problem?
   a. scratch marks on arms
   b. itching increases with stress
   c. bald patches on crown of head
   d. cuticles torn and reddened

21. Which of the following occupations increases one's risk for developing skin-related problems?
   a. secretary
   b. research scientist
   c. stock broker
   d. textile worker

22. The following is a partial client history. Discuss the significance these data have for an assessment of the integumentary system. Submit the completed exercise to the clinical instructor on a separate sheet.

   Female client, 67 years old, admitted from a nursing home. States that she began having pain 2 weeks ago. Pain is intense, burning, and limited to the left thorax. Several days after the pain began, client began to notice small blisters on her skin that coincided with where the pain was most intense. The blisters were filled with clear fluid. Client reports fatigue and feeling run down, so that she spends much of the day napping instead of socializing in the day room. Recalls having had most childhood illnesses. Denies any allergies to foods or medications.

Objective Assessment

23. List the objective client data relevant to assessment of the skin. Use a separate sheet.

24. Using the data in question 22, construct a physical assessment recording for the integumentary system. Submit the completed exercise to the clinical instructor on a separate sheet.

25. Which of the following is an abnormal finding in the assessment of the skin that should be reported to the physician immediately?
   a. yellow cast to skin on palms and soles and around mouth
   b. immediate capillary refill following nail bed blanching
   c. several brown macula on soles of feet
   d. nail bed angle is 180 degrees or less

26. Which of the following skin lesions is a normal finding in an elderly client?

    a. telangiectasis

    b. cherry angioma

    c. hematoma

    d. venous star

27. Which of the following assessment findings is abnormal in the client who has a fever?

    a. skin over abdomen flushed

    b. extremities moist and warm

    c. tenting of skin over forearm

    d. oral mucous membranes dry

28. Which part of the body should the nurse examine to identify the presence of cyanosis in a dark-skinned client?

    a. earlobes

    b. nail beds

    c. back of hands

    d. over the sacrum

29. Which part of the body should the nurse examine to identify the presence of jaundice in a dark-skinned client?

    a. conjunctiva

    b. sclera

    c. palms

    d. hard palate

Match the following primary skin lesions (30–39) with their descriptions (a–j).

_____ 30. bulla

_____ 31. cyst

_____ 32. macule

_____ 33. nodule

_____ 34. papule

_____ 35. patch

_____ 36. plaque

_____ 37. pustule

_____ 38. vesicle

_____ 39. wheal

   a. flat, less than 1 cm in diameter

   b. flat, larger than 1 cm in diameter

   c. elevated, firm, less than 1 cm in diameter

   d. elevated, plateau-like, more than 1 cm in diameter

   e. elevated, irregular shape, transient edema

   f. round, filled with fluid or semisolid material, less than 1 cm wide and deep

   g. filled with clear fluid, less than 1 cm in diameter

   h. filled with clear fluid, more than 1 cm in diameter

   i. filled with purulent fluid

   j. elevated, round, larger than 1 cm wide, and deep

Match the following secondary lesions (40–45) with their associated diseases or skin problems (a–f).

_____ 40. atrophy

_____ 41. crust

_____ 42. fissure

_____ 43. lichenification

_____ 44. scale

_____ 45. ulcer

   a. psoriasis

   b. chronic dermatitis

   c. fungal infection

   d. decubitus

   e. impetigo

   f. striae

46. Which of the following statements is correct about the collection of specimens for culturing infective skin organisms?

    a. bacterial cultures are transported on ice

    b. viral cultures are transported at room temperature

    c. fungal cultures are collected with a cotton-tipped applicator

    d. crusted lesions are opened and the exudate is cultured

47. The type of skin biopsy procedure most uncomfortable for a client is the

    a. punch biopsy

    b. shave biopsy

    c. excisional biopsy

    d. wedge resection

48. The test that is used to differentiate an allergic contact dermatitis is the

    a. diascopy

    b. patch test

    c. scratch test

    d. intradermal test

49. A skin lesion composed of multiple lesions that merge together is called

    a. diffuse

    b. clustered

    c. universal

    d. coalesced

CRITICAL THINKING EXERCISES

Case Study: Skin Assessment

S. A. is a 37-year-old housewife who recently went on vacation with her family. They visited many different areas, stopping to camp in national parks and forests. S. A. noticed a rash on her legs, left arm, and abdomen yesterday, the day after the family returned home. The rash is linear in configuration and is vesicular. S. A. tells the nurses, "I itch all over where the rash is. It's so bad that I didn't get much sleep last night. I finally got up and took a couple of Benadryl. That knocked me out. I don't want to take Benadryl during the day because it makes me too sleepy, but I need something to keep me from scratching. Please tell me what I can do!"

Address the following questions:

1. What further data should the nurse collect from S. A. about her rash?

2. Based on the above data, identify relevant nursing diagnoses for S. A.

3. Some of the lesions have opened and crusting adheres to the skin. The physician orders that a culture be taken of the lesions. Describe what the nurse should do to collect the specimens.

4. What information does S. A. need in preparation for the cultures being taken?

5. S. A. asks if her rash is contagious. She is concerned about infecting her children, ages 3 and 6 years. What should the nurse tell her?

6. S. A. is to go home and take tepid Aveeno Colloidal baths, tid. She may take Benadryl (diphenhydramine hydrochloride), 50 mg, PO, at bedtime. Develop a teaching/learning plan for S. A.

C H A P T E R 6 7

Interventions for Clients with Problems of the Skin and Nails

LEARNING OBJECTIVES

At the end of this chapter, the student will be able to

- Discuss collaborative management of minor skin irritations: dryness, pruritus, sunburn and urticaria
- Discuss trauma to the skin
- Discuss pressure ulcers
- Describe collaborative management of pressure ulcers
- Discuss common skin infections
- Describe collaborative management of common skin infections
- Discuss parasitic skin infections
- Discuss eczema and dermatitis
- Describe the collaborative management of clients with skin inflammations
- Describe the pathophysiology, etiology, and incidence of psoriasis
- Discuss the collaborative management of the client with psoriasis
- Discuss benign skin tumors
- Describe the various skin cancers
- Discuss collaborative management of the client with skin cancer
- Discuss the indications for plastic and reconstructive surgery
- Discuss the collaborative management of the client having plastic and reconstructive surgery
- Identify other skin problems

PREREQUISITE KNOWLEDGE

Prior to beginning this chapter, the student should review

- The anatomy and physiology of the skin and its appendages
- The principles of infection control
- The principles of general nutrition
- The principles of fluid and electrolyte balance
- The procedure for application of topical medications
- Pain management
- The principles of wound healing and wound care
- The concepts of body image and self-esteem
- The concept of human sexuality
- The concepts of loss, grief, death, and dying
- Perioperative nursing care
- Isolation techniques

STUDY QUESTIONS

Minor Irritations

1. A problem resulting from unrelieved pruritus in a skin lesion is

   a. vesicles

   b. infection

   c. plaque

   d. wheals

2. List factor that contribute to xerosis.

   a. _____

   b. _____

   c. _____

   d. _____

   e. _____

   f. _____

3. Interventions to rehydrate the skin include

   a. soaking in a warm tub of water for an hour

   b. applying emollient cream to dry skin surfaces

   c. bathing every day with warm water

   d. using an alkaline soap for washing

   e. maintaining an adequate fluid intake

4. Which of the following statements is correct about pruritus?

   a. Distribution and severity vary from person to person.

   b. Most clients report increased pruritus during the day.

   c. Symptoms remain relatively constant in any one client.

   d. Emotional stress distracts from pruritus and scratching.

5. List the interventions for pruritus management. Use a separate sheet.

6. Interventions for the management of prickly heat rash include

   a. using waterproof pads on the bedding under the client

   b. wearing loose-fitting cotton clothing

   c. patting cornstarch on the affected skin surfaces

   d. applying oil-based creams or lotions for lubrication

7. Sunburn, a common skin injury, is a

   a. first-degree burn

   b. second-degree burn

   c. third-degree burn

   d. fourth-degree burn

8. Preventive measures for sunburn include

   a. seeking shade whenever possible

   b. wearing light, mesh-weave clothing

   c. applying a sun screen with a sun protection factor (SPF) of 15 or less

   d. reapplying sun screen lotion after swimming

9. Interventions to relieve discomfort from sunburn include

   a. taking warm baths or showers

   b. applying antibiotic ointments

   c. applying cooled moisturizing lotions

   d. taking an oral nonsteroidal anti-inflammatory drug

10. List, in sequence, the events leading to urticaria.

    a. _____

    _____

    b. _____

    _____

    c. _____

    _____

    d. _____

    _____

11. The drug of choice to treat urticaria is

    a. a corticosteroid

    b. an antihistamine

    c. a nonsteroidal anti-inflammatory

    d. an analgesic

Trauma

Match the following descriptions of wound healing (12–14) with their related terms (a–c).

_____ 12. gradual filling in of dead space with connective tissue

_____ 13. wound left open initially, then closed with sutures

_____ 14. wound edges are approximated and sutured together

a. first intention

b. second intention

c. third intention

15. Put the following events of wound healing in the correct order.

____ a. cell injury or death

____ b. collagen and ground substance laid down

____ c. erythema, swelling, heat, and pain

____ d. fibrin network

____ e. granulation tissue

____ f. leakage of plasma into tissue

____ g. local accumulation of fluid

____ h. migration of fibroblasts to wound

____ i. phagocytosis

____ j. revascularization

____ k. scar no longer blanches with pressure

____ l. scar tissue remodeled

____ m. wound exudate formed

16. Which of the following statements is correct about wound healing?

a. Partial thickness wounds heal by filling in with granulation tissue and contraction.

b. Migration of epithelial cells is enhanced by tissue that is hydrated, oxygenated, and free of pathogens.

c. Full-thickness wounds heal by the reproduction of new skin cells or epithelialization.

d. A full-thickness wound covered by epithelial cell migration is less prone to reinjury.

17. Which of the following clients is at the greatest risk for impaired wound healing?

a. an 18-year-old teen with a closed fracture of the humerus

b. a 34-year-old woman who has had a cholecystectomy

c. a 56-year-old man with crush injuries to both lower legs

d. an 81-year-old woman who has a deep knife cut on her thumb

Pressure Ulcers

18. Identify the mechanical forces responsible for pressure ulcer formation.

a. _____

b. _____

c. _____

19. Pressure ulcer formation is enhanced by

a. turning and repositioning

b. excessive skin moisture

c. exposure to the air

d. massage and heat

20. List the subjective client data relevant to pressure ulcers. Use a separate sheet.

21. List the objective client data relevant to pressure ulcers. Use a separate sheet.

22. Which of the following is a normal finding in a healing wound?

a. creamy yellow drainage from a secondary lesion

b. pink-amber fluid from a second-day surgical wound

c. green-blue drainage from a puncture wound

d. gray-brown drainage from an abdominal wound

23. List three ways that a dressing can expedite wound healing.

a. _____

_____

_____

b. _____

_____

_____

c. _____

_____

_____

24. What factor determines the frequency of dressing changes?

_____

_____

_____

25. List categories of nonsurgical interventions other than dressings that assist in wound healing.

    a. _____

    _____

    b. _____

    _____

    c. _____

    _____

26. Which of the following foods offers the most benefit for wound healing?

    a. liver

    b. potatoes

    c. apple juice

    d. carrots

27. Interventions following skin grafting include

    a. turning the client frequently to prevent stasis

    b. changing the dressing tid to promote healing

    c. elevating the grafted area to decrease swelling

    d. soaking the graft to keep it moist

28. Interventions for a donor site include

    a. turning the client to the position of comfort

    b. wrapping the site to collect any exudate

    c. changing the dressing bid to promote healing

    d. exposing it to the air to promote drying

29. List interventions to prevent wound infections in the hospital setting and give examples of each.

    a. _____

    _____

    _____

    b. _____

    _____

    _____

Common Infections

30. Which of the following four statements is correct about skin infections?

    a. Bacterial lesions usually involve the hair and nails.

    b. Viral infections produce immunity and recurrence is rare.

    c. Fungal infections spread readily in dry, cracked skin.

    d. Lesion location helps determine the causative organism

31. List the subjective client data relevant to skin infection. Use a separate sheet.

32. List the objective client data relevant to skin infection. Use a separate sheet.

33. The client who is taking a board-spectrum antibiotic is prone to developing

    a. tinea corporis

    b. cellulitis

    c. herpes simplex

    d. candidiasis

34. Viral infections are confirmed by

    a. swab culture

    b. blood culture

    c. Tzanck's culture

    d. potassium hydroxide (KOH) preparation

35. Interventions for skin infections include

    a. warm compresses to furuncles or areas of cellulitis

    b. emollients applied to viral lesions to promote crusting

    c. occlusive wet dressings applied continuously

    d. aggressive oral or parenteral antibiotic therapy

36. The client with a skin infection who probably requires the most emotional support is one with

    a. candidiasis

    b. genital herpes

    c. folliculitis

    d. herpes zoster

Parasitic Disorders

37. Which of the following statements is correct about pediculosis?

    a. Pediculosis capitis is more commonly found in men.

    b. Pediculosis corporis commonly affects the pubic area.

    c. Pediculosis pubis is spread during sexual intercourse.

    d. Treating only the client for infestation is sufficient.

38. Which of the following statements is correct about scabies?

   a. Pruritus associated with scabies infestation is less intense than that associated with pediculosis.

   b. Scabies infection can be transmitted through infested bed linens.

   c. Scabies is an infection that is limited to the lower socioeconomic population.

   d. Pruritus usually resolves quickly following successful treatment for scabies.

Common Inflammations

Match the following descriptions (39–45) with their categories of skin inflammation (a–c). Answers may be used more than once.

_____ 39. genetic predisposition

_____ 40. antibiotic induced

_____ 41. contact with allergen

_____ 42. direct contact with irritant

_____ 43. respiratory allergy association

_____ 44. sulfa drugs

_____ 45. cell-mediated immune response

a. contact dermatitis

b. atopic dermatitis

d. drug eruption

46. List the subjective client data relevant to skin inflammation. Use a separate sheet.

47. List the objective client data relevant to skin inflammation. Use a separate sheet.

48. Interventions for skin inflammation include

   a. exposing one's self to gradually increasing amounts of an allergen for desensitization

   b. wearing protective clothing to provide a barrier to allergen contact

   c. applying topical ointments to inflamed areas in the antecubital fossa or popliteal space

   d. administering antihistamines on a regular schedule for maximal effectiveness

49. Self-care measures for the client with a skin inflammation include

   a. avoiding things that exacerbate the rash

   b. informing health care providers about drug allergies

   c. preventing excessive dry skin by using moisturizers

   d. keeping a log of activities and skin condition

   e. all of the above

Psoriasis

50. Which of the following statements is correct about psoriasis?

   a. It is a scaling disorder, limited to the epidermis.

   b. Epidermal cells multiply and migrate at a faster rate than normal.

   c. The disease tends to worsen in warm, sunny climates.

   d. The earlier in life the disease starts, the better the prognosis.

51. List the subjective client data relevant to psoriasis. Use a separate sheet.

Match the following objective data (52–59) with their types of psoriasis (a–c). Answers may be used more than once.

_____ 52. no obvious lesions

_____ 53. silvery white scales

_____ 54. pustules along with scaling

_____ 55. sharply defined plaque borders

_____ 56. generalized erythema and scaling

_____ 57 symmetric distribution of lesions

_____ 58. secondary infection

_____ 59. disturbed thermo-regulatory ability

a. vulgaris

b. exfoliative

c. pustular

60. List the major agents used in the treatment of psoriasis.

   a. _____

   _____

   b. _____

   _____

   c. _____

   _____

61. Interventions for anthralin therapy include

   a. applying the paste to active lesions to reduce spread

   b. leaving the paste on from one application to the next

   c. removing the paste carefully after 2 hours of contact

   d. spreading the paste over large, contiguous areas

62. The most severe and potentially threatening side effect of ultraviolet therapy for psoriasis is

    a. premature aging of the skin

    b. actinic keratosis

    c. Koebner's phenomenon

    d. cutaneous malignancy

63. Interventions to assist the client with psoriasis to cope include all of the following *except* encouraging the client to

    a. use relaxation techniques

    b. engage in physical exercise

    c. seek professional counseling

    d. develop new social contacts

64. Failure to comply with self-care activities for managing psoriasis is an indication that the client

    a. is immature

    b. requires further assessment

    c. is incapable of self-care

    d. is too dependent on others

Benign Tumors

Match the following descriptions of benign skin tumors (65–76) with their related terms. Answers may be used more than once.

_____ 65. port-wine stain

_____ 66. common in the elderly

_____ 67. difficult to treat cosmetically

_____ 68. firm nodule filled with liquid

_____ 69. infection of keratinocytes

_____ 70. may result in malignant melanoma

_____ 71. mobile upon palpation

_____ 72. mole

_____ 73. multiple pasted on plaques

_____ 74. overgrowth of scar tissues

_____ 75. treated topically

_____ 76. vascular neoplasm

a. cyst

b. hemangioma

c. keloid

d. nevus

e. seborrheic keratosis

f. wart

Skin Cancer

77. All of the following are malignant skin cancers *except*

    a. actinic keratoses

    b. squamous cell lesions

    c. basal cell lesions

    d. melanomas

78. Which of the following clients is at greatest risk of developing skin cancer?

    a. an 18-year-old Hispanic woman who is a lifeguard at a beach in southern California

    b. a 52-year-old Caucasian man who works for a lawn and tree service company

    c. a 36-year-old African-American man who works as a lineman for a power company

    d. a 65-year-old Caucasian woman who enjoys gardening, swimming, and sunbathing

79. List the warning signs of skin cancer. Use a separate sheet.

80. List the subjective client data relevant to skin cancer. Use a separate sheet.

81. List the objective client data relevant to skin cancer. Use a separate sheet.

82. Drug therapy in the management of skin cancer commonly includes

    a. systemic chemotherapy

    b. topical chemotherapy

    c. psoralen and light therapy

    d. systemic corticosteroids

83. The client with skin cancer is most likely to experience difficulty adjusting to an altered body image following

    a. cryosurgery

    b. curettage and electrodesiccation

    c. wide scalpel excision

    d. Moh's surgery

84. Discharge teaching of the client who has had surgery for skin cancer includes

    a. assisting the client in placing his or her concerns into perspective

    b. reviewing risk factors for skin cancer and assessing the client's personal risk

    c. suggesting alternatives for avoiding overexposure to sunlight

    d. emphasizing compliance with regular self-inspection of the skin as a preventive measure

    e. all of the above

Plastic and Reconstructive Surgery

85. Identify the main purposes of plastic or reconstructive surgery.

    a. _____

    _____

    b. _____

    _____

86. List the subjective client data relevant to plastic surgery. Use a separate sheet.

87. When taking the history of a client who wishes to have plastic surgery, the nurse

    a. assumes the reason for surgery is based on the client's physical appearance

    b. asks numerous questions to encourage the client to verbalize frustrations and embarrassment

    c. observes for nonverbal communication that reflects the client's emotional status

    d. reaffirms that the client's expectations for a successful outcome of surgery are realistic

88. Medications that the client who is scheduled for plastic surgery may be taking and that the nurse should specifically inquire about include

    a. acetaminophen (Tylenol)

    b. salicylic acid (Bufferin)

    c. multiple vitamins (Stresstab)

    d. magnesium hydroxide (Milk of Magnesia)

89. List the objective client data relevant to plastic surgery. Use a separate sheet.

90. Which of the following assessment findings of the client who has had plastic surgery should be reported to the physician immediately?

    a. swallowing after a rhinoplasty

    b. lip numbness after a rhytidectomy

    c. pain after a dermabrasion

    d. eye pain after a blepharoplasty

91. Which of the following interventions is therapeutic in the immediate postoperative period for the client who has had plastic surgery?

    a. encouraging the client to seek the assistance of a support group

    b. encouraging the client to go to a vacation resort for recovery

    c. encouraging the client to limit contacts to the immediate family

    d. referring the client for profession counseling

Other Disorders of the Skin and Nails

92. Which of the following statements are true about skin and nail problems?

    a. Insect bites often resolve spontaneously.

    b. Rabies is a neurological disease caused by a virus.

    c. Bite wounds are usually closed with sutures.

    d. Pemphigus vulgaris is an acute epidermal drug reaction.

    e. Toxic epidermal necrolysis is an autoimmune disease.

    f. Treatment in a burn unit is indicated for clients with toxic epidermal necrolysis.

    g. Lichen planus lesions in the mouth are sometimes mistaken for thrush.

    h. Cold injury to the skin depends on temperature, duration of exposure, and tissue hypoxia.

    i. Recommended treatment for frostbite consists of slow thawing.

    j. Leprosy is an infection of the peripheral nervous system.

    k. The mode of transmission of Hansen's disease is ingestion.

    l. Treatment of Hansen's disease is short term.

    m. Severe acne can lead to scarring.

    n. Retinoic acid (Accutane) has few serious side effects.

    o. Ingrown toenails can have serious consequences for the diabetic client.

    p. The treatment for nail hypertrophy is uncomplicated.

CRITICAL THINKING EXERCISES

Case Study: Pressure Ulcer

L. B. is a 35-year-old man who has been a paraplegic for the past 10 years since he sustained gunshot wounds to the lumbar spine. He is admitted to the nursing unit for treatment of two ischial ulcers in preparation for surgical closure of the wounds with myocutaneous flaps. On admission, the nurse notes that he is in a poorly maintained wheelchair and is wearing very tight jeans (which she presumed was restricting circulation to the lower extremities and buttocks). He is also obese, weighing 220 pounds at a height of 5 feet 6 inches. His general health has been good, but he does smoke 1-1/2 packs of cigarettes per day. The ulcers are 6 cm wide on both ischia and covered with a yellow-brown eschar.

Address the following questions:

1. The physician orders wet-to-dry dressing to both ulcers every 4 hours. He also orders Travase (sutilains) ointment bid. Discuss the purpose of the dressings and the ointment, and develop a plan of care of L. B. for the dressing changes. Consider the times of dressing changes, the position in which L. B. will need to be placed for the dressings to dry, and the risk of immobility for L. B.

2. Some of the nurses on the unit have been wondering if L. B. should be placed on a calorie reduction diet to assist him with weight loss. What needs to be considered in planning L. B.'s diet?

3. Three days later, L. B. is scheduled for surgery to debride the ulcers. A general anesthetic is planned for the surgery. L. B. asks the nurse why he needs a general anesthetic, since he has no feeling in the sites where the operation will be performed. How should the nurse respond?

4. Three days later, the wounds are clean and L. B. is scheduled for closure of the wounds with myocutaneous flaps. Discuss the advantages of this type of operation over a skin graft to close L. B.'s wounds. Consider the amount of tissue absent, the stress that will be placed on the sites, and the required blood supply for healing.

5. L. B. is placed on an air-fluidized bed after surgery. Describe the rational for the use of this type of bed after pressure ulcer repair.

6. What nursing assessments should be routinely performed on the flap and donor sites? Discuss the term *pedicle* and how it applies to L. B.'s surgery.

7. What instructions should L. B. be given about his smoking? Consider the impact on the flaps.

8. L. B. is to be dismissed to home care. What other health care team members should be involved in his discharge plans? Explain your answer.

Case Study: Psoriasis

E. C. is a 22-year-old man admitted to the general medical nursing unit with severe psoriasis. His major complaint is severe pruritus. Physical assessment reveals red and silver plaques on his scalp, limbs, elbows, knees and sacrum. On admission, E. C. states that he "knew it would just be a matter of time" because many members of his family have psoriasis and that he hopes that he will not be as sick as some of his family have been with the disease. E. C. is currently employed with a large business firm in the city and travels 2 or 3 days each week.

Address the following questions:

1. The physician has ordered that E. C. be treated with crude coal tar bid. Develop a plan of care for E. C. regarding the treatment plan. Consider techniques to apply the tar, clothing, timing of treatments, and side effects.

2. E. C. also has a systemic corticosteroid ordered. What is the purpose of this drug, and what side effects should be monitored for?

3. In addition to using medications for pruritus, what nursing interventions might be used to assist in control of itching?

4. Once the flare-up of E. C.'s psoriasis is over, the physician orders him to begin PUVA therapy. Describe the goals and rationale for this treatment.

5. Develop a teaching/learning plan for E. C.'s self-management of psoriasis.

Case Study: Malignant Melanoma

D. N. is a 44-year-old Caucasian woman admitted for wide local excision of a malignant melanoma on her upper thigh. Her past history is negative for serious illness. She was hospitalized for the birth of her three children. She admits to being an "avid sun worshipper" and is noted to have very dark brown skin and some premature aging in the facial skin.

Address the following questions:

1. Considering the possible etiology of melanoma, what effect does the exposure to sunlight have on this form of cancer?

2. During her preoperative instructions, D. N. asks why she is going to have a 4-inch circle of skin and tissue removed to get rid of this "little mole." What information should the nurse consider before responding to her question?

D. N. has a wide excision of the melanoma, and the surgical site is closed with a split-thickness skin graft from the opposite thigh. Following surgery, D. N.'s wound is dressed with a bulky dressing and the donor site is covered with a transparent dressing. When assessing D. N.'s dressings, the nurse notes that the bulky dressing is dry and intact, but the donor site has dark red blood trapped beneath the clear dressing.

3. How should the nurse respond? What is the significance of these findings?

4. The following morning, the clear dressing is removed from the donor site and the physician orders that the area be left "open to air" to dry. What equipment might facilitate this process for D. N.?

5. D. N. reports severe burning pain in the donor site. Is this finding normal or abnormal? Explain your answer.

On D. N.'s third day after surgery, the bulky dressing is removed. The wound appears wet and "soupy" with cloudy fluid oozing from it, and the skin graft is unattached to the wound. The surrounding tissues are red and swollen.

6. What is the likely cause of these features in D. N.'s wound?

7. What changes in the plan of care might the nurse anticipate for D. N.?

8. During the next few days, D. N. appears very depressed and sullen. Finally she asks if there is "any hope for her to live or should she just give up now?" How should the nurse respond?

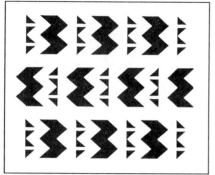

CHAPTER 68

Interventions for Clients with Burns

LEARNING OBJECTIVES

At the end of this chapter, the student will be able to

- Describe the classifications of burn injuries
- Discuss activation of compensatory responses following a burn injury
- Discuss the etiology and incidence of burn injuries
- Discuss emergency care of the client with a burn
- Describe assessment of the burned client
- Describe nursing interventions for the nursing diagnoses of Decreased Cardiac Output, Fluid Volume Deficit, and Altered Tissue Perfusion
- Describe nursing interventions for Ineffective Breathing Pattern and Ineffective Airway Clearance
- Identify nursing interventions for the client in Pain
- Describe nursing interventions for the client with Impaired Skin Integrity
- Discuss nursing interventions when there is High Risk for Infection
- Discuss nursing interventions for Altered Nutrition: Less than Body Requirements
- Discuss nursing interventions for Impaired Physical Mobility
- Identify the nursing interventions directed at Body Image Disturbance following a burn injury
- Discuss planning for the burned client's discharge

PREREQUISITE KNOWLEDGE

Prior to beginning this chapter, the student should review

- The anatomy and physiology of the skin and its appendages
- The principles of fluid and electrolyte balance
- The principles of acid–base balance
- The principles of general nutrition
- The principles of wound healing and wound care
- The principles of infection control
- The principles of intravenous therapy
- Pain management
- Isolation techniques
- The concepts of loss, grief, death, and dying
- The concepts of body image and self-esteem
- Perioperative nursing care
- The procedure for application of topical medications
- The principles of airway management
- The concept of human sexuality

STUDY QUESTIONS

Pathophysiology

1. The *true skin* is the
   a. dermis
   b. epidermis
   c. keratin layer
   d. basement membrane

2. Skin regeneration depends on the
   a. integrity of the peripheral nerves
   b. presence of the basement membrane
   c. ability of the epidermis to form scar tissue
   d. presence of sebaceous and apocrine glands

3. List the major functions of the skin. Use a separate sheet.

4. Which of the following statements is correct about tissue damage due to heat?
   a. Physical response to skin cell destruction varies depending on the cause.
   b. Skin damage is inversely proportional to the degree of heat applied and duration of exposure.
   c. Thin skin requires less heat and less time for damage to occur than does thick skin.
   d. Most burn injuries of significant size cause cell damage to an even depth through the skin layers.

5. Complete the following chart on the classification of burn injuries by identifying the associated level of cellular injury, appearance, and method of healing. Use a separate sheet.

Classification	Level of Injury	Appearance	Method of Healing
a. first-degree (superficial)			
b. second-degree (superficial partial thickness)			
c. second-degree (deep partial thickness)			
d. third-degree (full thickness)			

6. Eschar is
   a. usually dry and cold to the touch
   b. firm, thick, leathery, and black
   c. viable tissue with an adequate blood supply
   d. elastic, resilient, and flexible to tissue swelling

7. Blood flow to a third-degree burn area
   a. is reduced due to hypovolemic shock
   b. is reduced due to thrombosis of vessels
   c. reestablishes itself after skin grafting
   d. must be reestablished by vein grafts

8. A fourth-degree burn is
   a. extremely painful
   b. an inaccurate term
   c. covered with blisters
   d. burn to muscle and bone

9. List the sources of burn injury.
   a. _____
   b. _____
   c. _____
   d. _____
   e. _____
   f. _____

10. Which of the following thermal sources would produce the most severe burn injury?
    a. boiling milk from a spilled saucepan
    b. boiling coffee just removed from a microwave oven
    c. hot vegetable oil from an overturned frying pan
    d. an overheated glazed casserole dish filled with soup

11. A 35-year-old electrical lineman is brought to the emergency department after coming in contact with a live overhead wire. He has four quarter-sized burns on his left hand. Although his burn wounds are small, he is admitted to the hospital. What is the rationale for his admission?
    a. The skin provides the least resistance to the flow of electricity.
    b. The evident skin injury seldom represents the full extent of damage.
    c. Lethal arc burns may subsequently develop and observation is necessary.
    d. Ventricular fibrillation is a common fatal sequela of an electrical burn.

12. Which of the following four statements is correct about radiation burns?
    a. Damage is caused at the level of the cell cytoplasm and has little permanent effect.
    b. All organs have the same capacity to resist radiation-induced damage at the cellular level.

c. The severity of the burn is determined by the type and duration of radiation exposure.

d. Therapeutic radiation delivery is the most common source and usually causes extensive skin damage.

13. List three ways to prevent burn injury in the home.

a. _____

   _____

   _____

b. _____

   _____

   _____

c. _____

   _____

   _____

14. Describe factors in the elderly that increase their risk of severe burns.

a. _____

   _____

b. _____

   _____

c. _____

   _____

Collaborative Management

Match the following burn injuries (15–18) with their types of emergency care (a–d).

_____ 15. flame burn

_____ 16. chemical burn

_____ 17. electrical burn

_____ 18. radiation burn

a. irrigate with copious amounts of water; do not neutralize

b. decontaminate using special precautions

c. stop, drop, and roll; cool with tepid water

d. remove from power source safely; assess the ABCs (airway, breathing, and circulation)

19. Which of the following statements is correct about burn injuries?

a. Small, superficial burns may require as intensive therapy as larger, deeper burns.

b. Burns due to scalding, flames, and ionizing radiation have similar prognoses and outcomes.

c. Chemical burns require different initial treatment than do electrical or flame burns.

d. A burn injury to the hands or feet is associated with a greater risk of infection than a similar-sized burn elsewhere.

20. Which of the following statements is the rationale for obtaining a complete history of the burn client on admission?

a. The client's memory is clear because he or she is not in severe pain.

b. The client's family needs to be informed of the injury.

c. There are few other interventions necessary at this time.

d. The client is conscious, lucid, and usually able to talk.

21. List the pertinent information that should be included in the history of a burn accident. Use a separate sheet.

22. List the subjective client data relevant to burn injuries. Use a separate sheet.

23. List the psychosocial client data relevant to burn injuries. Use a separate sheet.

24. Explain the rationale for assessing past coping mechanisms used by the client with a burn injury. Use a separate sheet.

25. List the objective client data indicating burn injury to the respiratory tract. Use a separate sheet.

26. Which of the following statements is correct about pulmonary damage following a burn injury?

a. Carbon monoxide poisoning is a rare finding in burn victims.

b. Upper airway burns are most common in burns to the face, neck, and upper chest.

c. Damage to the lower respiratory tract is due to inhaled hot air.

d. Pulmonary parenchymal changes are temporary and resolved when steroids are administered.

27. List the objective client data relevant to the cardiovascular system in a burn injury. Use a separate sheet.

28. Hypovolemic shock occurs in burned clients as a result of

    a. erratic lymphatic drainage

    b. altered osmotic pressure in vessels

    c. albumin trapped in the interstitial spaces

    d. a marked increase in capillary permeability

29. Which of the following statements is correct about the hematological response to burn injury?

    a. The white blood cells are unaltered by burn injury.

    b. Some red blood cells are directly destroyed.

    c. Hematocrit levels fall due to hypovolemic shock.

    d. Thrombi can form due to decreased blood viscosity.

30. List the objective client data relevant to the renal system in a burn injury. Use a separate sheet.

31. Which of the following is *not* a cause of renal damage after burn injury?

    a. hemoglobin molecules

    b. myoglobin molecules

    c. hyperkalemia

    d. hypovolemia

32. Hyperkalemia is a common finding after burn injury. What is the cause of this imbalance?

    a. disruption in the sodium-potassium pump

    b. dilutional changes with hemoconcentration

    c. direct cellular release of potassium

    d. all of the above

33. List the objective client data relevant to the integumentary system in a burn injury.

    a. _____

    _____

    b. _____

    _____

    c. _____

    _____

34. A client has a 40% third-degree burn on the entire surface of the upper arms. Which of the following assessments should the nurse report?

    a black nonelastic eschar

    b. diminished or absent pulses

    c. swelling of the fingers

    d. absence of pain in burned tissue

35. List the objective client data relevant to the gastrointestinal system in a burn injury.

    a. _____

    b. _____

    c. _____

    d. _____

    e. _____

    f. _____

36. Which of the following gastrointestinal alternations are *not* typically seen after a burn injury?

    a. paralytic ileus

    b. peptic ulcers

    c. bowel obstruction

    d. Curling's ulcer

37. List the objective client data relevant to the neuroendocrine system in a burn injury.

    a. _____

    b. _____

    c. _____

    d. _____

    e. _____

    f. _____

38. Which of the following interventions would support the metabolic demand in a burned client?

    a. keeping the client's room cool

    b. keeping the wounds covered

    c. limiting protein consumption

    d. limiting fluid consumption

39. In response to a burn injury, the immune system is

    a. altered by toxins produced by the burned cells

    b. taxed by the pathogens present on the skin surface

    c. assisted by the impermeable barrier of the eschar

    d. responsible for the rapid rejection of homografts

40. List the objective client data relevant to the musculoskeletal system in a burn injury.

    a. _____

    _____

    _____

    b. _____

    _____

    _____

41. The following laboratory reports are taken by the nurse for a new client with a 20% total body surface area (TBSA) burn injury: hemoglobin = 15.5 g/100 mL; hematocrit = 52%; serum potassium = 4.6 mEq/L; serum glucose = 134 mg/100 mL. Which of the following actions is best for the nurse to take?

    a. Post the reports on the client's chart.

    b. Monitor the next series of data for comparison.

    c. Call the client's physician immediately with the reports.

    d. Have the laboratory redrawn and retest the specimens.

42. What is the purpose of using a fluid resuscitation formula for the initial management of burns?

    _____

    _____

43. a. Using Parkland's (Baxter's) formula, calculate the fluids needed for the first 24 hours after injury for a 70-kg man with a 50% TBSA burn. The time now is 11 a.m. and he sustained his burn injury at 9 a.m.

    _____

    _____

    _____

    b. How much fluid would be given in the first 8 hours? In the next 16 hours? When does the first 8-hour period end?

    _____

    _____

    _____

44. Identify the organs that are especially sensitive to inadequate tissue perfusion and whose parameters of function are monitored closely after a burn injury.

    a. _____

    b. _____

    c. _____

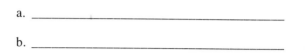

45. Compare and contrast the data that would indicate a client had received (1) adequate fluid resuscitation, (2) inadequate fluids, and (3) over-administration of fluids. Consider vital signs, urinary output, laboratory findings, and lung sounds. Submit the completed exercise to the clinical instructor on a separate sheet.

46. Maintenance of urinary output following burn injury is managed by

    a. administering a loop (high-ceiling) diuretic such as furosemide (Lasix)

    b. decreasing the amount and rate of administering fluids

    c. increasing the amount and rate of administering fluids

    d. administering the osmotic diuretic mannitol (Osmitrol)

47. An escharotomy is a procedure involving

    a. removing eschar to improve circulation

    b. incising eschar to release constriction

    c. fenestrating eschar to permit serous drainage

    d. draining eschar to decrease hydrostatic pressure

48. Airway maintenance for the client with a burn injury and respiratory involvement includes

    a. monitoring for signs and symptoms of upper airway edema during fluid resuscitation

    b. inserting a naso- or oropharyngeal airway if the airway is completely obstructed

    c. securing loose dressings for burns on the thorax with a rib binder instead of tape

    d. weighing the client three times a week to monitor for patterns of fluid overload

49. An elderly client has a 32% TBSA second-degree burn injury on his right anterior thorax and abdomen, right thigh, and lower leg. It has been 4 days since he was burned, and he is now scheduled to begin hydrotherapy followed by the application of occlusive dressings. The first therapy session is scheduled in 45 minutes. The client has order for both meperidine hydrochloride (Demerol), 25–50 mg IV every 3–4 hours prn, and oxycodone hydrochloride (Roxicodone) 5 mg PO every 4–6 hours prn. It has been 4 hours since he last received medication for pain. Which of the following interventions should the nurse implement?

    a. meperidine because the client still has severe pain from the burn injury

    b. meperidine because the oral medication will take longer than 45 minutes to be effecctive

    c. oxycodone because the client should be weaned off the stronger opioid medication

    d. oxycodone because the hydrotherapy and dressing changes are not especially painful procedures

50. Define the term *débridement* and give examples of this procedure as it is used in burn care management.

    _____

    _____

    _____

    _____

Match the following types of biological dressings (51–53) with their descriptions (a–c).

_____ 51. autograft

_____ 52. heterograft

_____ 53. homograft

    a. skin from a species other than human

    b. skin from another human, usually a cadaver

    c. skin from one's own body

54. What type of wound is created in the typical donor site?

    a. first-degree

    b. deep partial thickness

    c. superficial partial thickness

    d. full thickness, deep dermal

55. Drug therapy to reduce the risk of wound infection in the burn client includes

    a. tetanus toxoid given IM prophylactically once early in the hospitalization

    b. silver nitrate solution covered by dry dressings applied every 4 hours

    c. mafenide acetate (Sulfamylon) on partial thickness injuries every 4 hours

    d. silver sulfadiazine (Silvadene) on full thickness injuries every 4 hours

56. A 40-year-old woman is admitted with second-degree burns of the legs that occurred 24 hours ago. The nurse notes that on the previous shift, bowel sounds were hypoactive and the abdominal girth was 54 cm. The client reports mild abdominal pain. Bowel sounds are now absent, and abdominal girth is 55 cm. Which of the following actions is best for the nurse to take?

    a. Insert a nasogastric tube and begin immediate saline lavage.

    b. Give an ordered H_2 antagonist immediately to reduce gastric acid secretions.

    c. Notify the physician of the change and plan on inserting a nasogastric tube.

    d. Continue to assess the client's condition and report the findings in 4 hours if there is no change.

57. Physical mobility in the burn client is best maintained by

    a. assisting the client with passive ROM exercises twice per day

    b. positioning joints with minimal flexion and support

    c. ambulating the client when IV therapy is completed

    d. having the client wear elasticized garments during waking hours

58. Which of the following interventions best promotes a positive body image in a burn client?

    a. The dietitian selects the client's daily menus.

    b. The client's spouse plays cards with the client.

    c. The client's physician discusses future scar revision.

    d. The nurse applies the pressure garment upon discharge.

59. Identify the types of problems burn clients have during the recovery period following discharge from the hospital.

   a. _____

   _____

   b. _____

   _____

   c. _____

   _____

60. A client with which of the following burns would *not* require transfer to a burn center?

   a. a 10% TBSA burn of the face and hands

   b. a 40% TBSA burn in an elderly client

   c. a 10% TBSA third-degree burn

   d. a 12% TBSA burn in a diabetic client

61. A 70-year-old man sustains a 60% burn injury when his house burns. He also suffers inhalation burn injury. His wife is killed in the accident. How many factors are present that decrease the prognosis for his recovery?

   a. two

   b. four

   c. six

   d. eight

62. Identify the factors in question 61 that affect the client's recovery.

   a. _____

   b. _____

   c. _____

   d. _____

   _____

CRITICAL THINKING EXERCISES

Case Study: Acute Burn

K. L. is a 35-year-old electrician who was severely burned when he came in contact with "live" power lines. He fell 20 feet from the power line pole to the ground and sustained a fracture of the pelvis and left femur. He was in asystole when the paramedics arrived on the scene, although CPR had been initiated by his co-workers. On arrival to the hospital, he was in normal sinus rhythm with frequent PVCs and was comatose. He sustained evident second- and third-degree burns to his right hand and arm and left foot. The burns are over 18% of his body surface area.

Address the following questions:

1. Discuss the events that lead to K. L.'s asystole.

2. Considering electrical burn injury, why are K. L.'s visible burns like "the tip of the iceberg"?

3. In addition to the fall from the power line, what may have happened to K. L. during the contact with the power line that led to bone fracture?

K. L. is admitted to intensive care. His fluid orders are for lactated Ringer's solution at 200 mL per hours. K. L.'s weight is estimated at 72 kg.

4. Use Baxter's formula of weight (in kg) × 4 mL × percentage of burn area to calculate K. L.'s fluid needs for the first 24 hours. Is the order for fluids correct? If not, what should the nurse do?

5. Urine output was 15 mL for the past hour. Should K. L. be given more fluids or a diuretic (e.g., furosemide)?

K. L.'s laboratory values are RBCs 5.0, WBCs 6.1, Hgb 20.4, Hct 60.6, K+ 4.8, Na+ 138. Urine concentrated with specific gravity of 1.032, but otherwise normal. Chest x-ray normal with ET tube in place. ABGs on mechanical ventilation are PaO_2 121, $PaCO_2$ 45, bicarbonate 32, pH 7.35. A thallium scan reveals massive muscle injury in the arm and leg.

6. Which of these values are normal and which are expected results of a burn injury?

7. K. L. requires wound care, and because he is in critical condition, his wounds are cleaned and redressed in the room. The nurse uses sterile saline to remove old silver sulfadiazine. What assessments of the wound should be made before reapplying the ointment and dressings?

8. The nurse has been monitoring K. L.'s pedal pulses and leg circumference. Over the past hour, the pulses have diminished and the diameter of the leg has increased by 3.5 cm. The nurse notifies the physician. What procedure should the nurse expect to be required to restore normal circulation to the leg?

9. Mrs. L. visits her husband and asks the nurse how serious his injuries really are. How should the nurse respond? Even after explanations, Mrs. L. does not seem to realize the seriousness of her husband's burns. What type of assistance may she need?

10. K. L.'s urine is noted to be dark brown. What is the probable cause of this change and what should the nurse do? What should the nurse expect to be ordered to resolve this problem?

11. K. L.'s potassium soars to 7.5 mEq/L. What is the probable etiology of the hyperkalemia? What emergency treatments are required? What ECG changes might be noted during the hyperkalemia?

Three days after the burn, K. L. is breathing on his own and is extubated. He remains on oxygen by nasal cannula because cardiac studies show that he sustained heart damage during the injury. He also has open wounds appearing on his entire body.

12. What is the cause of these new wounds?

13. He is very confused and has no recall of what happened to him. He remains agitated, fearful, and in pain. He has orders for morphine IV for pain and Valium (diazepam) IV for severe agitation. He has had neither drug for some time; which agent would be preferable for him now?

14. On the fourth day after the injury, K. L. becomes less responsive. His respiratory rate rises to 28–32 breaths per minutes with marked dyspnea. He also has a sustained tachycardia of 120–130 beats per minute. His blood gases on 4 L of O_2 are PaO_2 65, PCO_2 50, pH 7.34, HCO_3 32. He is diagnosed with pulmonary embolism. K. L. has a cardiac arrest and is not able to be resuscitated. List at least two etiologies of pulmonary emboli in K. L.

15. What type of grief response might be expected from Mrs. L. when she is told that K. L. has died?

Case Study: Burn Rehabilitation

C. P. is a 76-year-old widow who was burned 3 days ago in a kitchen fire. She was using an electric frying pan, and when she turned her back, the corner of her apron caught on the pan. She sustained a second-degree burn on her back, side of her left chest, left axilla, and left upper arm. The burn equaled 24% of her body surface area. She has a past history of type II diabetes and hypertension. She controls her diabetes with diet and an oral hypoglycemic; her hypertension is controlled with hydrochlorothiazide and triamterene (Dyazide). Since she has recovered from the emergent phase of the burn, she is ready for aggressive wound care. The physician has prescribed hydrotherapy and silver sulfadiazine (Silvadene) dressing changes bid.

Address the following questions:

1. C. P. is scheduled for hydrotherapy in 30 minutes. She has requested "something for the pain" in anticipation of the treatment. Yesterday when she went for hydrotherapy, the nurse gave her 25 mg of meperidine hydrochloride (Demerol) intravenously. She appeared to have no side effects from the agent. She also has an order for oral oxycodone hydrochloride (Roxicodone). Which agent should be given to C. P. and why?

2. The nurse follows C. P. to hydrotherapy to inspect the wound. What signs of infection should be specifically assessed for?

3. The nurse prepares C. P.'s dressings while the client is in hydrotherapy. List at least three rationales for preparing the dressings in advance.

4. One of the potential risks of burns to the axilla is contracture. What nursing interventions are used to reduce this risk? What surgical intervention is required if contracture occurs?

C. P. has been noted not to have eaten much of the food on her trays. Yesterday's caloric intake was 850 calories. Her admission weight was 124 pounds, while her current weight is 117 pounds. She is 5 feet 5 inches tall.

5. Was her admission weight within normal limits for her height? What about her present weight?

6. In addition to not eating, what are some other possible causes of her weight loss?

7. What is her daily caloric need? What is her caloric need since she has been burned?

8. List nursing interventions that may improve C. P.'s intake. What methods may need to be used if oral intake is not adequate?

9. What is likely to happen to C. P.'s diabetes with her change in food intake? What is likely to happen to her wound healing? Her risk of infection?

C. P. spikes a fever to 101.6°F on the sixth day after her burn. The nurse inspects her wound and notices that its edges have changed from a flesh color, 2 days ago, to a bright red color.

10. Do these data mean that C. P.'s fever is from an infected wound?

11. How might the nurse assess for data that would rule out fever from other sources, such as the lungs and urinary tract?

C. P. is ready for skin grafting. She is scheduled to follow all the other cases for the day (some operating rooms call these cases "contaminated").

12. What is the rationale for scheduling her at that time?

13. C. P. will be NPO after midnight. Will she require some type of insulin on the morning of surgery? What routes might be used to give it?

She undergoes debridement of the axillary wound and has split-thickness skin grafting to the other burned areas. The physician orders C. P. on complete bed rest, with the head of the bed and arm elevated.

14. What is the rationale for the bed rest and elevation?

15. The donor sites are on the thigh. What assessments should the nurse make of the donor sites while they are dressed following surgery? After the dressings are removed? Explain why the donor sites temporarily increase the body surface area of the burn.

16. While C. P. was in surgery, the surgeon removed enough skin to graft her axilla once it was ready. The extra skin was wrapped around wet sterile gauze and placed in the refrigerator where it can remain for up to 21 days. Explain how the skin can survive in that environment.

17. What are some advantages to harvesting skin grafts in the above manner?

18. Three days following surgery, the dressings are removed from C. P.'s grafts. The surgeon records that the grafts have "taken." What do the skin grafts look like when they have taken versus not taken?

C. P. has the remaining skin grafts placed on the axilla in her room. The procedure is not painful. She has the arm immobilized for 72 hours, and these grafts "take" as well. It is time for discharge.

19. Her surgeon plans to send her home in a Jobst garment. Explain the purpose of this garment.

20. Develop discharge teaching plans for C. P. on graft and donor site care, nutritional needs, activities to prevent contractures, and care of the Jobst garment.

Case Study: The Man Who Wanted To Die

J. G. is a 76-year-old man who is badly injured when a leaking propane gas line explodes. His son is killed in the accident. J. G. has second- and third-degree burns over 68% of his body; his eyes, ears, and most of his face are burned away. His hands required amputation due to the injury. After many months of skin grafts, he is still susceptible to infections and has to be bathed daily in a Hubbard tank. Although J. G. accepts treatment, he says he wants to die. Eventually, J. G. refuses treatment and insists on going home. His wife opposes his decision, and a psychiatrist agrees to see J. G. after getting the impression that he is irrational and depressed. J. G.'s competency is uncertain and there is discussion of appointing a legal guardian who can authorize treatment. The psychiatrist finds J. G. to be bright, coherent, logical, and articulate. J. G. tells the psychiatrist, "I do not want to go on as a blind, crippled person." He wants his attorney to have him released from the hospital, by court order if necessary.

Address the following questions:

1. Are there circumstance in which a person has the right to refuse treatment?

2. Does J. G. have any responsibilities to others that should affect his decision? What are the responsibilities of the health care team to J. G.? Of his wife? Of his lawyer?

3. Are the rights of dying people different from those of the living? Is one of these rights the choice of whether to hasten the end of life?

4. Is there any justification for concealing medical facts from someone who is dying, especially the fact that death is imminent?

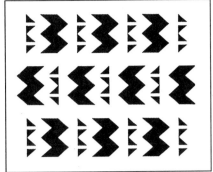

C H A P T E R 6 9

Assessment of the Renal/Urinary System

LEARNING OBJECTIVES

At the end of this chapter, the student will be able to

- Describe the location, structure, and function of the kidneys
- Describe the location, structure, and function of the ureters
- Describe the location, structure, and function of the urinary bladder
- Describe the location, structure, and function of the urethra
- Identify renal/urinary system changes that are associated with aging
- Identify history-taking and physical assessment data related to renal/urinary problems
- Describe diagnostic tools used to detect renal and urological disorders

PREREQUISITE KNOWLEDGE

Prior to beginning this chapter, the student should review

- The anatomy and physiology of the urinary system
- The anatomy and physiology of the nephron

- The principles of osmosis and diffusion
- Collection of laboratory specimens for urinalysis (UA), urine culture, and sensitivity
- The characteristics of normal urine and serum urine values of electrolytes
- The principles of acid–base balance
- The principles of fluid and electrolyte balance
- Normal growth and development

STUDY QUESTIONS

Anatomy and Physiology Review

1. List the structures that constitute the renal/urinary system.

   a. _____

   b. _____

   c. _____

   d. _____

Match the following terms related to the kidneys (2–25) with their descriptions (a–x).

_____ 2. afferent arteriole

_____ 3. Bowman's capsule

_____ 4. calyx

_____ 5. collecting duct

_____ 6. cortical nephron

_____ 7. distal convoluted tubule

_____ 8. efferent arteriole

_____ 9. glomerulus

_____ 10. hilum

_____ 11. juxtaglomerular apparatus

_____ 12. juxtaglomerular cell

_____ 13. juxtamedullary nephron

_____ 14. loop of Henle

_____ 15. macula densa

_____ 16. nephron

_____ 17. parenchyma

_____ 18. peritubular capillary

_____ 19. proximal convoluted tubule

_____ 20. renal capsule

_____ 21. renal cortex

_____ 22. renal medulla

_____ 23. renal pelvis

_____ 24. renin

_____ 25. ureteropelvic junction

a. functional renal tissue composed of several units

b. several join to form the renal pelvis

c. pyramid-shaped tissue lining inside of cortex

d. loop of Henle extends into renal medulla

e. special cells in afferent and efferent arterioles and distal convoluted tubules

f. outer surface of kidney

g. exist in renal cortex only

h. tunnels urine into ureter

i   carries blood away from glomerulus

j. structure located between Bowman's capsule and loop of Henle

k. where renal pelvis joins the ureter

l. area of kidney directly under the capsule

m. functional unit of kidney

n. supplies arterial blood to glomerulus

o. structure surrounding glomerulus

p. renin-releasing cell

q. carries urine into renal pelvis from nephron

r. channels urine into collecting duct

s. system for blood to leave efferent arteriole

t. series of special capillary loops

u. where renal vessels and ureter exit

v. structure located between proximal and distal convoluted tubule

w. cell in distal convoluted tubule sensitive to volume and pressure changes

x. hormone that helps regulate blood pressure

---

26. Draw and label a nephron unit. Include the tubular and vascular components. Use a separate sheet.

27. List the functions of the kidney essential to homeostasis.

   a. _____

   _____

   b. _____

   _____

   c. _____

   _____

Match the following nephron processes (28–30) with their descriptions (a–c).

_____ 28. glomerular filtration

_____ 29. tubular reabsorption

_____ 30. tubular secretion

a. restoration of plasma concentration and excretion of excess solutes

b. separation of plasma from protein molecules

c. removal of substances from plasma into filtrate

31. Put in correct order the following steps in the process of urine production by tracing the flow of blood and filtrate through the nephron.

_____ a. water reabsorption occurs due to the influence of antidiuretic hormone (ADH)

_____ b. urine enters the collecting ducts

_____ c. reabsorption of water, sodium, and chloride occurs in the proximal convoluted tubules

_____ d. sodium reabsorption occurs due to the influence of aldosterone

_____ e. filtration occurs across the glomerular basement membrane into Bowman's capsule

_____ f. chloride is actively reabsorbed and sodium is passively reabsorbed

32. Which of the following statements is correct about pressure and glomerular filtration.

a. Creation of a net negative pressure is responsible for glomerular filtration.

b. Plasma oncotic pressure is the primary force promoting ultrafiltration of the blood.

c. Filtration occurs when the hydrostatic pressure exceeds the sum of the plasma oncotic pressure and tubular filtrate pressure.

d. Blood pressure (hydrostatic pressure) is the force that opposes glomerular filtration.

33. Which of the following statements is correct about tubular reabsorption?

a. About 50–75% of sodium, chloride, and water reabsorption occurs in the loop of Henle.

b. About 50–70% of potassium is reabsorbed in the distal convoluted tubule.

c. About 50–75% of sodium, chloride, and water reabsorption occurs in the distal convoluted tubule.

d. Calcium reabsorption parallels water reabsorption in the proximal convoluted tubule.

34. Which hormone increases the permeability of the distal convoluted tubule to water?

a. ADH

b. renin

c. aldosterone

d. erythropoietin

35. Identify the functions of the following hormones produced by the kidney. Use a separate sheet.

a. active vitamin D

b. erythropoietin

c. kinins

d. prostaglandins

e. renin

Match the following terms relating to the ureter, bladder, and urethra (36–49) with their descriptions (a–n).

_____ 36. bladder neck

_____ 37. continence

_____ 38. detrusor muscle

_____ 39. external urethral sphincter

_____ 40. fundus

_____ 41. internal urethral sphincter

_____ 42. micturition

_____ 43. trigone

_____ 44. ureter

_____ 45. ureterovesical junction

_____ 46. urethra

_____ 47. urethral meatus

_____ 48. urinary bladder

_____ 49. urothelium

a. triangular area formed on posterior bladder wall by ureters and urethra

b. reservoir for urine

c. rounded sac portion of bladder

d. middle muscle layer of bladder

e. external opening of urethra

f. distal portion of ureter

g. propels urine from renal pelvis to urinary bladder

h. conveys urine from bladder to outside of body

i. ability to hold urine in bladder voluntarily

j. portion of posterior urethra

k. inner lining of ureter and bladder

l. smooth muscle of bladder neck encircling urethra

m. skeletal muscle surrounding urethra

n. voiding or emptying the bladder

50. Identify the changes that occur in the following urinary system structures and functions that are associated with aging and their possible causes. Use a separate sheet.

a. kidney size

b. glomerular and tubular basement membrane

c. glomerular quantity and surface area

d. length of tubules

e. glomerular filtration rate

f. ability to dilute and concentrate urine

g. renin production

h. vitamin D activation

i. urinary sphincter tone

j. bladder capacity

Subjective Assessment

51. List the subjective client data relevant to the renal/urinary system. Use a separate sheet.

52. List the psychosocial client data relevant to the renal/urinary system. Use a separate sheet.

Match the following terms on renal/urinary assessment (53–62) with their definitions (a–j).

_____ 53. anuria

_____ 54. dysuria

_____ 55. hematuria

_____ 56. hesitancy

_____ 57. oliguria

_____ 58. polyuria

_____ 59. renal colic

_____ 60. retention

_____ 61. uremia

_____ 62. urgency

a. urinary output of 100–400 mL per 24 hours

b. inability to void

c. urinary output more than 1500 mL per 24 hours

d. sudden need to void

e. blood in urine

f. urinary output less than 100 mL per 24 hours

g. accumulation of nitrogenous wastes in blood

h. painful urination

i. difficulty initiating urine stream

j. severe, spasmodic flank pain radiating into perineal area, groin, or genitals

63. The following is a partial client history. Discuss the significance these data have for an assessment of the renal/urinary system. Submit the completed exercise to the clinical instructor.

> *African-American female, 48 years old. Lives with husband, two children, and mother. Reports having problems with recurrent urinary tract infections "ever since I've had relations with my husband." Has burning and pain with urination, urine smells "strong and bad." "It's cloudy, too." Denies anorexia, weight change, or diarrhea. States that father is deceased; he had problems with "bloating and sugar" and had to take medicine for these problems. Currently has right flank pain described as a dull, continuous ache. Has taken aspirin (two tablets) every 4–6 hours for the past 2 days with some relief, but pain recurs and "never goes away for long." Difficulty sleeping at night, waking several times because of the pain and "in a cold sweat."*

Objective Assessment

64. List the objective client data relevant to the renal/urinary system. Use a separate sheet.

65. Using the data in question 63, construct a physical assessment recording for the renal/urinary system. Submit the completed exercise to the clinical instructor.

66. An elevation of the blood urea nitrogen (BUN) level definitively indicates that

    a. renal disease is present

    b. liver disease is present

    c. overhydration exists

    d. protein intake is high

67. An elevation of serum creatine level definitively indicates that

    a. muscle wasting is occurring

    b. dehydration is present

    c. renal disease is present

    d. liver disease is present

68. The BUN to serum creatinine ratio

    a. is used to determine the cause of acid–base imbalance

    b. increases with dehydration or kidney hypoperfusion

    c. decreases with dehydration or kidney hypoperfusion

    d. increases with liver disease or overhydration

69. Which of the following urinalysis results is abnormal?

    a. protein = 5 mg/100 mL, pH = 5.4, few casts

    b. clear, pale yellow, specific gravity = 1.015

    c. glucose = 10 mg/100 mL, pH = 5.7, ketones negative

    d. osmolality = 1080 mOsm/L, specific gravity = 1.028

70. What is the probable creatine clearance rate in an adult female client whose serum creatine level is elevated?

    a. 50 mL/minute

    b. 85 mL/minute

    c. 100 mL/minute

    d. 135 mL/minute

71. List classes of drugs that may decrease the creatinine clearance rate related to nephrotoxicity in the elderly.

    a. _____

    _____

    b. _____

    _____

    c. _____

    _____

72. Which of the following complications is most likely to result from taking a loop diuretic?

    a. hyperchloremia

    b. hypercalcemia

    c. hypoglycemia

    d. hypokalemia

73. The radiographic procedure most likely to result in a hypersensitivity reaction is a

    a. renogram

    b. intravenous pyelogram

    c. flat plate of the abdomen

    d. voiding cystourethrogram

74. List the radiographic procedures that are likely to cause acute renal failure in dehydrated clients.

    a. _____

    _____

    b. _____

    _____

    c. _____

    _____

    d. _____

    _____

CRITICAL THINKING EXERCISES

Case Study: Urinary Assessment

G. W. is a 74-year-old client who is scheduled to have a series of urological studies for diagnostic purposes. The physician orders the following: urinalysis, urine for culture and sensitivity, BUN serum creatine, and 24-hour urine for creatinine clearance. The tests will be conducted on an outpatient basis.

Address the following questions:

1. Describe what the nurse should do to instruct G. W. in the collection of these laboratory specimens.

2. Which specimens should be collected first?

3. G. W. returns the collection container with a 24-hour urine specimen to the physician's office. As he gives it to the nurse, he comments, "I had a hard time remembering to save it all. Actually, I think I missed some when I forgot and used a bathroom at the shopping mall yesterday." What should the nurse do?

4. Further tests are ordered for G. W., including a renal ultrasound and intravenous pyelography (IVP). These are scheduled at an outpatient radiology clinic. Design a teaching/learning plan for G. W. to prepare him for these studies.

5. Following the ultrasound and IVP, what assessments should be made for G. W.?

6. Explain what information the nurse should discuss with G. W. prior to his discharge from the radiology clinic.

C H A P T E R   7 0

Interventions for Clients with Urinary Problems

LEARNING OBJECTIVES

At the end of this chapter, the student will be able to

- Discuss infectious disorders of the lower urinary tract and corresponding treatment
- Identify the types of urinary incontinence and possible interventions
- Identify causes of and treatment for urinary tract obstruction

PREREQUISITE KNOWLEDGE

Prior to beginning this chapter, the student should review

- The anatomy and physiology of the kidneys and urinary system
- Normal growth and development
- Normal laboratory values for urinalysis, urine culture, and serum and urine electrolytes
- The principles of acid–base balance
- The principles of fluid and electrolyte balance
- The principles of skin care
- The concepts of body image and self-esteem
- The concepts of grief, loss, death, and dying
- Low-protein and low-calcium diets
- Catheter care and catheter insertion
- The principles of perioperative nursing management

STUDY QUESTIONS

Infectious Disorders

1. Which of the following statements is correct about urinary tract infections (UTI)?

   a. UTI primarily refers to infection of the ureter, bladders, and urethra.

   b. Accurate diagnosis of UTI requires a random voided urine specimen.

   c. A UTI is present when more than 100,000 organisms/mL are present.

   d. Bacteriuria always results in symptoms of fever, dysuria, and cloudy urine.

Match the following terms (2–4) with their correct definitions (a–c).

_____	2. cystitis	a. inflammation of urethra
_____	3. pyelonephritis	b. inflammation of urinary bladder
_____	4. urethritis	c. bacterial infection of kidney and its pelvis

5. List anatomical and physiological factors that contribute to the maintenance of urinary bladder sterility. Use a separate sheet.

6. List anatomical and physiological factors that contribute to cystitis development. Use a separate sheet.

7. Preventive measures for cystitis include

    a. routine mass screening of large groups of the population for detection of infections

    b. using povidone-iodine ointment at the urethral meatus for clients with in-dwelling catheters

    c. wearing cotton instead of nylon undergarments to reduce irritation of skin surfaces

    d. restricting fluids in clients with reduced mobility to prevent incontinent episodes

8. List the subjective client data relevant to cystitis. Use a separate sheet.

9. List the objective client data relevant to cystitis. Use a separate sheet.

10. Which of the following statements is correct about drug agents used to treat cystitis?

    a. Propantheline bromide (Pro-Banthine) can be safely given to clients with bladder neck obstruction.

    b. Nitrofurantoin (Macrodantin) should be administered on an empty stomach to promote absorption.

    c. Sulfisoxazole (Gantrisin) should be administered with food or milk to decrease gastrointestinal (GI) upset.

    d. Nalidixic acid (NegGram) is contraindicated for clients with low creatinine clearance.

11. List the self-care measures for the client with cystitis. Use a separate sheet.

12. The most common cause of urethritis in men is

    a. *Chalamydia*

    b. *Neisseria gonorrhoeae*

    c. *Trichomonas vaginalis*

    d. *Ureaplasma urealyticum*

Urinary Incontinence

Match the following types of urinary incontinence (13–17) with their causes (a–e).

_____ 13. stress

_____ 14. urge

_____ 15. over-flow

_____ 16. func-tional

_____ 17. total

a. physical, environmental, or psychological cause

b. when bladder pressure exceeds urethral resistance due to overfilling with urine

c. result of neurological disease and bladder nerve dysfunction

d. resistance of the urethra is overcome by pressure in the bladder

e. inability to suppress the signal to urinate resulting in a sudden contraction of the detrusor

18. Which of the following statements is correct about urinary incontinence?

    a. A reversible cause of urinary incontinence is injury to the spinal cord.

    b. An irreversible cause of urinary incontinence is prostate enlargement.

    c. Restricting caffeine and alcohol consumption may help prevent incontinence.

    d. The incidence of urinary incontinence is about equal in men and women.

19. List the subjective client data relevant to urinary incontinence. Use a separate sheet.

20. List the objective client data relevant to urinary incontinence. Use a separate sheet.

21. In addition to the nursing diagnoses specific to the type of incontinence, list additional diagnoses that may be present in the client with urinary incontinence.

    a. _____

    _____

    b. _____

    _____

    c. _____

    _____

Match the following medications (22–27) with the types of urinary incontinence for which they are commonly used (a–c). Answers may be used more than once.

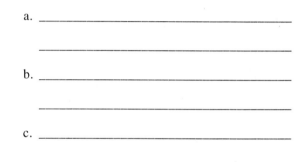

_____ 22. bethanechol chloride (Urecholine)

_____ 23. ephedrine sulfate (Efedron)

_____ 24. amitriptyline hydro-chloride (Elavil)

_____ 25. oxybutynin chloride (Ditropan)

_____ 26. dicyclomine hydro-chloride (Bentyl)

_____ 27. propantheline bromide (Pro-Banthine)

a. stress

b. urge

c. overflow

Match the following interventions for incontinence management (28-32) with the types of urinary incontinence for which they are prescribed. Answers may be used more than once.

____	28. bladder capacity training	a. stress
____	29. Credé's method	b. urge
____	30. double voiding	c. overflow
____	31. Kegel exercises	
____	32. Valsalva's maneuver	
____	33. habit training	
____	34. intermittent catheterization	

35. Briefly discuss why intermittent self-catheterization of the bladder is preferred to in-dwelling urinary catheters. Use a separate sheet.

Urolithiasis

Match the following terms (36–38) with their definitions (a–c).

____	36. nephrolithiasis	a. stones in the ureter
____	37. ureterolithiasis	b. stones in the urinary tract
____	38. urolithiasis	c. stones in the renal parenchyma

39. List the factors that contribute to urinary tract calculi formation. Use a separate sheet.

40. Define *hydroureter* and *hydronephrosis.*

hydroureter: _____

_____

_____

hydronephrosis: _____

_____

_____

41. List the subjective client data relevant to urologic calculi. Use a separate sheet.

42. List the objective client data relevant to urologic calculi. Use a separate sheet.

43. Identify the significant laboratory data for the client with urologic calculi. Use a separate sheet.

44. Which of the following four radiographic tests is preferable for clients at high risk for acute renal failure who have urinary tract stones?

a. intravenous pyelography

b. renal tomography

c. computed tomography with contrast

d. renal ultrasonography

45. Identify the common nursing diagnoses for the client with urinary tract stones.

a. _____

b. _____

_____

c. _____

_____

46. Nonsurgical management of the client with urinary tract stones includes

a. restricted activity such as bed rest

b. fluid restriction of 1000–1500 mL/day

c. oral opioid analgesics such as codeine

d. antispasmodics such as oxybutynin chloride (Ditropan)

47. Which of the following surgical procedures for urologic calculi removal results in a large flank incision?

a. cystoscopy

b. pyelolithotomy

c. percutaneous ultrasonic lithotripsy

d. extracorporeal shock wave lithotripsy

48. Discuss the rationale for changing dressings frequently following nephrolithotomy, pyelolithotomy, and ureterolithotomy. Use a separate sheet.

49. Identify the diet changes and pharmacological treatments of the following urologic calculi. Use a separate sheet.

a. calcium phosphate

b. calcium oxalate

c. uric acid

d. struvite

Urothelial Cancer

50. List the etiological agents associated with the development of bladder cancer. Use a separate sheet.

51. List the subjective client data relevant to bladder cancer. Use a separate sheet.

52. List the objective client data relevant to bladder cancer. Use a separate sheet.

Match the following types of urinary diversion surgery (53–58) with their descriptions (a–f).

_____ 53. cutaneous ureterostomy

_____ 54. ileal conduit

_____ 55. internal ileal reservoir

_____ 56. partial cystectomy

_____ 57. radical cystectomy

_____ 58. uretero-ureterostomy

a. complete removal of urinary bladder

b. continent pouch constructed for storing urine

c. both ureters anastomosed together but have only one external stoma

d. portion of ileum used to divert urine from ureters to an abdominal stoma

e. ureter drains to abdominal surface via a stoma

f. removal of a portion of the urinary bladder

59. Which of the following is a potential complication for the client who has a urinary diversion with an abdominal stoma?

a. alkalemia

b. hyponatremia

c. hyperkalemia

d. urinary calculi

CRITICAL THINKING EXERCISES

Case Study: Urinary Tract Infection

J. H. is a 21-year-old client who comes to the Urology Clinic with complaints of urinary frequency and dysuria. Her urine is cloudy, contains WBCs 1,000,000 bacteria/mL, and a trace of protein. A diagnosis of cystitis is confirmed. The physician orders co-trimoxazole (Bactrim), one tablet every 12 hours for 10 days. J. H. is also given a prescription for phenazopyridine hydrochloride (Pyridium) if it is needed.

Address the following questions:

1. Identify the relevant nursing diagnoses for J. H. based on the above data and discuss the related nursing interventions.

2. What instructions should be given to J. H. related to the co-trimoxazole (Bactrim)?

3. What would the indications be for J. H. to have the prescription for phenazopyridine hydrochloride (Pyridium) filled and to begin taking this medication? What instructions should the nurse discuss with J. H. about this medication?

4. What additional instruction is necessary for J. H. to manage her self-care?

J. H. returns to the clinic in 1 week with a temperature of 103°F, chills, left flank pain, and hematuria. She states that after 2 days of taking the Bactrim and Pyridium, she felt fine and stopped taking the medications. J. H. is now diagnosed with acute pyelonephritis. A clean catch urine specimen is obtained for culture and sensitivity. J. H. is begun on cefaclor (Ceclor), 500 mg, PO, every 8 hours. She is also scheduled for an IVP in 2 days.

5. Develop a teaching/learning plan for J. H. to prepare her for the IVP. Why is this procedure being scheduled? What assessments should the nurse make for J. H. prior to implementing this plan?

6. What additions to the original teaching/learning plan should the nurse make? Consider the new drug order and J. H.'s new symptoms.

7. J. H. asks if she can return to work tomorrow. What should the nurse tell her?

8. What follow-up measures are indicated for J.H.?

Case Study: Urinary Obstruction

T. R. is a 56-year-old widow admitted for severe pain the right flank and pelvic areas. She is nauseated and has been vomiting. A kidney stone is suspected. Admission vital signs are temperature = 103°F, pulse = 126, regular, respirations = 20.

Address the following questions:

1. Discuss what additional data the nurse should collect.

2. T. R. requests assistance to go to the bathroom to void. What should the nurse do with this and any other urine specimens produced by T. R.?

3. Identify the relevant nursing diagnoses for T. R. based on the known data and develop a care plan for her.

4. What medications should the nurse be prepared to administer to T. R. for pain management? For infection control? How are these medications best administered?

5. T. R. is unable to pass the stone and is scheduled for extracorporeal shock wave lithotripsy (ESWL). Prepare a perioperative teaching/learning care plan for her.

6. The ESWL is successful and T. R. is scheduled for discharge the next day. Develop a discharge teaching/learning care plan for her.

7. T. R. asks whether she will have to change her diet to remain free of future kidney stones. What should the nurse discuss with T. R.?

Case Study: Bladder Cancer

S. L. is a 58-year-old kindergarten teacher with a history of smoking. She is admitted for a radical cystectomy and ileal conduit procedure. Her husband died a year ago following a myocardial infarction. Her youngest daughter recently enrolled as a freshman at college out of state. Two older children are married and also live out of state.

Address the following questions:

1. Identify relevant nursing diagnoses for S. L. based on the above data.

2. Because of previous abdominal surgery, S. L. is not a candidate for a Kock or Indiana pouch procedure. Develop a perioperative teaching/learning care plan for S. L.

3. Following surgery, what observations should the nurse make about the urinary stoma? What interventions are indicated for skin care? Monitoring of fluid and electrolyte balance?

4. S. L. progresses rapidly postoperatively, but refuses to care for the ileal conduit. She calls it "that disgusting thing." What should the nurse do to assist S. L. in assuming self-care?

5. Discharge is planned. Develop a discharge teaching/learning care plan for S. L. that will allow her to care for the ileoconduit. Consider the probable location of her stoma and her occupation when discussing adaptations.

6. Identify community resources that may be beneficial to S. L. in learning to cope with her ileal conduit.

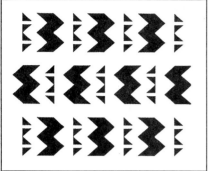

C H A P T E R 7 1

Interventions for Clients with Renal Disorders

LEARNING OBJECTIVES

At the end of this chapter, the student will be able to

- Compare and contrast congenital renal disorders
- Provide care for the client with a congenital renal disorder
- Discuss infectious disorders of the upper urinary tract and corresponding treatment
- Identify disorders associated with obstruction of urine outflow
- Compare and contrast the various immunological renal disorders and their management
- Describe the degenerative renal disorders and related management
- Discuss renal cell carcinoma
- Manage care for the client with renal trauma

PREREQUISITE KNOWLEDGE

Prior to beginning this chapter, the student should review

- The anatomy and physiology of the kidneys and urinary system
- The role of the immune system
- Normal growth and development
- Normal laboratory values for urinalysis, urine culture, and serum and urine electrolytes
- The principles of acid–base balance

- The principles of osmosis and diffusion
- The principles of skin care
- The concepts of body image and self-esteem
- The concepts of grief, loss, death, and dying
- Low-sodium, low-potassium, low-protein, and low-calcium diets
- Catheter care and catheter insertion
- The principles of perioperative nursing management
- The principles of shock management

STUDY QUESTIONS

Congenital Disorders

1. Identify the similarities that all clients with congenital kidney disorders have.

    a. _____

    _____

    b. _____

    _____

    c. _____

    _____

2. What other organs does polycystic kidney disease (PKD) affect?

   a. brain and lung

   b. lung and pancreas

   c. brain and liver

   d. liver and pancreas

3. PKD is genetically transmitted in a pattern that is

   a. autosomal dominant

   b. autosomal recessive

   c. sex-linked dominant

   d. sex-linked recessive

4. Which of the following statements is correct about PKD? This disease

   a. causes end-stage renal disease in 25% of Americans who require chronic dialysis or transplantation

   b. does not demonstrate clinical manifestations until the 20s or 30s

   c. is preventable with advanced techniques of genetic manipulation and transplantation

   d. is the cause of hypertension in over 50% of all clients who are hypertensive

5. List the subjective client data relevant to PKD. Use a separate sheet.

6. List the objective client data relevant to PKD. Use a separate sheet.

7. Laboratory findings for the client with PKD include

   a. hyperkalemia, hypercalcemia, and hyperphosphatemia

   b. hyperkalemia, hypocalcemia, and metabolic alkalosis

   c. proteinuria, hematuria, and increased creatinine clearance

   d. elevated blood urea nitrogen and serum creatinine levels and decreased creatinine clearance

8. List common nursing diagnoses for the client with PKD.

   a. _____

   b. _____

      _____

   c. _____

      _____

   d. _____

      _____

9. Which of the following agents would be used in the management of PKD?

   a. antibiotics such as gentamicin sulfate (Garamycin)

   b. analgesics such as acetylsalicylic acid (Ascriptin)

   c. antihypertensives such as hydralazine (Apresoline)

   d. diuretics such as urea (Ureaphil)

10. Self-care management for the client with PKD includes

    a. weighing one's self on a weekly basis

    b. consuming a diet high in potassium

    c. monitoring blood pressure for hypotension

    d. monitoring temperature for signs of infection

11. Which of the following statements is correct about horseshoe kidney?

    a. It results from fusion of the renal masses' upper poles.

    b. It increases the client's risk for infection and stones.

    c. It often leads to twisting and displacement of the urethra.

    d. It leads to compromised renal function and eventual failure.

Infectious Disorders

Match the following terms (12–14) with their definitions (a–c).

_____ 12. pyelonephritis

_____ 13. renal abscess

_____ 14. renal tuberculosis

a. collection of fluid and cells in or near kidney resulting from inflammatory response to bacteria

b. granulomatous nephritis

c. bacterial infection of kidney and its pelvis

15. Which of the following statements is correct about pyelonephritis?

    a. Postinflammatory scar tissue develops in the renal calyces.

    b. Fibrosis of the renal interstitial tissue impairs glomerular filtration.

    c. Acute pyelonephritis results from urinary reflux or obstruction.

    d. Chronic pyelonephritis results from direct bacterial contamination.

16. List the subjective client data relevant to pyelonephritis. Use a separate sheet.

17. List the objective client data relevant to pyelonephritis. Use a separate sheet.

18. Identify the surgical interventions that may be used to treat pyelonephritis.

a. _____

_____

b. _____

_____

c. _____

_____

d. _____

_____

19. Which of the following statements is correct about renal infections?

a. Symptoms of a renal abscess include dysuria and pus in the urine.

b. The client with renal tuberculosis will always have a positive tine test.

c. A renal abscess may not respond promptly to antibiotic therapy.

d. Treatment of renal tuberculosis includes percutaneous needle aspiration.

20. Define *hydroureter* and *hydronephrosis*. Use a separate sheet.

21. List the causes of hydronephrosis and hydroureter.

a. _____

b. _____

c. _____

d. _____

e. _____

f. _____

Immunologic Disorders

22. Which of the following statements is correct about acute glomerulonephritis (AGN)?

a. It is a sequela of infections of the eyes and ears.

b. It can result from both internal and external antigens.

c. It is preventable with management of existing infections.

d. It results in decreased tubular reabsorption and secretion

23. List the subjective client data relevant to AGN. Use a separate sheet.

24. List the objective client data relevant to AGN. Use a separate sheet.

25. List the abnormal findings on a urinalysis report associated with AGN.

a. _____

b. _____

c. _____

d. _____

e. _____

f. _____

g. _____

26. Clients with AGN who are oliguric are treated with

a. diuretic and antihypertensive medications

b. increased intravenous fluid administration

c. insertion of a permanent shunt for dialysis

d. low-sodium, high-potassium, high-protein diet

27. What is the result of chronic glomerulonephritis (CGN)?

_____

28. List the subjective client data relevant to CGN other than those it has in common with AGN.

a. _____

_____

b. _____

_____

c. _____

_____

29. List the objective client data relevant to CGN other than those it has in common with AGN.

    a. _____

    b. _____

    c. _____

    d. _____

    e. _____

    f. _____

    g. _____

30. In end-stage renal disease (ESRD),

    a. dilutional hyponatremia may occur

    b. creatinine clearance is 50–75 mL per minute

    c. base excess leads to metabolic alkalemia

    d. arterial pH is normal with renal compensation

31. The primary laboratory finding in nephrotic syndrome is

    a. hyperalbuminemia

    b. hyperlipidemia

    c. proteinuria

    d. hematuria

32. Dietary protein intake in nephrotic syndrome is

    a. normal if the glomerular filtration rate (GFR) is 75 mL per minute

    b. increased if the GFR is 105 mL per minute

    c. decreased if the GFR is 50 mL per minute

    d. eliminated if kidneys are nonfunctioning

Degenerative Disorders

33. Which of the following statements is correct about nephrosclerosis?

    a. Renal arteries become narrowed, reducing blood flow to the renal parenchyma.

    b. Vessels in afferent and efferent arterioles and glomerulus thicken and narrow.

    c. Resulting benign essential hypertension is difficult to control with medication.

    d. Compliance with medication therapy is high in clients with nephrosclerosis.

34. Which of the following four statements about renal artery stenosis is correct?

    a. Renal artery stenosis results in kidney hypertrophy and eventual ischemia.

    b. Effective control of hypertension will preserve kidney function over the years.

    c. Renal artery bypass surgery requires less recovery time than angioplasty.

    d. Clients with renal artery stenosis are at increased risk of acute renal failure.

35. Which of the following statements about diabetic nephropathy is correct?

    a. Nephropathy occurs as a result of type I diabetes mellitus but not type II.

    b. Proteinuria is present within 16–21 years of onset of type I diabetes mellitus.

    c. Diabetic nephropathy is definitively diagnosed following a renal biopsy.

    d. Clients with diabetic nephropathy may require more insulin for adequate control.

Tumors

36. Which of the following statements is correct about benign renal tumors?

    a. Most benign renal cysts are symptomatic.

    b. Benign renal cysts do not result in kidney damage.

    c. Preventive measures include limiting caffeine intake.

    d. Malignant growths may occur within cystic structures.

Match the extent of involvement of renal tumors (37–40) with their classifications (a–d).

_____ 37. extending into renal vein or nodes   a. stage I

                                                b. stage II

_____ 38. extending beyond renal capsule but within Gerota's fascia   c. stage III

                                                d. stage IV

_____ 39. invasion of adjacent organs or distant metastases

_____ 40. within the renal capsule

41. List the subjective client data relevant to renal tumors. Use a separate sheet.

42. List the objective client data relevant to renal tumors. Use a separate sheet.

43. The preferred treatment of renal tumors includes

    a. chemotherapy

    b. hormonal therapy

    c. local excision

    d. radical nephrectomy

44. The client who has had a radical nephrectomy is monitored postoperatively for
    a. development of hypertension
    b. diuresis and sodium loss
    c. respiratory depression
    d. secondary hepatic failure

45. Discharge instruction for the client who has had a radical nephrectomy includes
    a. explaining the need for continued bed rest
    b. cautioning against lifting heavy objects
    c. limiting physical activity such as walking
    d. teaching about leaving the flank dressing on

Trauma

46. Describe the three classifications of renal trauma. Use a separate sheet.

Match the following causes (47–52) with their resultant renal trauma (a or b). Answers may be used more than once.

_____ 47. being thrown from a horse
_____ 48. hunting arrow
_____ 49. fall from tree
_____ 50. stab wound
_____ 51. shotgun pellet
_____ 52. football tackle

a. blunt
b. penetrating

53. List the subjective client data relevant to renal trauma. Use a separate sheet.

54. List the objective client data relevant to renal trauma. Use a separate sheet.

55. Identify the nursing diagnosis that is of highest priority for clients with renal trauma.

_____

_____

56. Management of the client with renal trauma includes
    a. replacement therapy with platelets
    b. rapid infusion of solutions such as D_5W
    c. administration of dobutamine (Dopamine)
    d. treatment of the resulting renin-induced hypertension

57. Which is more common, ureteral trauma or bladder trauma, and why?

_____

_____

_____

_____

_____

_____

CRITICAL THINKING EXERCISES

Case Study: Polycystic Kidney Disease

J. W. is a 48-year-old teacher who has polycystic kidney disease (PKD). He now has end-stage renal disease (ESRD) and needs hemodialysis. J. W. and his wife have two children, an 18-year-old son who is starting college and a 16-year-old daughter. Although the parents know that the disease is genetically transmitted, the son and daughter have not been told the nature of their father's disease. The parents insist that their children should not be told because the information would frighten them unnecessarily and inhibit their social lives. Mr. and Mrs. W. do not want the children to feel hopeless about their futures. The parents are firm in instructing the hospital staff not to tell their children about J. W.'s reason for needing hemodialysis. The information is privileged and to be kept confidential. The staff are uncomfortable with this burden of confidentiality and worry about the children. The staff have concerns about the children innocently involving future spouses and victimizing future offspring.

Address the following questions:

1. Do the parent have the right to choose whether or not to tell their children about the disease?

2. Whose rights should be considered in making such a decision?

3. As funding and medical resources become scarcer, is it ethical to "waste" these resources on people who have congenital terminal defects?

4. Screening for congenital defects such as PKD comprises 2–5% of the cost of health care maintenance. Is this a preferable course of action in these types of cases?

5. If Mr. and Mrs. W. decide that the children should be told about their father's PKD, how would the nurse explain what PKD is, how it is transmitted, and what the eventual outcome is for their father?

6. Identify the laboratory findings that would be present with J. W.

7. Identify the relevant nursing diagnoses for J. W. based on the known data. Plan the nursing interventions for him for the identified diagnoses.

8. J. W. develops bleeding in the left kidney, which necessitates surgical removal. Develop a perioperative care plan for J. W. as he undergoes a nephrectomy.

9. Why is only the left kidney removed and not the right one?

J. W. recovers uneventfully postoperatively. He will continue to be on a low-sodium, low-potassium, low-protein diet with fluid restrictions of 500 mL per day. Medications include hydralazine hydrochloride (Apresoline) for hypertension.

10. Design a discharge teaching/learning plan for J. W. for his diet and medications.

11. Discuss what resources are available to J. W. and his family to assist with his care management at home.

Case Study: Acute Glomerulonephritis

C. T. is a 22-year-old male college student admitted to the medical nursing unit with a diagnosis of acute glomerulonephritis (AGN). Three weeks ago, C. T. was treated with oral antibiotic therapy for strep throat.

Address the following questions:

1. What data should the nurse collect from C. T.?

C. T.'s urinalysis reveals the presence of RBCs, protein, and white cell casts. His glomerular filtration rate (GFR) is 50 mL per minute, his serum creatinine is 1.7 mg/dL, and his total 24-hour protein secretion is 2 g. A renal biopsy is scheduled to confirm the diagnosis.

2. Develop a teaching/learning plan for C. T. about the renal biopsy.

3. Identify the nursing interventions that should be implemented both pre- and post-biopsy.

4. The biopsy confirms a diagnosis of acute post-streptococcal glomerulonephritis (APSGN). Identify the relevant nursing diagnoses for C. T. based on the known data. Develop a care plan for these diagnoses.

5. Cefamandole nafate (Mandol) 1 g, IV, every 4 hours is ordered. Set up a dosage schedule for C. T.

6. After 4 days intravenous antibiotic therapy, C. T. is scheduled for discharge. He will continue the intravenous antibiotic therapy at home. Develop a discharge teaching/learning plan for C. T. about the antibiotic administration.

Case Study: Renal Tumor

C. C. is a 68-year-old retired mail carrier who lives with his wife. They spend six months living in their midwestern home state and the other six months during the winter living in Arizona. C. C. is admitted with a diagnosis of suspected renal cell carcinoma. Laboratory tests and a nephrotomogram confirm the diagnosis.

Address the following questions:

1. Identify the probable nursing diagnoses for C. C. based on the known data.

2. A radical nephrectomy is scheduled for C. C. Develop a perioperative teaching/learning plan for him.

3. Postoperative analgesia orders include meperidine hydrochloride (Demerol) 100 mg, with hydroxyzine hydrochloride (Vistaril) 25 mg, to be given IM. The Vistaril is supplied in vials containing 100 mg/2 mL. The Demerol is available only in prefilled cartridges containing 50 mg/mL. How many milliliters of medication should C. C. receive? How should the medications be administered?

4. Describe the postoperative assessments the nurse should make for C. C. for pain management, vital signs, surgical dressings, drainage tubes, and urine output.

5. C. C. recovers uneventfully and discharge is scheduled. No radiation or chemotherapy is planned. Develop a teaching/learning care plan for him.

6. Mr. and Mrs. C. are planning to travel to Arizona where C. C. can continue to recover from the surgery. They usually drive, and Mrs. C. tells the nurse that Mr. C. does the driving since she does not know how. What should the nurse discuss with them about their travel plans?

CHAPTER 72

Interventions for Clients with Chronic and Acute Renal Failure

LEARNING OBJECTIVES

At the end of this chapter, the student will be able to

- Compare and contrast chronic and acute renal failure
- Describe the stages of chronic renal failure (CRF)
- Identify pathological alterations associated with CRF
- Manage care for the client with end-stage renal disease (ESRD)
- Describe the special dietary considerations for clients with ESRD
- Discuss the hemodialysis process
- Discuss the peritoneal dialysis procedure
- Discuss renal transplantation
- Explain the three types of acute renal failure (ARF)
- Describe the phases of ARF
- Manage care for the client with ARF

PREREQUISITE KNOWLEDGE

Prior to beginning this chapter, the student should review

- The anatomy and physiology of the kidneys and urinary system
- The principles of osmosis and diffusion
- The principles of fluid and electrolyte balance
- The principles of acid–base balance
- Normal laboratory values for urinalysis and serum and urine electrolyte levels
- Low-sodium, low-potassium, and low-protein diets
- The principles of skin care
- The principles of perioperative nursing management
- The concepts of body image and self-esteem
- The concepts of grief, loss, death, and dying
- The role of the immune system
- The principles of intravenous therapy

STUDY QUESTIONS

Chronic Renal Failure

1. Complete the following chart by comparing the characteristics of chronic renal failure (CRF) with acute renal failure (ARF). Use a separate sheet.

Characteristic	CRF	ARF
a. onset		
b. reversible pathology		
c. nitrogen waste build-up		
d. need for dialysis		

Match the following changes in CRF (2–8) with their stages of disease progression (a–c). Answers may be used more than once.

_____ 2. fatal unless dialysis is begun

_____ 3. no metabolic waste build-up

_____ 4. partial compensation with careful management

_____ 5. renal function loss of 50%

_____ 6. renal function loss of 75%

_____ 7. renal function loss of 95%

_____ 8. severe fluid and electrolyte imbalances

a. diminished renal reserve

b. renal insufficiency

c. end-stage renal disease (ESRD)

9. Which percentage of kidney function loss leads to an insufficient glomerular filtration rate (GFR)?

 a. 25%

 b. 50%

 c. 65%

 d. 80%

10. Hyposthenuria is

 a. decreased urinary output

 b. increased urinary output

 c. urine with a fixed osmolality

 d. loss of the ability to concentrate urine

11. Increased concentrations of blood urea nitrogen (BUN) and serum creatinine constitute a condition called

 a. uremia

 b. azotemia

 c. osteodystrophy

 d. hyperproteinemia

12. The most accurate indicator of renal function is

 a. BUN level

 b. creatinine clearance

 c. serum creatinine level

 d. GFR

13. Which of the following metabolic alterations is seen in CRF?

 a. hypokalemia

 b. hypocalcemia

 c. hypophosphatemia

 d. metabolic alkalosis

14. Skeletal demineralization seen in CRF is known as renal

 a. hypocalcemia

 b. osteomalacia

 c. osteodystrophy

 d. hyperphosphatemia

15. Cardiovascular changes seen in the client with CRF include

 a. hyperemia

 b. hypotension

 c. palpitations

 d. pericarditis

16. List the types of treatment for prolonging life that are available to clients with ESRD.

 a. _____

 b. _____

 c. _____

17. The most common cause of ESRD is

 a. glomerulonephritis

 b. hyperparathyroidism

 c. diabetic nephropathy

 d. hypertensive renal disease

18. List the subjective client data relevant to CRF. Use a separate sheet.

19. List the changes that occur in the neurological system related to CRF. Use a separate sheet.

20. List the changes that occur in the cardiovascular system related to CRF. Use a separate sheet.

21. List the changes that occur in the respiratory system related to CRF. Use a separate sheet.

22. List the changes that occur in the hematological system related to CRF. Use a separate sheet.

23. List the changes that occur in the gastrointestinal (GI) system related to CRF. Use a separate sheet.

24. List the changes that occur in the urinary system related to CRF. Use a separate sheet.

25. List the changes that occur in the integumentary term related to CRF. Use a separate sheet.

26. Which of the following radiographic tests is usually done initially when evaluating the kidneys?

    a. computed tomography with contrast

    b. plain abdominal film

    c. intravenous pyelography

    d. aortorenal angiography

27. Identify two of the more common nursing diagnoses for CRF.

    a. _____

    _____

    b. _____

    _____

    _____

28. Identify the principles that guide dietary management of CRF.

    a. _____

    _____

    b. _____

    _____

    c. _____

    _____

    d. _____

    _____

    e. _____

    _____

    f. _____

    _____

29. Protein consumption in the client with CRF is monitored by measuring serum levels of

    a. creatinine and total protein

    b. total protein and urea nitrogen

    c. creatinine and urea nitrogen

    d. albumin and urea nitrogen

30. Explain why the client on peritoneal dialysis is encouraged to eat more protein than the client on hemodialysis.

    _____

    _____

    _____

31. Which of the following statements is correct about drug therapy for CRF?

    a. Diuretics are often used in clients in the late stages of renal insufficiency.

    b. Insulin-dependent diabetics often require more insulin as kidney function diminishes.

    c. Antibiotics that are excreted by the kidneys necessitate reduced dose adjustment.

    d. Antihypertensives such as propranolol (Inderal) must be discontinued in ESRD.

32. Which of the following is the correct intervention in drug therapy for the client with CRF?

    a. The daily digoxin (Lanoxin) dose is administered prior to the beginning of dialysis.

    b. Folic acid is administered after hemodialysis because it is removed in that process.

    c. Antidiarrheals are often necessary because of adverse effects from antacids.

    d. The dose of opioids must be reduced by one-half to prevent further nephrotoxicity.

33. Briefly describe what hemodialysis does for the client with ESRD.

    _____

    _____

    _____

    _____

    _____

    _____

    _____

    _____

Match the following terms relating to hemodialysis (34–41) with their definitions (a–h).

_____ 34. arterio-venous fistula

_____ 35. arterio-venous catheter

_____ 36. bruit

_____ 37. dialysate

_____ 38. dialyzer

_____ 39. diffusion

_____ 40. hemo-dialysis machine

_____ 41. thrill

a. mixture of electrolytes and water for waste removal from blood

b. palpable sensation produced by blood flowing through arteri-ovenous (AV) connection

c. movement of molecules from higher to lower area of concentration

d. sound produced by blood flow in AV connection

e. anastomosis of artery and vein

f. monitors hemodialysis

g. artificial kidney

h. external cannula connecting artery and vein

42. List the factors that determine the duration and frequency of hemodialysis treatments.

a. _____

_____

_____

b. _____

_____

_____

c. _____

_____

_____

43. Anticoagulant therapy for the client on hemodialysis is necessary because

a. blood tends to clot when it comes in contact with foreign surfaces

b. the increased erythropoietin tends to cause problems with thrombus formation

c. there is considerable variability between individuals in coagulation response

d. there is an increased risk for hemorrhage or bleeding during dialysis

44. Identify the antidote used to neutralize heparin.

_____

45. Assessments the nurse should make for an AV shunt or fistula include

a. palpating for a bruit over the site

b. checking skin temperature proximal to the site

c. assessing movement and paresthesia distal to the site

d. checking the blanche response by compressing the site

46. The effectiveness of dialysis treatment is monitored by evaluating

a. BUN level

b. serum potassium level

c. serum creatinine level

d. creatinine clearance

47. Which of the following findings is abnormal after hemodialysis?

a. headache

b. muscle cramps in legs

c. temperature elevation of 2°F

d. decreased level of consciousness

48. Identify the infectious diseases that the client who requires hemodialysis is at increased risk of acquiring.

a. _____

_____

b. _____

_____

49. Compared with hemodialysis, peritoneal dialysis

a. is complex and difficult to manage

b. takes less time per dialysis session

c. requires more dialysate for one dialysis

d. results in readily predictable waste removal

50. Identify two factors that affect the efficiency of peritoneal dialysis.

a. _____

_____

_____

b. _____

_____

_____

51. The major difference between the composition of dialysate used for peritoneal dialysis and that used for hemodialysis is the

    a. type of fluid used

    b. glucose concentration

    c. magnesium concentration

    d. phosphorus concentration

52. List the types of peritoneal dialysis.

    a. _____

    _____

    b. _____

    _____

    c. _____

    _____

    d. _____

    _____

    e. _____

    _____

Match the following assessments (53–63) with their complications from peritoneal dialysis (a–d). Answers may be used more than once.

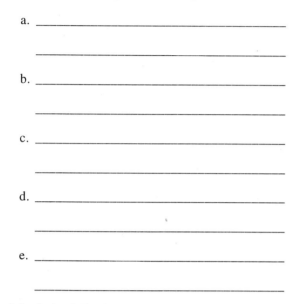

_____ 53. brown drainage   a. catheter integrity

_____ 54. cloudy return   b. outflow character

_____ 55. cold dialysate   c. pain

_____ 56. decreased   d. peritonitis
          outflow volume

_____ 57. fever

_____ 58. inflow discomfort

_____ 59. kinked tubing

_____ 60. leakage of
          dialysate

_____ 61. leukocytes in
          outflow

_____ 62. malaise

_____ 63. nausea and
          vomiting

64. Which of the following four findings indicates that a client on peritoneal dialysis has developed an acute complication?

    a. pulse = 86, blood pressure = 112/74

    b. respirations = 30, bibasilar rales

    c. sleeping intermittently throughout dialysis run

    d. dressing around catheter saturated with clear fluid

65. Which of the following statements is correct about renal transplantation?

    a. The principal histocompatibility system used to match recipients with donors is ABO typing.

    b. Candidates for transplantation should be free from major metabolic diseases including cancer.

    c. Kidneys for transplantation must be matched for age, race, and sex of the donor and recipient.

    d. The size of the transplanted kidney should be about the same as that of the recipient's.

66. Which of the following statements is correct about living related donor renal transplants?

    a. Kidney donors may be of any age.

    b. Donors are usually children or young adults.

    c. They have the lowest graft survival rates.

    d. Donors must express a clear understanding of the procedure.

67. After transplantation, the transplanted kidney should function immediately. Which of the following findings should the nurse report to the physician immediately?

    a. urine pink and bloody

    b. intake = 2500 mL, output = 2000 mL

    c. blood pressure = 104/68

    d. weight gain of 2 pounds in 1 day

68. List the three types of kidney rejection and discuss when they occur and how they are diagnosed and treated. Use a separate sheet.

69. Which of the following statements is correct about immunosuppressive drug therapy in renal transplantation?

    a. Cyclosporine has relatively few serious side effects.

    b. Corticosteroids are used as anti-inflammatory agents.

    c. Reactions from monoclonal antibodies increase with use.

    d. Antilymphocyte drugs provide long-term immunosuppression.

70. Describe the stages that the client with CRF goes through over the course of treatment for the disease process. Use a separate sheet.

Acute Renal Failure

71. Compare the causes of the three types of acute renal failure (ARF) and the changes that occur in each disease process. Use a separate sheet.

72. Compare the duration and clinical manifestations of the following phases of ARF. Use a separate sheet.

    a. onset

    b. oliguria

    c. diuresis

    d. recovery

73. The most common cause of ARF is

    a. pyelonephritis

    b. glomerulonephritis

    c. prolonged hypotension

    d. disseminated intravascular coagulation

74. Causes of ARF include all of the following *except*

    a. radiographic contrast media

    b. prolonged dehydration

    c. analgesic toxicity

    d. cystitis

75. One prerenal cause of ARF is

    a. glomerulonephritis

    b. urethral stricture

    c. analgesic toxicity

    d. severe hemorrhage

76. One postrenal cause of ARF is

    a. glomerulonephritis

    b. urethral stricture

    c. analgesic toxicity

    d. severe hemorrhage

77. List the subjective client data relevant to ARF. Use a separate sheet.

78. List the objective client data relevant to ARF due to prerenal causes. Use a separate sheet.

79. List the objective client data relevant to ARF due to intrarenal causes. Use a separate sheet.

80. List the objective client data relevant to ARF due to postrenal causes. Use a separate sheet.

81. Identify the nursing diagnosis that is common in the client with ARF but is not found in the client with CRF.

    _____

    _____

82. Briefly discuss why the care plan may change frequently for the client with ARF.

    _____

    _____

    _____

83. Which of the following statements is correct about drug management of the oliguric phase of ARF?

    a. Fluids are restricted to prevent fluid overload and potential cardiac failure.

    b. Diagnostic laboratory specimens are collected once administration of diuretics and fluid challenges has been initiated.

    c. Controlled fluid challenges with normal saline and a loop diuretic may potentiate a diuretic response.

    d. Vascular competency and intravascular status are continuously monitored with intra-arterial pressures.

84. List the types of dietary support that are used for the client with ARF who is in a catabolic state.

    a. _____

    _____

    _____

    b. _____

    _____

    _____

85. Identify the sites used for temporary external vascular access when the client with ARF requires hemodialysis.

    a. _____

    b. _____

    c. _____

86. Which of the following statements is correct about continuous arteriovenous hemodialysis and filtration (CAVHD)?

    a. CAVHD is the most common renal replacement therapy for clients with ARF.

    b. CAVHD often results in problems with hypotension.

    c. Highly specialized equipment is required for CAVHD.

    d. Clotting of the filter and tubing is a possibility.

CRITICAL THINKING EXERCISES

Case Study: Hemodialysis

H. D. is a 32-year-old female client with chronic glomerulonephritis. She is married and has three children. H. D. is in chronic renal insufficiency and nearing ESRD. She is to have an arteriovenous (AV) fistula created and is scheduled for surgery tomorrow.

Address the following questions:

1. Develop a perioperative teaching/learning plan for H. D.

2.   What assessments should the nurse make postoperatively about the fistula?

3. What teaching is indicated for H. D. prior to her discharge to encourage "ripening" of the fistula? What should H. D. be told about preventing clotting of the fistula?

H. D. returns to the hospital 8 months after the initial surgery to begin hemodialysis on an outpatient basis.

4. Develop a care plan for H. D. that includes her dialysis "runs" and self-care in between sessions.

5. During a hemodialysis session, what should the nurse monitor?

6. What are the potential complications that H. D. may incur from hemodialysis?

H. D. is dialyzed every Monday, Wednesday, and Friday. After 2 months of outpatient dialysis, H. D. and her husband inquire about home dialysis.

7. What assessments should be made by the nurse and other health care team members to determine whether H. D. is a suitable candidate for home hemodialysis?

8. Develop a teaching/learning care plan for H. D. and her husband about home hemodialysis.

9. What support systems will H. D. and her family need to manage home hemodialysis?

10. What are the potential complications H. D. may incur while on home dialysis?

Case Study: Peritoneal Dialysis

P. N., a 68-year-old African-American male client, is currently being treated with outpatient peritoneal dialysis 3 days per week for ESRD secondary to hypertensive nephrosclerosis. He is anorectic, weak, and hypertensive. A low-sodium diet and antihypertensive drugs have failed to control his blood pressure. P. N. was placed on hemodialysis 5 years ago. He had several fistula failures requiring revisions in both arms and the left leg. Following the clotting of the last fistula in his right arm, a Tenckhoff peritoneal catheter was inserted 1 year ago. P. N. has been on peritoneal dialysis since that time. During dialysis sessions, he has episodes of cramping, nausea, and diarrhea.

P. N. also had a pacemaker inserted 2-1/2 years ago because of a dysrhythmia. He was placed on disopyramide (Norpace) 100 mg, qd, and digoxin (Lanoxin) 0.125 mg, on M-W-F. P. N. also takes a multivitamin, thiamine, folate, iron, and a stool softener. P. N. is on a 2 g sodium, 50–60 g protein, 50 mEq potassium diet. He lives alone and finds it difficult to follow the dietary restrictions. His dry weight is 148 pounds.

Address the following questions:

1. Identify the relevant nursing diagnoses for P. N.
2. Develop a care plan for P. N. including care of the Tenckhoff catheter, medications, and care during dialysis sessions.
3. What assessments should the nurse make about P. N.'s dietary habits?
4. What resources are available to assist P. N. in being more compliant with his dietary restrictions?
5. On this admission, P. N. weighs 154 pounds. The dialysate order is for a 30% solution if he is 0–3 pounds above dry weight or a 50% solution if he is 4–5 pounds above dry weight. An additional 250 mL of D_{50} in water is to be added if he is more than 6 pounds above dry weight. What dialysate should the nurse use?

Case Study: Continuous Ambulatory Peritoneal Dialysis (CAPD)

G. D. is a 36-year-old female client who is married and has two adopted children. She is diagnosed with polycystic kidney disease (PKD). G. D. will soon have to go on dialysis or consent to a renal transplant.

Address the following questions:

1. Develop a teaching/learning care plan for G. D. that explains hemodialysis, peritoneal dialysis, CAPD, and renal transplantation.
2. What additional data should the nurse collect to help G. D. make the best decision for herself?
3. Due to long distance G. D. lives from the medical center, she elects to begin CAPD. Develop a plan of care for G. D. for this procedure.
4. Develop a teaching/learning care plan for CAPD management.

Case Study: Renal Transplantation

K. T. is a 22-year-old college student with diabetic nephropathy. He has an older brother (D. T.) who matches well for a living related donor kidney.

Address the following questions:

1. What assessments must be made for both K. T. and his brother before the transplantation is performed? Consider both the physiological and psychological data.

2. Develop preoperative teaching/learning plans for both K. T. and his brother.

3. Develop postoperative teaching/learning plans for both K. T. and his brother.

4. What data should the nurse assess to monitor for rejection in K. T.? What would be done if K. T. went into rejection?

5. K. T. recovers and discharge is planned. Medication orders include prednisone (Deltasone) 20 mg, qod, PO; cyclosporine (Sandimmune) 750 mg, qd, PO; and azathioprine (Imuran) 150 mg, qd, PO. What should his teaching/learning plan include for these medications?

6. If K. T. is on 750 mg of cyclosporine per day and his dose is calculated at 10 mg/kg per day, how much does he weigh in kilograms? In pounds? How many milligrams per kilogram per day is K. T. receiving of the Imuran?

7. Discuss why K. T. must take these drugs for the remainder of his life.

8. Develop discharge instructions for both K. T. and D. T.

Case Study: Acute Renal Failure

T. C. is an 80-year-old retired farmer who is diabetic. His history includes smoking for 50 years (but not in the past 10 years), angina, hypertension, and atrial fibrillation. T. C. has been on nifedipine (Procardia) 20 mg, qid, and digoxin (Lanoxin) 0.375 mg, qd. He adjusts his insulin (regular and Lente) depending on his activity (he occasionally helps his sons with livestock and field work). T. C. underwent triple coronary bypass surgery yesterday. The postoperative course was uncomplicated until it was determined in the post-anesthesia recovery area that he was bleeding. T. C. was returned to surgery, and five units of blood were administered during the second surgery. Today, T. C.'s urine output is less than 5 mL per hour and he is diagnosed with acute tubular necrosis (ATN).

Address the following questions:

1. Since T. C.'s blood pressure never dropped below 80/50 in the recovery area and in surgery, what contributed to the poor kidney perfusion that led to ATN? Consider his original medical problems.

2. Identify the relevant nursing diagnoses for T. C. based on the above data.

3. Develop a care plan for T. C.

T. C.'s serum creatinine climbs to 5.4 mg/dL and his BUN to 101 mg/dL. He is becoming more irritable and lethargic. The family, which includes his wife, five children and their spouses, and numerous grandchildren and great-grandchildren, maintain a vigil at the hospital.

4. What can the nurse do to help the family?

The laboratory values indicate that dialysis is necessary. But before the initial surgery, T. C. indicated that he wanted no heroic measures taken if the surgery did not go well. He refuses dialysis. His family supports his decision.

5. What can the nurse do to comfort both the client and family?

6. Is it feasible that the ATN will reverse itself?

7. Is dialysis considered a heroic measure in this situation?

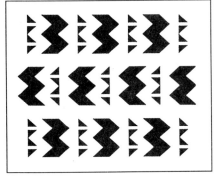

CHAPTER 73

Assessment of the Reproductive System

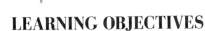

LEARNING OBJECTIVES

At the end of this chapter, the student will be able to

■ Describe the structure and function of the female reproductive system

■ Describe the structure and function of the breasts

■ Discuss the normal menstrual cycle

■ Define *climacteric* and *menopause*

■ Describe the structure and function of the male reproductive system

■ List changes of the reproductive system associated with aging

■ Identify the data to be collected by the nurse when obtaining a reproductive system history

■ Identify information to be obtained during a physical assessment of the client with genito-reproductive system dysfunction

■ List diagnostic assessment studies for the reproductive system

PREREQUISITE KNOWLEDGE

Prior to beginning this chapter, the student should review

■ The anatomy and physiology of the male and female reproductive systems

■ The effect of the endocrine system on genito-reproductive tissue

■ The concept of human sexuality

■ The concepts of body image and self-esteem

■ Normal growth and development

STUDY QUESTIONS

Anatomy and Physiology Review

Match the following terms related to the female reproductive system (1–25) with their descriptions (a–y).

_____	1.	breasts
_____	2.	cervix
_____	3.	climacteric
_____	4.	clitoris
_____	5.	Döderlein's bacilli
_____	6.	endometrium
_____	7.	fallopian tube
_____	8.	fourchette
_____	9.	hymen
_____	10.	labia majora
_____	11.	labia minora
_____	12.	lactation
_____	13.	menopause
_____	14.	menstruation
_____	15.	mittelschmerz
_____	16.	mons pubis
_____	17.	myometrium
_____	18.	ovary
_____	19.	perineum
_____	20.	peritoneum
_____	21.	prepuce
_____	22.	prolactin
_____	23.	uterus
_____	24.	vagina
_____	25.	vestibule

a. hood of clitoris

b. occludes vaginal opening

c. receives penis during intercourse

d. middle uterine layer

e. outer layer of uterus

f. covers symphysis pubis

g. area between clitoris, labia minora, and fourchette

h. homologous to penis

i. stimulates milk production

j. cyclic shedding by endometrium

k. protect inner vulvar structures

l. nourishes and expels fetus

m. area between fourchette and anus

n. normal vagina flora

o. duct between ovary and uterus

p. develops and releases ova and hormones

q. pain corresponding with follicle rupture

r. tissue at posterior ends of labia minora

s. expression of milk or colostrum

t. mammary glands

u. lie inside labia majora

v. inner mucosal layer of uterus

w. biological end of reproductive ability

x. canal for sperm entry to uterus

y. decline of estrogen production

26. Which of the following statements is correct about female external genitalia development?

   a. Pubertal development begins at about age 14 years.

   b. The mons pubis becomes covered with hair.

   c. Presence of a hymen conclusively determines virginity.

   d. The clitoris is insensitive to stimulation in prepuberty.

27. Identify two factors about uterine anatomy that have implications for migration of malignant cells.

   a. _____

   _____

   _____

   b. _____

   _____

   _____

Match the following terms (28–31) with their definitions (a–d).

_____	28.	amenorrhea
_____	29.	menarche
_____	30.	menses
_____	31.	menstrual cycle

a. first menstrual flow

b. repetitive process of ovum development and uterine lining changes

c. absence of menstrual flow

d. flow of sloughed endometrial tissue

Match the following events of the menstrual cycle (32–49) with their phases (a–c). Answers may be used more than once. (*Continues on next page.*)

_____	32.	corpus luteum secretes estrogen
_____	33.	edema in stroma increases
_____	34.	estrogen secreted by follicles
_____	35.	follicles begin to develop
_____	36.	follicle-stimulating hormone (FSH) released
_____	37.	FSH secretion suppressed

a. hypothalamic-pituitary cycle

b. ovarian cycle

c. uterine cycle

_____ 38. gonadotropin-releasing factor secreted

_____ 39. graafian follicle grows

_____ 40. increased endometrial vascularity

_____ 41. ischemia and sloughing of endometrium

_____ 42. layers of endometrium definable

_____ 43. luteinizing hormone (LH) released

_____ 44. LH secretion increased

_____ 45. prolactin-inhibiting factor secreted

_____ 46. rapid growth of endometrial layer

_____ 47. release of mature ovum

_____ 48. stroma disintegrates

_____ 49. uterine lining proliferates

50. Menopause is the cessation of menstrual function. One of the causes is

a. decreased amount of circulating gonadotropic hormones

b. increased progesterone secretion from ovarian follicles

c. decreased production of prostaglandins from the ovaries

d. inability of ovaries to respond to gonadotropic hormones

51. Ovulation occurs when

a. oxytocin levels are high

b. progesterone levels are high

c. the endometrial wall is sloughed

d. circulating levels of FSH and LH are high

52. A high concentration of estrogens in the blood

a. causes ovulation

b. stimulates lactation

c. contributes to the development of osteoporosis

d. inhibits FSH secretion by the anterior pituitary

53. Which of the following statements is correct about the female climacteric and menopause?

a. Ovarian follicles begin to atrophy between the ages of 40 and 50 years.

b. Estrogen and progesterone production ceases abruptly with menopause.

c. Women with more body fat have lower estrone levels following menopause.

d. The exact date of menopause is determined after 1 year of amenorrhea.

Match the following terms related to the female breast (54–62) with their descriptions (a–i).

_____ 54. alveoli

_____ 55. ampulla

_____ 56. areola

_____ 57. Cooper's ligaments

_____ 58. lactiferous ducts

_____ 59. lobes

_____ 60. lobules

_____ 61. Montgomery's glands

_____ 62. nipple

a. erectile tissue in middle of breast

b. pigmented tissue near breast midline

c. sebaceous glands on areola

d. radially arranged structures separated by adipose tissue

e. structures attaching breast to chest wall

f. structures consisting of secretory tissue

g. Sac-like structures lined with epithelium

h. structures that combine and empty out at nipple

i. reservoir to collect milk

63. Which of the following statements about female breast development is correct?

a. Breast tissue develops symmetrically during puberty.

b. Both breasts are usually symmetric by adulthood.

c. For one breast to be slightly larger than the other is abnormal.

d. Premenstrual increase in breast size is abnormal.

64. Which of the following statements is correct about male external genitalia development?

a. Pubertal development begins at about age 14 years.

b. Public hair grows in a triangular-shaped pattern.

c. One testis being lower than the other is abnormal.

d. The scrotum has fewer rugae and hangs lower with aging.

65. List the secondary signs of puberty related to testosterone production in boys.

a. _____

_____

b. _____

_____

c. _____

_____

d. _____

_____

Match the following terms related to the male reproductive system (66–78) with their descriptions (a–m).

_____ 66. Cowper's glands

_____ 67. ejaculation

_____ 68. ejaculatory duct

_____ 69. emission

_____ 70. epididymis

_____ 71. foreskin

_____ 72. penis

_____ 73. prostate gland

_____ 74. scrotum

_____ 75. seminal vesicle

_____ 76. seminiferous tubule

_____ 77. testes

_____ 78. vas deferens

a. organ for urination and copulation

b. ductal system transporting sperm from testes to vas deferens

c. secrete mucus to mix with other secretions to form semen

d. transports sperm from epididymis to ejaculatory ducts

e. largest accessory gland in male reproductive system

f. produce spermatozoa and testosterone

g. protects testes, epididymis, and vas deferens

h. functional unit of testis that produces sperm

i. formed by joining of seminal vesicle and vas deferens

j. second stage of male orgasm

k. glands that secrete major portion of ejaculate

l. skin covering glans penis

m. first stage of male orgasm

79. Which of the following statements is correct about changes that occur with aging?

a. Pubic hair becomes gray and sparse.

b. Breast tissue remains firm and elastic.

c. Support connective tissue retains tone.

d. The endometrium and prostate gland hypertrophy.

Subjective Assessment

80. List the subjective client data relevant to the reproductive system. Use a separate sheet.

81. List the subjective client data that should be collected from a female client. Use a separate sheet.

82. List the subjective client data that should be collected from a male client. Use a separate sheet.

83. List psychosocial data relevant to the reproductive system. Use a separate sheet.

84. Identify factors that affect libido.

a. _____

_____

b. _____

_____

c. _____

_____

85. Identify three classes of drugs that may affect fertility.

a. _____

_____

b. _____

_____

c. _____

_____

86. Severe infection with which one of the following may result in reproductive problems?

a. mumps virus at age 3 years

b. *Neisseria gonorrhoeae*

c. *Streptococcus* (throat infection)

d. *Staphylococcus aureus* (osteomyelitis)

87. A diet history is often critical to the correct interpretation of symptoms involving the reproductive system because

    a. obesity minimizes one's risk of developing breast and uterine cancer

    b. anemia and a nutritionally poor diet may contribute to lack of sexual interest

    c. low-fat diets have been linked with cancer of the breast and prostate

    d. women who use oral contraceptives have deficiencies in vitamins A and D

88. Which of the following subjective data may have an effect on the reproductive system?

    a. religious belief explains vegetarian diet

    b. admits to 12 sexual partners in the past 2 years

    c. Caucasian

    d. woman, age 56

    e. gets 8–9 hours of sleep per night

    f. swims 45 minutes, three times per week

    g. uses hot tub daily for 1 hour to relax (man)

    h. smokes two packs of cigarettes per day

    i. drinks a six-pack of beer every 2 days

    j. had mumps at age 30 years (man)

    k. had rubella while pregnant

    l. mumps, measles, and rubella vaccine current

    m. has type I diabetes mellitus

    n. takes methyldopa for hypertension

    o. ruptured appendix at age 22 years

    p. gravida 3, para 2

    q. consumes a balanced diet

    r. training for a marathon (woman)

    s. works in a dry-cleaning shop

89. The following is a partial client history. Discuss the significance these data have for assessment of the reproductive system. Submit the completed exercise to the clinical instructor.

    Caucasian male client, age 67. Lives with wife of 42 years. Four children. Reports difficulty with urination that has become increasingly more bothersome in past 2 months. Feels urge to urinate almost continually but produces only small amounts with a weak stream. Nocturia (three or four times per night). Occasional dribbling. Tends to be constipated, relying on prune juice for bowel movements. Denies impotence, but admits that feelings of bladder fullness interfere with positions assumed during intercourse and frequency of intercourse. "I guess I'm getting old; my dad had this same problem and it nearly killed him to pee. He was afraid of doctors and never did anything about it!"

Objective Assessment

90. List the objective client data relevant to the female productive system. Use a separate sheet.

91. List the objective client data relevant to the male reproductive system. Use a separate sheet.

92. Using the data from question 89, construct a physical assessment recording for the reproductive system. Submit the completed exercise to the clinical instructor.

93. A female pelvic examination is recommended

    a. for girls beginning at age 14 years

    b. to assess localized abdominal pain

    c. for every sexually active woman

    d. to assess regular menstrual cycles

94. A male pelvic examination is recommended

    a. for boys beginning at age 16 years

    b. to assess for incontinence

    c. for every man over the age of 30 years

    d. to teach about testicular self-examination

95. The Papanicolaou (Pap) test

    a. is recommended only for women who are sexually active

    b. may be scheduled for a time during the menstrual flow

    c. requires special preparation as a douche

    d. involves analysis of specimens from the vagina, cervix, and endocervix

96. Describe what each classification of the Papanicolaou test results mean. Use a separate sheet.

Match the following laboratory tests for the reproductive system (97–103) with their descriptions (a–g).

____ 97. enzyme-linked immunosorbent assay	a. elevation indicates possible uterine cancer, cystic breast disease, corpus luteum cyst
	b. diagnostic of herpes simplex
____ 98. FSH levels	c. decrease indicates infertility, anorexia nervosa, neoplasm
____ 99. potassium hydroxide	
____ 100. progesterone	d. decrease indicates inadequate luteal phase, amenorrhea
____ 101. prolactin	e. test for AIDS antibody
____ 102. total estrogens	f. elevation indicates hypothyroidism, disease of pituitary or hypothalamus
____ 103. Tzanck's test	g. diagnostic of candidiasis, gardnerella vaginitis

104. The Venereal Disease Research Laboratory
     (VDRL) test

     a. is highly specific for diagnosis of syphilis

     b. results do not vary with the stage of syphilis

     c. will be negative during the first week of infec-
        tion

     d. will remain positive even if primary syphilis
        is treated

Match the following diagnostic procedures for the reproductive system (105–119) with their descriptions on the right (a–o).

_____ 105. breast biopsy

_____ 106. cervical biopsy

_____ 107. colposcopy

_____ 108. computed
           tomography

_____ 109. culdocentesis

_____ 110. culdoscopy

_____ 111. endometrial biopsy

_____ 112. hysterosalpingogram

_____ 113. hysteroscopy

_____ 114. KUB

_____ 115. laparoscopy

_____ 116. mammography

_____ 117. prostate biopsy

_____ 118. ultrasonography

_____ 119. xeromammography

a. study of soft breast tissue by x-ray

b. abdominal x-ray of kidneys, ureters, bladder

c. x-ray of breast with low-dose radiation

d. endoscopic examination of interior uterus

e. differentiates solid masses from cysts or hemorrhagic masses

f. x-ray of cervix, uterus, and fallopian tubes
   following injection of contrast medium

g. endoscopy to visualize pelvic contents

h. removal of tissue for cervical cytological study

i. endoscopy to visualize pelvic cavity

j. allows assessment of pelvic structures without
   radiation

k. examination under magnification of cervix,
   vulva, and vagina

l. needle aspiration of fluid from posterior cul-de-
   sac

m. method to obtain cells from uterine lining

n. removal of tissue from a breast mass for study

o. needle aspiration of cells from prostate gland
   for study

CRITICAL THINKING EXERCISES

Case Study: Infertility

A. S. is a 30-year-old woman who has been trying to conceive a child for the past 2 years. She has not used any form of contraception since her marriage 4 years ago. Her husband wore condoms during the first 2 years of their marriage. Prior to marriage, A. S. states that she had 15 different sexual partners and was treated for pelvic inflammatory disease. She used oral contraceptives during that time. A hysterosalpingogram (HSG) is scheduled.

Address the following questions:

1. Why is an HSG being ordered for A. S.?

2. Develop a teaching/learning plan for A. S. about the HSG. Include her husband in the plan.

3. The nurse gives A. S. a perineal pad after the procedure. Why is this necessary? How long will the pad be needed?

Following the procedure, A. S. reports shoulder pain. The physician orders acetaminophen with codeine (Tylenol with codeine) #3, one or two tablets every 3–4 hours as needed for pain.

4. What is the cause of A. S.'s pain?

5. What should the nurse teach A. S. about her prescription?

6. The HSG shows no anatomical reason for A. S.'s infertility. Discuss what other diagnostic tests may be necessary for A. S. and her husband to determine whether conception is possible for them.

CHAPTER 74

Interventions for Clients with Breast Disorders

LEARNING OBJECTIVES

At the end of this chapter, the student will be able to

- Discuss breast self-examination (BSE)
- List the various kinds of benign breast disease
- Describe fibroadenoma and related treatment
- Discuss fibrocystic breast disease (FBD)
- Describe ductal ectasia and intraductal papilloma
- List the problems experienced by large-breasted women and describe the related treatment
- Discuss gynecomastia
- Discuss the pathophysiology, etiology, and incidence of breast cancer
- Manage care for the client with breast cancer

PREREQUISITE KNOWLEDGE

Prior to beginning this chapter, the student should review

- The anatomy and physiology of the male and female breast
- The concept of human sexuality
- The concepts of body image and self-esteem
- The effect of the endocrine system on breast tissue
- Normal growth and development of breast tissue

- The concepts of grief, loss, death, and dying
- Care of the client undergoing chemotherapy and radiation therapy
- The principles of perioperative nursing management

STUDY QUESTIONS

Breast Self-Examination

1. Identify the goal of breast self-examination (BSE).

   _____

   _____

2. Which of the following statements is correct about BSE?

   a. All woman over the age of 20 years should practice BSE.

   b. Approximately 80% of all women practice BSE regularly.

   c. Most women who practice BSE do so competently.

   d. Self-taught BSE results in a higher level of proficiency.

3. Motivation to practice BSE is affected by

   a. women's lack of knowledge about the technique

   b. women not understanding the benefits of early detection

   c. the adequacy of a physician's yearly examination

   d. BSE begin an excellent method of prevention

4. Risk factors for increased incidence of breast cancer include being

   a. sterile

   b. underweight

   c. under age 25 years

   d. on a low-cholesterol diet

5. BSE should be performed by premenopausal women

   a. at the midpoint of the menstrual cycle

   b. during the time of the menstrual flow

   c. 1 week after menstrual flow begins

   d. the same calendar day of each month

6. When examining a client's breasts, the nurse

   a. begins palpating the breast having a reported abnormality first

   b. lightly palpates both breasts simultaneously first then individually for comparison

   c. compresses the breast tissue laterally and medially between both hands

   d. includes the axillae, infraclavicular, and supraclavicular areas in the examination

Benign Breast Disorders

Match the following benign breast disorders (7–10) with their age-related times of occurrence (a–d).

____ 7. ductal ectasia

____ 8. fibroadenoma

____ 9. fibrocystic breast disease (FBD)

____ 10. intraductal papilloma

a. most common in teenage years

b. occurs mainly in 40–55 age group

c. seen in women nearing menopause

d. most common in early 20s to 50s

11. Which of the following statements is correct about fibroadenoma?

   a. Most fibroadenoma become malignant.

   b. The lesion is composed of glandular tissue.

   c. Most fibroadenomas are discovered during annual check-ups.

   d. Lesions are firm, moveable, and delineated.

Match the following stages of fibrocystic breast disease (FBD) (12–21) with their descriptions (a–c). Answers may be used more than once.

____ 12. bilateral multinodularity

____ 13. premenstrual bilateral breast tenderness

____ 14. three-dimensional lesion

____ 15. indistinguishable borders of lesion

____ 16. lesions painful and tender

____ 17. symptoms resolve after menses

____ 18. cysts appear suddenly

____ 19. lesions present throughout menstrual cycle

____ 20. symptoms cyclical with menses

____ 21. two-dimensional lesions

a. first

b. second

c. third

22. Which of the following statements is correct about FBD?

   a. Estrogen and progesterone levels do not affect symptom occurrence.

   b. Most women with FBD seek professional help to cope with their symptoms.

   c. Risk factors associated with FBS are controllable with careful management.

   d. Oral contraceptives may decrease a woman's risk of developing FBD.

23. List the measures used to treat FBD.

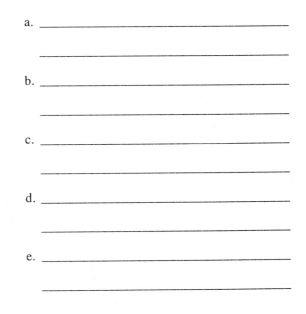

   a. _____

   _____

   b. _____

   _____

   c. _____

   _____

   d. _____

   _____

   e. _____

   _____

24. Which of the following statements is correct about ductal ectasia?

    a. Masses feel firm with regular borders.

    b. There often is a yellow drainage from the nipple.

    c. Masses are often difficult to distinguish from cancer.

    d. Ductal ectasia is an autoimmune disease.

25. Which of the following statements is correct about papilloma?

    a. Papillomas arise from glandular tissue.

    b. Green-brown nipple discharge is present.

    c. Tenderness over the lesion is usually absent.

    d. Diagnosis must determine if a mass is malignant.

26. Which of the following statements is correct about women with large breasts?

    a. They are usually grossly overweight.

    b. They have difficulty finding clothes that fit.

    c. Their breasts are in proportion to their bodies.

    d. Bilateral mastectomies are required to resolve their problems.

27. Which of the following statements is correct about gynecomastia?

    a. It is a problem found in both sexes.

    b. Breast enlargement is usually unilateral.

    c. It is cause by glandular tissue proliferation.

    d. Etiology includes underlying cardiopulmonary disease.

Breast Cancer

28. Which of the following statements is correct about breast cancer?

    a. It is the leading cause of breast masses.

    b. The risk of a breast lump being cancerous is 40%.

    c. Breast cancer is preventable by controlling risk factors.

    d. Early detection and treatment increase survival rates.

29. Which of the following four statements is correct about breast cancer pathophysiology?

    a. The most common type of breast cancer is intraductal papilloma.

    b. Invasive tumors grow irregularly, resulting in poorly defined lesions.

    c. Blockage of lymphatic channels causes the characteristic skin dimpling.

    d. Breast cancer rarely metastasizes to distant sites by seeding.

30. Identify the common sites where breast cancer metastasizes.

    a. _____

    b. _____

    c. _____

    d. _____

31. Compared with breast cancer in women, breast cancer in men

    a. has a similar incidence rate

    b. results in similar symptoms

    c. has a poorer prognosis

    d. is treated only with a mastectomy

32. Risk of breast cancer is greatest in women

    a. with a familial history of breast cancer

    b. who are between the ages of 45 and 50 years

    c. who have had multiple pregnancies

    d. with over-sized breasts

33. List the subjective client data relevant to breast cancer. Use a separate sheet.

34. List the two major psychosocial issues faced by women with breast cancer.

    a. _____

    b. _____

35. List the areas of distress that contribute to psychosexual morbidity of clients with breast cancer and give an example of each.

    a. _____

    b. _____

    c. _____

36. List the objective client data relevant to breast cancer. Use a separate sheet.

37. The most sensitive screening procedure to detect breast cancer is

    a. ultrasonography

    b. mammography

    c. chest radiography

    d. thermography

38. Which of the following indicates a better prognosis for a woman with breast cancer? Involvement of

    a. the supraclavicular node

    b. the infraclavicular node

    c. three axillary nodes

    d. none of the nodes

39. Breast tumors that respond best to adjuvant therapy are those that are

    a. estrogen-receptor positive

    b. estrogen-receptor negative

    c. poorly differentiated

    d. locally infiltrating

40. List the nursing diagnoses common to clients with breast cancer.

    a. _____

    _____

    _____

    b. _____

    _____

    _____

41. Which of the following statements is correct about anxiety expressed by the women who have a breast lump?

    a. Many women have no intuitive feelings about the potential diagnosis.

    b. The probability that a lesion is cancerous is irrelevant to the level of fear experienced.

    c. Acceptance of the diagnosis of cancer is easy, especially if a women feels well otherwise.

    d. Clients and their families react to a diagnosis of breast cancer in predictable ways.

42. List items about which the client who is having a mastectomy should be knowledgeable (in addition to basic perioperative information).

    a. _____

    _____

b. _____

_____

c. _____

_____

d. _____

_____

e. _____

_____

f. _____

_____

43. Briefly describe the surgical difference between a radical-radical and a modified-radical mastectomy.

_____

_____

_____

44. List procedures that should be avoided postoperatively in the arm on the operative side of the client who has had a mastectomy.

    a. _____

    _____

    b. _____

    _____

    c. _____

    _____

45. Following a mastectomy, the client should be encouraged to exercise the arm on the operative side by doing which of the following?

    a. flex and extend the fingers and wrist of the operative side periodically

    b. circumduct the arm on the operative side at the shoulder periodically

    c. position the arm on the operative side with the elbow flexed and shoulder adducted

    d. position the arm on the operative side so that it is dependent and in straight alignment

46. The client who is having breast reconstruction should be informed that

    a. the reconstructed breast will be identical to the natural remaining breast

    b. optimum appearance will occur within 3–6 months of surgery

    c. usual daily activities may be resumed as soon as the client feels ready

    d. she may sleep in any position that is most comfortable for her

47. Interventions to promote a positive body image following a mastectomy include encouraging the client to

    a. discuss the effects of her breast loss on herself and others

    b. discouraging visitors from coming and to take no phone calls

    c. obtain a permanent prosthesis as soon as she is dismissed from the hospital

    d. arrange for reconstructive surgery after determining that tumor recurrence is minimal

48. List factors that are considered when determining whether to initiate adjuvant therapy following surgery for breast cancer.

    a. _____

    b. _____

    c. _____

    d. _____

    e. _____

    f. _____

49. Identify two purposes of adjuvant therapy for breast cancer.

    a. _____

    _____

    _____

    b. _____

    _____

    _____

50. Treatment of estrogen-dependent breast tumors includes

    a. medroxyprogesterone (Provera)

    b. diethylstilbestrol (DES)

    c. tamoxifen (Nolvadex)

    d. clomiphene (Clomid)

51. Discharge plans for the client following a mastectomy include

    a. modifying the home environment to allow for increased mobility

    b. minimizing activities that involve reaching for lightweight objects

    c. wearing an underwire brassiere for its maximal support and comfort

    d. having a soft breast form to wear with a loose fitting brassiere

CRITICAL THINKING

Case Study: Breast Cancer

C. W. is a 34-year-old woman who was admitted to the nursing unit following a modified-radical mastectomy. The evening following the operation, her vital signs are stable and she seems to be recovering from the effects of the operation and anesthetic. The tumor was found to be an infiltrating ductal carcinoma.

Address the following questions:

1. Is this tumor a common or uncommon type of breast cancer?

2. What symptoms in the breast might indicate, even before surgery, that the tumor was in an advanced state?

The following morning the nurse is caring for C. W. when the surgeon makes morning rounds. He explains that, as was expected, her breast did need to be completely removed, but he is fairly sure that all of the tumor was removed during the operation. He answered her questions about future care.

3. After the surgeon leaves, C. W. says to the nurse, "Why did I wait so long to schedule that mammogram? Maybe I wouldn't have needed to lose a breast." How should the nurse respond?

4. What precautions are required for her arm on the operative side? Can she lie on that side?

During the course of the day, C. W. relates how she went in for a mammogram on Tuesday and by Thursday she has had her operation. "It all happened so fast," she says. "I hope this is all just a dream and I will wake up soon." Then she cries.

5. How should the nurse respond? Are these later comments expected or are they indicative of an early coping problem? What nursing diagnoses can be formulated?

6. The next day C. W. asks the nurse what she "did" to get this cancer. What additional data might the nurse assess before replying?

7. C. W.'s pathological reports return and indicate that the tumor was 4.5 cm, with involvement of six axillary nodes, but no supraclavicular or infraclavicular nodes were evident in the specimen. Using the chart in the textbook, at what stage is C. W.'s breast cancer? What can the nurse expect to be the prescribed course of therapy for her?

8. When C. W. sees the oncologist, she becomes very upset and cries almost continuously, "I thought they got it all! Am I going to die?" She also talks a lot about her two daughters at home, ages 5 and 3 years. "I won't live to see them grow up!" Is her response normal? Therapeutic? Nontherapeutic? What facts may be helpful for C. W. to know? What would be wrong to say to her at this point?

9. C. W. has the dressings removed and looks at her wound for the first time. She says nothing to the nurse about the appearance of her chest and turns her head to the other side during later wound assessments. Should the nurse try to get her to look at the wound?

10. Saturday, C. W. glances again at her chest and says, "My husband will never want me now! I am deformed!" What response from the nurse would be therapeutic?

11. On Sunday morning the surgeon tells C. W. that she will be going home Monday. She has expressed acceptance of the plans for adjuvant therapy and asks about breast reconstruction. What information could the nurse share with her at this time? When would she be a candidate for surgery? Would reconstruction impair her ability to undergo adjuvant treatment? Would it guarantee that her husband would "want" her again?

12. Should the nurse encourage her to have regularly scheduled mammography on the remaining breast? Why or why not?

CHAPTER 75

Interventions for Clients with Gynecologic Problems

LEARNING OBJECTIVES

At the end of this chapter, the student will be able to

- Discuss problems related to menstruation
- Discuss endometriosis
- Manage care for the client with endometriosis
- Discuss dysfunctional uterine bleeding (DUB)
- Manage care for the client with DUB
- Discuss inflammatory and infectious conditions of the vagina
- Discuss cervicitis and vulvitis
- Discuss toxic shock syndrome (TSS)
- Discuss uterine displacement
- Discuss fistulas involving the female reproductive tract
- Discuss ovarian cysts
- Discuss the pathophysiology, etiology, and incidence of uterine leiomyomas
- Manage care of the client with uterine leiomyomas
- Discuss Bartholin cysts
- Discuss cervical polyps
- Discuss the pathophysiology, etiology, and incidence of endometrial cancer
- Provide care for the client with endometrial cancer
- Discuss the pathophysiology, etiology, and incidence of cervical cancer
- Manage care for the client with cervical cancer
- Discuss the pathophysiology, etiology, and incidence of ovarian cancer
- Manage care of the client with ovarian cancer
- Discuss vulvar cancer
- Describe management of the client with vulvar cancer
- Discuss vaginal and fallopian tube cancer

PREREQUISITE KNOWLEDGE

Prior to beginning this chapter, the student should review

- The anatomy and physiology of the female reproductive system
- The effects of the endocrine system on the female reproductive system
- The concept of human sexuality
- The concepts of body image and self-esteem
- The concepts of grief, loss, death, and dying
- Normal human growth and development
- Perineal care
- Sitz baths
- Enema administration
- Care of the client undergoing chemotherapy and radiation therapy
- The principles of perioperative nursing management

STUDY QUESTIONS

Menstrual Cycle Disorders

Match the following menstrual cycle disorders (1–6) with their descriptions (a–f).

_____ 1. amenorrhea

_____ 2. dysfunctional uterine bleeding (DUB)

_____ 3. dysmenorrhea

_____ 4. endometriosis

_____ 5. postmenopausal bleeding

_____ 6. premenstrual syndrome (PMS)

a. painful menstrual flow

b. collection of symptoms occurring during luteal phase each month

c. absence of menstrual periods

d. vaginal bleeding 12 months after menses cease and menopause

e. uterine tissue implant outside the uterus

f. excessive or abnormal bleeding in amount or frequency

7. Which of the following statements is correct about primary dysmenorrhea?

a. Symptoms become more severe in multigravida women.

b. It is associated with an underlying pelvic pathology.

c. Spasmodic lower abdominal pain begins with menses onset.

d. The probable cause is endometrial prostaglandin deficit.

8. Management of primary dysmenorrhea includes

a. withdrawal from oral contraceptive medications

b. increasing dietary intake of sodium and vitamin C

c. reducing activity and elevating lower extremities

d. taking prostaglandin synthetase inhibitors (ibuprofen)

9. Which of the following statements is correct about PMS?

a. Severity of symptoms tends to increase over time.

b. Symptoms are predictable and similar in most women.

c. Diagnosis is confirmed with objective laboratory tests.

d. Although PMS causes discomfort, activities are usually not affected.

10. Management of PMS focuses on

a. stimulating ovulation to occur

b. initiating estrogen replacement therapy

c. limiting intake of caffeine, sugar, and alcohol

d. supplementing the diet with vitamin C and zinc

11. Which of the following statements about amenorrhea is correct?

a. A common cause is pregnancy.

b. It usually does not affect fertility.

c. Most women are relieved not to have regular menses.

d. Surgical intervention is the first line of treatment.

12. Which of the following statements is correct about postmenopausal bleeding?

a. Its occurrence signifies gynecological cancer in 50% of cases.

b. Exploratory surgery is required to confirm a diagnosis and plan treatment.

c. Cervical polyps are a precursor to endometrial cancer and should be surgically removed.

d. All women should be counseled that any postmenopausal bleeding should be evaluated.

13. Which of the following statements is correct about endometriosis?

a. It often progresses to endometrial cancer.

b. Implants produce hormones that mimic the ovaries.

c. Trapped hematomas cause scarring and adhesions.

d. There is no known familial tendency of occurrence.

14. Symptoms reported by women with endometriosis include

a. melena

b. amenorrhea

c. dyspareunia

d. constipation

15. Management of endometriosis includes

a. ice pack application to the abdomen during menses

b. medicated douches during the menstrual flow

c. continuous high-dose oral estrogen therapy

d. surgical removal of endometrial implants

16. Discuss the disadvantages of treating endometriosis with danazol (Danocrine).

_____

_____

_____

17. Which of the following statements is correct about DUB?

    a. Bleeding often results from vaginal dysfunction.

    b. A breakdown of hormonal events and imbalances occur.

    c. Episodes tend to occur during the reproductive years.

    d. It can be prevented by pregnancy or oral contraceptives.

18. List the subjective client data relevant to DUB. Use a separate sheet.

19. List the objective client data relevant to DUB. Use a separate sheet.

20. Identify the drugs used for hormonal management of DUB.

    a. _____

    b. _____

    c. _____

    d. _____

21. The client who is taking oral contraceptives should also take vitamin

    a. B_2

    b. B_6

    c. C

    d. K

22. Preparation for a dilation and curette (D & C) includes

    a. perineal shave

    b. vaginal douche

    c. enemas until clear

    d. bladder catheterization

    e. none of the above

23. Instructions for the client who has had a D & C include

    a. avoiding sexual intercourse for 1 week postoperatively

    b. taking oral opioid analgesics for several days

    c. soaking in a warm tub bath 20 minutes daily

    d. reporting bleeding lasting more than 2 weeks

Inflammation and Infections

Match the following problems of the female reproductive tract (24–31) with their descriptions (a–h).

_____ 24. atrophic vaginitis

_____ 25. _Candida albicans_

_____ 26. cervicitis

_____ 27. _Gardnerella vaginalis_

_____ 28. simple vaginitis

_____ 29. toxic shock syndrome

_____ 30. _Trichomonas vaginalis_

_____ 31. vulvitis

a. causes a gray-white discharge with fishy odor

b. dry vaginal mucosa seen in post-menopausal women

c. inflammation of vulva

d. fungus causing odorless, cottage cheese–like vaginal discharge

e. infection of endo-cervix

f. parasitic protozoa causing green-yellow vaginal discharge

g. caused by _Staphylococcus aureus_ and related to tampon use

h. inflammation of lower genital tract

32. Identify hygienic practices that are recommended for simple vaginitis and vulvitis.

    a. _____

    _____

    _____

    b. _____

    _____

    _____

    c. _____

    _____

    _____

    d. _____

    _____

    _____

Pelvic Support Problems

Match the following pelvic support problems (33–37) with their descriptions (a–e).

_____ 33. cystocele

_____ 34. fistula

_____ 35. rectocele

_____ 36. uterine displacement

_____ 37. uterine prolapse

a. variation of cervix and uterus from usual location

b. various grades of the uterus falling through the vagina

c. abnormal opening between two adjacent structures

d. protrusion of bladder through the vaginal wall

e. protrusion of rectum through the vaginal wall

38. Surgical treatment of the client with a rectocele and a cystocele includes

a. anterior colporrhaphy

b. posterior colporrhaphy

c. abdominal hysterectomy

d. anteroposterior colporrhaphy

Benign Neoplasms

Match the following types of benign ovarian cysts (39–45) with their descriptions (a–g).

_____ 39. corpus luteum cyst

_____ 40. cystadenoma

_____ 41. dermoid cyst

_____ 42. fibroma

_____ 43. follicular cyst

_____ 44. polycystic ovaries

_____ 45. theca-lutein cyst

a. seen with elevated levels of luteinizing hormone

b. associated with increased progesterone secretion

c. connective tissue tumor

d. mature follicle fails to rupture or immature follicle fails to reabsorb

e. result of prolonged stimulation by human chorionic gonadotropin

f. benign germ cell tumor

g. epithelial ovarian tumor

46. List the interventions for benign ovarian masses.

a. _____

b. _____

c. _____

d. _____

_____

e. _____

_____

47. Which of the following statements is correct about leiomyomas?

a. They usually develop from the endometrium.

b. Leiomyomas are the most common pelvic tumors.

c. Tumor growth is related to progesterone stimulation.

d. Incidence of leiomyoma is highest in Caucasian women.

48. Common findings on assessment of the client with a leiomyoma include

a. dyspareunia and fertility

b. pelvic pressure and diarrhea

c. abnormal bleeding and diarrhea

d. abnormal bleeding and pelvic pressure

Match the following surgical procedures (49–51) with their definitions (a–c).

_____ 49. hysterectomy

_____ 50. myomectomy

_____ 51. oophorectomy

a. local removal of leiomyomas with preservation of the uterus

b. removal of the uterus

c. removal of the ovaries

52. Discharge teaching of a client following vaginal hysterectomy includes

a. advising that warm tub baths may be relaxing

b. reassuring that feelings of depression are uncommon

c. teaching that strenuous physical activity is inadvisable

d. counseling that sexual intercourse can be resumed at anytime

53. Which of the following statements is correct about Bartholin's cysts?

    a. A large cyst may cause difficulty walking or sitting.

    b. Swelling is under the skin anteriorly on the vulva.

    c. These cysts are usually treated even if asymptomatic.

    d. Postoperative management includes avoiding tub baths.

54. Management of Bartholin's abscess includes

    a. encouraging moderate upright activity for drainage

    b. applying cold packs to the vulva to reduce swelling

    c. obtaining a culture of any drainage for analysis

    d. having the client wear support briefs to reduce skin irritation

55. Which of the following statements is correct about cervical polyps?

    a. Cervical polyps are most common in nulliparous women.

    b. Surgical removal is performed using local anesthesia.

    c. Tampons are used as pressure dressings after surgery.

    d. Postoperative douching removes accumulated debris.

Malignant Neoplasms

56. Which of the following statements about endometrial cancer is correct?

    a. It is the least frequently occurring reproductive cancer.

    b. The tumor grows rapidly and thus has a poor prognosis.

    c. The Papanicolaou test is only about 25% effective for detection.

    d. Risk factors include obesity, nulliparity, and sterility.

57. Estrogen replacement therapy may increase a woman's risk of developing endometrial cancer. The client on estrogen replacement therapy should

    a. take the highest effective dose possible

    b. take the medication daily for maximum benefit

    c. include a progesterone agent as part of the therapy

    d. have appointments for breast examinations twice a year

58. List the subjective client data relevant to endometrial cancer. Use a separate sheet.

59. List the objective client data relevant to endometrial cancer. Use a separate sheet.

60. Which organs are examined and which radiographic tests are used to determine whether metastases from the uterus have occurred?

    a. _____

    _____

    b. _____

    _____

    c. _____

    _____

    d. _____

    _____

    e. _____

    _____

    f. _____

    _____

    _____

61. List the common nursing diagnoses for the client with endometrial cancer.

    a. _____

    _____

    b. _____

    _____

62. Discuss why the radiologist does not insert a radioactive isotope into a uterine applicator until after the client has returned to her room postoperatively. Use a separate sheet.

63. Preoperative preparation of the client who is to have insertion of an intrauterine radioactive isotope includes

    a. instruction about deep breathing and coughing

    b. demonstrating leg exercises such as bicycling

    c. explaining why a bedside commode must be used

    d. applying thigh-length antiembolic stockings

64. List the types of drug agents administered to the client who has an intrauterine radioactive isotope in place.

    a. _____

    b. _____

    c. _____

    d. _____

    e. _____

    f. _____

65. Postoperative interventions for the client with an intrauterine radioactive isotope include

    a. routinely administering an antidiarrheal drug to prevent bowel movements

    b. a high-residue diet to avoid constipation and accidental dislodgement of the isotope

    c. restricting fluids to decrease the number of times the client must get up to void

    d. encouraging the client to have visitors to help pass the time and prevent boredom

66. Side effects of the antiestrogen agent tamoxifen citrate (Nolvadex) include

    a. hypocalcemia

    b. corneal opacity

    c. chilling and fever

    d. restlessness and anxiety

67. Hot flashes are caused by

    a. hormonal stimulation of the sympathetic nervous system

    b. overreaction of the ovaries in producing progesterone

    c. decreased production of pituitary gonadotropins

    d. overstimulation of the adrenal medulla

68. Which of the following procedures results in surgically induced menopause?

    a. tubal ligation

    b. panhysterectomy

    c. total hysterectomy

    d. bilateral salpingectomy

69. A 36-year-old client who is 3 months pregnant is scheduled for an exploratory abdominal laparotomy. She has had three previous miscarriages. She is informed that there are many risks involving this surgery. She signs the operative permit for exploratory laparotomy. During surgery, endometrial cancer is found and the surgeon performs a panhysterectomy. When the client is told that her uterus was removed, she

calls her lawyer and files a lawsuit against the surgeon, the hospital, and the nurse who witnessed the operative permit. The legal decision in this situation will be based on the fact that

    a. the surgeon had a legal right to remove the uterus to do what was in the client's best interest

    b. consent for exploratory surgery implies permission for removing diseased organs if they are life threatening

    c. general consent forms signed by a client on admission give consent for extenuating circumstances

    d. the client received inadequate information preoperatively and was unable to give an informed consent

70. Following radiation treatment for endometrial cancer, the client should be instructed to

    a. use a contraceptive method to prevent pregnancy and any further complications

    b. continue on a low-residue diet to reduce irritation to the rectogenital area

    c. advise her sexual partner to use a condom to prevent penile irritation from the radiation

    d. use a dilator and water-soluble lubricant to help stretch the vagina prior to resuming intercourse

Match the following terms related to cervical cancer (71–74) with their descriptions (a–d).

____ 71. carcinoma in situ

____ 72. dysplasia

____ 73. invasive

____ 74. preinvasive

    a. earliest premalignant change

    b. limited to the cervix

    c. in cervix and other pelvic structures

    d. most advanced premalignant change

75. Which of the following are risk factors associated with squamous cell cervical cancer?

    a. early sexual activity and multiple sex partners

    b. venereal disease and vitamin E deficiency

    c. nulliparity and cigarette smoking

    d. Caucasian and late marriage

76. A woman 40 years or older should have a Papanicolaou smear done

    a. only if she is sexually active

    b. every year following a hysterectomy

    c. along with a pelvic examination once a year

    d. every 3 years if negative for 3 consecutive years

77. If a Papanicolaou smear report is abnormal, the next step in evaluating the client for cervical cancer is

   a. an endocervical curettage

   b. a repeat Papanicolaou smear

   c. a colposcopy

   d. a conization

78. Which of the following surgical procedures is the most disruptive to the client's body image and self-concept?

   a. radical hysterectomy

   b. pelvic exenteration

   c. laser therapy

   d. cryosurgery

79. Which of the following statements is correct about the client who has a pelvic exenteration?

   a. The client should be permitted to chose the location of the stoma sites.

   b. Postoperative depression, denial, hostility, and anger often occur.

   c. The client may resume vaginal intercourse once all the tissues heal.

   d. Sexual counseling is not indicated for the unmarried, older client.

80. Which of the following statements is correct about ovarian cancer?

   a. Ovarian cancer is leading cause of mortality in female reproductive malignancies.

   b. Ovarian tumors grow slowly, are unilateral, and have a good prognosis for recovery.

   c. Risk factors include a high dietary fat intake such as omega-3 fatty acids.

   d. The best means of prevention is the surgical removal of ovaries prior to tumor formation.

81. Diagnosis of an ovarian tumor is by

   a. pelvic examination

   b. CA-125 analysis

   c. exploratory surgery

   d. Papanicolaou smear

82. Surgical management of ovarian cancer consists of

   a. pelvic exenteration

   b. bilateral oophorectomy

   c. intraperitoneal chemotherapy instillation

   d. total hysterectomy with salpingo-oophorectomy

83. Define *second-look procedure*.

   _____

   _____

   _____

84. Which of the following statements is correct about vulvar cancer?

   a. This type of cancer grows rapidly.

   b. It may spread directly to the uterus.

   c. Its causes include sexually transmitted diseases.

   d. Premalignant changes may occur between the ages of 20 and 30 years.

85. Physical examination of the client with vulvar cancer will reveal

   a. labial lesions filled with yellow-green exudate

   b. severe labial and perineal excoriation

   c. white, pinpoint lesions near the introitus

   d. multifocal white-red labial lesions

86. Which structures are removed in a radical vulvectomy that are left intact in a simple vulvectomy?

   a. vulvar skin and clitoris

   b. labia majora and minora

   c. inguinal and femoral nodes

   d. urethra and clitoris

87. Discomfort during sexual intercourse following a vulvectomy can be minimized by the couple

   a. using a side-lying position

   b. starting with the woman on top

   c. using a vibrator for arousal

   d. using the "missionary position"

88. Chronic leg edema following a radical vulvectomy may be minimized by

   a. avoiding standing and walking

   b. wearing support panty hose

   c. applying vitamin E oil daily

   d. taking a diuretic daily

89. Which of the following statements is correct about vaginal cancer?

   a. Most tumors develop in the lower part of the vagina.

   b. Adenocarcinoma is linked with intrauterine diethylstilbestrol exposure.

   c. Metastases tend to occur late in the disease process.

   d. Early symptoms include a foul-smelling vaginal discharge.

90. List the predisposing factors associated with the development of vaginal cancer.

a. _____

_____

_____

b. _____

_____

_____

c. _____

_____

_____

91. Interventions for the client being treated for vaginal cancer nonsurgically include

a. a Papanicolaou smear and colposcopic examination every 3 months

b. daily application of 5-fluorouracil cream to the vulva

c. external radiation therapy used alone

d. laser therapy for early-stage tumors

92. Fallopian tube cancer

a. is the rarest form of gynecological cancer

b. most often begins as a primary tumor

c. presents with easily recognizable symptoms

d. is caused by chronic salpingitis

CRITICAL THINKING EXERCISES

Case Study: Dilatation and Curettage (D & C)

E. H. is a 48-year-old woman with dysfunctional uterine bleeding (DUB). She has one 26-year-old daughter, and she reports no other pregnancies. E. H. and her husband both work in a small town. She used oral contraceptives for 6 years before undergoing a tubal ligation.

Address the following questions:

1. What subjective data should the nurse collect from E. H.?

2. Identify data that should be collected during the physical examination.

3. E. H. states that she had a colectomy 2 years ago for a malignant tumor. What diagnostic testing would probably be indicated in determining the cause of E. H.'s DUB?

4. After laboratory and x-ray test results return negative, an outpatient D & C is scheduled. Develop a perioperative teaching/learning plan for E. H. and her husband.

5. Following the procedure, E. H. is returned to the outpatient unit. What assessments should the nurse make?

6. E. H. is scheduled for discharge. Provide discharge instructions for her.

Since the D & C and endometrial biopsy results were negative, the physician tells E. H. that surgery may correct the DUB. If not, hormonal therapy will be prescribed. E. H. asks the nurse, "What does the doctor mean by hormonal therapy? I've heard that estrogen therapy increases the risk of getting cancer."

7. How should the nurse respond?

Case Study: Leiomyoma and Hysterectomy

M. T. is a 42-year-old woman who has had multiple leiomyomas that have been conservatively managed for the past 5 years. In the past 4 months, she has become anemic from the excessive bleeding. M. T. and her husband have three children and are happy with their family. Although M. T. fears losing her femininity, she agrees to have a hysterectomy.

Address the following questions:

1. Develop a perioperative teaching/learning plan for M. T. and her family.

2. What can the nurse do to help M. T. cope with the loss of her uterus?

3. The leiomyomas have enlarged the uterus to the size of a 16-week pregnancy. Which type of hysterectomy will M. T. have performed? Discuss why this procedure is indicated.

4. What should the preoperative preparation for M. T. include?

5. Beside the routine postoperative care for a client having abdominal surgery, what specific interventions are indicated for M. T.?

6. Identify postoperative interventions that would minimize the development of complications for M. T.

7. M. T.'s recovery is uncomplicated and she is scheduled to be dismissed to home care. Develop a discharge teaching/learning plan.

8. M. T. is an elementary school teacher and asks when she can return to work. How should the nurse respond?

9. M. T. states that she cannot wait to get home and relax in her hot tub. What should the nurse discuss with M. T. about this?

CHAPTER 76

Interventions for Male Clients with Reproductive Problems

LEARNING OBJECTIVES

At the end of this chapter, the student will be able to

▌ Discuss the pathophysiology, etiology, and incidence of benign prostatic hyperplasia (BPH)

▌ Manage care for the client with BPH

▌ Discuss cancer of the prostate

▌ Manage care of the client with cancer of the prostate

▌ Discuss impotence

▌ Describe management of the client with erectile impotence

▌ Discuss the pathophysiology, etiology, and incidence of testicular cancer

▌ Discuss management of the client with testicular cancer

▌ Identify other problems affecting the testes and adjacent structures

▌ Describe problems of the penis

▌ List infections of the male genitoreproductive system

PREREQUISITE KNOWLEDGE

Prior to beginning this chapter, the student should review

▌ The anatomy and physiology of the male genito-reproductive system

▌ The effects of the endocrine system on the male reproductive tissue

▌ Normal growth and development

▌ The concept of human sexuality

▌ The concepts of body image and self-esteem

▌ The concepts of grief, loss, death, and dying

▌ Perineal care

▌ Sitz baths

▌ Enema administration

▌ Care of the client undergoing chemotherapy and radiation therapy

▌ The principles of perioperative nursing management

STUDY QUESTIONS

Benign Prostatic Hyperplasia

1. Prostatic hyperplasia arises from the
   a. bladder neck
   b. glandular tissue
   c. prostatic capsule
   d. prostatic urethra

2. *Hyperplasia* means
   a. containing abnormal cells
   b. enlargement in the size of cells
   c. proliferation of interstitial cells
   d. an increased number of normal cells

3. List the subjective client data relevant to benign prostatic hyperplasia (BPH). Use a separate sheet.

4. The nurse should suspect BPH when a client voices which of the following symptoms?
   a. hesitancy, postvoid dribbling, nocturia
   b. intermittency, dysuria, postvoid dribbling
   c. frequency, dysuria, diminished urine stream force
   d. increased urine stream force, hesitancy, nocturia

5. List the objective client data relevant to BPH. Use a separate sheet.

6. Preparation of the client for a prostate examination includes
   a. explaining that the prostate gland may be palpated during an abdominal examination
   b. assisting the client to a knee-chest position or having him bend over the examining table
   c. explaining that the prostate gland will be massaged gently if a mass is felt
   d. instructing the client to bear down and push while gland is palpated

7. The extent of urinary obstruction by prostatic enlargement is determined by
   a. a cystogram
   b. a cystometrogram
   c. rectal examination
   d. flow rate analysis

8. Identify the common nursing diagnosis for the client with BPH.

   _____

   _____

   _____

9. Nonsurgical management of BPH includes
   a. taking a prescribed diuretic agent
   b. doing Kegel exercises with each voiding
   c. engaging in frequent sexual intercourse
   d. drinking 3000–4000 mL of fluids per day

Match the following characteristics (10–23) with their surgical approaches for prostatectomy (a–d). Answers may be used more than once and more than one answer may apply to each.

_____ 10. bladder problems treated simultaneously

_____ 11. greatest risk of postoperative infection

_____ 12. low abdominal incision

_____ 13. medical lobe enlargement

_____ 14. no bladder problems but prostate large

_____ 15. possible regrowth of prostate tissue

_____ 16. potential urethral trauma

_____ 17. prostate enucleation via bladder incision

_____ 18. prostatic calculi, abscess

_____ 19. pudendal nerve damage

_____ 20. repair of lacerated prostate capsule

_____ 21. resectoscope used

_____ 22. short hospital stay

_____ 23. suprapubic tube used postoperatively

a. transurethral resection of prostate (TURP)

b. suprapubic (travesical) prostatectomy

c. Retropubic (extravesical) prostatectomy

d. perineal prostatectomy

24. List the major preoperative concerns often expressed by a client who is to have a prostatectomy.

   a. _____

   _____

   _____

   b. _____

   _____

25. Preoperative instructions for the client who is to have a prostatectomy include explaining

    a. the need to use a urinal or bedside commode for urination immediately after surgery

    b. that an in-dwelling catheter will be in place and will drain blood-tinged urine

    c. that the client's urine should be clear and light amber in color following surgery

    d. that the client should not have to a continual urge to urinate while the catheter is in place

26. Following a TURP, the client has a continuous bladder irrigation (CBI). When checked, the catheter drainage tubing is full of thick, bright red clots and tissue shreds. The nurse should

    a. clamp the drainage tube and take the client's pulse and blood pressure

    b. irrigate the catheter until clear and increase the flow rate of the intravenous infusion

    c. irrigate the catheter until clear and take the client's vital signs

    d. clamp the drainage tube and notify the physician of the bleeding

27. A client with CBI reports feeling the urge to urinate. Which of the following should be the nurse's first action?

    a. remove the traction on the catheter

    b. empty the drainage collection bag

    c. assist the client with a bedpan

    d. assess the patency of the catheter

28. A client with CBI asks the nurse to check the catheter for leaks; he tells the nurse that his leg is wet. The sheet under the client's buttocks is saturated with pink-tinged urine. The nurse should further assess for

    a. urinary tract infection

    b. autonomic dysreflexia

    c. bladder spasms

    d. atonic bladder

29. The clients who has had a suprapubic prostatectomy and has postoperative bleeding will need

    a. frequent irrigation by hand of the Foley catheter

    b. continuous gravity irrigation via the Foley catheter

    c. gentle gravity irrigation of the suprapubic catheter

    d. brisk continuous irrigation via the suprapubic catheter

30. Which of the following medications is prescribed to alleviate bladder spasms after prostatectomy?

    a. meperidine hydrochloride (Demerol)

    b. belladonna and opium (B and O) suppositories

    c. docusate sodium (Colace)

    d. sulfamethoxazole-trimenthoprim (Bactrim)

31. Discharge instructions for the client who has had a prostatectomy include telling the client to

    a. drink 12–14 cups of liquid each day, including soft drinks, coffee, tea, and water

    b. resume activities such as driving the car, taking long walks, and golfing as soon as the client feels up to it

    c. expect that there may be some blood in the urine but it should subside with rest and more fluids

    d. plan on returning to work after a 6-week recovery period at home with restricted activity

Prostate Cancer

32. Prostate cancer is

    a. inhibited by the administration of androgens

    b. associated with recurrent prostatitis

    c. a rapidly growing and aggressive tumor

    d. more common in men over the age of 50 years

33. One of the earliest symptoms that a client with prostatic cancer may have is

    a. recurrent bladder infections

    b. hydronephrosis

    c. bone pain

    d. painful urination

34. The most frequently occurring complication from radical perineal prostatectomy is

    a. priapism

    b. impotence

    c. phimosis

    d. nocturia

35. List the types of hormones used in the management of prostate cancer.

    a. _____

    _____

    b. _____

    _____

Impotence

36. Which of the following statements is correct about impotence?

    a. It has a psychological cause 90% of the time.

    b. It is experienced by most men at least once in their lives.

    c. It has an underlying physical cause about 75% of the time.

    d. It is an inevitable consequence of the aging process.

37. List the psychological factors contributing to impotence.

    a. _____

    _____

    b. _____

    _____

    c. _____

    _____

    d. _____

    _____

    e. _____

    _____

    f. _____

    _____

38. List the physiological factors contributing to impotence and give an example of each.

    a. _____

    _____

    b. _____

    _____

    c. _____

    _____

    d. _____

    _____

    _____

39. List the subjective client data relevant to impotence. Use a separate sheet.

40. Complete the following chart by comparing the subjective data typical of psychological impotence with those typical of physical impotence. Use a separate sheet.

	Psychological	Physical
a. onset		
b. erectile ability		
c. nocturnal erections and emissions		
d. sexual desire, interest, libido		
e. testicular sensitivity		

41. Which the following is *not* associated with male impotence?

    a. Alzheimer's disease

    b. multiple sclerosis

    c. chronic alcoholism

    d. migraine headaches

42. Which of the following medications can render a man impotent?

    a. testosterone

    b. ampicillin

    c. methyldopa

    d. pyridium

43. List the objective client data relevant to impotence.

    _____

    _____

    _____

44. In relationship to systemic systolic blood pressure, penile systolic blood pressure should be

    a. greater

    b. less

    c. equal

45. Which of the following statements is correct about nocturnal erections?

    a. Nocturnal erections occur randomly throughout the night.

    b. Normal men have one or two erections per night.

    c. Each nocturnal erection lasts approximately 10 minutes.

    d. Nocturnal erections closely parallel rapid eye movement (REM) sleep cycles.

46. Postoperative care for the client who has a penile implant includes

    a. observing for urinary incontinence

    b. applying ice packs to the scrotum and penis

    c. inflating the prosthesis every 4 hours

    d. measuring penile systolic blood pressure daily

47. Discharge instructions for the client who has had a penile implant include

    a. advising him that he will continue to have some pain or discomfort once he has returned home

    b. suggesting that the penis and incision be exposed to the air several times during the day to promote healing

    c. informing him that mild activity such as playing golf is permissible after the first week postoperatively

    d. telling him to stay home from work for about 6 weeks until the incision has healed

Testicular Cancer

48. Which of the following statements is correct about testicular cancer?

    a. Incidence is higher in men with cryptorchidism.

    b. This type of cancer represents 30% of all male cancers.

    c. Incidence is highest in men over the age of 40 years.

    d. Primary testicular cancer often occurs bilaterally.

49. Nurses can promote early detection of testicular cancer by

    a. instructing wives and girlfriends in how to perform testicular examination on their partners

    b. promoting local education and screening programs in school systems, boys' and mens' clubs, and the military

    c. performing a complete physical examination, including a testicular examination, on each male client

    d. encouraging all male clients to have baseline radiography of the testes at age 18 and yearly thereafter

50. List the subjective client data relevant to testicular cancer. Use a separate sheet.

51. List the objective client data relevant to testicular cancer. Use a separate sheet.

52. Serum laboratory tests commonly performed in the client with testicular cancer include

    a. acid phosphatase measurement

    b. alpha fetoprotein measurement

    c. alkaline phosphatase measurement

    d. alpha human chorionic gonadotropin measurement

53. Preoperative care of the client with testicular cancer includes

    a. reassuring the client that the various treatments rarely result in sterility

    b. discussing the option of sperm banking in case future offspring are desired

    c. informing the client that testicular implants are not recommended in most cases

    d. telling the client that the loss of one testis is unimportant and that the second testis will make up for it

54. When retroperitoneal lymph node dissection for testicular cancer is required, the client should be informed that

    a. he may have two incisions

    b. the surgery will last about 2–6 hours

    c. he will return to his room postoperatively

    d. his ability to experience orgasm should remain

Other Problems Affecting Male Reproductive Structures

Match the following terms related to the male reproductive system (55–64) with their descriptions (a–j).

_____ 55. cryptorchidism

_____ 56. epididymitis

_____ 57. hydrocele

_____ 58. orchitis

_____ 59. phimosis

_____ 60. priapism

_____ 61. prostatitis

_____ 62. spermatocele

_____ 63. torsion

_____ 64. varicocele

a. twisting of spermatic cord

b. maintained erection in absence of sexual desire

c. constricted foreskin unable to retract over glans

d. cluster of dilated veins near the testis

e. undescended testis

f. sperm-containing cystic mass

g. acute testicular inflammation

h. cystic fluid-filled mass that forms around testis

i. infection of the epididymis

j. infection of the prostate gland

Match the following terms related to male reproductive surgery (65–71) with their definitions (a–g).

_____ 65. circumcision

_____ 66. hydrocelectomy

_____ 67. orchidopexy

_____ 68. penectomy

_____ 69. spermatocelectomy

_____ 70. varicocelectomy

_____ 71. vasectomy

a. excision of a spermatocele

b. placement of testis into scrotum

c. removal of varicocele

d. removal of prepuce

e. correction of hydrocele

f. ligation of vas deferens

g. partial or total removal of the penis

CRITICAL THINKING EXERCISES

Case Study: Benign Prostatic Hyperplasia (BPH)

P. H. is a 62-year-old man who lives with his wife on a farm. They are both very active with the farming operation. P. H. has BPH, which has been managed nonsurgically for several months. Treatment has been unsuccessful, and P. H. elects to have a transurethral resection of the prostate (TURP) during December so that he will be able to plant spring crops. A son is helping to manage the cattle while P. H. is unable to do so.

Address the following questions:

1. Preadmission testing is scheduled at the local hospital 1 week before the surgery. What diagnostic tests will probably be completed prior to his TURP?

2. What information should the nurse discuss with P. H. and his wife about the surgery, anesthesia (a spinal is planned), the admission procedure the morning of surgery, and the postoperative catheter and urine characteristics?

3. All of P. H.'s preadmission tests are normal and he is admitted to the hospital the morning of surgery. What are the nurse's responsibilities for P. H. at this time?

The surgery is uneventful and P. H. returns to his room with an intravenous infusion of D$_5$W and 1/2 NS with 20 mEq of potassium chloride infusing at a rate of 100 mL per hour. The infusion may be discontinued once P. H. has a sufficient oral intake. There is a three-way Foley catheter with a 30 mL retention balloon connected to a normal saline continuous irrigation. The Foley catheter is to traction. P. H.'s urine is medium cherry-red in color.

4. What assessments should the nurse make postoperatively?

5. What is the purpose of the continuous bladder irrigation?

6. Should the nurse be concerned about the color of the urine?

7. Four hours after P. H. is returned to his room, he begins to report that he has the urge to void. What should the nurse tell him? What is probably causing P. H. to have this urge?

P. H.'s urine continues to change from red to light pink. He requests pain medication. Analgesia orders include acetaminophen with codeine #3 (Tylenol #3), PO, one or two tablets every 2–4 hours as needed, and belladonna and opium (B & O) suppositories, prn, every 8 hours as needed.

8. What should the nurse administer?

9. Should the nurse change the flow rate of the irrigation?

Two hours after being medicated, P. H.'s blood pressure goes up and he reports severe discomfort and cramping in his lower abdomen. Urine output diminishes and clots are noted in the drainage collection bag. Urine color is redder than it was 2 hours ago.

10. What should the nurse do with the three-way irrigation? Which of the analgesics may provide relief from the bladder spasms?

11. What should the nurse do to provide Foley catheter care?

The day after surgery, P. H. gets up to sit in a chair with minimal problems. He is tolerating a regular diet and no longer requires pain medication. His urine is still pink, with the irrigation running very slowly. However, when P. H. is ambulated in his room, the urine becomes red. The physician orders that the three-way irrigation be maintained for one more day. On postoperative day 2, the urine is almost clear and the irrigation is discontinued. The Foley catheter is attached to straight drainage.

12. Discuss why the Foley catheter was probably left in place. How long will the catheter remain in place?

13. If P. H. should pull his catheter out, what should the nurse do?

On postoperative day 4, the Foley catheter is discontinued and P. H. is voiding 150 mL of clear yellow urine every 3–4 hours. He is scheduled for discharge even though he has difficulty with postvoid dribbling.

14. What should the nurse tell P. H. about the dribbling?

15. What should the nurse include in the discharge instructions?

16. How should the nurse respond to a question about impotence?

17. How long will it be before P. H. is able to begin farming fulltime again?

Case Study: Cancer of the Prostate

B. W. is a 72-year-old widowed man who lives alone. He has had symptoms of bladder neck obstruction: hesitancy, urgency, and urinary retention. A TURP was performed and a malignancy was found. B. W. has remained hospitalized for staging of the cancer and a probable perineal prostatectomy.

Address the following questions:

1. What diagnostic tests will probably be performed to determine the staging of B. W.'s disease?

2. B. W.'s serum acid phosphatase and alkaline phosphatase levels are 40 U/dL and 28 U/dL, respectively. What do these levels indicate?

3. A perineal prostatectomy and bilateral simple orchiectomies are planned. What effect will this surgical approach have on B. W.'s sexual functioning?

4. Develop a perioperative teaching/learning plan for B. W.

Following the surgery, B. W. returns to his room with a three-way Foley catheter with a 30-mL balloon tip in place. The catheter is to traction.

5. When assessing B. W., how will the nurse distinguish between arterial and venous bleeding?

6. Why are rectal temperatures and enemas contraindicated postoperatively?

7. What perineal exercises should the nurse instruct B. W. to perform to facilitate the return of urinary continence once the Foley catheter is removed?

8. External beam radiation is planned following B. W.'s discharge from the hospital. Identify measures the nurse can take to facilitate B. W.'s daily trips to the hospital for the therapy.

9. Develop a discharge teaching/learning plan for B. W.

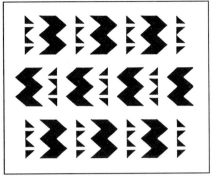

CHAPTER 77

Interventions for Clients with Sexually Transmitted Diseases

LEARNING OBJECTIVES

At the end of this chapter, the student will be able to

▪ Discuss sexually transmitted diseases (STDs) associated with ulcer formation and related management

▪ Discuss condylomata acuminata, gonorrhea, and *Chlamydia trachomatis* infection and related management

▪ Discuss the pathophysiology, etiology, and incidence of pelvic inflammatory disease (PID)

▪ Provide care for the client with PID

PREREQUISITE KNOWLEDGE

Prior to beginning this chapter, the student should review

▪ The anatomy and physiology of the male and female genitoreproductive systems

▪ The principles of infection transmission

▪ The concept of human sexuality

▪ The concepts of body image and self-esteem

▪ Perineal care

▪ The principles of perioperative nursing management

STUDY QUESTIONS

Infections Associated with Ulcers

Match the following causative organisms (1–8) with the diseases they produce (a–h).

_____ 1. *Calymmato-bacterium*

_____ 2. *Chlamydia trachomatis*

_____ 3. *Haemophilus ducreyi*

_____ 4. human papillomavirus

_____ 5. *Neisseria gonorrhoeae*

_____ 6. *Pediculus pubis*

_____ 7. *Sarcoptes scabiei*

_____ 8. *Treponema pallidum*

a. syphilis

b. gonorrhea

c. scabies

d. granuloma inguinale

e. crab lice

f. lymphogranuloma

g. genital warts

h. chancroid

9. Complete the following chart by comparing the stages of syphilis. Use a separate sheet.

	Primary	Secondary	Latent	Late
a. onset				
b. degree of localization				
c. type of infectious lesions				

10. Of the following drugs, which is *not* used in the treatment of syphilis?

   a. benzathine penicillin G

   b. tetracycline

   c. podophyllin

   d. doxycycline

11. The most severe reaction that may occur following an injection of penicillin is

   a. hemorrhage

   b. anaphylaxis

   c. distributive (septic) shock

   d. Jarisch-Herxheimer reaction

12. Which of the following statements is correct about genital herpes?

   a. Type 1 (herpes simplex virus 1, or HSV 1) causes only cold sores.

   b. Type 2 (HSV 2) causes only genital lesions.

   c. Recurrent episodes are usually due to reinfection.

   d. Either type of virus can cause oral or genital lesions.

13. Which of the following statements is correct about genital herpes?

   a. Blisters in the perineal area cause a tingling sensation when they erupt.

   b. Genital herpes can be cured permanently with aggressive acyclovir treatment.

   c. Infected clients are at increased risk for developing cervical cancer and contracting human immunodeficiency virus (HIV).

   d. The virus stays active in nerve ganglia until stimulated by stress, fever, or sexual activity.

14. Identify nursing diagnoses and develop a plan of care for the client with genital herpes. Submit the completed exercise to the clinical instructor.

15. Lymphogranuloma venereum is

   a. becoming an epidemic in the United States

   b. characterized by painful primary lesions

   c. treated with one dose of benzathine penicillin G

   d. associated with complications such as fistulas

16. Which of the following statements is correct about chancroid?

   a. It is rarely seen in tropical or subtropical climates.

   b. It is characterized by an irregular, deep ulcer.

   c. It is treated with one dose of benzanthine penicillin G.

   d. It is another name for syphilis.

17. Which of the following statements is correct about granuloma inguinale. It is

   a. endemic in the United States and Europe

   b. characterized by inguinal node ulcers

   c. treated with one does of benzathine penicillin G

   d. aggravated by pregnancy but not transmitted to the fetus

Infections of Epithelial Surfaces

18. Genital warts are

   a. characterized by some growths that form cauliflower-like masses

   b. associated with pelvic inflammatory disease and infertility

   c. often confused with genital carcinoma

   d. difficult to contract, but hard to cure

19. Treatment of genital warts includes

   a. podophyllin applied internally after protecting the surrounding tissue

   b. cryotherapy performed using general anesthesia on an inpatient basis

   c. biannual Papanicolaou smear and endometrial biopsy for infected female clients

   d. recommending that condoms be used to reduce transmission

20. Symptoms of gonorrhea include all of the following *except*

   a. penile or vaginal discharge

   b. urinary frequency

   c. chancres

   d. dysuria

21. The recommended treatment for penicillin-resistant gonorrhea is

   a. ceftriaxone is a single dose

   b. ceftriaxone plus doxycycline

   c. amoxicillin plus probenecid

   d. doxycycline in a single dose

22. Disseminated (systemic) gonococcal infection includes
    a. meningitis
    b. endocarditis
    c. systemic arthritis
    d. all of the above

23. Safe sexual practices include
    a. using a spermicide as a lubricant
    b. abstinence from all forms of sexual contact
    c. sexual contact with familiar, selected partners
    d. substituting oral-anal for vaginal intercourse

24. Proper use of condoms includes
    a. purchasing multiple-use condoms
    b. applying a condom after emission occurs
    c. leaving space at the tip to collect semen
    d. using petroleum jelly as a lubricant

25. Infection with *Chlamydia trachomatis* is
    a. the second most commonly transmitted bacterial infection in the United States
    b. responsible for 75% of nongonococcal urethritis and epididymitis in men
    c. responsible for about 40% of pelvic inflammatory disease cases
    d. transmitted to the newborn from the mother regardless of delivery method

26. In men, *C. trachomatis* infection results in
    a. urinary retention
    b. watery discharge
    c. hesitancy
    d. pyuria

27. In women, *C. trachomatis* infection results in
    a. foul-smelling green vaginal discharge
    b. markedly elevated temperature
    c. lymphadenopathy
    d. no symptoms

28. List the tests used to confirm a diagnosis of chlamydial infection.

    a. _____

    _____

    b. _____

    _____

c. _____

_____

d. _____

_____

29. The drug of choice to treat chlamydial infection is
    a. gentamicin
    b. clindamycin
    c. doxycycline
    d. erythromycin

Pelvic Inflammatory Disease

30. Briefly discuss pelvic inflammatory disease (PID). Use a separate sheet.

31. Of the following organisms, which is *not* responsible for PID?
    a. *Treponema pallidum*
    b. *Neisseria gonorrhoeae*
    c. *Chlamydia trachomatis*
    d. *Mycoplasma hominis*

32. One risk factor for PID is
    a. being sexually active with multiple partners
    b. using a barrier method for contraception
    c. maintaining celibacy in heterosexual relationships
    d. using a spermicide foam for contraception

33. List the subjective client data relevant to PID. Use a separate sheet.

34. List the objective client data relevant to PID. Use a separate sheet.

35. List nursing diagnoses common to clients with PID.

    a. _____

    b. _____

36. Care of the client with PID includes
    a. strict bed rest in a supine position
    b. avoiding tub baths and showering instead
    c. heat application to the lower abdomen
    d. a full liquid diet as tolerated

37. Outpatient instructions for the client with PID include which of the following statements?

    a. "Return to see your doctor in 7 days for a recheck."

    b. "Ask your partner to come into the clinic to be tested."

    c. "Resume sexual intercourse whenever you feel up to it."

    d. "Take the medicine with Maalox if your stomach is upset."

38. Briefly explain why it is important to treat all sexual partners of the client who is infected with a sexually transmitted disease.

    _____

    _____

    _____

    _____

CRITICAL THINKING EXERCISES

Case Study: Syphilis

B. B., a 20-year-old single male, reports to the family practice clinic with a chancre on his penis. He went on a fishing trip with friends about 3 weeks ago. After an evening of drinking, the men went into a local town looking for "some action." Although a believer in safe sex, B. B. did not have a condom with him and engaged in unprotected sexual intercourse. He tells the clinic nurse, "I guess I've learned a lesson."

Address the following questions:

1. What diagnostic tests should be done on B. B.? Give rationales for your answers.
2. The VDRL and FTA-ABS tests are positive. What does this mean?
3. Identify relevant nursing diagnoses for B. B. based on the above data and develop a plan of care.
4. What information must B. B. provide about his sexual partners?
5. Benzathine penicillin G is ordered to be given intramuscularly in a dose of 2.4 million units. What should the nurse do before administering the injection?
6. The penicillin comes in a pre-mixed syringe with 0.6 million units/mL. How should the nurse prepare and administer the prescribed dosage?
7. Formulate a teaching/learning plan for B. B.
8. Three hours after leaving, B. B. calls the clinic and reports "being hot and aching all over." He asks what to do. How should the nurse respond?
9. Why must the nurse report B. B.'s diagnosis of syphilis to the local health department?

Case Study: Pelvic Inflammatory Disease (PID)

L. L. is a 26-year-old divorced women with no children. She reports to the outpatient clinic with "chills, fever, fatigue, lower abdominal pain, and tenderness." L. L. has stayed home from her job the past 3 days because she thought she had the flu. Now she has dysuria and is seeking medical attention for what she feels is a urinary tract infection. The pelvic examination reveals uterine tenderness with motion, swollen fallopian tubes, and bilateral ovarian enlargement. A culture of the vaginal discharge is taken. Her vital signs are temperature = 101.4°F orally; pulse = 124, regular; respirations = 20, regular; and blood pressure = 134/86. L. L.'s urine is clear. A diagnosis of PID is made and outpatient management is selected.

Address the following questions:

1. Ceftriaxone (Rocephin) 250 mg, IM, and doxycycline (Vibramycin) 100 mg, PO, are ordered to be administered stat. Identify appropriate nursing interventions for administering these medications.

L. L. will be sent home on doxycycline 100 mg, PO, bid, for 2 weeks. She is instructed to remain on bed rest in a semi-reclining position until afebrile. A heating pad and sitz baths are recommended for comfort. Acetaminophen with codeine #3 (Tylenol #3), one tablet, PO, every 4 hours is also ordered for pain.

2. Develop a teaching/learning plan for L. L.
3. What information should the nurse discuss with L. L. about her self-care?
4. L. L. asks the nurse when she will be able to return to work. How should the nurse reply?

Case Study: Ruptured Ectopic Pregnancy

A. B. is a 26-year-old woman who is brought to the Emergency Department (ED) by her husband. She reports lower right quadrant abdominal pain. Although not confirmed, A. B. believes that she may be pregnant because her last menstrual period was 8 weeks ago and the couple has not been using any means of contraception. Her vital signs are pulse = 90, regular; blood pressure = 120/72 sitting and 104/60 standing; respirations = 18; and temperature = 36.9°C orally. A. B.'s abdomen is slightly distended, tender to light palpation, and positive for rebound tenderness. Bowel sounds are faint. The ED physician orders an intravenous infusion of D_5W and lactated Ringer's solution, blood to be drawn for type and cross-match for 5 units of packed cells, Rh factor and pregnancy test, and a urinalysis. After the blood specimens are drawn, A. B.'s pulse is 124, her blood pressure is 84/50, and respirations are 20. A. B. is restless, has cool, clammy skin, and says that her right shoulder hurts. There has been a small amount of brown vaginal discharge. The pregnancy test confirms a pregnancy. A. B.'s hemoglobin is 8.5% and her hematocrit is 26 g/100 mL. A ruptured tubal pregnancy is suspected.

Address the following questions:

1. What should the nurse do immediately?

2. What should the nurse explain to A. B. and her husband before A. B. signs a surgical consent form and goes to surgery?

3. The surgery is successful and the right fallopian tube was removed during the procedure. One unit of packed cells was infused intraoperatively. Identify the relevant nursing diagnoses for A. B. postoperatively.

4. Describe the postoperative care for A. B.

5. A. B. is scheduled for discharge. Develop a teaching/learning plan for her.

6. What should be discussed with the couple about future attempts to conceive? Consider any possible effects from the blood transfusion and the increased risk of infertility.

ANSWER KEY

CHAPTER 1

Definitions of Health and Illness

1. a. prevailing levels of knowledge

    b. philosophical theories

    c. cultural and religious beliefs

2. High-level wellness is the optimal level at which a person can function given his or her environment (internal and external). It is an active, dynamic state.

3. a. biological: structure of body tissues, organs, biochemical interactions, and functions

    b. psychological: mood, emotions, personality

    c. sociological: interaction between individual and environment

4. See p. 4 in the textbook for discussion

5. Disease: altered body function resulting from a disturbance in the biological or psychological state

    Illness: an individual's perception of and response to not being well. May also refer to the perceptions of people around the individual. See also p. 6 for further discussion

6. Refer to Figure 1-1 on p. 4 of the textbook for assistance with drawing and labeling the diagram. Submit the completed exercise to the clinical instructor for evaluation and feedback.

7. Genetic influences (diabetes mellitus, hemophilia); cognitive abilities (educational level, decision-making ability); demographic characteristics (age, sex); environment and lifestyle (smog, recreation-related trauma); geographic location (sun exposure, dampness); culture (diet, hygiene); spirituality and religion (viewing illness as punishment); economics (ability to afford health care); health beliefs and practices (trust or mistrust of health care workers); previous health experiences (positive or negative); support systems (internal coping ability, external support from significant others)

Assessment

8. b	12. b
9. a	13. a
10. a	14. a
11. b	15. b

16. Changes in the following:

    a. body appearance

    b. body function

    c. body emissions

    d. the senses

    e. emotional state

    f. relationships with others

    g. any uncomfortable physical symptoms

17. a. taking action (self-medicating; seeking professional help)

    b. taking no action (because of fear, expense, or unavailability of care)

    c. taking counteraction (type of denial, e.g., trying to disprove existence of symptoms)

18. a. availability of health care

    b. affordability of health care

    c. failure or success of self-prescribed treatment

    d. client's perception of the problem

    e. others' perception of the illness

19. The "sick role" is a set of behavior patterns that may be observed in ill clients. Four typical aspects of the sick role are exemption from normal social role responsibilities; the sick person is not viewed as being responsible for causing the illness; being ill is viewed as undesirable; and there is believed to be an obligation to seek competent help. The sick role does not apply to all circumstances.

20. d	25. b
21. b	26. a
22. e	27. e
23. a	28. d
24. c	29. c

30. a. which family member is ill

    b. seriousness and length of illness

    c. social and cultural customs of the family

Prevention

31. b

32. c

33. a

34. a

35. c

36. b

37. a. eating three balanced meals per day

    b. eating in moderation to prevent obesity

    c. regular, moderate exercise

    d. regular sleep in sufficient quantity

    e. moderate alcohol consumption

    f. no smoking

    g. minimal exposure to the sun

CHAPTER 2

Definitions of Nursing

1. a. Legal definitions are stated in the various nurse practice acts.

    b. Professional nursing organizations such as the American Nurses' Association have stated a more global definition.

    c. Nursing theorists also have defined nursing.

2. Definitions vary because the purposes of different definitions also vary. Nursing is a dynamic profession and the scope of practice continues to change. New definitions arise to help explain the nature and purpose of nursing.

Roles of the Nurse

3. b	12. c
4. a	13. a
5. b	14. e
6. a	15. b
7. a	16. f
8. a	17. d
9. d	18. a
10. f	19. b
11. e	20. c

21. a. client's educational level

    b. socioeconomic level

    c. support system

    d. age

    e. transcultural considerations

Practice Settings

22. a. hospitals

    b. long-term care facilities

    c. community health settings

    d. physicians' offices

    e. schools of nursing

    f. occupational health settings

    g. self-employment (including private duty)

Professional Development

23. Submit the completed exercise to the clinical instructor for evaluation and feedback.

24. Nurses have a responsibility to society to keep their knowledge base and skills current to be safe practitioners. This can be accomplished via several routes, including workshops, inservice programs, formal classes, and professional journals.

25. a. to promote growth of the science of nursing

    b. to develop nursing theories and the scientific basis for nursing practice

26. Communicating nursing research results helps the profession to grow and to adapt. By continually validating and updating nursing practice, the profession remains viable and recognized as a service to society.

CHAPTER 3

Problem-Solving Approaches

1. Refer to Table 3-1 in the textbook on p. 26.

Assessment

2. The purpose of assessment is to identify client health-related problems, both actual and potential.

3. *Subjective* data consist of verbal information provided by the client about himself or herself. These data cannot be directly measured by anyone other than the client.

   Objective data consist of information about a client that can be observed by others. These data are measurable.

4. a. interviewing

    b. observation

    c. physical examination

5. c
6. a
7. b
8. a
9. b
10. b
11. c
12. a
13. c
14. the nursing history
15. a
16. b

17. b
18. c
19. a
20. a
21. c
22. b
23. c
24. b
25. a
26. c

27. a. family members or significant others

    b. medical records

    c. other health team members who have dealt with the client

28. A *nursing history* is a tool used to collect data regarding the meaning that illness and hospitalization have for the client. It is used to plan the client's nursing care. A *medical history* is a tool used to collect client data to assist the physician in formulating a medical diagnosis. It is used to plan medical care for the client.

Analysis

29. The purpose of analysis is to summarize and organize client data to determine whether the client's needs are being met.

30. Submit the completed exercise to the clinical instructor for evaluation and feedback. Also refer to Table 3-2 and p. 32 in the textbook for further information.

31. a. P (problem, either actual or high risk)

    b. E (etiology or risk factor)

    c. S (symptom or defining characteristic)

32. b

33. Submit the completed exercise to the clinical instructor for evaluation and feedback. Also see p. 32 in the textbook for discussion.

Planning

34. a. Setting priorities

    b. setting goals

    c. planning nursing actions (interventions)

    d. identifying available resources

    e. establishing criteria for evaluation

35. Priority setting helps the nurse to organize and plan care to resolve the client's most urgent problems.

36. d

37. The purpose of goal setting is to provide guidelines for evaluating whether a client's identified health problems have been resolved.

38. a. goals should be client-centered and realistic for both the client and the nurse

    b. goals should be written clearly and concisely

    c. goals should be measurable using observable behaviors

39. a

40. a

Implementation

41. a. characteristics of the nursing diagnosis
    b. research knowledge associated with specific interventions
    c. choosing for the greatest possibility of success
    d. the client's acceptance of the specific intervention
    e. minimizing the risk and discomfort for the client
    f. the nurse's capabilities
42. a. intellectual (problem solving, critical thinking, making judgments)
    b. interpersonal (communicating, listening, showing interest and compassion)
    c. technical (performing procedures, using equipment)

Evaluation

43. Evaluation reveals the degree to which the other steps in the nursing process have been accurate and effective. Evaluation is essential in determining whether the client's goals have been attained.
44. Refer to p. 35 in the textbook for discussion.

Documentation

45. a. specialty nursing practice forms
    b. focus charting
    c. charting by exception
46. b

CHAPTER 4

Theories of Adult Development

1. Adulthood has no definite beginning or predictable end point. There is disparity among the dimensions of chronological, psychological, and physiological age. Other factors to consider are the individual rate of aging, genetic and environmental factors, and how aging affects organisms at various levels. Consequently, each discipline favors certain theories that best represent its current level of knowledge.
2. d
3. b
4. a
5. c

Theories of Aging

6.	b	10.	d
7.	c	11.	e
8.	a	12.	b
9.	f	13.	d

Stages of Adulthood

14.	c	26.	c
15.	b	27.	b
16.	b	28.	a
17.	a	29.	c
18.	c	30.	b
19.	a	31.	c
20.	c	32.	d
21.	b	33.	a
22.	a	34.	b
23.	c	35.	b
24.	c	36.	c
25.	b		

CHAPTER 5

Health Issues

1. a
2. a. self-responsibility and self-management
   b. nutritional awareness
   c. physical fitness and mobility
   d. stress management
   e. environmental sensitivity

3.	d	9.	c
4.	a	10.	b
5.	d	11.	d
6.	b	12.	a
7.	a	13.	b
8.	d		

14. a. edema   g. weakness
    b. nausea   h. dizziness
    c. vomiting   i. urinary retention
    d. anorexia   j. diarrhea
    e. dry mouth   k. constipation
    f. fatigue   l. confusion

15. a. They may forget to take medications at the correct times.

b. They may not understand the correct way to safely take their medications.

c. They may either overmedicate or undermedicate themselves because of attitudes or feelings about taking medications.

16. a. loss of income

b. loss of health

c. lack of comprehensive health and social services

d. loss of social roles

e. deaths of significant others

17. *Dementia* is a change of mental status resulting in impaired orientation, memory, judgment, and intellectual functioning. It is unrelated to a major, focal neurological deficit and more likely a result of cerebral arteriosclerosis. It is less common in the elderly than popularly believed.

Depression, in contrast, may develop in response to multiple life stresses. Symptoms may go unnoticed until the elderly person can no longer cope.

18. b

19. a

Economic Issues

20. a. declining financial resources

b. fixed assets

c. rising expenses

d. inflation

e. more out-of-pocket health care costs

f. need for special housing

21. d

22. a

23. c

24. b

CHAPTER 6

Key Definitions

1.	a, c, d, e, g, h	7.	c
2.	c	8.	d
3.	c	9.	a
4.	b	10.	c
5.	d	11.	a
6.	d		

Ethical Decision Making and Resources

12. a. nurse (gender, age, maturity level, assumptions)

b. task (time available, complexity, perceived cost/benefit ratio)

c. environmental (institutional policies, time limitations, conflicting loyalties)

13. a. Identify the ethical problem.

b. Identify and consider alternatives.

c. Implement a choice.

d. Evaluate the decision-making process and its outcome.

14. a. They do not perceive that an ethical situation is occurring.

b. They do not identify possible options themselves.

c. They often cannot satisfactorily resolve ethical issues.

15. d

16. Submit the completed exercise to the clinical instructor for evaluation and feedback.

17. c

CHAPTER 7

Key Definitions

1. c
2. e
3. a
4. d
5. b

Stress Theories

6. a. stress as a physiological response

b. stress as a stimulus

c. stress as a transaction between a person and the environment

7. a. The body's response to stress is nonspecific

b. Stress is a physiological response

c. Both "good" and "bad" events can cause stress

8.	b	12.	a
9.	a	13.	b
10.	a	14.	a
11.	c	15.	c

16. Refer to pp. 102–103 and Figure 7-1 in the textbook for discussion. Many basic fundamentals nursing textbooks also include discussion of stress and adaptation models. Answers follow:

    a. stressor

    b. posterior pituitary

    c. ACTH

    d. epinephrine and norepinephrine

    e. water and sodium, urinary output

    f. cortisol and aldosterone

    g. gluconeogenesis, protein and fat

    h. water and sodium, potassium

    i. fight-or-flight

    j. ACTH

    k. recovery

    l. exhaustion

17. a. death

    b. divorce

    c. monetary concerns

    d. health concerns

18. Daily stressors resulting in minor annoyances (hassles)

19. a. depth of feeling about the event

    b. personal beliefs

    c. belief that one has control over one's world

20. a. unpredictability of events

    b. uncertainty about an event

    c. timing of an event for the individual

    d. duration of events (long term vs. short term)

    e. ambiguity about elements of an event

Coping Theories

21. Problem-focused coping style: a, c, f

    Emotion-focused coping style: b, d, e

22. d

23. a

24. g

25. h

26. f

27. c

28. i

29. k

30. j

31. e

32. b

33. *Event rehearsal* is a coping strategy used *before* a stressful episode happens. It is the mental or physical practicing of what the individual plans to do when faced with a stressor. *Event review* is a coping strategy used *after* a stressful episode. It provides an opportunity for the individual to understand what has happened.

Adaptation Theories

34. *Morale* is the psychological outcome of coping and is related to emotional equilibrium or a sense of well-being.

35. *Psychophysiologic disease* is a process in which the mind (psyche) influences the body's (somatic) response to disease. The individual's response to stress is believed to be a factor in psychophysiologic diseases.

36. a. commitment that provides a sense of satisfaction and motivation

    b. looking at life's events as challenges, not threats

    c. having a sense of control over one's life

Collaborative Management

37. a. physiological signs manifested by the client (hypersecretion of gastric acid)

    b. psychosocial signs manifested by the client (anger, denial)

    c. client's appraisal of stress-provoking events (reality testing)

    d. coping ability of the client (constructive problem solving)

38. Submit the completed exercise to the clinical instructor for evaluation and feedback. Consider the variability of individual responses to stress when formulating an answer.

39. e

40. g

41. a

42. h

43. b

44. i

45. d

46. c

47. f

48. a. biofeedback

    b. progressive muscular relaxation

    c. meditation

    d. guided imagery

49. The client should experience a sense of psychological and physical well-being.

50. a. resentment toward supervisors or co-workers

    b. loss of temper at small incidents

    c. constant fatigue

    d. reluctance to go to work

    e. withdrawal from work relationships

CHAPTER 8

Definitions of Pain

1. c
2. b
3. c
4. a
5. b
6. b
7. c
8. a

Pain Theories, Anatomy, and Physiology

9. b
10. c
11. a
12. b
13. c

14. a. superficial receptors in the skin and subcutaneous tissue

b. deep somatic receptors in bone, blood vessels, muscles, and connective tissue

c. visceral receptors in body organs

15. *Referred pain* is visceral pain that is perceived in a part of the body distant from the original site of painful stimulation. It occurs because the visceral fibers converge (synapse) in the spinal cord close to fibers that innervate other subcutaneous tissues.

16. a. cutaneous: well localized and defined; sharp, pricking, piercing

b. deep somatic: poorly localized; dull, achy, burning

c. visceral: poorly localized, diffuse; achy, more continuous

17. *Neuropathic pain* is perceived pain even though there is no obvious physiological cause. It is often unrelieved by analgesics. Phantom limb pain is an example.

18. a. *A delta fibers* are myelinated. They transmit rapid, sharp, pricking, or piercing sensations that are well localized and intermittent.

b. *C fibers* are unmyelinated or poorly myelinated. They transmit diffuse, dull, burning, or achy sensations that are more continuous.

19. Stimulation of peripheral receptors is transmitted to the spinal cord where impulses are conveyed to neurons that cross to the opposite side of the cord. Impulses continue up the ascending lateral spinothalamic tract via either the neospinothalamic or the paleospinothalamic pathways. At the level of the thalamus, synapses relay the impulses to the midbrain where the reticular activating system (RAS) signals the cortex to increase awareness of incoming noxious stimuli. The cortex is involved in discriminating the location of pain stimulus. It also affects the cognitive aspects of pain.

20. b
21. c
22. a
23. a. Endorphins and enkephalins exert analgesic effects on the brain.

b. Endorphins have a more prolonged effect.

24. Age; sex; sociocultural background; personality characteristics; affect/mood state (anxiety, depression)

25. *Psychosomatic pain* has no detectable physical cause and is believed to derive from a person's mental (psychic) reaction to the pain experience.

26. Little personal experience with pain (cannot relate it to self); lack of appreciation for the degree of pain associated with procedures; expectation that clients with chronic pain will react as clients with acute pain do; expectation that clients with pain will react within a certain behavior pattern; concern that age may affect a client's reaction to prescribed doses of analgesics (undermedication)

27. See pp. 125–128 in the textbook for discussion. Submit the completed exercise to the clinical instructor for evaluation and feedback.

Collaborative Management

28. There may be an absence of observable or documented physiological changes to support the client's subjective report of pain. Chronic pain may be too diffuse to permit description of localization. The client's fears and the length of time that chronic pain has persisted affect the client's perception, verbalization, and expression of pain, as well as his or her coping abilities.

29. Precipitating factors; aggravating factors; relieving factors; localization of pain, character, and quality of pain; intensity; duration; chronology (pattern over time); psychosocial factors such as meaning of pain to the individual, feelings of anger, powerlessness, hostility, depression, withdrawal, and fear of death or mutilation

30. Client self-rating using analog scales and diagrams to locate, describe, and quantify pain; crying; writhing; grimacing; tachycardia; tachypnea; increased blood pressure; diaphoresis; guarding; splinting; restlessness; apprehension

31. Advantages: simple; understandable; economical; easier to use; improvement over subjective reporting alone; variety of types of scales (word and numerical) available

Disadvantages: rate only the intensity of pain; biased against clients with low verbal or visual discrimination abilities related to level of education or interference from severe pain

32. a. Pain
    b. Chronic Pain
33. a. Anxiety
    b. Fear
    c. Powerlessness
    d. Altered Role Performance
    e. Altered Sexuality
    f. Impaired Physical Mobility
    g. Self-Care Deficit
    h. Activity Intolerance
    i. Altered Health Maintenance
    j. Sleep Pattern Disturbance
34. Relief of pain
35. a. reduction, relief, or modification of the pain
    b. prevention of pain recurrence or worsening
36. Near or complete pain relief with analgesia and other modalities designed to interrupt the pain cycle
37. a. nonopioid agents (acetylsalicylic acid, acetaminophen)
    b. opioids (morphine, meperidine)
    c. opioid adjuvants (hydroxyzine, promethazine)
    d. nonsteroidal anti-inflammatory agents (ibuprofen, indomethacin)
38. Undermedication may be due to underprescription by the physician or a reluctance on the part of the nurse to administer potentially dangerous drugs. Delays in achieving effective analgesia may be a result of a client not requesting medication in a timely manner or the nurse not responding to the request promptly.
39. Opioid adjuvants enhance the sedation effect of opioids, as well as help relieve anxiety and act to calm a client. These effects augment the analgesic properties of opioids.
40. Monitoring vital signs for tachycardia, low blood pressure, and respiratory depression; observe for altered level of consciousness; assess bowel sounds and monitor for abdominal distention and constipation; monitor urinary output for signs of retention
41. Maintenance of aseptic technique is essential to prevent infection when administering analgesics. All catheter connections are secured, and an occlusive sterile dressing is kept over the catheter insertion site. Care is taken to secure the catheter to the skin to prevent dislodging.
42. Efficacy is influenced by a client's belief that something will help relieve the pain. This belief is enhanced by the release of endogenous opiates.

43. Clients can self-administer analgesics whenever they feel a need with reduced risk of over-medicating themselves.
44. Gate control theory postulates that stimulation of fibers in skin and subcutaneous tissues blocks transmission of painful stimuli to the spinal cord.
45. a. TENS
    b. local heat/cold application
    c. pressure
    d. massage
    e. vibration
46. a. benefits are unpredictable and may vary
    b. relief is not sustained when stimulation ceases
    c. desired effects may be attained only after trial and error with application and intensity
    d. stimulation may aggravate pain or produce new pain
47. See pp. 136–137 in the textbook for discussion.
48. d
49. d
50. Advantages: anti-inflammatory effects and prostaglandin inhibition, which reduce the need for opioid analgesics

    Disadvantages: gastric disturbances (hyperacidity and potential ulceration) and thrombocytopenia, which may lead to bleeding tendencies

51. c	61. c
52. a	62. b
53. b	63. b
54. c	64. d
55. a, c	65. a
56. a	66. c
57. b	67. a
58. c	68. d
59. b	69. b
60. b	70. c

71. a. anesthesia
    b. pain control
72. *Rhizotomy* is a neurosurgical procedure used to control chronic pain. An open rhizotomy necessitates a laminectomy to resect the posterior nerve root before it enters the spinal cord. Cutting the nerve interrupts transmission of pain stimuli from the periphery to the cerebral cortex. A closed rhizotomy achieves similar results without an extensive open surgical procedure; the nerve roots are destroyed with chemicals, coagulation, or cryodestruction.
73. Submit the completed exercise to the clinical instructor for evaluation and feedback.

CHAPTER 9

Key Definitions

1. d
2. e
3. b
4. c
5. a

Arousal Mechanism

6. The RAS is primarily responsible for activating central nervous system arousal. All sensory input stimulates the cerebral cortex through the RAS, and the cerebral cortex stimulates the RAS via descending pathways.

7. a. *Sensory overload* is a condition in which the cerebral cortex is unable to regulate overwhelming incoming stimuli.

   b. *Sensory deprivation* is a condition resulting from the failure of the RAS to recognize incoming stimuli.

Sensory Deprivation and Sensory Overload

8. a. absolute reduction or absence of sensory stimuli in external environment (solitary confinement)

   b. reception deprivation (loss of hearing, sight, taste, smell, or touch)

   c. perceptual deprivation (agnosia resulting from a cerebral vascular accident)

   d. technologic deprivation (critical care unit environment)

   e. confinement deprivation (hospitalization in a location other than one's own familiar locale)

   f. immobility deprivation (prolonged bed rest)

9. a. lack of color simulation

   b. dim lighting

   c. bland food

   d. confinement to a limited physical space

   e. few visitors

10. a. client's age (alteration in perception related to aging)

    b. type of health problem or illness (bed rest, traction)

    c. type of treatment procedure (isolation)

11. a. lack of affect

    b. confusion

    c. depression

12. a. confusion

    b. inaccurate perception

    c. faulty reasoning

    d. impaired memory

    b. hallucinations

13. a. cognitive (confusion, disorientation)

    b. emotional (anxiety, depression)

    c. perceptual (visual or auditory distortion

    d. physical (drowsiness, sleep)

14. Critical care unit psychosis is a syndrome of associated behaviors observed in clients who have been in critical care units. Changes include altered cognitive function, confusion ,disorientation, and inability to maintain attention. It may be the result of sensory overload.

15. Observed behavior changes are similar. The major difference is that sleep is used less often as a compensating mechanism for sensory overload due to frequent interruptions and stimulation.

Collaborative Management

16. Age; developmental level; alterations in reception; corrective devices for sensory impairments; alteration in mobility; any neurological impairment; cognitive status; communication ability; previous hospitalization; recent surgery; length of hospital stay; medications; substance abuse; type of physical environment prior to hospital admission; psychological status; psychosocial factors such as alteration in thought processes or emotional responses (increased irritability, mood swings, fear, anger, depression, daydreaming, decreased attention span)

17. Alteration in activity; dry mouth; difficulty breathing; heart palpitations; decreased appetite; laboratory data regarding fluid, electrolyte, and nutritional status; medication side effects

18. a. amount and intensity of stimuli present

    b. patterning and meaningfulness of stimuli

    c. degree of social isolation experienced by the client

    d. familiarity of the surroundings

19. a. unfamiliar environment

    b. sleep deprivation

20. Submit the completed exercise to the clinical instructor for evaluation and feedback. Also see pp. 156–159 in the textbook for further discussion.

21. a. receives optimal level of stimulation

    b. interprets sensory stimuli meaningfully

    c. is oriented to time, place, and person.

CHAPTER 10

Key Definitions

1. c
2. a
3. b

Factors Affecting Body Image

4. a. cultural norms and influences (beauty favored over plain features)

   b. normal aging process (youth preferred to aging)

   c. societal sex roles (behaving and dressing according to assigned sexual stereotype)

   d. technologic developments (artificial limbs, organs transplants)

Theories of Body Image Development

5. g	13. f
6. e	14. g
7. h	15. h
8. a	16. c
9. c	17. f
10. e	18. a
11. d	19. d
12. b	20. b

Alterations in Body Image

21. Submit the completed exercise to the clinical instructor for evaluation and feedback.

22. A chronic illness is a long-term process requiring that a client continually adjust to its effects. Reintegration of body image is a never-ending process.

23. b	30. c
24. d	31. d
25. a	32. e
26. c	33. a
27. a	34. c
28. d	35. b
29. b	

Collaborative Management

36. Client's view of self; client's and family's perception of the body changes; client's developmental level; past successful coping strategies used by client and family; occupation and work history; past and current experience with pain; physical environment; social and community support of environmental needs

37. Change in current life style or role; fears related to rejection or reaction by significant others; focusing on the past; negative feelings verbalized about the body, helplessness, hopelessness, or powerlessness; preoccupation with body change; overemphasis on residual strengths and achievements; personalization or depersonalization of body part or loss; incorporation of environmental objects within the body boundary; refusal to verify actual body change; current coping behavior; client's family role; client and family support systems

38. Missing or changed body part; avoiding body part by look or touch; hiding or overexposing body part intentionally or unintentionally; trauma to nonfunctioning part; change in social relationships; change in ability to estimate spatial relationships of body

39. a. Anxiety

    b. Ineffective Individual Coping

    c. Ineffective Family Coping

40. a. preparatory teaching before body-altering surgery

    b. light touch

    c. verbalization

    d. encouragement of client participation in planning care

41. Submit the completed exercise to the clinical instructor for evaluation and feedback.

42. Family members and significant others need support so that they, in turn, can support the client. They must resolve feelings (both past and current) related to the client and to the body changes the client has experienced.

43. a

CHAPTER 11

Key Definitions

1. b
2. a
3. a
4. b
5. a
6. b
7. a
8. b

Theoretical Perspectives

9. a. internal reproductive organs (ovaries, testes)

   b. external anatomical structures associated with sexuality (breasts, external genitalia)

   c. the endocrine system's effects on reproductive organ structure and function (estrogen, progesterone, testosterone)

10. c
11. a
12. b
13. c
14. a
15. d
16. a
17. d
18. b
19. c
20. a
21. c
22. a
23. d
24. b

25. a. homosexuality

    b. bisexuality

    c. transsexuality

    d. transvestism

    e. pedophilia

26. pedophilia

27. Submit the completed exercise to the clinical instructor for evaluation and feedback. Refer to chart 11-1 in the textbook for discussion.

28. See Table 11-2 in the textbook for discussion.

    a. discouragement of sexual activity; identification of clients by the sick role versus gender identity

    b. physical inability to engage in sexual activity due to fatigue, pain, anxiety, presence of tubes, catheters, or machinery

    c. rejection by others; others' fears of contagion

    d. side effects from antihypertensive medications including decreased libido, impotency, ejaculatory problems

    e. inability to assume or maintain positions during sexual intercourse; side effects of corticosteroid therapy such as weight gain and mood swings

    f. changes in body boundary and body image due to surgical procedures; physical reactions to radiation and chemotherapeutic agents such as nausea, vomiting, fatigue, anorexia, and alopecia

    g. client's or partner's fears of myocardial infarction or sudden death during sexual activity

    h. chronic vaginal infections resulting in dyspareunia; impotency resulting from neuropathy and microvascular changes

    i. changes in body boundary and body image as the disease progresses, such as edema, jaundice, and pruritus; impotency; depression

29. See p. 183 and Table 11-3 in the textbook for discussion.

30. See p. 184 in the textbook for discussion.

31. a. skills in verbal and nonverbal communication

    b. sensitivity to one's own needs and desires

    c. sensitivity to the needs and desires of another person

    d. ability to communicate sensitivity

    e. ability to trust another person

    f. ability to give and receive affection

    g. ability to listen openly to another

32. a. possession of open attitudes and positive values about sexuality

    b. development of skills in physical and psychosocial assessment

    c. ability to educate and counsel clients with diverse needs

    d. adequate preparation and a broad knowledge base of the complex factors that affect sexual health

Collaborative Management

33. Changes in self-image; disruption in usual sex role; change in sexual functioning or desire for sexual activity (decline in libido); dyspareunia; vaginismus; orgasmic dysfunction; erectile dysfunction; ejaculatory dysfunction (either premature, delayed, or retrograde); sexual aversion; use of vaginal creams, foams, douches, deodorants; intrauterine device; hormonal replacement therapy; use of contraceptives, antihypertensives, barbiturates, tranquilizers, sedatives, amphetamines; eating disorder; weight gain or loss; substance use or abuse; chronic illness; insomnia; fatigue; prostatic surgery; decreased vaginal lubrication

34. Client's description of problem including specific behaviors, thoughts, feelings, or attitudes; client's perception of the cause of the problem and contributing factors; environmental or situational factors present at problem onset; any change in the problem over time; measures taken by client to seek help from others, as well as self-help measures; client's expectations and goals for resolution of the problem; changes in self-concept; changes in functioning as a sexual partner; anticipated changes in sexual activity; beliefs that medications or treatments contribute to sexual activity alterations; rape trauma; unwanted or unsatisfactory sexual experiences including incest; physical or psychological abuse; marital discord; depression; anxiety; fear; negative parental or religious teachings; homosexual experimentation; guilt; knowledge deficit; poor communication skills; fear of interruption; confusion about gender identify; fear of rejection; resentment of partner; fear of pregnancy

35. External appearance; palpation of internal reproductive structures; examination of discharges, including laboratory tests; genitalia assessment; breast assessment; acting-out behaviors; intact hymen; venereal warts; STDs; irritation or infection of vulva or vagina (female); inflammation or infection of penis, prostate, urinary bladder, urethra, or testes (male); obstetric trauma including episiotomy scarring; clitoral adhesions; lax pubococcygeal muscles; spinal cord injury; structural defects of urethra and bladder neck; known pathological conditions of uterus, cervix, ovaries, or fallopian tubes

36. a. impairment of the adult sexual response cycle

    b. deficits in coping skills

    c. knowledge deficits

    d. change in or loss of body parts

    e. physiological limitations

37. a. Sexuality is a natural human function that must be addressed by health care professionals.

    b. Interventions for sexual dysfunctions are based on affirmation of sexuality as an important part of the individual's health.

    c. A major aspect of intervention includes teaching clients about the anatomy and physiology related to sexual functioning.

    d. Counseling or referral to another health professional (physician, psychotherapist, psychiatrist, or clinical nurse specialist) is indicated when a client's sexual problem cannot be resolved through specific interventions and suggestions or teachings.

    e. Underlying physical and psychological problems may need to be resolved first.

38. Dialogue between partners throughout all the steps

CHAPTER 12

Key Definitions

1. b

2. d

3. a

4. c

5. See p. 196 in the textbook for discussion.

Dying, Death, and Grieving

6. Submit the completed exercise to the clinical instructor for evaluation and feedback. See p. 196 in the textbook for discussion.

7. a. cessation of respiration

   b. cessation of heartbeat

   c. lack of corneal reflexes

8. *Brain dead* is a term used to describe a client whose heart and lungs remain functional with the support of a respirator, but whose respiratory center in the brain stem is incapable of sustaining spontaneous breathing.

9. The determining factor is the ability to maintain sustained spontaneous breathing and heartbeat. In brain death, the ability is lacking, whereas in a persistive vegetative state, it is still present, although the individual shows no evidence of cortical or cerebral functioning.

10. Cessation of the heartbeat causes circulation to stop, and with it, organ perfusion ceases as well. Vital organs that could be used for tissue transplantation would be rendered nonfunctional and necrotic.

11. A clear definition of death would assist the health care team to determine whether interventions for a specific client constitute ordinary or extraordinary treatment. Depending on the individual's circumstances, even "ordinary" interventions such as providing food and water could be considered "extraordinary" if it means subjecting the client to repeated needle sticks for intravenous therapy or intubation with feeding tubes (sometimes going against the client's preferences.)

12. a. shock and disbelief

    b. denial

    c. anger

    d. bargaining

    e. depression

    f. acceptance

13. See p. 197 in the textbook for discussion. The models of response to dying may be used as a guide in evaluating individuals' responses since each person may adapt in specific or unique ways. Nurses should be aware of what may occur in order to enhance their ability to observe, assess, and intervene in a timely manner, including assisting with coping measures.

14. a. remissions (indicators of hope) and exacerbations (threats to hope of recovery) in a disease process (leukemia)

    b. diminishing levels of functioning with periods of stability (cerebral vascular accidents)

    c. continuous, rapid decline in level of health (postmyocardial infarction with extensive damage)

    d. gradual decline in level of health over time (Alzheimer's disease)

15. b

16. a. fully acknowledge the loss and be able to remember the lost person without undue pain

    b. being able to participate in life without losing the capacity to love

17. Muscular weakness; tremors; chest pain; throat tightness; diaphoresis; deep sighing; hot or cold sensations; anorexia; nausea; fatigue and exhaustion; insomnia; sense of longing for what was lost; extremes of mood and behavior; depression; difficulty concentrating

18. e	24. b
19. c	25. e
20. a	26. c
21. d	27. b
22. c	28. c
23. a	29. e

30. Delayed grief manifested by carrying on with life as if nothing has happened; pathology of delayed grief extending beyond 2 years after the loss by death of a loved one; uncontrollable weeping and high levels of distress soon after the death of a loved one; exaggerated expressions of guilt and self-reproach; prolonged anger and hostility; having frequent occurrences of illness or complaints for more than 2 years after the loss; threatening suicide

31. a. elderly people who have sustained multiple losses in a brief period

    b. the significant others of those who die from AIDS and who belong to the gay community

    c. the survivors of victims of suicide or those who die in social disgrace

Collaborative Management

32. Previous and current reactions such as headaches, appetite loss, insomnia, behavior changes; coping behaviors used; past experiences with loss or death (successful or unsuccessful resolution); quantity of losses over time; age, level of maturity, and intelligence; cultural and ethical background factors affecting the grief response; spirituality support system

33. Type, nature, and meaning of the loss to the individual; nature and qualities of the lost relationship; physical or symbolic loss; characteristics of the deceased person and his or her relationship to the survivors; timeliness of death; anticipated (expected) or sudden death

34. See Chart 12-1 on p. 202 in the textbook.

35. a. High Risk for Dysfunctional Grieving

    b. Anticipatory Grieving

    c. Fear

36. c	40. e
37. d	41. d
38. b	42. c
39. a	

43. Getting and providing information; encouraging expression of feelings; assisting with plans for funerals or after-death services; discussing organ donation (if appropriate); showing acceptance by being with client and significant others; encouraging participation in decision making; providing pain control measures

44. c, e, f, g, i, k

45. d

46. a

47. b

48. c

49. Submit the completed exercise to the clinical instructor for evaluation and feedback on a separate sheet. Also see p. 210 in the textbook for discussion.

CHAPTER 13

Key Definitions

1. a. duration longer than 3 months

    b. residual disability

    c. caused by nonreversible pathology

    d. need for special training of the client

    e. expectation that it will require a long period of supervision, observation, or care

2. d

3. d

4. c

5. b

6. a

Theories

7. Perceived inability to be involved in or influence self-care and quality of life

8. c

9. b

10. d

11. d

12. Submit the completed exercise to the clinical instructor for evaluation and feedback.

13. a. acting

    b. guiding

    c. supporting

    d. teaching

14. c

15. c

16. How the family responses to the client's disability; how decisions are made; who is the family's spokesperson; usual coping style; structure and roles; communication patterns; problem-solving skills; client's status and role in the family; economic status; religious and cultural influences

Rehabilitation and the Health Care System

17. a

18. a. prevention of deterioration or further injury

    b. restoration of as much function as possible

19. e	24. g
20. j	25. i
21. f	26. c
22. a	27. b
23. h	28. d

Assessment

29. a. general background data

    b. health history with a rehabilitation focus

    c. general data about physical abilities and limitations

    d. functional assessment

    e. psychosocial assessment

    f. vocational assessment

30. History of present condition; current medications; in any current special treatment program; financial status; occupation; educational level; cultural background; home situation; usual activity patterns with ADL; dietary habits; elimination habits; sexuality habits; sleep history; food allergies

31. b

32. Submit the completed exercise to the clinical instructor for evaluation and feedback.

33. d

34. Submit the completed exercise to the clinical instructor for evaluation and feedback.

35. e

36. Submit the completed exercise to the clinical instructor for evaluation and feedback.

37. Baseline urinary patterns (number of times voids per day, nocturia); fluid intake including types, when taken, and amounts; past problem with incontinence or retention; if client is catheterized for residual urine volumes; presence of any urinary tract infection

38. d

39. Submit the completed exercise to the clinical instructor for evaluation and feedback.

40. a. client's response to any impairment

    b. home, work, and school environments

    c. endurance level

    d. extent of active and passive ROM

    e. muscle strength ratings

41. Food intake; hydration status (intake and output); oxygen balance; waste removal mechanisms (functioning metabolic waste removal by the kidneys and liver); sensation; functional level of mobility; presence of friction and shearing forces; nutritional status indicators (serum albumin level, serum total protein level)

42. Depth and diameter of broken skin area; grading of any pressure sore areas; the client's ability to understand the cause and necessary treatment of the skin breakdown; ability to self-inspect the skin; ability to participate in maintaining skin integrity

43. Functional assessment is a systematic attempt to measure objectively the level at which a person is functioning in a number of areas. A person's abilities are measured against a predetermined evaluation tool.

44. c

45. a. body image

    b. self-esteem

    c. loss

    d. grief

    e. coping mechanisms

    f. family theory

    g. powerlessness

46. The purpose of vocational assessment is to help the client find meaningful training, education, or employment following dismissal.

Planning and Implementation

47. d	57. e
48. a	58. b
49. c	59. c
50. d	60. e
51. b	61. b
52. c	62. d
53. c	63. c
54. b	64. a
55. b	65. d
56. c	66. b

CHAPTER 14

Anatomy and Physiology Review

1. a
2. b
3. b
4. b
5. a
6. b
7. Refer to textbook Figures 14-3 and 14-4 on pp. 245 and 247. In *osmosis* (Figure 1), the water (solvent) moves across the membrane until the concentration of particles to water is equal on both sides; the particles cannot pass through the membrane. In *diffusion* (Figure 2), the particles (solute) move across the membrane until they are equally distributed on either side and water levels are equal.
8. *Filtration* is seen in the kidney as urine is produced. It is also evident in right-sided congestive heart failure in which peripheral tissue edema results.
9. c
10. *Facilitated diffusion* is the use of a carrier or transport system to move a substance across a membrane. Glucose for cell energy is carried into the cells by insulin. The client with insulin-dependent diabetes mellitus lacks sufficient endogenous insulin to transport glucose into the cells. The glucose remains in the extracellular fluid and continues to increase in concentration. Hyperglycemia results, and the cells quickly deplete their energy stores.

11. Refer to question 7. Osmosis involves movement of water across a semipermeable membrane due to a concentration gradient from solute that cannot cross the membrane. If the membrane were permeable to the solute, diffusion of both water and solute would occur.
12. Osmotic pressure
13. a
14. c
15. b
16. b
17. Active transport, or pumping (cellular sodium–potassium pump, phagocytosis, and pinocytosis)
18. a. pressure of blood
    b. dynamic ejection of blood from the heart
    c. blood vessel patency
19. d, c, a, e, b
20. a
21. e
22. d
23. b
24. f
25. a
26. c
27. c
28. b
29. c
30. a
31. a. They act as a *solvent* for electrolytes (ionized salts).
    b. They are a *transport medium* for hormones, blood cells, and nutrients.
32. a. imbibed fluids (1500 mL)
    b. water in food (800 mL)
    c. cellular oxidation (300 mL)
33. 2600 mL
34. a. ECF osmolarity
    b. ECF compartment's volumes and pressures
    c. ADH regulation
    d. aldosterone regulation
35. d
36. a. urine
    b. skin
    c. lungs
    d. gastrointestinal tract
37. a. excessive salivation
    b. fistulas and wound drains
    c. gastrointestinal suction
    d. hypermetabolic states (e.g., thyroid crisis, trauma, burns, extreme stress)
    e. fever

f. hot, dry weather

g. excessive sweating

h. diarrhea

38. a. dietary intake

b. renal excretion or reabsorption

39. d   43. b

40. f   44. e

41. a   45. b

42. c

Subjective Assessment

46. Fluid intake (amount, types); fluid output (urine, emesis, diaphoresis, conditions leading to increased IWL); diarrhea; medications taken (especially diuretics and laxatives); neuromuscular symptoms (heart palpitation, muscle weakness); body weight changes; diet history; thirst sensation; excessive drinking; exposure to environmental heat; history of medical disorders such as renal or endocrine diseases; level of consciousness; reliability

47. Psychosocial assessment includes both psychological and cultural factors that may influence balance. Confusion, anger, hostility, and hypochondriacal tendencies affect the client's reliability as a historian. Psychiatric, social, and cultural behaviors can endanger the client's maintenance of homeostasis.

Objective Assessment

48. Alert; moist eye conjunctiva; moist mucous membranes; volume of urine output with specific gravity of approximately 1.015; resilient skin turgor; skin not excessively dry; body weight; absence of tearing from eyes; pulse volumes; pulse deficit; heart rate; blood pressure; venous filling; peripheral perfusion; body temperature; general sympathetic nervous system arousal; blood chemistry values such as serum sodium, hematocrit, and hemoglobin levels; observable degree of client thirst; any fluid loss from wounds, gastrointestinal tube drainage, fistulas, and blood loss; amount of IWL; neurological examination; muscle tone, strength, movement, and tremors; cardiac dysrhythmias; bowel sounds

49. a. standardized normal ranges of electrolyte values

b. changes from standardized normal ranges

c. changes from client's previous levels

50. **Intake:**

Tube feeding (100 mL/hour) × (24 hours)
    = 2400 mL

Free water (120 mL) × (4 doses) = 480 mL

Water with medications (60 mL) × (6 doses)
    = 360 mL

Supplement KCl (240 mL) × (4 doses) = 960 mL

Residual tube feeding volumes are returned to the stomach via the nasogastric tube.

Total = 4200 mL

Output:

Stools (300 mL) × (6 times) = 1800 mL

Urine (200 mL) × (3 shifts) = 600 mL

Total = 2400 mL plus the IWL

CHAPTER 15

Dehydration

1. b   8. c

2. c   9. a

3. a   10. c

4. c   11. b

5. a   12. a

6. b   13. c

7. c   14. a

15. a. age

b. body size

c. metabolic rate

d. degree of fluid loss experienced

16. Age; height; weight; change in fit of clothing, rings, or shoes; reports of abnormal or excessive fluid loss (perspiration, diarrhea, bleeding, vomiting, urination, salivation, or wound drainage); reports of palpitations or lightheadedness; chronic illness or recent acute illness; surgery; medication use; frequency and amount of urination; usual fluid intake in a 24-hour period; recent strenuous physical activity and temperature and humidity conditions at that time; psychosocial factors such as affect, feelings of apprehension, restlessness, lethargy, and confusion

17. Increased heart rate; weaker peripheral pulses; decreased blood pressure, especially systolic; orthostatic hypotension; flat or collapsed neck and hand veins; increased respiratory rate; skin color; degree of skin moisture; skin turgor; presence of edema; change in mental status; fever; decreased urinary output

18. c

19. Submit the completed exercise to the clinical instructor for evaluation and feedback.

20. Identifying clients at risk so that necessary interventions can be instituted; educating clients about the need for adequate intake of fluids and electrolytes; assisting clients to maintain sufficient intake of fluids and electrolytes; assessing frequently the parameters that indicate the state of hydration

21. c

22. b

23. a. They tend to dry the oral mucosa further.

   b. They may cause increased discomfort by stinging or burning open fissures in the mucosa.

24. b

Overhydration

25. a

26. c

27. c

28. Age; height; weight, especially recent sudden gain; noticeable swelling; tight rings, shoes, or clothing; frequency and amount of urination; use of medications (diuretics, antacids, laxatives, and morphine); presence of disease or recent therapy; diet history; headaches, behavior changes, increased somnolence, decreased alertness, decreased attention span, anorexia, diarrhea, or increased fatigue; psychiatric disorder, especially compulsive behavior (polydipsia, alcoholism)

29. Increased pulse rate with bounding quality; very strong peripheral pulses; elevated diastolic or systolic blood pressures; decreasing pulse pressure; increased venous pressure; distended veins (neck, hand); increased central venous pressure; enlargement of hemorrhoids or other varicosities; pulmonary edema (moist rales upon inhalation); increased respiratory rate; shortness of breath; pitting edema; altered cerebral functions, e.g., decreased level of consciousness, disorientation, ease with which client is aroused, decreased attention span; any headache, visual disturbance, or hearing disturbance; muscle cramps, skeletal muscle weakness; paresthesias; weight gain; increased gastrointestinal motility

30. a. polyuria

   b. diarrhea

   c. nonpitting edema

   d. cardiac dysrhythmias (related to electrolyte dilution)

   e. projectile vomiting

31. Submit the completed exercise to the clinical instructor for evaluation and feedback.

Principles of Intravenous Therapy

32. d

33. a. medication administration (continuous or intermittent)

   b. correction of an existing fluid or electrolyte imbalance

   c. prevention of a fluid or electrolyte imbalance

   d. long-term nutritional support

34. a. avoid inserting IV line over a joint—joint immobilization is difficult to achieve, is uncomfortable, and may lead to complications; needle may become dislodged

   b. initiate IV line in upper extremity—better venous return than in lower extremities; less risk of thrombus or embolus formation

   c. initiate IV line in nondominant arm—allows client better motor control and participation in activities

   d. initiate IV line in arm veins rather than hand veins—using hand veins limits client's use of the hand; site is more painful; risk of tissue damage is greater; more prone to dislodgment

   e. begin venipuncture in distal portion of arm—allows use of proximal sites later; dorsal veins are preferred to ventral veins

   f. select a healthy vein—it is elastic and less prone to developing complications

   g. select arm with intact venous and lymphatic drainage—permits sufficient blood flow to decrease incidence of vein irritation

35. b

36. c

37. a. flow rate

   b. equipment function

   c. site condition

38. Refer to pp. 284–288 and Table 15-5 and Charts 15-7 and 15-9 in the textbook for discussion.

39. 31 gtt per minute

CHAPTER 16

Hypokalemia

1. d
2. c
3. b
4. Age; mediation use (especially diuretics, steroids, and digitalis); presence of any disease state; any recent illness; diet history; method of food preparation; psychosocial factors including usual mental status, mood, behavior changes, lethargy, and confusion
5. a
6. Shallow, ineffective respirations; diminished breath sounds; cyanotic nail beds and mucosa; thready, weak peripheral pulses; variable heart rate; postural hypotension; ECG changes (ST depression, flat/inverted T waves, prominent U waves, heart block); mental status changes (transient irritability or anxiety, lethargy, confusion, coma); decreased sensory perception; muscle weakness including weak hand grasps; hyporeflexia; flaccid paralysis; decreased peristalsis; nausea or vomiting; constipation; abdominal distension; decreased bowel sounds; polyuria; low urine specific gravity
7. b
8. a, b, e h, i, j, l
9. b. Potassium elixir should be given after meals to decrease gastric irritation.
10. d
11. b

Hyperkalemia

12. d
13. a
14. b
15. c
16. Age; presence of risk factors such as debilitating or chronic illness (renal disease); any recent medical or surgical treatment; urinary output; use of medications; diet history; use of salt substitute; any palpitations or irregular heartbeat; muscle twitching; weak leg muscles; tingling or numbing in extremities or face; explosive diarrhea; decrease in activity level; fatigue; weakness; psychosocial factors including compliance with prescribed dietary restrictions or limitations, knowledge of foods to avoid, use of medications, and details about food preparation

17. Cardiovascular changes including slow, weak peripheral pulses; low blood pressure; ECG changes (tall, peaked T waves, prolonged PR interval, flat/absent P waves, widening of QRS complexes), complete heart block, or ventricular dysrhythmias; neuromuscular symptoms including muscle twitching, paresthesia, numbness, progressive ascending muscle weakness, and paralysis in arms and legs; increased respiratory rate; hyperactive bowel sounds; watery, explosive diarrhea
18. a
19. c
20. d
21. b

Hyponatremia

22. a
23. d
24. a
25. b
26. Age; medication usage; presence of risk factors such as kidney or liver disease or congestive heart failure; recent medical treatment or surgery; vomiting; diarrhea; fever; draining wounds; burn injury; urinary output; fluid intake; height; usual weight and any recent weight changes; diet history; recent engagement in strenuous physical activity and the environmental temperature and humidity at the time; behavior changes; headaches; increased somnolence; decreased alertness and attention span; difficulty awakening; muscle weakness, anorexia; abdominal cramping; increased fatigue; signs of edema
27. Presenting behavior; altered mental status including level of consciousness, orientation, attention span, memory, and fund of knowledge; headache; muscle weakness; decreased muscle tone; depressed deep tendon reflexes; increased GI motility; nausea; diarrhea; abdominal cramping; hyperactive bowel sounds; visible peristalsis; explosive, watery stools; rapid, weak, thready pulse; decreased peripheral pulses; flat neck veins at 90 degrees and possibly when supine; decreased blood pressure (especially diastolic); orthostatic hypotension; variable central venous pressure; full, bounding peripheral pulses; shallow respirations; variable respiratory rate; rales or rhonchi; edema; urine specific gravity; urine color; daily weight
28. c
29. a
30. c
31. c

Hypernatremia

32. d	38. c
33. a	39. b
34. c	40. a
35. b	41. c
36. a	42. b
37. b	

43. Age; presence of renal disease or conditions promoting excessive water loss (fever, vomiting, diarrhea, heavy diaphoresis); urinary output; fluid intake in past 24 hours; recent weight change; medication use; diet history including use of sodium-containing condiments; recent strenuous physical activity as well as temperature and humidity conditions at the time; insomnia or mental irritability; edema; changes in skin texture or turgor; change in activity level; mental status; weakness; fatigue; psychosocial factors including behavior change, agitation, and manic excitement

44. Attention span; recall of recent events; ability to perform cognitive functions; agitation; confusion regarding the sequence of events; lethargy; drowsiness; stupor or coma; convulsions; sporadic muscle twitches; progressive muscle weakness; diminished or absent deep tendon reflexes; variable pulse rate; variable blood pressure; changes in peripheral pulse intensity and quality; changes in skin color and turgor; dry mucous membranes and skin; coated tongue and gums; oral fissures; decreased urine output; concentrated urine

45. b
46. a
47. c
48. d
49. c

Hypocalcemia

50. c	58. b
51. b	59. a
52. b	60. d
53. d	61. b
54. a	62. a
55. a	63. a
56. c	64. d
57. d	

65. Age; sex; race; skin exposure to sunlight; activity level (especially weight bearing); diet history; use of calcium supplements; reports of frequent leg cramps ("charley horses"); recent orthopedic surgery or episodes of bone healing; thyroid surgery, neck radiation, or recent anterior neck injury; abdominal cramping; taking medications such as calcium channel blockers; psychosocial factors including subtle behavior changes (anxiety), increasing sensitivity to extraneous environmental stimuli, progressive irritability, irrational thinking, and frank psychosis; ability to understand medication and diet regimen; ability to afford dietary supplements

66. Progressive paresthesia in hands or feet (distal to proximal); tingling; numbness; muscle twitching, cramps, or spasms, tetany; presence of Trousseau's or Chvostek's sign; convulsions; hyperactive deep tendon reflexes; hyperactive bowel sounds; diarrhea; hypotension; diminished pulse quality

67. b
68. b
69. a
70. a
71. d

72. a. continuous assessment of cardiovascular status via ECG monitoring

    b. frequent assessment of Chvostek's and Trousseau's signs;

    c. frequent monitoring of serum calcium levels

    d. assessment of the infusion site for infiltration at least every 15 minutes

73. c

74. The purpose of drug therapy is to decrease intestinal motility so that more calcium can be absorbed and to prevent dehydration from excessive fluid loss through diarrheal stools.

75. d

Hypercalcemia

76. b
77. c
78. b

79. Immobility and the absence of weight bearing cause bone demineralization and resorption of calcium.

80. Excessive intake of vitamins can lead to increased absorption of calcium if a large amount of the active form of vitamin D is ingested.

81. a

82. Age; presence of other illnesses including malignancy, renal disease, heart disease, and endocrine disorders; medication use, especially antacids, thiazide diuretics, glucocorticoids, thyroid replacements, calcium supplements, and vitamin D supplements; activity level; diet history; nausea; abdominal pain; anorexia

83. Bradycardia; full peripheral pulses; ECG changes (shortened QT interval, widened T wave); profound muscle weakness; diminished deep tendon reflexes; altered level of consciousness (lethargy, drowsiness, time or place disorientation); decreased or absent bowel sounds; increased abdominal girth; vomiting; constipation; renal stone formation

84. d

85. a

86. d

87. Submit the completed exercise to the clinical instructor for evaluation and feedback. See pp. 310–311 in the textbook for reference.

88. b

Phosphorus Imbalances

89. c		95.	b
90. a		96.	a
91. d		97.	a
92. b		98.	a
93. a		99.	b
94. a		100.	a

101. Easily obliterated peripheral pulses; generalized muscle weakness; ineffective respiratory movements; prolonged bleeding after slight trauma; bruising; bleeding gums; increased irritability; seizures; coma; spontaneous fractures; renal calculi

102. b

Magnesium Imbalances

103. b

104. a. malnutrition or starvation

    b. prolonged nasogastric suctioning

    c. diarrhea or steatorrhea

    d. destruction of intestinal villi

    e. alcoholism

    f. liver disease

    g. excess phosphorus in the GI tract

105. a. diuretic therapy including loop (high-ceiling) or osmotic diuretics

    b. aminoglycoside therapy

    c. ECF volume expansion

    d. hypoparathyroidism

    e. hyperaldosteronism

106. Hyperactive deep tendon reflexes; painful paresthesia; tetanic muscle contractions; positive Chvostek's and Trousseau's signs; skeletal muscle weakness; increased central nervous system irritability associated with depression or psychosis; decreased GI motility; anorexia; nausea; abdominal distention; paralytic ileus

107. c

108. d

109. Bradycardia; hypotension; prolonged PR interval; widened QRS complex; widening of pulse pressure; lethargy; coma; diminished or absent deep tendon reflexes; progressive muscle weakness including respiratory insufficiency

110. d

CHAPTER 17

Anatomy and Physiology Review

1. d		6.	e
2. a		7.	c
3. j		8.	b
4. g		9.	f
5. h		10.	b

11. a. structure and function of many proteins are altered

    b. fluid and electrolyte imbalances

    c. altered excitable membrane responses

    d. altered uptake, activity, and distribution of drugs and hormones

12. a. strong acid—frees up all of its hydrogen ions when dissolved in water

    b. weak acid—frees up only a small portion of its hydrogen ions when dissolved in water

13. a

14. c

15. c

16. b

17. Refer to the diagrams in the textbook on p. 322.

18. a. production of carbonic acid, bicarbonate, and hydrogen ions during cell metabolism

    b. catabolism of food resulting in formation of fixed acids

    c. anaerobic metabolism leading to formation of lactic acid

    d. incomplete oxidation of fatty acids leading to ketoacidosis

    e. release of lysosomal fluid (acidic) into the ECF when cell membranes are disrupted

19. b

20. b

21. d

22. c

23. a

24. b

25. c

26. a. chemical buffers

    b. lungs

    c. kidneys

27. Chronic airflow limitation—the kidneys excrete excess hydrogen ions and reabsorb bicarbonate to counter the retained carbon dioxide unable to be released via the lungs

28. Lactic acidosis resulting from anaerobic metabolism (e.g., running)—excess hydrogens ions in the ECF lead to an increase in the carbon dioxide concentration, which in turn leads to increased depth and rate of respiration in attempts to exhale the excess

29. *Full compensation* exists when either the lungs or kidneys are able to correct for changes in pH when the other system is unable to manage or is contributing to the cause of the acid–base imbalances. *Partial compensation* exists when the lungs or kidneys are unable to correct completely for pH changes and the pH is not within the normal range.

Changes with Aging

30. a. less alveolar membrane available for gas exchange

    b. vascular thickening that impairs gas diffusion

    c. retention of carbon dioxide that increases hydrogen ion concentration

31. a. reduced ability to excrete hydrogen ions

    b. reduced ability to synthesize bicarbonate ions

32. c

CHAPTER 18

Pathophysiology Review

1. d

2. a. indirect—conditions that increase the concentration of acids or bases at a rate beyond the body's capacity to regulate

   b. direct—pathological conditions that directly impair specific regulatory mechanisms

3. *Acidosis* is the process that causes blood pH to decrease.

   Acidemia is the result of acidosis when there are too may hydrogen ions in the extracellular fluid and the arterial pH drops below 7.35.

4. *Alkalosis* is the process that causes blood pH to increase.

   Alkalemia is the result of alkalosis when there are too few hydrogens ions in the extracellular fluid and the arterial pH rises above 7.45.

5. c   12. a

6. b   13. a

7. d   14. b

8. a   15. a

9. a   16. b

10. b   17. a

11. b   18. b

19. a. metabolic disturbances

    b. respiratory disturbances

    c. combined metabolic and respiratory disturbances

20. b

21. c

22. a

23. c; The lactic acid (product of lactose breakdown) sours the milk.

24. c   34. a

25. c   35. d, e

26. e   36. b

27. f   37. e

28. f   38. c

29. a   39. b

30. b   40. a

31. b   41. b

32. e   42. d

33. b

Collaborative Management

43. Age; urinary output and frequency; fluid intake; use of over-the-counter (OTC) or prescribed medications (especially diuretics, aspirin, or alcohol): diet history of calorie intake, nutrients ingested, or fasting; headache; behavior changes; increased somnolence; decreased alertness and attention span; lethargy; anorexia; abdominal distention; nausea or vomiting; muscle weakness; fatigue; psychosocial factors including data from significant others about mental status

44. Age; recent history of prolonged vomiting, fever, severe pain, licorice ingestion, or respiratory problems; use of OTC or prescribed medications (especially antacids, thiazide diuretics, antihypertensives, aspirin, or salicylates); urinary output and frequency; recent weight loss; muscle cramping, twitching, or weakness; insomnia; sleep pattern disturbance; anxiety; behavior changes; psychosocial factors such as increased sensitivity to environmental noise or activity, irritability, belligerence, irrational behavior, or psychosis

45. Lethargy; confusion; stupor; unresponsiveness; orientation to time, person, or place; decreased muscle tone; decreased tendon reflexes; decreased muscle strength; flaccid paralysis; increased rate and depth of respiration (Kussmaul's); difficulty talking or eating; skin and mucous membranes warm, dry, or pink; shallow respirations with variable rate; skin and mucous membranes pale or cyanotic; increased heart rate (early); bradycardia (late); electrocardiographic changes; peripheral pulses of low amplitude; hypotension

46. Agitation; confusion; hyperreflexia; seizures, paresthesias; positive Chvostek's and Trousseau's signs; skeletal muscle cramps or twitches; hyperactive tendon reflexes; tetany of localized muscle groups; muscle weakness; increased heart rate without increased blood pressure; thready pulse; increased minute respiratory volume and rate

47.	a	56.	b
48.	a	57.	b
49.	a	58.	a
50.	a	59.	d
51.	a	60.	c
52.	b	61.	b
53.	a, b	62.	a
54.	b	63.	b
55.	b	64.	a

65. Submit the completed exercise to the clinical instructor for evaluation and feedback. Refer to textbook pp. 340–341 and 344 for discussion.

66. Bronchodilators act to relax the smooth muscle of constricted bronchioles, allowing air to reach the alveoli. Administering other agents to the client who has bronchospasm without first opening the constricted air passages is less than effective. The medications will be unable to penetrate past the level of the bronchioles.

67. b

68. c

69. c

70. Refer to pp. 339–340 in the textbook for discussion.

71. a

72. c

CHAPTER 19

Surgical Settings

1.	b	5.	c
2.	f	6.	e
3.	d	7.	b
4.	a	8.	b

Collaborative Management

9. Age; tobacco or cigar use; medical problems; medication use; alcohol and illicit substance use; previous surgical procedures; experience with anesthetic agents; allergies; record of autologous blood donation; environment; self-care capabilities; support systems; family medical history; psychosocial factors such as anxiety or fear about the surgery, effects and outcomes of the surgery, coping abilities, and ability to learn and cooperate

10. Vital signs; peripheral pulses; heart sounds; capillary refill; edema; respiratory excursion; lung sounds; arterial blood gases; posture; clubbing; respiratory depth and rhythm; urinary frequency and characteristics; urinalysis; level of consciousness; orientation; attention span; ability to follow commands; ambulatory ability; motor or sensory deficits; skin and nails; hair texture; muscle mass and tone; skin turgor; joint deformities

11. c

12. b

13. d

14. Refer to pp. 355–357 in the textbook for discussion.

15. b	20. c
16. c	21. a
17. b	22. c
18. a, e, h	23. d
19. a	

24. Refer to pp. 370–371 in the textbook for discussion.

CHAPTER 20

Surgical Team and Environment

1. d
2. b
3. e
4. b
5. a
6. d
7. b
8. c
9. b
10. a. blood bank
    b. pathology
    c. radiology
    d. central supply
11. a. unrestricted
    b. semirestricted
    c. restricted
12. a. cap or hood
    b. frequent handwashing, covering clothes, and daily bath or shower
    c. mask
    d. do not wear
13. b, e, g

Anesthesia

14. a. block transmission of nerve impulses
    b. suppress reflexes
    c. promote muscular relaxation
    d. achieve a controlled level of unconsciousness
15. Anesthesia begins with selection and administration of preoperative medication.

16. d	21. a
17. b	22. b
18. c	23. a
19. a	24. b
20. c	25. b

26. a. type of anesthetic agent administered
    b. length of time client is anesthetized
    c. administration of a reversal agent for neuro-muscular blockade
27. c
28. b
29. d
30. a. tachycardia or other dysrhythmias
    b. continual increase in body temperature
    c. cyanosis
    d. hypotension
    e. muscle rigidity
    f. tachypnea
    g. dark urine
31. Height and weight are used by the anesthesiologist to calculate the amount of anesthetic agent needed for the client. Inaccurate or lack of recording may result in overdose.
32. a. hypnosis
    b. analgesia
    c. muscle relaxation
    d. relaxation of reflexes with minimal disturbance of the client's physiological function
33. a. site of application
    b. total volume administered
    c. concentration of drug
    d. penetrating ability of drug
34. Restlessness; excitement; incoherent speech; headache; blurred vision; metallic taste; nausea; vomiting; tremors; seizures; increased pulse, respirations, and blood pressure

35. c	40. d
36. f	41. b
37. a	42. d
38. e	43. d
39. b	

44. a. level of consciousness
    b. oxygen saturation
    c. ECG status
    d. vital signs

Collaborative Management

45. a. to prevent identifying the client incorrectly

    b. to assess if the client's perception, permit, and operative schedule agree

46. See pp. 399–401 in the textbook for discussion.

47. a. High Risk for Injury;

    b. Impaired Skin Integrity

    b. Impaired Tissue Integrity

48. a. age

    b. size

    c. weight

    d. type of physical limitation

49. b

50. a. prevent tearing of the surgical incision

    b. prevent migration of bacteria into the wound

51. d

52. a. protect wound from contamination

    b. absorb drainage

    c. provide support to the incision

53. a

54. c

55. b

56. a. circulating nurse

    b. anesthesiologist

    c. surgeon

57. Client's preanesthesia level of anxiety; type and length of surgical procedure; location of incision and drains; past reactions to anesthesia; respiratory dysfunction; blood loss; intravenous fluids given; medications given; joint or limb immobility; primary language; special client requests

CHAPTER 21

Assessment

1. a. age

    b. type and length of procedure

    b. anesthesia used

    b. client's physical health

    b. postoperative complications

2. a. medical history

    b. presurgical physical and emotional status

3. Age; medical history; surgical procedure; effect of the procedure on the client's recovery, body image, roles, and life style; anxiety level

4. d

5. a

6. e

7. b

8. a

9. b, c, g

10. b

11. c

12. d

13. f

14. a

15. b, d

16. g

17. c

18. c, f

19. d

20. a

21. c, f

22. g

23. e

24. c

25. b

26. c, g

27. f

28. a

29. d

30. b

31. g

32. a

33. a. increased pulse

    b. increased blood pressure

    c. increased respiratory rate (hyperventilation)

    d. diaphoresis

    e. restlessness

    f. wincing

    g. moaning

    h. crying

34. Multiple factors are considered based on client condition both intra- and postoperatively and the type of surgical procedure performed. Factors include, but are not limited to, fluid and electrolyte status, serum glucose levels, presence of infectious process, renal functioning, level of consciousness, degree of tissue oxygenation, and effects of medications and IV fluids; previous health status; complications during surgery; unanticipated change in client status

35. a. stable vital signs

    b. normothermic

    c. no overt bleeding

    d. return of gag and swallow reflexes

    e. adequate respiration

    f. cough reflex present

    g. arousable

    h. intact peripheral circulation

    i. ability to move extremities on command

Analysis

36. a. Impaired Gas Exchange

    b. Impaired Skin Integrity

    c. Pain

37. a. smoking

  b. history of respiratory disease (asthma, chronic airway limitation)

  c. being elderly

Planning and Implementation

38. See pp. 420–422 in the textbook for discussion.

39. c

40. Promote lung expansion; decrease joint and muscle stiffness; increase circulation; prevent bone demineralization; prevent urinary stasis

41. a. prevention of infection

  b. care and assessment of the surgical wound

  c. diet therapy

  d. drug therapy

  e. progressive activity

42. b

CHAPTER 22

General Concepts

1. a

2. a, c, e, g, h, i

3. b

4. c

5. Recognition of self versus nonself; phagocytosis of foreign cells, cellular debris, and abnormal self cells; lytic destruction of foreign invaders and unhealthy self cells; production of antibodies; activation of complement; production of hormones that stimulate increased leukocyte production in bone marrow; production of hormones that increase specific leukocyte growth and activity

6. b

7. g

8. f

9. h

10. j

11. i

12. a

13. e

14. c

15. b

16. d

17. a. inflammation

  b. antibody-mediated immunity

  c. cell-mediated immunity

Inflammation

18. a. Nonspecific response to invasion or injury rather than specific antigen–antibody reactions

  b. Provides immediate, short-term protection against effects of injury or foreign invaders rather than long-term, sustained immunity against repeated exposure to the same foreign invader

19. d

20. b

21. c

22. b

23. a

24. c

25. c

26. a

27. a

28. The same tissue level responses occur as a result of any type of injury or invasion regardless of location or specific initiating agent. The extent of the body's reaction to inflammation depends on the intensity, severity, and duration of its exposure to injury or invasion.

29. a. neutrophils

  b. macrophages

  c. eosinophils

  d. basophils

30. a, d, e, f

31. b

32. a

33. c

34. *Phagocytosis* is the process by which leukocytes engulf cellular debris or foreign proteins and then destroy them through a series of intracellular degradative events.

35. a. exposure and invasion

  b. attraction

  c. adherence

  d. recognition

  e. cellular ingestion

  f. phagosome formation

  g. degradation

36. c, g, e, i, b, f, a, h, d

37. a. increased warmth

  b. redness

  c. swelling

  d. altered sensation (pain)

  e. altered function

38. a	46. c
39. b	47. a
40. a	48. b
41. a	49. a
42. c	50. c
43. b	51. b
44. a	52. a
45. b	

Antibody-Mediated Immunity

53. a. neutralize foreign proteins
    b. eliminate foreign proteins
    c. destroy foreign proteins

54. c	74. e
55. c	75. b
56. f	76. a
57. b	77. d
58. f	78. b
59. c	79. b
60. f	80. c
61. a	81. a
62. c	82. c, d
63. e	83. a
64. g	84. d
65. b	85. b
66. c	86. a, b
67. f	87. c
68. b	88. b
69. d	89. c, d
70. b	90. a
71. f	91. d
72. d	
73. c	

Cell-Mediated Immunity

92. d	99. b
93. c	100. b
94. b	101. a
95. c	102. c
96. a	103. a
97. a	104. c
98. c	

105. a. Phagocytosis is only a minor function of cells involved in cell-mediated immunity.

b. Some of the leukocytes involved in cell-mediated immunity require prior sensitization to nonself cells before being able to exert cytotoxic or cytolytic effects.

106. a	113. c
107. c	114. b
108. d	115. b
109. b	116. a
110. a	117. c
111. b	118. b
112. a	119. c

CHAPTER 23

Degenerative Joint Disease

1. c
2. d
3. g, e, b, h, f, a, d, c
4. a
5. a
6. Age; sex; occupation and type of work; history of trauma; current or previous involvement in sports; history of obesity; family history of arthritis; medical diagnosis with joint manifestations; history of symptoms (onset, character, duration, aggravating and relieving factors); presence of joint pain; nature of pain; psychosocial factors such as anger, depression, change in body image, self-esteem, role changes
7. Crepitus; pain with palpation or motion; joint stiffness with range of motion; bony hypertrophy; joint effusion; Heberden's nodes; Bouchard's nodes; muscle atrophy adjacent to affected joint; radiating pain and stiffness; muscle spasms in extremities if cervical or lumbar spine involved; level of mobility; ability to perform activities of daily living (ADL)
8. b
9. a. Chronic Pain
   b. Impaired Physical Mobility
10. c
11. b
12. c

13. Infecting organisms from the primary source can seed the replaced joint, resulting in infection at the operative site. The resulting joint infection leads to inflammation, tissue changes, and an unstable prosthesis (prothesis failure).

14. b

15. c

16. a. increased hip pain

    b. shortening of the operative leg

    c. rotation of the operative leg

17. d

18. c

19. a

20. c

21. d

Rheumatoid Arthritis

22. c

23. a

24. Age; sex; family history of RA; previous viral infections; use of oral contraceptives; ability to cope with stress; fatigue; weakness; anorexia; psychosocial factors such as life style changes due to the crippling effects of the disease, change in self-esteem, body image, depression, grieving, suicidal thoughts, helplessness, support systems

25. Weight loss; low-grade fever; joint redness, warmth, stiffness, swelling, tenderness, or pain; bilateral and symmetrical involvement of joints; morning stiffness; muscle atrophy; decreased range of motion; joint deformity; carpal tunnel syndrome; Baker's cysts; tendon rupture; subcutaneous nodules; vasculitis of body systems (ischemic skin, pericarditis, myocarditis, pleurisy, pneumonitis, lung nodule, foot drop, paresthesias, dry eyes, dry mouth, dry vagina, liver or spleen enlargement)

26. b

27. a. Chronic Pain

    b. Impaired Physical Mobility

    c. Self-Care Deficit

    d. Fatigue or Activity Intolerance

    e. Body Image Disturbance, also Altered Role Performance and Self-Esteem Disturbance

28. a

29. c

30. b

31. d

32. c

Lupus Erythematosus

33. c

34. a

35. Sex; age; family history of lupus or other connective tissue diseases; reaction to ultraviolet light such as burning or splotching; medication history; fatigue; generalized weakness; anorexia; abdominal pain; psychosocial factors such as altered self-esteem, body image changes, avoidance of social gatherings, fear, anxiety, coping ability, support systems

36. Dry, scaly raised rash of the face or upper arms; butterfly rash across bridge of nose and cheeks; photosensitivity; ulcerations of extremities; mottling of the extremities; arthritis-like involvement of joints (pain, decreased mobility); muscle atrophy; fever; weight loss; nephritis; dyspnea; arterial blood gas changes; tachycardia; chest pain; Raynaud's phenomenon; psychoses; paresis; seizures; migraine headache; palsies; liver enlargement; splenomegaly

37. d

38. It is difficult to typify a client with SLE because no two clients have the same clinical problems or disease progression. Because of this variability, the relevant nursing diagnoses may vary greatly from one client to another.

39. d

40. b

41. c

Progressive Systemic Sclerosis

42. b

43. c

44. CREST syndrome is a group of clinical manifestations that often occur in PSS and can be diagnostic for the disease. The letters stand for the following terms: C, calcium deposits; R, Raynaud's phenomenon; E, esophageal dysmotility; S, sclerodactyly; T, telangiectasis.

45. d

46. c

Gout

47. b	53. d
48. b	54. a
49. c	55. c
50. d	56. d
51. a	
52. b	

57. Age; sex; family history of gout; complete medical history including use of medications such as diuretics; excruciating pain in joint; psychosocial data including fear of painful attacks

58. Joint inflammation; inability to palpate affected joint without increasing discomfort to client; tophi under skin; flank pain; decreased urinary output; fever

59. c

60. a. Pain

   b. Altered Urinary Elimination

61. b

62. c

63. d

Other Connective Tissue Diseases

64. d	69. e
65. h	70. f
66. c	71. b
67. a	72. d
68. g	73. a

CHAPTER 24

Immunodeficiencies

1. a. missing a component of immune system (primary or congenital)

   b. having a damaged immune system component (secondary or acquired)

2. c

3. b

4. A retrovirus reproduces itself by using the genetic material from its host cell. This results in an abnormal host cell but more virus when cell replication occurs.

5. c

6. d

7. e

8. c

9. d

10. b

11. Age; sex; occupation; residence; reason for admission; complete details about the current illness (nature, onset, symptoms and their severity, related problems, interventions taken); pain; whether a diagnosis of AIDS has been made; when diagnosis was made; infections, clinical problems, or treatment to date; history of blood transfusion or treatment with clotting factors; sexual practices and history of sexually transmitted diseases; taking any medications; past or present drug use or needle sharing; allergies; level of knowledge about AIDS; psychosocial data including family structure and significant others, ADL and changes, anxiety, mood, cognitive ability, employment status, social activities, hobbies, current living arrangements, financial resources, problems with discrimination, level of self-esteem, coping ability, depression, suicidal ideation, and support systems

12. Shortness of breath; cough; fevers; night sweats; fatigue; nausea; vomiting; weight loss; lymphadenopathy; diarrhea; visual changes; headache; memory loss; confusion; seizures; personality changes; dry skin; rashes (Kaposi's sarcoma, herpes)

13. a	20. d
14. d	21. b
15. a	22. d
16. b	23. a
17. c	24. c
18. c	25. b
19. a	26. c

Hypersensitivities

27. *Hypersensitivity* is a condition in which the immune system overreacts to an antigen to which it has been previously exposed. This overreaction may result in damage or disease in the host rather than the expected protective action.

28. a	36. d
29. a	37. c
30. d	38. d
31. a	39. c
32. a	40. c
33. d	41. d
34. a	42. b
35. b	43. e

44. Description of symptoms (what they were, what provoked them, nature of onset, and resolution); history of allergic symptoms or tendencies (urticaria, angioedema, tingling around mouth, throat swelling, vomiting, diarrhea, abdominal swelling, rhinorrhea, wheezing, shortness of breath, and hypotension); known allergens and the symptoms they provoke; family history of allergies; current medications; reactions to medications taken in past; variation of symptoms according to time of day, month, or year; change in symptoms over time and from episode to episode; prior skin testing for allergies and results; any desensitization therapy; level of knowledge for self-care; expressed feelings of uneasiness, apprehension, or weakness; itching; psychosocial factors such as anxiety and its effect on daily activities, ability to take action if symptoms occur

45. Scratching; urticaria; erythema; angioedema of eyes, lips, or tongue; rhinorrhea; dyspnea; audible wheezing; crackles; diminished breath sounds; hoarseness; stridor; hypotension; rapid, weak pulse; irregular pulse; syncope; diaphoresis; confusion; decreasing level of consciousness; cardiac dysrhythmias; shock; cardiac arrest; diarrhea; vomiting

46. a. Ineffective Breathing Pattern

    b. Ineffective Airway Clearance

    c. Altered Tissue Perfusion: cardiopulmonary, cerebral, renal, peripheral

    d. Anxiety

47. c
48. b
49. b
50. c
51. d
52. a
53. a. control of exacerbating factors

    b. treatment of acute episodes

    c. maintenance drug therapy

54. c
55. b
56. c
57. d
58. d
59. a

Autoimmunities and Gammopathies

60. b
61. c
62. d

CHAPTER 25

Key Definitions

1.	h	11.	f
2.	e	12.	d
3.	d	13.	b
4.	i	14.	e
5.	k	15.	a
6.	b	16.	c
7.	j	17.	c
8.	a	18.	b
9.	g	19.	c
10.	c		

20. Cell division is rapid; differentiated function of the parent cells is lost; cells are able to migrate; cells are loosely adherent; cells do not recognize or respect tissue borders; cells are not contact inhibited; growth rate is not well regulated; there is a large nucleus to cytoplasm ratio

Cancer Development

21. *Oncogenes* are genes that are supposed to be repressed in embryonic development but later become active after stimulation by an initiator.

22. c

23. d, g, b, f, h, c, a, e

24. a. Local seeding via distribution of shed cancer cells from the primary tumor into the local area (e.g., ovarian cancer spreading to peritoneal cavity)

    b. Blood-borne metastases via tumor cells released into the blood steam and circulating to distant sites (e.g., prostate cancer)

    c. Regional spread via lymphatics and lymph nodes (e.g., bowel cancer)

25. b

26. a. to help standardize cancer diagnosis, prognosis, and treatment among various institutions

    b. grading is done to classify a cancer's cellular properties

    c. staging is done to classify the clinical aspects of tumor location and degree of metastasis

27. a. to determine appropriate treatment

    b. to evaluate the results of management of the cancer

    c. to be able to compare statistics reported from various sources

28. b

29. d

30. c

31. d

32. b

33. a. exposure to carcinogens environmentally

    b. genetic predisposition

    c. immune function status

34. c

35. A *carcinogen* is an agent that elicits malignant changes in any tissue type.

36. d

37. e

38. a

39. d

40. c

41. b

42. a

43. a

44. Very few viruses have been identified as being carcinogenic in humans. It is thought that viruses infect the DNA of cells and cause cell mutation, activating oncogenes.

45. b

46. d

47. a. immunocompetence

    b. age

    c. genetic predisposition

48. b

49. c

50. Lifelong accumulation of DNA alterations or cell mutations that result in cell transformation and neoplasia; the body may no longer be capable of repairing the mutated cells; the immune system's effectiveness is decreased as the thymus becomes involved and atrophied, resulting in loss of ability to differentiate T-cells; elderly people may overlook malignant changes and attribute such findings to the aging process

51. a. inherited predisposition for specific cancers

    b. inherited conditions associated with malignancies

    c. familial clustering

    d. chromosomal aberrations

52. c

53. b

54. b

55. b

56. a

57. a

58. a. cultural or ethnic behaviors

    b. geographic location

    c. diet

    d. socioeconomic factors such as availability of health care services

59. a

60. b

61. a

CHAPTER 26

Consequences of Cancer and its Treatment

1. a. impaired immune and hematopoietic function (infection, anemia, bleeding tendency)

    b. altered GI structure and function (obstruction, malnutrition, anorexia, cachexia)

    c. motor and sensory deficits (bone fractures, nerve compression, pain)

    d. decreased respiratory function (airway obstruction, pulmonary edema, dyspnea, altered gas exchange)

2. e

3. d

4. c

5. c

6. d

7. b

8. a. to prolong client's survival time

    b. to improve client's quality of life

9. a. surgery

    b. radiation

    c. chemotherapy

    d. hormonal manipulation

    e. immunotherapy

10. A client's cancer therapy is determined by the specific type of cancer present, the extent of the cancer, and the client's health status. An established protocol is often used to guide the therapy.

11. e	15. f
12. c	16. b
13. g	17. d
14. a	18. a

19. a. Body Image Disturbance

    b. Anxiety

    c. Anticipatory Grieving

20. To destroy malignant cells while limiting damage to surrounding normal cells

21. b

22. a. tumor location

    b. size and depth of tumor from body surface

    c. stage of the cancer

    d. radiosensitivity of the cancer

    e. client's health and physical condition

23. d

24. c

25. a. amount of time exposed to radiation

    b. distance of client from the source of radiation

    c. amount and type of shielding afforded the client from the radiation source

26. b	30. c
27. d	31. a
28. d	32. d
29. e	33. d

34. a. to cure the specific cancer

    b. to increase the client's mean survival time

    c. to decrease the incidence of life-threatening complications

35. b

36. a. right drug

    b. delivered to the right cells

    c. in the right concentration

    d. at the right time

37. a	46. d
38. c	47. b
39. a	48. b
40. b	49. d
41. a	50. a
42. c	51. e
43. d	52. c
44. d	53. c
45. a	

54. To modify the client's biological responses to tumor cells. Actions include enhancing the effectiveness of the immune system and inducing more rapid recovery of the bone marrow following cancer chemotherapy suppression.

55. b

Oncologic Emergencies

56. b	61. a
57. d	62. c
58. e	63. a
59. a	64. c
60. c	

CHAPTER 27

The Infectious Process

1. a	7. i
2. d	8. c
3. d	9. a
4. j	10. e
5. g	11. f
6. h	12. b

13. a. reservoir

    b. pathogen

    c. susceptible host

    d. portal of entry

    e. mode of transmission

    f. portal of exit

14. b	23. a
15. b	24. h
16. c	25. d
17. a	26. b
18. f	27. c
19. e	28. b
20. g	29. b
21. i	30. a
22. c	

31. a. respiratory tract

    b. gastrointestinal tract

    c. genitourinary tract

    d. skin or mucous membrane breaks

    e. blood stream

32. e

33. f

34. a

35. g

36. c

37. b

38. d

39. c

40. b

41. b

42. a

43. b

44. a

45. a

46. a

47. a

48. a

49. a

50. a

51. a

52. c

53. c

54. b

55. a. category-specific isolation

b. disease-specific isolation

c. universal precautions

d. body substance precautions

56. d

57. d

58. a

59. a. relapse of the infection

b. emergence of resistant strains of the microorganism

c. cellulitis and abscess formation

d. sepsis

Collaborative Management

60. Age; history of cigarette smoking or alcohol use; current illness or disease; past and current medications; family history of infectious diseases; diet history; recent exposure to someone with possible infectious disease; exposure to contaminated food or water; when any exposure to known pathogens occurred; exposure to animals, pets, or insects; travel history; sexual history; IV drug use; any blood transfusions; detailed explanation of symptom type, location, and onset

61. Frustration; anxiety; prolonged feeling of malaise and easy fatiguability; degree of family and social interactions; effects of illness on interpersonal interactions; life style activities; guilt related to being stigmatized

62. Localized pain, swelling, heat, redness, and pus; fever; chills; malaise; lymphadenopathy; photophobia; pharyngitis; gastrointestinal disturbances; possible change in mental status

63. d

64. c

65. a. Hyperthermia

b. Fatigue

c. Social Isolation

66. a. antimicrobial therapy

b. antipyretic drug therapy

c. external cooling

d. fluid administration

67. d

68. a. delivery of the appropriate agent

b. sufficient dosage

c. proper route of administration

d. sufficient duration of therapy

69. b

70. d

71. c

72. b

73. a

74. d

75. c

76. d

77. e

78. a. when to take the medication

b. the importance of completing all the doses prescribed

c. how the medication should be taken, e.g., with or without food

d. any expected or unexpected side effects

e. adverse reactions to the medications and what to do for these

CHAPTER 28

Anatomy and Physiology Review

1. b

2. b

3. a

4. a

5. b

6. j

7. e

8. i

9. m

10. c

11. n

12. k

13. l

14. a

15. o

16. b

17. f

18. g

19. d

20. h

21. j

22. d

23. f

24. a

25. b

26. k

27. e

28. i

29. c

30. g

31. h

32. b

33. c

34. a

35. Refer to Chart 28-1, Nursing Focus on the Elderly, and pp. 613–614 in the textbook for discussion.

Subjective Assessment

36. Age; sex; race; childhood illnesses; adult illnesses; immunizations; operations; injuries; hospitalizations; last chest radiograph; PFTs; environmental data such as home and living conditions; exposure to environmental irritants; smoking habits; travel outside of local area; area of residence; current and past medication use; allergies; family history of genetically transmitted respiratory disorders; diet history especially for food allergies; occupational history; current health problems; hobbies; leisure activities; current problem with cough, sputum production, chest pain, shortness of breath, dyspnea on exertion, paroxysmal nocturnal dyspnea, orthopnea; recent weight loss; night sweats; psychosocial factors such as effect of stress on respiratory conditions, coping ability, effect of illness on family, financial status, and support systems

37. b	44. b, ii
38. a	45. e, v
39. a	46. a, i
40. a, i	47. b, ii
41. e, v	48. d, iv
42. c, iii	49. d, iv
43. d, iv	50. c, iii

51. Submit the completed exercise to the clinical instructor for evaluation and feedback.

Objective Assessment

52. Cough (productive, nonproductive); sputum production (color, consistency, amount); hemoptysis; external nose deformity or mass; nostril symmetry; nasal flaring; nasal polyps; deviated septum; color of nasal mucosa; septal perforation; sinus tenderness; decreased sinus transillumination; movement of soft palate and uvula with phonation; color and symmetry of posterior oral cavity; postnasal drainage; tonsilar enlargement; pharyngeal edema or ulceration; neck symmetry; use of neck muscles for respiration; palpable lymph nodes; tracheal deviation from midline; tracheal swelling; abnormal voice; thorax skin color, lesions, and masses; spinal deformities; respiratory rate, rhythm, and depth; symmetry of thoracic movement; inspiratory to expiratory ratio; ratio of anterior–posterior to lateral diameter of chest; chest movement with respiration; muscle retraction with respiration;

respiratory excursion; crepitus; vocal fremitus (increased, decreased, or absent); diaphragmatic excursion; chest percussion note resonant over lung fields; decreased, diminished, or absent breath sounds, adventitious breath sounds, (crackles, ronchi, wheezes, pleural friction rubs); bronchophony; whispered pectoriloquy; egophony

53. Submit the completed exercise to the clinical instructor for evaluation and feedback.

54. c	65. d
55. d	66. h
56. b	67. d
57. f	68. d
58. j	69. c
59. e	70. a
60. i	71. e
61. c	72. b
62. a	73. d
63. g	74. d
64. b	

CHAPTER 29

Disorders of the Nose and Sinuses

1. c
2. c
3. d
4. d
5. b
6. d
7. d
8. A *moustache dressing* is a 2 × 2 inch gauze pad placed under the nose, giving the appearance of a moustache. Its purpose is to collect any wound drainage from the nose following nasal surgery.
9. b
10. c
11. d
12. a

Facial Trauma

13. d
14. c
15. c
16. a

Disorders of the Pharynx and Tonsils

17. a

18. a

19. a. acute glomerulonephritis

    b. rheumatic fever

20. b	25. d
21. d	26. d
22. c	27. b
23. c	28. c
24. d	29. b

Disorders of the Larynx

30. d

31. a. steam inhalation

    b. voice rest

    c. increased liquids

    d. topical throat lozenges (Note: treatment with antibiotics and bronchodilators must be ordered by the physician.)

32. a

33. Nodules occur more frequently in teachers, coaches, sports fans, and singers, whereas polyps occur more often in smokers, people with many allergies, and those who live in dry climates.

34. a

35. a. slate board and chalk

    b. pen or pencil and paper

    c. magic slate

    d. alphabet board

36. c

37. The edema can occlude the airway, leading to respiratory arrest.

38. c

39. d

40. a. knife wounds

    b. gunshot wounds

    c. traumatic accidents

Head and Neck Cancer

41. c

42. d

43. Tobacco abuse; alcohol abuse; voice abuse; chronic laryngitis; industrial chemical or hard wood dust exposure; neglect of oral hygiene. The combination of tobacco and alcohol abuse results in an even greater risk.

44. Color change in mouth or tongue; sore that does not heal; lump in mouth or neck; unexplained persistent bleeding; hoarseness. Also persistent or recurring pain in ears or face; numbness in mouth or lips; difficulty swallowing

45. a

46. c

47. d

48. c

49. a. mechanical devices

    b. esophageal speech

    c. tracheoesophageal fistula

50. a

51. c

52. Prolonged intubation or mechanical ventilation; acute upper airway obstruction; obstructive sleep apnea; retention of secretions; decreased airway dead space; also airway protection for large aspirations; prophylaxis against airway obstruction during surgery or as a result of severe injury; laryngectomy

53. Tube displacement; airway obstruction; aspiration; cuff leak and rupture; tracheomalacia; tracheal stenosis; tracheoesophageal fistula; trachea-innominate artery fistula

54. d	64. a
55. c	65. j
56. b	66. b
57. c	67. f
58. d	68. c
59. d	69. a
60. e	70. b
61. h	71. a
62. i	72. d
63. g	

73. i, e, g, a, d, k, b, f, m, j, c, h, l, n,

74. One person secures the tube while a second person changes the neck ties. If one person is changing the ties alone, the old neck ties are not removed until the new ties are in place and secured.

75. g, b, i, n, c, a, f, d, k, m, q, j, e, o, h, l, p

76. a

77. d

78. d

79. a

CHAPTER 30

Chronic Airflow Limitation

1. a
2. b
3. a, b
4. b
5. c
6. c
7. b, c
8. b
9. b, c
10. a
11. b
12. b, c
13. a
14. a
15. a
16. c
17. a
18. c
19. a
20. b, c
21. c
22. a
23. b
24. b

25. Age; sex; ethnic background; family history of asthma and emphysema; smoking history; type of cigarettes smoked; cough pattern and sputum production described; dyspnea episodes; activity tolerance; wheezing; orthopnea; feet swelling; diet history; practice of special breathing maneuvers; current medications; emergency plan; exposure to environmental irritants in home or work setting; psychosocial factors such as isolation, hobbies, pets, coping abilities, anxiety, fear, support systems, and significant others; financial circumstances

26. a

27. Smoking paralyzes the ciliary motion of the lungs; mucus secretion cannot be mobilized and removed from the lungs effectively during sleep. Upon awakening and with increased inspiratory effort, the smoker has excess mucus, which triggers the cough reflex to remove the local irritant.

28. c

29. Ability to answer questions lucidly, with or without breathlessness; weight; respiratory rate; breathing pattern; use of accessory muscles; anteroposterior diameter relative to lateral diameter of chest; presence of cyanosis; capillary refill; clubbing; decreased fremitus; abnormal percussion note; auscultation for breath sounds; chest wall retractions and tenderness; heart rate and rhythm; pedal edema

30. d
31. f
32. b
33. e
34. a
35. c
36. b
37. d
38. c
39. d
40. a
41. c

42. e
43. g
44. b
45. f
46. a

47. Impaired Gas Exchange; Ineffective Breathing Pattern; Ineffective Airway Clearance; Anxiety; Altered Nutrition (Less than Body Requirements); Activity Intolerance; High Risk for Infection; Powerlessness

48. b
49. d
50. b
51. b

52. Concentration of oxygen required by the client; concentration of oxygen achieved by a delivery system; importance of accuracy and control of oxygen concentration; client comfort; client expense; importance of humidity; client mobility

53. b
54. b
55. a
56. a
57. a
58. a
59. b
60. b
61. b
62. a
63. b
64. a

65. a. bronchodilators
    b. anticholinergics
    c. corticosteroids
    d. cromolyn sodium
    e. mucolytics

66. a. methylxanthines: relax smooth muscles of bronchial tubes
    b. sympathomimetics (adrenergics): mimic the sympathetic nervous system and cause bronchodilation

67. c
68. a
69. Refer to Chart 30-7 on p. 703 in the textbook for discussion.
70. a
71. b
72. c
73. d
74. d
75. a
76. b
77. c

Pneumonia

78. d

79. c

80. l, e, g, j, b, h, c, a, k, i, d, f

81. b

82. b

83. a

84. c

85. c

86. a

87. Age; environmental factors such as home, work, school; diet; exercise patterns; sleep patterns; use of cigarettes or alcohol; medications; known drug abuse; past respiratory-related illnesses; recent exposure to flu, viruses, or pneumonia; rashes or insect bites; exposure to animals; known neurological deficits; use of respiratory equipment; vaccinations for flu or pneumococcus; chest pain; myalgia; headache; chills; reported fever; dyspnea; sputum production (and characteristics); psychosocial factors such as anxiety

88. Anxious expression; flushing; bright eyes; coughing; splinting with respirations; breathing pattern; use of accessory muscles with respiration; cyanosis of lips or nail beds; depth and symmetry of thoracic wall expansion; adventitious sounds; decreased breath sounds; tactile fremitus increased; dullness to percussion; sputum characteristics; pulse rate and quality; mental status; rashes; nausea

89. d

90. a

91. a. Ineffective Airway Clearance
    b. Impaired Gas Exchange

92. c

93. b

94. a

95. b

Tuberculosis

96. b

97. c

98. d, b, g, h, f, c, e, a

99. c

100. Past exposure to someone with TB; foreign travel or residence; past skin testing for TB and results; vaccination with BCG; diffuse anxiety or nervousness

101. a

102. b

103. Multidrug regimens destroy organisms as quickly as possible and minimize emergence of drug-resistant organisms.

104. d

105. d

Pulmonary Abscess and Empyema

106. c

107. b

108. b

109. a

Influenza and Sarcoidosis

110. c

111. The vaccine is altered every year based on the specific viral strains that are predicted to be prevalent that year during the flu season.

112. b

113. a

114. b

115. c

Occupational Pulmonary Disease

116. e

117. d

118. g

119. f

120. a

121. c

122. b

123. a

CHAPTER 31

Pulmonary Embolism

1. a

2. d

3. a

4. a

5. d

6. b

7. b

8. a

9. b

Lung Cancer

10. d
11. b
12. d
13. c
14. b
15. a. Pain
    b. Ineffective Airway Clearance
    b. Impaired Gas Exchange

16. b	27. f
17. a	28. d
18. a	29. a
19. b	30. e
20. c	31. b
21. d	32. c
22. a	33. c
23. f	34. c
24. b	35. d
25. g	36. e
26. e	37. d

Acute Respiratory Failure

38. b	50. a
39. a	51. b
40. b	52. a
41. a	53. a
42. c	54. c
43. b	55. b
44. a	56. a
45. a	57. a
46. b	58. b
47. c	59. d
48. b	60. a
49. a	

Adult Respiratory Distress Syndrome

61. c
62. a
63. c
64. c

Mechanical Ventilation

65. a. maintain a patent airway
    b. reduce the work of breathing
    c. provide a way to remove secretions
    d. provide ventilation and oxygen
66. c
67. a
68. d
69. b
70. a. resuscitation bag with face mask
    b. source for 100% oxygen
    c. suction equipment
    d. oral airway

71. c	81. h
72. c	82. c
73. a	83. b
74. b	84. e
75. b	85. g
76. a	86. j
77. b	87. f
78. a	88. a
79. a	89. i
80. b	90. d

91. a. no problem, but low oxygen: give oxygen
    b. metabolic acidosis: correct metabolic cause
    c. respiratory acidosis: increase ventilations, especially length of expiration with pursed-lip breathing
    d. respiratory alkalosis: decrease ventilations or have client rebreathe ventilations
    e. no problem: no treatment needed
    f. respiratory acidosis: give oxygen, increase length of expirations and ventilations

92. b	104. c
93. c	105. b
94. e	106. a
95. a	107. a
96. d	108. d
97. b	109. d
98. c	110. b
99. b	111. d
100. e	112. b
101. a	113. a
102. b	114. b
103. c	115. c

CHAPTER 32

Anatomy and Physiology Review

1.	c	13.	d
2.	b	14.	m
3.	d	15.	e
4.	e	16.	c
5.	c	17.	b
6.	a	18.	a
7.	d	19.	k
8.	l	20.	g
9.	h	21.	j
10.	n	22.	i
11.	o	23.	b
12.	f		

24. The sequence is SA node (rate = 60–100 beats per minute), intranodal tracts, junctional area, AV node (rate = 40–60 beats per minute), bundle of His, bundle branches, Purkinje fibers (rate = 20–40 beats per minute), and ventricles.

> SA node to AV node = 0.04 second
>
> AV node delay = 0.07–0.1 second to allow for atrial contraction
>
> AV node to ventricular contraction = 0.08–0.12 second

25.	c	29.	f
26.	a	30.	a
27.	c	31.	d
28.	e	32.	b

33. a. autonomic nervous system via the chemoreceptors and baroreceptors through stimulation of the vasomotor center

   b. kidneys via the renin-angiotensin-aldosterone mechanism

   c. endocrine system via the release of various hormones that stimulate the sympathetic nervous system at the target tissue level

34.	b	40.	a
35.	a	41.	c, d, f
36.	a	42.	a
37.	a	43.	a
38.	b	44.	b
39.	b		

Subjective Assessment

45. Age; sex; ethnic origin; height; weight; major illness (e.g., diabetes mellitus, kidney disease, anemia, high blood pressure, stroke, bleeding disorders, connective tissue diseases, chronic pulmonary disease, heart disease, thrombophlebitis); history of streptococcal infection or rheumatic fever; congenital heart defects; drug allergies; habits (e.g., alcohol consumption, use of drugs, caffeine intake, smoking, activity level and type); family history; diet history (especially intake of sodium, sugar, cholesterol, and fat); household members (spouse, children, others); living environment; occupation; hobbies; history of obesity or weight gain; estrogen intake; emotional stress; details of current health problems such as chest pain, dyspnea, fatigue, palpitations, weight gain, syncope, pain in extremities; psychosocial factors such as support systems, coping abilities, fear about pain, disability, self-esteem, physical dependence, change in family role dynamics

46. a

47. One-half pack/day × 2 years = 1 pack-year

   One pack/day × 4 years = 4 pack-years

   Two packs/day × 20 years = 40 pack-years

   Total = 45 pack-years

The greater the number of pack-years, the greater the risk a client has of developing arteriosclerosis or pulmonary diseases (e.g., chronic airflow limitation). By stopping smoking, the adverse physiologic effects gradually reverse themselves and the client's risk level decreases.

48. Submit the completed exercise to the clinical instructor for evaluation and feedback.

Objective Assessment

49. General build and appearance; skin color; distress level; level of consciousness; shortness of breath; position (posture); verbal responses; pallor; cyanosis; cool skin temperature; clubbing; capillary fill delay; edema; paresthesia; muscle fatigue; loss of hair; blood pressure; orthostatic hypotension; paradoxical blood pressure; pulse pressure; jugular venous pressure; presence of hepatojugular reflux; quality of peripheral arterial pulsations; pulsus alternans; pulsus bisferiens; carotid bruit; tachypnea; use of accessory muscles for breathing; dyspnea; shallow respirations; Cheyne-Stokes respirations; hemoptysis; adventitious breath sounds (crackles or wheezes); precordial vibration or movement except at PMI; heaves; lifts; thrills; auscultation for rate, rhythm, murmurs, extrasystolic sounds, and rubs; abnormal splitting of S_2; presence of S_3 or S_4

50. Submit the completed exercise to the clinical instructor for evaluation and feedback.

51. b
52. b
53. c
54. c
55. d
56. b
57. c
58. d
59. c
60. b
61. b
62. c
63. a
64. d
65. a

CHAPTER 33

Electrocardiography

1. d
2. a. atrial tissue

   b. junctional tissue (AV node, intraventricular tissue, bundle of His, Purkinje fibers)

   c. ventricular tissue

3. b
4. d
5. a
6. c
7. f
8. e
9. b
10. d
11. c
12. e
13. a
14. f
15. b
16. b

17. 1500/25 = 60 beats per minute

18. Analyze the P waves, analyze the QRS complexes, determine the atrial rhythm or regularity, determine the ventricular rhythm or regularity, determine the heart rate, measure the PR interval, measure the QRS duration, and interpret the rhythm

19. *Arrhythmia* means a complete absence of a cardiac rhythm, which is the electrical conduction and mechanical contraction that results in a heartbeat. *Dysrhythmia* is a disorder or irregularity in the cardiac cycle. There is still a heartbeat, but it may not be effective in producing a cardiac output sufficient to sustain life.

20. c
21. c, d, e, h, i, j, o, p
22. Ischemia of cardiac tissue, digitalis toxicity, increased catecholamine release, hypoxia, electrolyte imbalances, overuse of stimulants, lack of sleep, and anxiety

Collaborative Management of Dysrhythmias

23. History of cardiac arrest; coronary artery disease; heart failure; congenital defects; rheumatic fever; cardiac medications; diuretics; supplemental electrolyte therapy; palpitations; shortness of breath; chest pain; weakness; dizziness; confusion; black-outs; diaphoresis; caffeine and alcohol intake; smoking history; and psychosocial factors such as fear of incapacitation or death and fear of recurrence of an MI

24. Heart rate; rhythm; hypotension; confusion, restlessness, or anxiety; dyspnea; oliguria; irregularity of apical or radial pulse; pulse deficit; delayed capillary refill; pale, ashen, or cyanotic skin color; cool, clammy skin; adventitious lung sounds such as crackles; weakness; fatigue

25. Decreased Cardiac Output
26. a. type of dysrhythmia

    b. cause of the dysrhythmia

    c. effect on cardiac output

    d. risks to the client

27. a
28. b
29. *Demand mode* means that a cardiac pacemaker is set so that it produces an electrical impulse to trigger a contraction only if the client's own intrinsic rhythm is less than a targeted range. If the client's heart is capable of producing and conducting its own impulses, the demand pacemaker does not function.

30. a. discomfort, skin irritation, and diaphoresis

    b. loss of capture

    c. inappropriate pacing

31. d
32. b
33. c

ECG Strip Exercise

Strip 1. Normal sinus rhythm with first-degree A-V block and multifocal PVCs > 6 per minute

Strip 2. Second-degree A-V block I (Wenckebach)

Strip 3. Ventricular tachycardia

Strip 4. Normal sinus rhythm with ST elevation and unifocal PVCs

Strip 5. Third-degree (complete heart block), apical rate 80, ventricular rate 50

Strip 6. Normal sinus rhythm with a PVC on a T wave and ventricular fibrillation

Strip 7. Idiojunctional rhythm, rate 75

Strip 8. Normal sinus rhythm, rate 75, PR interval 0.20

Strip 9. Atrial fibrillation

Strip 10. Sinus bradycardia, rate 50, PR interval 0.12

Strip 11. Atrial flutter with a 2:1 block

Strip 12. Ventricular (VVI) pacer rhythm

CHAPTER 34

Heart Failure

1. d
2. b
3. a
4. History of high blood pressure, angina, MI, rheumatic heart disease, valvular disorders, endocarditis, pericarditis; description of breathing patterns (dyspnea, exertional dyspnea, orthopnea, paroxysmal nocturnal dyspnea, cough); noticed fluid retention (peripheral edema, weight gain); response to activity (ability to perform activities of daily living, climb stairs without dyspnea, weakness or fatigue while at rest); knowledge of heart failure; change in mental status (insomnia, memory loss, confusion); irregular heart rhythm; nausea; anorexia; nocturia; use of salt in diet; psychosocial factors such as fear of death, anxiety, frustration, and coping ability
5. d
6. Breathlessness; weakness; fatigue; confusion; dizziness; hypotension; irregular cardiac rhythm; displacement of the point of maximal impulse to the left; tachycardia; pulsus alternans; S_3 gallop; S_4; crackles (rales); wheezes; jugular venous distention; hepatomegaly; dependent edema; ascites
7. d
8. a
9. d
10. c
11. c
12. a. low salt, low fat diet
    b. weight loss
    c. smoking cessation
    d. exercise
    e. prompt treatment of infections
13. b

Valvular Heart Disease

14. d
15. b
16. c
17. Family health history including any valvular or other heart disease; history of rheumatic heart fever and use of prophylactic antibiotic therapy; fatigue level; level of activity tolerated; reports of orthopnea, paroxysmal nocturnal dyspnea (PND), dyspnea on exertion, palpitations, dizzi-

ness, syncope, and angina; psychosocial factors such as fear of heart surgery, frustration, and coping skills
18. Dyspnea on exertion; orthopnea; PND; dry cough; hemoptysis; hepatomegaly; neck venous distention; pitting edema; variable pulse rate and rhythm; murmurs; S_3; clicks; syncope, especially with exertion; bounding arterial pulses; widened pulse pressure
19. a
20. Decreased Cardiac Output
21. b
22. c
23. c
24. d

Inflammations and Infections

25. a
26. a
27. Fever; chills; malaise; night sweats; fatigue; heart murmurs; peripheral edema; weight loss or gain; anorexia; shortness of breath; crackles; sudden abdominal pain radiating to left shoulder and rebound tenderness; flank pain radiating to groin with hematuria or pyuria; transient ischemic attacks; cerebrovascular accident; confusion; aphasia; dysphagia; pleurisy; dyspnea; cough; petechiae; splinter hemorrhages; Osler's nodes; Janeway's lesions; splenomegaly; finger clubbing
28. b
29. b
30. c
31. d
32. c
33. a
34. a, d, e, f

Cardiomyopathy

35. a, c, d, e, g, h
36. a

CHAPTER 35

Arteriosclerosis and Atherosclerosis

1. *Arteriosclerosis* is a thickening or hardening of the arterial wall resulting in a loss of elasticity. *Atherosclerosis* is a form of arteriosclerosis that involves the formation of plaque within the arterial wall, which leads to eventual interference with blood flow through the artery.
2. b, d, a, c

3. c

4. d

5. Age; sex; race; weight; height; exercise habits; smoking habits; diet; family diseases and client's previous health problems (diabetes, hypertension, hyperlipidemia); previous vascular diseases such as cerebrovascular accident, myocardial infarction, and peripheral vascular disease; previous surgical procedures (coronary bypass, carotid endarterectomy, lower extremity revascularization); previous angioplasty or thrombolytic therapy; medications; pain and its characteristics; psychosocial factors such as denial of need for assessment or intervention, fear, stressors and stress management, and social support systems

6. Areas of dry skin; atrophic changes (hair loss, muscle atrophy, thickened or clubbed nails, circumoral pallor, pale nail beds, reddened skin); cellulitis and distended veins; varicosities; edema; ulcerations of peripheral extremities; shortness of breath; lethargy; irregular heart rate; murmur; pericardial rub; bruits; arterial pulse rates, rhythms, and quality; temperature difference between comparable extremities; nail bed capillary refill delay; pain upon palpation of extremities; positive Homan's test

7. d   11. b

8. b   12. c

9. c   13. b

10. a

Hypertension

14. c

15. a. peripheral resistance

    b. heart rate

    c. stroke volume

16. b

17. d

18. b

19. Age; race; genetic disposition to hypertension; obesity; weight changes in past year; cigarette smoking; excessive alcohol intake; increased salt intake; exercise routines; history of renal or cardiovascular disease; medications; baseline sexual history; headaches; dizziness; fainting; vision changes; psychosocial factors such as competitiveness, impatience, work addiction, aggressiveness, hostility, excessive ambition, abruptness of speech or gesture, response to stress, types of current stressors, and coping strategies

20. Edema; nocturia; lethargy; nosebleeds, supine, sitting, and erect blood pressures; rate, rhythm, and quality of peripheral arterial pulses; funduscopic examination for hemorrhage, exudates, papilledema, and arteriovenous compression; bruits; enlarged organs or abdominal masses

21. b

22. c

23. a

24. d

25. d

26. False assumption that the hypertension is under control because there are no symptoms; false assumption that the disease has been "cured" because blood pressure is normal; unpleasant side effects from the medications; cost of the medications

27. a

Peripheral Arterial Disease

28. d

29. Reported discomfort in lower back, buttocks, and thighs; leg or foot pain that develops with walking; reported pain relief with cessation of activity; rest pain; psychosocial factors such as depression, anxiety, limited mobility, fear of limb loss or death, and coping style

30. c

31. Hair loss on lower calf, ankle, and foot; dry, scaly skin; thickened toenails; extremity cool and gray-blue; elevational pallor; dependent rubor; mottling of extremity; delayed capillary filling; gangrene; areas of ulceration; decreased or absent peripheral arterial pulses; asymmetric limb temperature

32. c

33. d

34. a. segmental systolic blood pressure measurements

    b. exercise tolerance testing

    c. plethysmography

35. d   39. a

36. b   40. d

37. b   41. c

38. b   42. d

43. Emboli that originate in the heart following acute myocardial infarction or atrial fibrillation

44. b

Aneurysms

45. a

46. c

47. Age; sex; race; cigarette smoking; history of hypertension; hypercholesterolemia, obesity, stress, or familial predisposition; history of diabetes mellitus; reported deep, aching chest pain that may radiate to neck, back, or shoulders; psychosocial factors such as altered activity levels, fear of impending death, and occupational and financial concerns

48. Prominent pulsation in upper abdomen, left of midline; abdominal or lower back pain; abdominal tenderness or rigidity with palpation; sudden severe abdominal pain or back pain; possible hoarseness or coughing; pulsating mass in popliteal space or over femoral artery; pulmonary edema; diminished heart sounds; varying blood pressure in upper extremities; bruit over aneurysm; sudden hypotension; diaphoresis; decreased level of consciousness; oliguria; dysrhythmia

49. d

50. a

51. c

52. b

53. b

Other Arterial Disorders

54. c	58. c
55. b	59. e
56. d	60. a
57. b	

Venous Disorders

61. b

62. b

63. Age; history of previous thrombophlebitis; recent surgery or trauma; recent immobilization, e.g., prolonged travel requiring sitting; pregnancy; estrogen therapy such as oral contraceptives; history of intermittent leg swelling; psychosocial factors such as interruption of customary role functions, anxiety, stress, fear of pulmonary embolus, prolonged treatment regimen, depression, and hopelessness

64. Calf or groin tenderness or pain; leg swelling; warmth or edema in affected limb; pitting edema; stasis dermatitis; lower leg discoloration; ulcer formation; positive Homan's sign

65. a. white blood cell count

    b. PTT

    c. PT

66. d

67. a. bed rest

    b. elevation of the affected extremity

    c. anticoagulation therapy

68. b

69. c

70. a

71. a. inferior vena caval interruption

    b. ligation or external clips

72. d

73. a. edema (swelling)

    b. venous ulcers

    c. cellulitis

74. b

75. a

76. c

77. c

Vascular Trauma

78. a. puncture

    b. laceration

    c. transection

79. b

80. c

81. a. establishment of a patent airway

    b. control of bleeding

    c. restoration of blood flow

CHAPTER 36

Anatomy and Physiology Review

1. b

2. a. total blood volume

    b. cardiac output

    c. vascular bed size

3. d

4. c

Pathophysiology

5. b

6. c

7. a. **Initial:** Loss of 5–10 mmHg MAP. Minimal change of heart rate from baseline

   b. **Nonprogressive:** Decrease of 10–15 mmHg MAP. Release of renin, ADH, aldosterone, epinephrine, and norepinephrine; kidneys decrease glomerular filtration rate and increase sodium reabsorption; urinary output decreases; heart rate and vasoconstriction increase; pulse pressure decreases

   c. **Progressive:** Sustained decrease greater than 20 mmHg of MAP. The same changes occur as in nonprogressive shock; hypermetabolism of the kidneys and peripheral arterioles; increasing anoxia and ischemia; cell damage and death

   d. **Refractory:** MAP change same as in progressive shock. The same changes occur as in progressive shock; widespread tissue anoxia and cell death and continued anaerobic metabolism; myocardium deteriorates

8. c

9. a, b

10. b

11. a

12. a

13. a. **Hypovolemic:** Causes include hemorrhage (loss of blood volume); total fluid volume loss (dehydration). Primary prevention includes treatment and correction of hemorrhage before shock occurs and replacement of fluid volume loss.

   b. **Cardiogenic:** Causes include inadequate pumping ability of heart from direct causes. Primary prevention includes early detection, rapid and accurate diagnosis, and treatment of cardiac disorders.

   c. **Distributive:** Causes include loss of sympathetic tone causing vasodilation and blood pooling, increased vascular permeability, anaphylactic reactions, sepsis, and capillary leak syndrome. Primary prevention includes avoiding known allergens and wearing a Medic Alert tag; using strict aseptic technique; maintenance of the mucous membranes and skin integrity; treatment of the underlying condition such as pain, psychologic stress, excessive nerve block anesthesia, and burn injury; trauma; and numerous pathologic disorders.

   d. **Obstructive:** Causes include cardiac tamponade, pulmonary embolism and hypertension, arterial stenosis, constrictive pericarditis, and aortic aneurism. Primary prevention includes early detection, rapid and accurate diagnosis, and treatment of the underlying condition.

14. d

15. b

16. c

17. b

18. d

19. a

20. c

Collaborative Management

21. Age; recent illness, trauma, procedures, or chronic conditions; allergies; use of medications including over the counter medications; fluid intake and output during previous 24 hours; height; weight; psychosocial factors such as manner in which client responds to questions, anxiety, and fear

22. Early increase in pulse rate; weaker distal peripheral pulses; progressive disappearance of superficial peripheral pulses; diminished pulse pressure from an initial increased diastolic pressure; gradual decrease of systolic pressure; eventual disappearance of diastolic pressure as systolic pressure continues to fall; skin clammy and cool or cold; pallor; cyanosis

23. c

24. b

25. Increased respiratory rate (except with head injury); increase depth of respiration; crackles on auscultation

26. a

27. Decreased or absent urinary output; increased specific gravity; hematuria; foaming

28. Decreased level of consciousness; disorientation; restlessness and agitation; expressed feelings of anxiety; confusion; lethargy; somnolence; eventual loss of consciousness

29. Muscle weakness and pain; diminished or absent deep tendon reflexes

30. d

31. a. Fluid Volume Deficit

    b. Decreased Cardiac Output

    c. Altered Thought Processes

32. c

33. b

34. c

35. c

36. d

37. b

38. d

39. d

40. a

41. b

42. a

43. d

44. b

45. c

46. c

CHAPTER 37

Pathophysiology

1. b
2. a. atherosclerosis of a coronary artery
   b. coronary artery spasm
   c. platelet aggregation
   d. emboli from mural thrombi
3. d
4. d
5. a
6. b
7. c
8. a
9. a. collateral circulation to the myocardium
   b. anaerobic metabolism
   c. myocardium workload demand
10. c
11. a
12. c
13. b

Collaborative Management

14. Description of chest discomfort, including pain in upper back, jaw, and arms and type of sensation, location, radiation, and duration; prior hospitalization for angina or MI; medications; family history; modifiable risk factors, including eating habits; life style; physical activity levels; nausea during pain episodes; dizziness; weakness; palpitations; psychosocial factors such as denial, fear, anxiety, and anger

15. Chest pain that lasts longer than 30 minutes; vomiting; diaphoresis; shortness of breath; blood pressure; apical pulse; presence of dysrhythmias; weakened distal peripheral pulses; cool skin temperature; diaphoretic skin; S_3 gallop; increased respiratory rate; breath sounds for crackles or wheezes; S_4; elevated temperature

16. b   22. b
17. d   23. c
18. b   24. b
19. c   25. a
20. b   26. c
21. d

27. a. hemodynamic compromise
    b. increase myocardial oxygen demand
    c. risk of lethal ventricular dysrhythmia
28. c   32. d
29. a   33. d
30. b   34. d
31. a   35. b

CHAPTER 38

Anatomy and Physiology Review

1. c
2. d
3. a
4. b
5. c
6. a
7. c
8. b
9. b
10. d
11. a
12. b
13. b
14. a. destroys aged or imperfect RBCs
    b. catabolizes hemoglobin released from destroyed RBCs
    c. stores platelets
    d. filters antigens
15. a. helps in erythropoiesis if RBC production is abnormal
    b. produces blood coagulant substances
    c. converts bilirubin to bile
    d. stores iron as ferritin
16. e, j, h, f, a, c, d, i, b, g
17. a. foreign substances such as collagen
    b. antigen–antibody reactions
    c. circulating debris
    d. platelet clumps on damaged vessels
    e. bacterial endotoxins
18. d
19. c

Subjective Assessment

20. Age; sex; occupation; hobbies; geographic location of residence; inherited hematologic disorders (hemophilia, sickle cell trait); allergies; current medications; family history (episodes of excessive bleeding or bruising, known jaundice, anemia, or gallstones); use of anticoagulants, antibiotics, or cytotoxic drugs; previous radiation therapy; diet history; alcohol consumption; recent weight loss; noted swelling of glands; bruising; bleeding; excessive fatigue; malaise; dyspnea on exertion; palpitations; frequent infections; fevers; diarrhea; menorrhagia; headaches; paresthesias; vertigo; tinnitus; angina; anorexia; dysphagia; sore tongue; perception of health status; identified stressors; psychosocial factors such as coping style, social support systems, community resources, self-concept, self-esteem; financial resources

21. b

22. d

23. Submit the completed exercise to the clinical instructor for evaluation and feedback.

Objective Assessment

24. Pallor; jaundice; pale or cyanotic mucous membranes or nail beds; pale gums, conjunctivae, or palmar creases; lesions or draining wounds; petechiae; confluent ecchymoses; overt bleeding; covert bleeding from any drainage tubes, central or peripheral intravenous lines, or catheters; turgor; scratching; dry skin; smooth tongue; red tongue; circumoral fissures; jaundiced sclerae; any lymph node enlargement and/or tenderness; fatiguability; shortness of breath; orthopnea; location of the point of maximal impulse; heaves; distended neck veins; edema; murmurs; gallops; irregular cardiac rhythms; hypertension; hypotension; hematuria; rib or sternal tenderness; palpable spleen; palpable liver, especially in the epigastrium; cranial nerve function; fever; chills; night sweats

25. Submit the completed exercise to the clinical instructor for evaluation and feedback.

26. c
27. c
28. d
29. c
30. c
31. d
32. a
33. c
34. b

CHAPTER 39

Red Blood Cell Disorders

1. b
2. a
3. c
4. d
5. c
6. b
7. c
8. b
9. a. maintaining adequate hydration to prevent cellular debris precipitation in renal tubules

   b. administering osmotic diuretics to promote diuresis and renal clearance

   c. transfusing RBCs in the presence of anemia when renal function is adequate

10. d	15. b
11. b	16. a
12. d	17. c
13. a	18. c
14. b	19. d

20. Age; sex; occupation; hobbies; duration of symptoms; family member who is anemic or family history of anemia; recent blood loss (trauma, melena, hematemesis, hematuria, menorrhagia); history of alcohol or drug abuse; medication history; exposure to household or industrial toxins; diet history; chronic fatigue; shortness of breath; infections; anorexia; weight loss; sore mouth or tongue; indigestion; bone pain or deformity; chronic depression; headaches; behavior changes; increased somnolence; decreased alertness and attention span; lethargy; muscle weakness; increased fatigue; activity intolerance; psychosocial factors such as altered self-concept, feeling of loss, changes in role function

21. Tachycardia; murmurs; orthostatic hypotension; angina; increased respiratory rate; exertional dyspnea; orthopnea; pallor; shortness of breath; weight loss; vertigo; loss of consciousness; bounding arterial pulses; vascular bruits; PMI shift; dependent edema; jaundice; spider angiomas; delayed wound healing; growth abnormalities

22. a	26. c
23. b	27. d
24. c	28. b
25. a	29. d

White Blood Cell Disorders

30. b

31. a. anemia

    b. thrombocytopenia

    c. leukopenia

32. The bone marrow produces an abnormally large number of a specific type of leukocyte, which results in a suppression of the bone marrow's ability to produce other cell types (e.g., RBCs, other types of WBCs, and platelets). The WBCs that are produced are immature and incapable of functioning normally. Consequently, the client is subject to infection and hemorrhage.

33. b

34. Age; demographic information (occupation, hobbies); previous illnesses and medical history (exposure to ionizing radiation or specific medications known to increase risk); frequency and severity of infections (colds, flu, pneumonia, bronchitis, fever of unknown origin); history of bleeding episodes (bruises, epistaxis, menor-rhagia, bleeding gums, rectal bleeding, hema-turia, prolonged bleeding after injury); weakness; fatigue; nausea; headaches; behavior change; somnolence; decreased alertness; decreased attention span; lethargy; muscle weakness; decreased appetite; weight loss; bone pain; joint pain; psychosocial factors such as anxiety, fear of death, and coping patterns

35. d

36. a

37. Pale, cool skin; petechiae; ecchymoses; gum bleeding; oral lesions; tachycardia; orthostatic hypotension; palpitations; delayed capillary filling; murmurs; bruits; shortness of breath; adventitious breath sounds; dyspnea on exertion; increased respiratory rate; weight less; rectal fissures; melena; diminished bowel sounds; constipation; hepatosplenomegaly; abdominal tenderness; papilledema; seizure activity; coma; fever; enlarged lymph nodes or masses

38. b

39. d

40. c

41. Induction therapy is initiated at the time of diagnosis and is intensive. It usually consists of aggressive combination chemotherapy aimed at producing a rapid, complete remission.

    Consolidation therapy occurs early in remission and attempts to cure the client. It uses the same agents as were used in induction but the duration of therapy may vary.

Maintenance therapy is prescribed after successful induction and consolidation occur. It attempts to sustain remission and may be necessary for long periods.

42. b	50. b
43. c	51. c
44. c	52. b
45. d	53. d
46. a	54. c
47. d	55. d
48. d	56. b
49. b	

Coagulation Disorders

57. a, c, e, f, g

58. High Risk for Injury

59. d

60. b

61. c

62. c

63. a. hepatitis B infection

    b. cytomegalovirus infection

    c. infection with human immunodeficiency virus

64. The client's blood is cross-matched with that of the donor; each unit to be transfused is checked by two registered nurses for the physician's order for the blood product and the client's identity; the identification numbers of the client and the blood product are ascertained to be identical; and the blood product's labeling is checked to be sure it agrees with the requisition slip and the client's blood type for compatibility.

65. d

66. d

67. c

68. a

69. c

70. a. hemolytic

    b. allergic

    c. febrile

    d. bacterial

71. d

CHAPTER 40

Anatomy and Physiology Review

1. f
2. i
3. b
4. e
5. h
6. d
7. j
8. a
9. c
10. g
11. c
12. The all-or-nothing principle refers to the reaction of the nerve cells in a nerve fiber to a stimulus. A stimulus must be of sufficient strength to provoke the cell membrane to depolarize. However, once the cell depolarizes, it transmits the impulse all along the nerve fiber membrane. Either the entire nerve fiber reacts or it does not, depending on the initial depolarization.

13. b
14. a
15. a
16. b
17. b
18. a
19. b

20. a
21. a
22. b
23. a
24. a
25. b

26. a. spinal nerves
    b. cranial nerves
    c. autonomic nervous system
27. d
28. d
29. a. spinal cord
    b. brain
30. b
31. d
32. c
33. c
34. d
35. a
36. c
37. b

38. h
39. f
40. b
41. d
42. c
43. a
44. g
45. e

46. a. control and direct voluntary movement
    b. maintain equilibrium

47. d
48. c
49. k
50. a
51. j
52. f
53. h

54. e
55. b
56. g
57. i
58. b
59. b
60. c

61. a. pia mater
    b. arachnoid
    c. dura mater
    d. cranium
    e. vertebrae
62. a

Subjective Assessment

63. Age; sex; history of injury, congenital problems, chronic disease (hypertension, diabetes mellitus, lung diseases); previous neurological problem (headache, seizures, trauma to head or spine, eye problems); allergies; current medications; pain tolerance and usual self-treatment for pain; recreational activities; ingestion of alcohol or other chemicals; sleep habits and any changes; usual bladder and bowel habits and any changes; hand dominance; occupation; financial resources; complete details about any current neurological health problems (onset, signs and symptoms, aggravating and relieving factors, effect on activities of daily living, level of understanding); changes in any of the senses or inability to perform motor skills.

64. d
65. b
66. Submit the completed exercise to the clinical instructor for evaluation and feedback.

Objective Assessment

67. Mental status including speech and behavior; ability to cooperate with the examination; level of consciousness; orientation to person, place, time; memory (remote, recent, new); attention span; ability to follow directions; speech hesitancy; reading comprehension; writing ability; copying ability; general fund of information or knowledge; abstract reasoning ability; judgment; olfaction; central and peripheral vision; funduscopic examination; eye movements; ability of pupils to constrict (direct and consensual); accommodation; eyelid position; nystagmus; sensation perception to the face; jaw clench ability; corneal reflex; ability to frown, smile, wrinkle forehead, puff out cheeks; ability to keep eyelids closed against resistance; hearing acuity;

sound lateralization with Weber's test; air conduction versus bone conduction of sound; taste sensation perception; rise of uvula and palate with phonation; gag reflex; swallowing ability; phonation; ability to turn head and shrug shoulders against resistance; ability to stick our tongue and push tongue against a tongue blade; perception of pain, temperature, light touch, touch discrimination, two-point discrimination, position, vibration over trunk and extremities; graphesthesia; stereognosis; involuntary tremor or movement; hand grip strength; arm drift; muscle group strength against resistance; gait; balance and equilibrium; ability to run heel of one leg down opposite shin; rapid alternating pronation and supination of hands; finger-to-nose pointing; deep tendon reflexes; plantar reflex; abdominal reflexes

68. Submit the completed exercise to the clinical instructor for evaluation and feedback.

69.	e	86.	c
70.	d	87.	b
71.	e	88.	c
72.	a	89.	b
73.	c	90.	d
74.	b	91.	d
75.	e	92.	b
76.	a	93.	d
77.	d	94.	a
78.	f	95.	c
79.	c	96.	b
80.	b	97.	d
81.	d	98.	a
82.	e	99.	d
83.	d	100.	b
84.	f	101.	d
85.	a		

CHAPTER 41

Headaches

1. b

2. c

3. Sex; age; onset of menses; use of contraceptive hormones; age at onset of first headache; sequence of events during headaches (including precipitating factors, presence of an aura, time between the aura and onset, accompanying nausea or vomiting, length of attack); use of medications to treat headaches; relieving factors; foods known to client that precipitate headache; alcohol intake; job-related activities; family history of migraines; numbness or tingling of lips or tongue before an attack; psychosocial factors such as client's work ethic, perceived ability to cope with stress, means of relaxation, degree to which attacks are incapacitating, self-image

4. Slowness or slight confusion; aphasia; vertigo; drowsiness; nausea or vomiting; distention and pulsation of frontotemporal vessels over affected side; nasal congestion; conjunctival congestion; obvious discomfort in client

5. a

6. a. consistent sleep patterns

   b. avoiding triggers such as monosodium gluconate, chocolate, ripened cheese, sausage, citrus fruits, and red wine

   c. discontinuing contraceptive pills

   d. coping with stress

7. b

8. d

9. c

10. c

11. c

Epilepsy

12. b

13. d

14. Description of the seizure activity and surrounding events (frequency, activity during seizures, sequence of events, duration, last occurrence, presence of an aura, post-seizure knowledge or recall of seizure, incontinence during seizure, activity after seizures, return to pre-seizure status); current medications; psychosocial factors such as fear, potential for job loss, rejection by friends, denial, coping ability

15. During seizure activity: all physical signs exhibited, especially eye fluttering; head or eye deviation; pupil size; movement and progression of motor activity; automatisms; LOC; cyanosis; salivation; incontinence; behavior following seizure including drowsiness

16. b

17. c

18. c

19. a

20. d

21. d

Infections

22. a. by crossing the blood–brain barrier

    b. directly from penetrating trauma

    c. inadvertently during surgical procedures

    d. from a ruptured cerebral abscess

    e. directly via a basilar skull fracture

23. b

24. History of head trauma or recent infection (respiratory, ear, nose, sinus); history of heart disease, diabetes mellitus, cancer; immunosuppressive therapy; recent surgical procedure, especially neurological, ear, or nose; headache; recent occurrence of a communicable disease, rash, bites; recent foreign travel; psychosocial factors such as subtle changes in personality, behavior, mental status, fear, anxiety

25. a

26. LOC; orientation; pupil reaction; extraocular movements; motor response; lethargy; memory changes; short attention span; bewilderment; behavior change; increasing stupor; photophobia; nystagmus; facial paresis; difficulty hearing; progressive hemiparesis, hemiplegia; decreased muscle tone; nuchal rigidity; nausea; vomiting; fever; chills; tachycardia; macular rash; increased ICP; seizures; bleeding; intravascular coagulation

27. d

28. b

29. c

30. d

31. b

32. a. cerebrum

    b. brain stem

    c. cerebellum

33. d

34. a

35. a

36. Compromise of pulmonary function such as atelectasis or pneumonia leads to hypoxia. Hypoxia, in turn, affects cerebral perfusion so that cerebral vessels dilate to provide an increased blood flow to the brain and more oxygen. The increased flow results in increased ICP. The benefit of preventing this from occurring outweighs the disadvantage of the temporarily increased ICP that occurs with suctioning and coughing.

37. c

38. b

39. a

Parkinson's Disease

40. d

41. Time and progression of symptoms; noted gait problems; noted change in posture (stooping); slow movements; reported difficulty performing two movements at once; noted tremor and the associated circumstances; reported problems with speech, swallowing, bladder or bowel continence; noted excess perspiration; dizziness upon arising; eye muscle spasms; oily skin and scalp; change in handwriting (cramped); psychosocial factors such as emotional liability, depression, paranoia, mood swings, slowness in finishing tasks

42. b

43. Rigidity (cogwheel, plastic, lead pipe); mask-like faces (wide-eyed staring); difficulty chewing or swallowing; drooling; decreased respiratory excursion; decreased breath sounds; soft, low voice; dysarthria; echolalia; stooped posture; flexed trunk; decreased or absent arm swing with walking; slow, shuffling gate; propulsive gait; reverse propulsion; inability to move; freezing; tremor at rest; pill rolling; flushing; orthostatic hypotension; change in skin texture; severe constipation

44. b

45. b

46. d

Alzheimer's Disease

47. Reduced brain weight; marked cerebral atrophy; enlargement of the ventricles, cerebral sulci, and fissures; microscopic changes including neurofibrillary tangles, senile (neuritic) plaques, and granulovascular degeneration

48. a

49. Memory changes; increasing forgetfulness; employment status; work history; ability to fulfill household duties; changes noted in ability to drive, handling routine financial affairs, and language and communication skills; personality or behavior changes; history of head trauma, viral illness, exposure to metal or toxic waste; family history of Alzheimer's; psychosocial factors such as social isolation, loss of interest in hobbies or current events, irritability, anxiety, suspiciousness, paranoia, abusiveness; hallucinations; delusions

50. a. client may be unaware of any problems

    b. client may deny problems exist

    c. client may try to cover up problems

51. Refer to Key Features of Alzheimer's Disease on p. 1155.

52. c
53. d
54. b
55. d
56. d
57. d

Huntington's Chorea

58. b
59. d

CHAPTER 42

Back Pain

1. **Cervical:** herniation of the nucleus pulposus in an intervertebral disk; osteophyte formation pressing on intervertebral foramen; muscle strain; ligament sprain

   Lumbosacral: herniation of nucleus pulposus; ligament sprain; disk injury from hyperflexion or degeneration; muscle strain or spasm

2. See Chart 42-5 on p. 1171 in the textbook.

3. Precipitating event leading to back pain; age; sex; occupation; client or family history of arthritis; current weight and weight history; smoking history; related medical problems, treatment, or spinal surgery; psychosocial factors such as financial concerns, changes in lifestyle (job, leisure), frustration, depression, family reaction

4. Posture; gait; vertebral alignment; local muscle spasm; pain, especially if it radiates down arm or leg; tenderness with palpation; sensory changes in an extremity; muscle tone and strength in extremities; pain with straight leg raises

5. a. drug therapy

   b. back exercises

   c. heat or ice therapy

   d. bracing

   e. diet therapy

   f. traction

   g. positioning and rest

   h. transcutaneous electrical nerve stimulation; also distraction, imagery, and music therapy

6. c
7. b
8. b

Spinal Cord Injury

9. b
10. c
11. c
12. b
13. d
14. a
15. a
16. How accident occurred; probably mechanism of injury; client's position immediately following injury; symptoms noted after injury; changes occurring since time of injury; type of immobilization device used; problems during retrieval and transport; nature of treatment given at the scene; medical history including arthritis of the spine, congenital deformities, osteoporosis, osteomyelitis, cancer, or neck or back injury; problems noted with respiration; psychosocial factors such as usual coping methods, level of independence or dependence on others, religious and cultural beliefs, changes in body image, self-esteem, role relationships, sexuality, family support systems, financial security, job status

17. d

18. Respiratory pattern; bleeding around fracture site; hypotension; tachycardia with weak, thready pulse; level of consciousness; determination of the level of injury by testing sensory and motor function in the dermatomes surrounding the area noted by client to be deficient; voluntary muscle movement and strength in major muscle groups; deep tendon reflexes (especially biceps, triceps, patellar, and Achilles'); bradycardia; inability to control body temperature; severe hypertension; severe headache; nasal stuffiness; flushing; vital capacity; minute volume; abdominal distention; decreased bowel sounds; urinary retention; muscle tone and size; skin integrity over pressure points

19. d
20. c
21. c
22. d
23. b
24. e
25. a
26. a. deep venous thrombosis

   b. pulmonary emboli

   c. pressure sores

   d. contractures

27. a

28. a. physical mobility and activity skills
    b. ADL skills
    c. bowel and bladder program
    d. skin care
    e. medication regimen
    f. sexuality

Spinal Cord Tumors

29. d
30. a. pain
    b. motor deficits
    c. sensory losses
    d. loss of bladder control
    e. loss of bowel control
    f. impaired sexual function
31. b

Multiple Sclerosis

32. a
33. History of changes in vision, motor skills, or sensations, especially if intermittent or transient; aggravating factors (fatigue, stress, overexertion, temperature extremes, hot bath or shower); personality or behavior change; family history of MS; diplopia; blurred vision; reported decreased visual acuity; fatigue and stiffness of extremities; reported flexor spasms at night; tinnitus; vertigo; noted loss of hearing; feelings of numbness, tingling, burning, crawling sensation; psychosocial factors such as anxiety, apathy, emotional lability, depression, giddiness, coping ability
34. b
35. Complete neurological assessment including visual acuity; visual filed; nystagmus; increased or hyperactive deep tendon reflexes; clonus; positive Babinski's reflex; absent abdominal reflexes; unsteady gait; intention tremor; dysmetria; dysdiadochokinesia; clumsiness; loss of balance; hearing loss; facial weakness; difficulty swallowing; dysarthria; ataxia; slow, scanning speech; hypalgesia; paresthesia; altered rectal tone; constipation; bowel incontinence; areflexic bladder; urinary frequency, urgency, nocturia; impotence; difficulty sustaining an erection; frigidity; decreased vaginal secretions; memory loss; decreased ability to perform calculations; inattentiveness; impaired judgment
36. d
37. b
38. c

Amyotrophic Lateral Sclerosis

39. c
40. c

Other Neurological Problems

41. a
42. b
43. c
44. c

CHAPTER 43

Guillain–Barré Syndrome

1. c
2. Recent illness 3 to 4 weeks prior to onset of symptoms; description of symptoms accurately as they occurred in sequence; paresthesia; pain; facial weakness; difficulty walking; motor weakness; loss of bladder or bowel control; pattern of symptoms occurring from distal to proximal usually, although the reverse is possible; diplopia; psychosocial factors such as fear, anxiety, panic, anger, depression, motivation, coping ability, support systems
3. b
4. Orthostatic hypotension; labile blood pressure; tachycardia; decreased or absent deep tendon reflexes; facial weakness (inability to smile, frown, whistle, drink from straw); dysphagia; inability to cough, gag, or shrug shoulders; dyspnea; decreased breath sounds; decreased tidal volume and vital capacity; ophthalmoplegia; severe ataxia
5. d
6. d
7. b
8. b
9. Monitoring for incontinence provides for timely cleaning of soiled skin surfaces to prevent irritation and potential breakdown of integrity. Taut bed linens provide a smooth surface under the client, free from wrinkles, which are a source of uneven pressure on skin surfaces or over bony prominences; this also reduces shearing. Adequate fluids promote hydration and turgor, making the skin less prone to drying and cracking. Enteral feedings may be necessary to provide sufficient calories for a positive nitrogen balance, tissue repair, and normal maintenance.

10. a

11. e

Myasthenia Gravis

12. c

13. b

14. Reported rapid onset of fatigue; muscular weakness that increases with exertion and improves with rest; specific muscle groups affected; inability to perform ADL; ptosis; diplopia; difficulty chewing, swallowing, or choking; respiratory difficulty; weak voice; diet changes to accommodate chewing or swallowing difficulties; difficulty holding up head, brushing teeth, shaving or combing hair; aching muscles; history of thymus gland tumor; recent infection, emotional upset, pregnancy, or anesthesia; psychosocial factors such as altered body image, feelings of loss, fear, helplessness, and grief, coping methods, and support systems, developmental level

15. d

16. Progressive paresis resolved by rest; ocular palsies; ptosis; incomplete eyelid closure; asymmetric smile; lax jaw; tongue fissures; difficulty chewing and swallowing; weight loss; voice weakening after extended conversation; proximal limb weakness; inability to sit or walk upright; muscle atrophy; decreased respiratory excursion; loss of bladder or bowel function; facial paresthesias; decreased sense of smell and taste

17. c

18. a

19. b

20. c

21. a. participate in activities early in the day

    b. engage in activities during energy peaks following medication administration

    c. plan rest periods

    d. avoid excess fatigue

22. b

23. Regular and timely administration maintains therapeutic blood levels of the medications. This prevents fluctuating levels, which lead to increased weakness and other symptoms.

24. a

25. b

26. c

27. d

28. b

29. a

30. d

Polyneuritis and Polyneuropathy

31. Muscle weakness with or without atrophy; pains; paresthesias; loss of sensation; impaired reflexes; autonomic manifestations such as orthostatic hypotension, abnormal sweating, miosis

32. c

33. a

34. c

Peripheral Nerve Trauma

35. b

36. a

37. Ability of inability to perform range of motion in an extremity; abnormal movement; tremor; atrophy; contractions; paresis; paralysis; weak or absent deep tendon reflexes; temperature and skin color of extremity; edema; scaling of skin; nail brittleness; loss of body hair

38. c

39. d

40. c

Diseases of the Cranial Nerves

41. b

42. d

43. d

44. b

45. c

CHAPTER 44

Cerebrovascular Accident

1.	a	7.	a
2.	d	8.	b
3.	b	9.	c
4.	b	10.	d
5.	b	11.	a
6.	a		

12. Age; sex; activity engaged in when stroke began; symptom progression (e.g., onset, severity); reports of loss of consciousness, intellectual impairment, memory loss, difficulty with speech, hearing loss, visual problems, change in reading or writing ability, motor or sensory changes, loss of balance, gait change; past history of head trauma, diabetes, hypertension, cardiac disease,

anemia, obesity, or headache; current medications (especially aspirin, anticoagulants, vasodilators, illegal drugs); education level; employment status; travel; type of leisure activities; habits such as smoking, diet, exercise, alcohol; psychosocial factors such as reaction to illness, body image, self-concept, ability to perform ADL, coping mechanisms, personality changes, financial status, emotional lability

13. d

14. Level of consciousness; change in level of consciousness (LOC); cognitive problems (denial; hemiparesis neglect; spatial and proprioceptive dysfunction; impaired memory, judgment, and problem-solving ability; decreased attention span); hemiplegia; decreased muscle tone; loss of balance; incoordination of gait; bladder or bowel incontinence; agraphia; alexia; agnosia; apraxia; neglect syndrome; pupil abnormalities; ptosis; visual field deficits (hemianopsia); difficulty chewing; facial paralysis or numbness; dysphagia; absent gag reflex; impaired tongue movement; cardiac murmur or dysrhythmia; hypertension

15. c

16. c

17. d

18. b

19. a

20. a. complete bed rest with head elevated 30–45 degrees

    b. quiet, darkened room with minimal distractions

    c. avoid stimulating beverages (caffeine) and liquids of extremely hot or cold temperature

    d. limit visitors

    e. avoid straining and coughing

    f. sedation as ordered

21. b

22. c

23. b

24. d

25. a

26. d

27. a. medication schedule and all pertinent information related to prescribed medications

    b. mobility transfer skills

    c. self-care skills

28. *Respite care* is for the caregivers (family members) of clients who are homebound and dependent on others for their well-being. These caregivers need "timeout" away from the client to maintain their own emotional and physical health. Respite caregivers take over for the family for a period of time. Respite care is most beneficial if it occurs on a regular basis.

Head Injury

29. b	36. f
30. l	37. a
31. h	38. b
32. d	39. k
33. i	40. e
34. j	41. c
35. m	42. g

43. a. edema

    b. hemorrhage

    c. impaired cerebral autoregulation

    d. hydrocephalus

    e. hypoxemia

    f. hypercapnia

    g. systemic hypotension

44. As ICP rises, cerebral blood flow decreases because of vessel compression. The decreased blood flow leads to brain tissue hypoxia from insufficient oxygen delivery and continued tissue metabolism. The serum pH decreases while the carbon dioxide level rises, resulting in a local tissue acidosis. Cerebral vasodilation then occurs, leading to cerebral edema, and further increases in ICP. The cycle continues, eventually causing brain herniation toward the brain stem.

45. a. vasogenic

    b. cytotoxic or cellular

    c. interstitial

46. b

47. c

48. a

49. c

50. a

51. *Herniation* is a shifting of brain tissue due to ICP. Because the rigid cranial vault (skull) cannot expand, the rising pressure pushes the brain toward the area of lesser resistance, i.e., downward. This results in pressure on structures such as the cranial nerves, brain stem, diencephalon, and medulla. The pressure affects the ability of vital centers of autoregulation (respiration, cardiovascular, thermoregulatory) to function.

52. Details about when, where, and how the injury occurred; loss of consciousness and duration; change in LOC; events following injury (e.g., responsiveness and unresponsiveness patterns); reported seizure activity; history of seizures; detailed information about falls; hand dominance; history of eye disease or trauma; allergies; alcohol or drug use; headache; nausea; psychosocial factors such as personality changes, memory loss, learning ability, problem-solving ability, coping strategies, family dynamics

53. b

54. Determination of spinal cord injury; breathing patterns; changes in blood pressure or pulse; LOC; orientation; decreased arousability; sleepiness; coma; restlessness; irritability; pupillary size and reaction to light; loss of vision; decreased EOMs; diplopia; visual field deficit; hemiparesis; deterioration in motor function; posturing; flaccidity; ataxia; change in muscle tone or weakness; cranial nerve dysfunction; speech difficulties; vomiting; seizures; papilledema; leakage of CSF from nose or ears; neck stiffness; skull fractures; ecchymosis; lacerations to scalp; tender areas

55. a. establishment of baseline data

    b. early detection of or prevention of increased ICP, systemic hypotension, hypoxia, and hypercapnia

56. b

57. c

58. b

59. c

60. a

61. d

62. c

Brain Tumor

63. a. lungs

    b. breast

    c. kidney

    d. colon

    e. pancreas

64. b

65. Identification of risk factors (e.g., radiation exposure or chemical agents); generalized headache, more severe in the morning; emesis shortly after awakening unrelated to nausea; decreased visual acuity; diplopia; loss of peripheral vision; reported personality of behavior changes; depression; forgetfulness; complete details about symptoms including any self-medication; psychosocial factors such as inappropriate behavior, impulsiveness, difficulty with decision making, wide mood swings, anxiety, fear

66. c

67. Complete neurological assessment; papilledema; altered visual acuity; decreased peripheral vision; inability to move eyes laterally; hemiparesis; hemiplegia; seizure activity; sensation changes (hyperesthesia, paresthesia, loss of tactile discrimination); astereognosis; agnosia; apraxia; agraphia; loss of body half awareness; inattention to personal grooming; aphasia; abnormalities of cranial nerve function (facial pain, weakness, hearing loss, dysphagia, decreased taste, loss of gag reflex, nystagmus, hoarseness); ataxia; dysarthria; possible signs of endocrine dysfunction

68. b

69. b

70. c

71. a. client's age

    b. neurological status

    c. stage of the disease process at time of diagnosis

    d. tumor type

72. d

73. d

74. b

75. a

76. b

Brain Abscess

77. a. extradural

    b. subdural

    b. intracerebral

78. a. ear infection

    b. sinus infection

    c. osteomyelitis (mastoid infection)

    d. septic emboli

    e. penetrating trauma to the skull

79. b

80. d

81. a

CHAPTER 45

Anatomy and Physiology Review

1. c	19. l
2. d	20. j
3. c	21. a
4. a	22. s
5. b	23. d
6. c	24. i
7. d	25. b
8. c	26. h
9. m	27. n
10. q	28. b
11. f	29. d
12. c	30. a
13. p	31. c
14. g	32. d
15. k	33. a
16. o	34. e
17. e	35. b
18. r	36. c

37. a. lens loses elasticity, hardens, become more dense

    b. loss of subcutaneous fat, skin elasticity, and muscle tone

    c. decreased strength of the levator muscle

    d. fatty globule deposits around cornea

    e. cornea flattens, resulting in an irregular curvature

    f. accumulation of fatty deposits

    g. decreased ability of iris to dilate

    h. lens yellows and absorbs light waves

    i. continued growth of lens' epithelial layers and water loss from lens

    j. weakened ciliary muscles produce loss of accommodation

Subjective Assessment

38. Age; sex; ethnic background; family history of eye problems; previous accidents, injuries, or blows to the head; previous laser treatment to the eye; sports activities; presence of systemic conditions (diabetes mellitus, hypertension, lupus erythematosus, sarcoidosis, cardiac or thyroid disease, sexually transmitted disease, sickle cell anemia, AIDS, multiple sclerosis); medications currently taken; allergies; diet history, especially lack of vitamins A and B; occupational hazards; current health problem details, especially whether symptoms are present in one or both eyes and if any treatment administered; psychosocial factors including anxiety, fear, disruption in ADLs, loss of self-esteem, dependency, coping abilities, support systems

39. Contact sports (football, lacrosse, boxing) may result in direct or indirect injury to the eye. Examples are hyphema (hemorrhaging into the anterior chamber) and retinal detachment.

40. a. pruritus

    b. foreign body sensation

    c. redness

    d. tearing

    e. photophobia

    f. cataracts

    g. glaucoma

    h. diplopia

41. Submit the completed exercise to the clinical instructor for evaluation and feedback.

Objective Assessment

42. Posture; squinting; symmetry; exophthalmos or enophthalmos; eyebrow hair distribution; ability to raise eyebrows; drooping of eyelids; inspect lids and lashes for redness, tenderness, swelling; ability to close lids; position of lids when eyes are open; palpebral conjunctiva color and moisture; lacrimal gland swelling; nasolacrimal duct obstruction; sclera color; degree of corneal transparency; presence of corneal reflex; pupil shape and size; pupillary response to light (direct and consensual) and accommodation; convergence ability; visual acuity (distant and near); peripheral vision; extraocular muscle strength and function; color vision; ophthalmoscopy results, including appearance of optic disk, retinal vessels, and backgrounds; macula

43. Submit the completed exercise to the clinical instructor for evaluation and feedback

44. e

45. c

46. a

47. f

48. d

49. b

50. a

51. c

52. d

53. b

CHAPTER 46

External Eye Disorders

1. f
2. d
3. b
4. a
5. c
6. e
7. c
8. a
9. a. explain any diagnostic tests

   b. assess eye for dryness

   c. suggest ways to increase moisture in environment (humidifier)

   d. assess client's ability to instill eye medication

   e. counsel client regarding eye irritants to avoid
10. c
11. b
12. d
13. a
14. b
15. c
16. a
17. d
18. b
19. a. *Pneumococcus*

    b. *Pseudomonas*

    c. *Staphylococcus*
20. a, c, d, f, g
21. Thorough description of eye pain (location, quantity, quality, timing, setting, aggravating and relieving factors, associated signs and symptoms); visual history including surgery or injury; visual environment; concurrent medical conditions; current and past use of medications; psychosocial data, including age, any loss of vision and accompanying grieving, anxiety, involuntary change of vocation, loss of self-esteem or role identity, change in lifestyle, feelings of isolation
22. Decreased visual acuity; photophobia; eye secretions; hazy or cloudy cornea; altered corneal reflex; changes in integrity of cornea
23. d
24. c
25. b
26. c

Intraocular Disorders

27. b
28. Age; presence of other factors such as trauma to the eye; exposure to radioactive materials or x-rays; systemic diseases (diabetes mellitus, hypoparathyroidism, Down's syndrome, atopic dermatitis); use of medications, such as corticosteroids, miotics, chlorpromazine; presence of intraocular disease (recurrent uveitis); description of client's vision; psychosocial factors such as denial of visual loss, fear of losing eyesight, anxiety, interference with activities of daily living
29. Slightly blurred vision; decreased color perception; double blurred images; decreased visual acuity; difficulty or inability to visualize retina with the ophthalmoscope; inability to elicit red reflex
30. d
31. Coughing; bending at waist; vomiting; sneezing; lifting more than 15 pounds; squeezing eyelids shut; Valsalva maneuver; sleeping or lying on operative side; bumping or rubbing eye; tight collars; sexual intercourse
32. **Eyeglasses:**

    Advantage—less expensive

    Disadvantages—distorted images; reduced peripheral vision; diplopia; increased risk for injury related to falls or stumbling

    Contact lenses:

    Advantage—more normal visual field without distortion

    Disadvantages—requires manual dexterity to manipulate; need for adequate lubrication by tears; cost
33. b
34. Age; race; familial tendency to eye disorders; previous or existing ocular conditions (recent surgery, uveitis, iritis, tumors, eye trauma, degenerative diseases); history of diabetes, hypertension, severe myopia, retinal detachment, central retinal vein occlusion; use of antihistamines; visual disturbances; date of last eye examination (was tonometry done?); foggy vision; diminished accommodation; aching eyes; frontal headaches; frequent eyeglass prescription changes; loss of visual fields; decreased visual acuity even with eyeglasses; halos around lights; photophobia; nausea; psychosocial factors such as anxiety about vision loss, grieving behavior (denial, anger, bargaining, depression, acceptance), coping ability and its effectiveness

35. Atrophy and cupping of the optic disk; firm eyeball; nasal and superior visual field deficits; blind spots; sudden, excruciating eye pain that may radiate to the forehead, cheek, and jaw; headache; browache; vomiting; reddened sclera; clouding of the cornea; large eyes

36. Refer to pp. 1333–1335 in the textbook for discussion.

37. c

38. d

39. b

40. a

Retinal Disorders

41. Arteriole narrowing; arteriovenous nicking; soft exudates (cotton wool patches); flame hemorrhages; papilledema; retinal detachment

42. b

43. c

44. Increased age; history of myopia; reported sudden decrease in vision; history of ocular surgery or injury; absence of pain; reports of seeing bright light flashes or floating dark spots; psychosocial factors such as anxiety, frustration, coping ability

45. Direct visualization of the retina showing gray bulges or folds

46. d

Refractive Errors

47. e

48. d

49. a

50. c

51. b

52. c

Traumatic Disorders

53. d

54. c

55. a

56. b

57. a

Ocular Melanoma

58. a, b, d, g, h, k

59. *Enucleation* is the surgical removal of the entire eyeball.

60. a

61. Submit the completed exercise to the clinical instructor for evaluation and feedback. Refer to pp. 1345–1346 in the textbook for discussion.

Ocular Manifestations of HIV

62. a

63. b

64. a

65. c

66. c

67. a

68. b

69. b

70. a

Blindness

71. d

72. **Orientation:** converse in a normal tone of voice; inform client as to size of room; use one object in room as a focal point; describe all other objects in relation to the focal point; accompany client to other areas; allow client to touch objects in room; permit client to set up location of personal objects; assist with meal trays

Ambulation: allow client to grasp nurse's elbow; allow client to remain one step behind; alert client to objects in path; client may use a cane in a sweeping motion

Self-Care: allow client to control surrounding environment; knock on room door before entering; state name and reason for visiting; provide a means of distraction and orientation such as radio; talking books, or large-print books; magnifiers and special lighting

73. Refer to p. 1348 in the textbook for discussion.

CHAPTER 47

Anatomy and Physiology Review

1. a

2. c

3. b

4. c

5. a

6. b

7. c

8. c

9. a, b

10. b

11. b

12. c

13. a

14. c

15. b

16. a

17. c

18. b

19. b

20. c

21. a

22. a. hearing
    b. maintaining balance
23. e, b, g, a, c, f, d
24. c

Subjective Assessment

25. Sex; age; ear pain; ear discharge; vertigo; tinnitus; hearing change; hearing environmental noises; history of ear trauma, surgery, infections; excessive ear wax; ear itch; use of instruments for cleaning the ears (especially ear canal); type and pattern of ear hygiene; exposure to loud noise or loud music; air travel; swimming habits; use of protective ear devices while swimming or in noisy environments; use of a hearing aid (how well it works); last hearing test, type of test, and results; allergies; URI; hypothyroidism; arteriosclerosis; diabetes; hypertension; head trauma; recent head, facial, or dental surgery; familial hearing loss; medication history; socioeconomic status; occupation; hobbies; use of instruments that are inserted into the ear; balance problems; dizziness; psychosocial factors such as irritability, depression, sense of isolation, frustration, denial

26. d
27. Submit the completed exercise to the clinical instructor for evaluation and feedback.

Objective Assessment

28. Redness or swelling of mastoid process; tenderness over mastoid, with compression of the tragus, or manipulation of the pinna; placement, shape, and symmetry of the pinnae; nodules or lesions on helix or antihelix; redness, scaliness, or accumulated cerumen in the external meatus; drainage from ear; presence of foreign object; otoscopic examination for color of ear canal, lesions, amount and consistency of cerumen and hair; tympanic membrane for intactness, color, lesions, mobility, presence and location of malleus, short process, umbo, light reflex, pars tensa, pars flaccida; whispered voice test discrimination; ability to hear a watch ticking; Weber's test for lateralization; Rinne's test for air versus bone conduction

29. b
30. c
31. d
32. a
33. b
34. a
35. a. culture and sensitivity for bacteria
    b. dextrostick for presence of cerebrospinal fluid

36. f
37. d
38. e
39. a
40. b
41. c
42. a. The singer is exposed to intense sound for long periods and does not wear protective gear during performances. The percussionist is exposed to sound of varying intensity for short periods. The baggage handler most likely wears protective gear owing to occupational health standards. The logger is exposed to sound that is less intense than the sound a singer is exposed to and for intermittent periods.

43. c
44. **Speech reception threshold:** the minimal hearing level (intensity) at which a client can repeat simple words correctly at least 50% of the time.

    Speech discrimination: the ability to distinguish between short words (monosyllabic) that are phonemically balanced to represent common sounds in the language. Testing is done at an intensity level above that of the speech reception threshold.

45. d

CHAPTER 48

External Ear Conditions

1. a. congenital malformation (pinna, auricle, auditory canal)

    b. hematoma of the auricle or in the canal

    c. growths blocking the canal

    d. infectious or allergic response in ear canal

2. Current review of client's symptoms, including onset, duration, possible injury or trauma to external ear, level of discomfort; change in ability to hear; family history of similar problems; age; general physical condition; presence of other medical problems (e.g., diabetes mellitus); use of a hearing aid or earphones; psychosocial factors such as difficulty with compliance with self-care of ear infections

3. Pain, especially with manipulation of tragus or pinna; redness; swelling; drainage; enlarged tender preauricular or postauricular lymph nodes

4. d
5. b

6. Located on outer half of external canal; area swollen and pink; intense local pain upon light touch; drainage only if ruptured; hearing impairment if canal occluded

7. Solutions that are either too warm or too cool trigger the caloric reflex, and the client may experience vertigo, nausea, vomiting, and nystagmus.

Middle Ear Conditions

8. b

9. c

10. c

11. a

12. b

13. a

14. History of recent upper respiratory infections; allergic response affecting the upper respiratory tract; previous diagnosis of otitis media and client's compliance with treatment regimen; age; pain; tinnitus; headache; nausea; vertigo or dizziness; psychosocial factors such as ability to cope with ear pain, interference with interpersonal relationships, lost time from work, hearing loss and its meaning; fear

15. Pain on manipulation of the external ear; malaise; fever; vomiting; retracted tympanic membrane; dilation of blood vessels over tympanic membrane; reddened or thickened membrane with bulging and loss of landmarks; reduced mobility of the membrane; fluid line behind membrane; membrane perforation (and relief of pain); mucoid otorrhea; sound changes; bubbles behind the membrane

16. a, c, d

17. Myringotomy is a surgical perforation of the pars tensa.

18. b

19. b

20. d

21. a. infection

　　b. direct damage to the structures

　　c. rapid changes in the middle ear cavity pressure

22. a

23. d

24. Time of onset of hearing loss and its progress; positive family history; age; sex; changes in hearing during pregnancy; history of ear infections; constant tinnitus; psychosocial factors such as fear of permanent deafness, coping ability, ability to manage hearing loss

25. Bilateral, slowly progressive conductive hearing loss; initial hearing loss in lower frequencies, becoming progressive; pink tympanic membrane; bone conduction greater than air conduction (Rinne's); lateralization to the most affected ear (Weber's)

26. b, c, e

Inner Ear Conditions

27. a. presbycusis

　　b. otosclerosis

　　c. Ménière's syndrome

　　d. ototoxic drugs

　　e. exposure to loud noise

28. *Dizziness* is a disturbed sense of one's relationship to the surrounding space. *Vertigo* is a sense of whirling or turning in space. It may be subjective (the person is moving) or objective (the surroundings are revolving).

29. a. eyes provide visual input

　　b. vestibular apparatus (cochlea and semicircular canals)

　　c. proprioceptive nerve endings in muscle

30. d

31. b

32. Length, intensity, and time between episodes; history of viral or bacterial infection; allergies; exposure to drugs or chemicals; tinnitus; vertigo; hearing loss; feeling of fullness in affected ear; nausea; headache; psychosocial factors such as client's stressors and coping style, activities used to relax, loss of control

33. Low-frequency tone loss progressing to include all levels with repeated episodes; loss of hearing during attacks; vomiting; nystagmus; rapid eye movements; low-tone tinnitus in affected ear (upon audiometry)

34. c

35. c

Hearing Loss

36. Refer in the textbook to pp. 1379–1380, Figure 48-7 on p. 1379, and Table 48-2 on p. 1380, for discussion.

37. Cerumen blocking ear canal; foreign body obstructing ear canal; changes in the tympanic membrane; edema of ear canal related to infection of external or middle ear; tumors; otosclerosis; scar tissue build-up on ossicles

38. Prolonged exposure to loud noise; presbycusis; ototoxic substances; Ménière's syndrome; acoustic neuroma; diabetes mellitus; labyrinthitis; infection; metabolic and circulatory disorders

39. c

40. *Presbycusis* is hearing loss associated with the aging process.

41. b

42. c

43. a. autogenous cartilage or bone

    b. cadaver ossicles

    c. stainless steel wire

    d. Teflon materials

44. d

45. b

46. See pp.1382–1388 and Chart 48-8 on p. 1388 in the textbook for discussion.

CHAPTER 49

Anatomy and Physiology Review

1. Bone undergoes continuous formation and resorption throughout the life cycle. Its growth and metabolism are affected by numerous factors including minerals and hormones. See p. 1395 in the textbook for further discussion.

2. d	13. m
3. b	14. o
4. d	15. i
5. g	16. q
6. r	17. a
7. b	18. l
8. t	19. c
9. e	20. k
10. n	21. h
11. p	22. s
12. j	23. f

24. a. long bones (femur, humerus)

    b. short bones (phalanges)

    c. flat bones (sternum)

    d. irregular bones (carpals)

25. a. provides body framework

    b. supports surrounding tissues

    c. assists movement

    d. protects vital organs

    e. manufactures blood cells

    f. stores mineral salts

26. a. completely immovable (cranium)

    b. slightly movable (pelvis)

    c. synovial or freely movable (elbow)

27. d, v

28. a, iv

29. e, i

30. b, iii

31. c, ii

32. a. **striated:** movement of the body and its parts

    b. **nonstriated:** contractions of organs and blood vessels

    c. **cardiac:** contraction of the heart

33. See Chart 49-1, Nursing Focus on the Elderly, and p. 1397 in the textbook for discussion.

Subjective Assessment

34. Age; sex; previous or concurrent illnesses or accidents; familial or genetic tendency; previous hospitalizations; complications of previous treatment; medications; dietary intake of calcium, protein, and vitamin C; obesity; amount of sunlight exposure; occupation; leisure activities; ethnic and cultural background; current health problems including pain; psychosocial factors such as sensory deprivation, employment status, coping ability, body image, and self-concept

35. Submit the completed exercise to the clinical instructor for evaluation and feedback.

Objective Assessment

36. Posture; muscle mass, gait; mobility; ability to perform activities of daily living; inspect and palpate major bones, joints, and muscles; ROM; muscle strength, symmetry, tenderness; pain; masses swelling; crepitus

37. Submit the completed exercise to the clinical instructor for evaluation and feedback.

38. c

39. d

40. Refer to Chart 49-2 on p. 1403 in the textbook for discussion. Normal values may vary from laboratory to laboratory according to the test used.

41. a. myelography

b. arthrography

c. computed tomography

42. b

43. b

CHAPTER 50

Metabolic Bone Diseases

1. b, iii	14. c
2. c, i	15. b
3. a, ii	16. a
4. c	17. b
5. a	18. c
6. b	19. c
7. a	20. a
8. a	21. b
9. c	22. a
10. b	23. b
11. a	24. a
12. b	25. c
13. a	

26. a. metabolic bone activity

b. actual or impending fracture

c. secondary arthritis

d. nerve impingement

27. a. alkaline phosphatase, serum phosphate, serum calcium, parathyroid hormone, and vitamin D metabolite measurements

b. alkaline phosphatase, 24-hour urine hydroxy-proline, serum calcium, urine calcium, and serum uric acid measurements

c. 24-hour hydroxyproline measurement

28. a. spinal x-ray films

b. computed tomographic scan of spine

c. long bone x-ray films

29. a. High Risk for Injury (fracture) related to trivial trauma or falls

b. Impaired Physical Mobility related to decreased muscle tone, dysfunction secondary to previous fractures, or pain secondary to recent fractures

c. Pain related to effects of fracture

30. a

31. b

32. a

33. b

34. a

35. a

36. a. monitor for drug side effects (drowsiness and incoordination)

b. keep bed at lowest height

c. reduce clutter in surrounding environment

d. provide extra lighting while avoiding glare

37. a. diuretics

b. phenothiazines

c. tranquilizers

38. Refer to the textbook, Chart 50-1 on pp. 1418–1419, as well as a pharmacology textbook for discussion. Submit the completed exercise to the clinical instructor for evaluation and feedback.

39. **Consume:** vitamin D–fortified milk and milk products (hard cheeses, cottage cheese, yogurt), dark green leafy vegetables (kale, broccoli collard greens), rhubarb, sardines with bones

Avoid: alcohol, caffeine-containing beverages (coffee, tea, soft drinks, hot chocolate), chocolate

40. a

Osteomyelitis

41. a. **acute:** an infection lasting less than 4 weeks

b. **chronic:** infection lasting longer than 4 weeks

42. A *sequestrum* is a fragment of necrotic bone tissue that has been separated or "walled off" form the underlying living bone. It may be completely detached, loosely attached, or partially detached and remaining in place.

43. Bone and often the surrounding tissue are invaded by one or more pathogenic microorganisms. The bone and soft tissue become inflamed, leading to increasing vascularity and edema. Vessels in the area occlude, resulting in ischemia and eventual bone necrosis. The necrotic bone tissue forms a sequestrum, which the delays healing and causes superimposed infection. The cycle of inflammation, thrombosis, and necrosis is repeated.

44. a. **hematogenous spread:** infection spreads via the blood stream from another part of the body to bone tissue

b. **direct inoculation:** bone tissue is infected directly with pathogenic microorganisms, such as in a contaminated compound fracture or puncture wound

c. **contiguous spread:** tissue surrounding bone is infected and the pathogenic microorganisms spread to the bone

45. a. bacteremia (urinary tract infection, long-term intravenous catheter placement); underlying disease (chronic hemodialysis, intravenous drug abuse, gastrointestinal tract salmonella infection); nonpenetrating trauma resulting in hemorrhage or small vessel occlusion

b. penetrating trauma (animal bites, puncture wounds, bone surgery)

c. poor dental hygiene; radiation therapy; malignant external otitis media; diabetes mellitus; peripheral vascular disease (foot ulcer)

46. Age; drug abuse; previous infections; concurrent medical conditions; nonpenetrating trauma; penetrating wounds; surgical procedures, especially of bone; tubes or catheters used; radiation therapy; overall health status; psychosocial factors such as fear of amputation, isolation

47. Fever; localized swelling, erythema, heat, and tenderness on palpation; bone pain; draining ulcers; sinus tract formation; neurovascular status in extremities

48. d

49. d

Bone Tumors

50. d	57. c
51. e	58. a
52. b	59. b
53. a	60. c
54. f	61. d
55. c	62. a
56. d	63. b

64. a. prostate
    b. breast
    c. kidney
    d. thyroid
    e. lung

65. a. vertebrae
    b. pelvis
    c. femur
    d. ribs

66. a. compression of peripheral nerves by soft tissue that has been invaded by tumor cells

    b. as a result of pathological fractures

67. Age; sex; incidence of trivial trauma, fractures, or neoplasms; family history of neoplasms; previous radiation therapy for cancer; general health status; psychosocial factors including pain

68. Local swelling, muscle atrophy or spasm; tenderness upon palpation; palpable mass; ability to perform ADLs; degree of mobility. In systemic disease: low-grade fever, fatigue, pallor

69. **Benign**
    a. fear of malignancy
    b. fear of surgery
    c. altered body image
    Malignant
    a. feeling loss of control
    b. fear of illness' outcome
    c. anxiety
    d. grieving

70. b

71. a

72. b

73. b

74. a

75. b

76. a

77. a. analgesics
    b. NSAIDs
    c. chemotherapy
    d. radiation therapy
    e. surgical excision or resection
    f. bracing and immobilization

78. c

79. d

Disorders of the Hand

80. a	86. b
81. c	87. a
82. a	88. b
83. b	89. a
84. c	90. a
85. a	

91. Submit the completed exercise to the clinical instructor for evaluation and feedback.

Disorders of the Foot

92. Metatarsophalangeal joint of great toe

93. a. corns on dorsal side of toe

    b. calluses on plantar surface of toe

94. A neuroma (tumor) forms in a digital nerve of the foot causing acute pain in the third and fourth toes. Tarsal tunnel syndrome results from compression of the posterior tibial nerve and causes decreased sensation and pain in the sole as well as distal phalanges.

Other Musculoskeletal Disorders

95.	b	101.	a
96.	c	102.	b
97.	a	103.	b
98.	b	104.	a
99.	a	105.	a
100.	b		

106. Submit the exercise to the clinical instructor for evaluation and feedback.

CHAPTER 51

Fractures

1. Refer to pp. 1450–1451 and Figure 51-1 on p. 1450 in the textbook for discussion.

2. d

3. c

4. a

5. b

6. a. acute compartment syndrome

    b. shock

    c. fat embolism syndrome

    d. thromboembolitic complications

    e. infection

    f. avascular necrosis

    g. delayed union or malunion

7. Increased pressure within one or more muscle compartments of an extremity causes reduced circulation to the area. This may lead to the ischemia-edema cycle, which, if untreated, can cause irreversible neuromuscular damage and permanent loss of function in the extremity.

8. Pallor of extremity; weakened peripheral pulses; swollen and tense skin surface; cyanosis; tingling; numbness; paresthesia; severe pain unrelieved by analgesics

9. a. infection

    b. persistent motor weakness

    c. contractures

    d. myoglobinuric renal failure

10. a. muscle tissue ischemia

    b. acidosis

    c. hyperkalemia

    d. shock

    e. myoglobinuria

    f. renal failure

    g. death if untreated

11. Hypovolemic shock related to hemorrhage

12. a. catecholamine-induced mobilization of free fatty acids in the serum, which leads to platelet aggregation and fat globule formation

    b. release of fat cells directly from the yellow marrow due to the pressure gradient between the bone marrow and the capillaries

13. a. long bones (hip)

    b. multiple fractures

    c. pelvis

14. a. smokers

    b. obese clients

    c. clients with a history of heart disease

    d. clients with a history of thromboembolitic complications

15. Death of bone tissue due to disrupted blood supply leading to ischemia

16. c

17. a

18. b

19. Age; sex; recall of specific events leading to the time of injury; medication history (including substance abuse); previous medical problems; occupation; leisure activities; nutrition history; psychosocial factors such as disruption in lifestyle, financial loss, fear of permanent disability, strained interpersonal relationships, coping ability, body image change, sexuality

20. Bone alignment; altered length of an extremity; change in bone shape; pain with movement; decreased range of movement; crepitus; skin integrity; ecchymosis; subcutaneous emphysema; swelling; neurovascular status distal to fracture site; bleeding; pain at or adjacent to fracture site; muscle spasm

21. a. extent of the injuries

    b. location of the fracture(s)

    c. if other body systems are affected

    d. medical complications

22. Assess and treat first: respiratory distress, bleeding, and head injury; remove any clothing over suspected fracture site; control bleeding from fracture site with applied pressure; assess vital signs; position in supine; keep warm; assess fracture site using inspection and palpation; assess distal pulses and motor function; immobilize fracture by splinting

23. a. bandages and splints

    b. casts

    c. traction

    d. internal fixation

    e. external fixation

24. Neurovascular status including color; temperature; presence of sensation; motor ability; peripheral pulses or skin blanching; swelling; snugness of device

25. Promote air drying of wet cast (leave uncovered); handle wet cast with palms of hands; use a firm mattress under cast; use cloth-covered pillow for extremity elevation if cast is wet; inspect cast for drainage, cracking, crumbling, alignment, and fit; prevent cast contamination with urine or feces; petal cast edges when dry

26. Infection; circulation impairment; peripheral nerve damage; joint contracture; degenerative arthritis in joint(s); muscle atrophy; other complications of prolonged immobility (skin breakdown, thromboembolism, constipation, pneumonia, atelectasis)

27. Never remove weights, lift weights, or let them rest on the floor; weights must hang freely. Instruct other caregivers and colleagues regarding the weights. Inspect skin integrity and condition every 8 hours, especially at pin sites. Perform pin care according to agency's protocol. Maintain body alignment and countertraction. Check all equipment for proper functioning.

28. Refer to p. 1463 in the textbook for discussion of pin site care and protocols.

29. a. hot or cold therapy applications depending on source of pain

    b. warm bath

    c. back rub

    d. therapeutic touch

    e. distraction

    f. imagery

    g. music therapy or other forms of relaxation therapy

30. a. thromboembolic disease

    b. respiratory complications (pneumonia, atelectasis)

    c. contractures or muscle atrophy

    d. skin breakdown

    e. elimination problems (constipation, urinary retention)

    f. cerebral dysfunction

31. c

32. a. remove objects in the walking path

    b. clean up spills

    c. use ambulatory aids prn

    d. place call bell within reach

    e. instruct client to remain in bed until help arrives

33. d

34. b

35. a

36. d

Amputations

37. **Open**

    a. preferred technique if infection is a consideration

    b. stump wound open with drains or packing material in place until infection resolves; skin flaps then sutured together

    Closed

    a. technique used if extremity or stump is at minimal risk for developing an infection

    b. skin flaps pulled together over bone end and sutured together at the time of the amputation

38. a. hemorrhage

    b. infection

    c. phantom limb pain

    d. problems of immobility

    e. neuroma formation

    f. flexion contractures

39. a. ischemia

    b. trauma

    c. thermal injuries

    d. tumors

    e. infections

    f. metabolic disorders

    g. congenital anomalies

40. Age; sex; historical events leading to tissue destruction; concurrent illness; smoking habits; neurovascular impairment in distal extremity; skin changes

41. Circulation in other body parts: color; warmth; sensation; pulses; capillary refill

42. Amputation is permanent loss. Assess client's psychological preparation. Expect client to go through a grieving process. It may result in loss of a job, leisure time activity, or a personal relationship. Body image and self-esteem are affected. The client's ability to make life changes is important. The family's reaction may affect the client's progress.

43. Submit the completed exercise to the clinical instructor for evaluation and feedback.

44. b

Sports-Related Injuries

45. a. torn meniscus

    b. ligament sprain

    c. patellar tendon rupture

    d. dislocation or subluxation of the joint

46. c

47. b

48. d

49. a

CHAPTER 52

Anatomy and Physiology Review

1. q	12. p
2. e	13. u
3. k	14. h
4. n	15. a
5. i	16. t
6. m	17. d
7. s	18. g
8. b	19. f
9. j	20. o
10. l	21. c
11. r	

22. a. *Transport* of water and food along the GI tract permits the eventual utilization of ingested foodstuffs.

    b. *Digestion* is the mechanical and chemical degradation of foodstuffs that can be used by the body.

    c. *Absorption* is the passage of nutrients through the intestinal walls into the circulatory system for eventual dissemination to individual cells.

23. a. **mucosa:** innermost layer, secretes mucous and digestive enzymes

    b. **submucosa:** middle layer, contains main blood vessels and additional exocrine gland cells

    c. **muscle layer:** outermost layer of circular and longitudinal smooth muscle, aids in propelling GI contents along

24. b

25. a

26. Refer to textbook pp. 1491–1496 and Tables 52-1 and 52-2 on pp. 1492 and 1494 for discussion.

27. Foodstuffs contain many different types of nutrients, each of which requires specific chemical digestive action before absorption and utilization by the body can occur.

28. Refer to Chart 52-1 on p. 1497 in the textbook. Submit the completed exercise to the clinical instructor for evaluation and feedback.

Subjective Assessment

29. Age; sex; culture; occupation; previous GI disorders or surgeries in self or family members; medications taken; travel history; diet history including religious or cultural influences; socioeconomic status; in-depth exploration of diarrhea, constipation, flatus, bloating, bowel habits and any changes; melena; urine changes; weight gain or loss; smoking history; complete description of pain; skin changes (itching, jaundice, bruising, bleeding); heartburn, hematemesis; nausea or vomiting; psychosocial factors such as effect of current problem on lifestyle, interference with job or leisure activities, job-related stress, financial status

30. See pp. 1502–1503 in the textbook for discussion.

31. Submit the completed exercise to the clinical instructor for evaluation and feedback.

Objective Assessment

32. Height; weight; triceps skinfold thickness; midarm circumference; midarm muscle circumference; inspect and palpate mouth (lips, oral mucosa, gums, teeth or dentures, tongue, odors, tonsils, uvula movement); inspect, auscultate, percuss, and palpate abdomen (skin, contour and symmetry, movement, edema, bowel sounds,

bruits, friction rub, venous hum, percussion notes elicited, liver span, spleen size, masses, tenderness); spider telangiectases on upper torso and neck; presence of leg edema and peripheral pulses; asterixis

33. Submit the complete exercise to the clinical instructor for evaluation and feedback.

34. Aggressive abdominal physical assessment (palpation) of clients with these pathologies could result in harm to the client from unintentional organ rupture. Hemorrhage, shock, and ensuing abdominal infection (peritonitis) could occur.

35. b

36. a. Barium solutions are either drunk by the client or instilled via catheter or enema.

    b. Iodine-based dyes are either taken orally or injected directly into an organ by catheter or intravenously.

37. Barium must be evacuated from the GI tract to avoid constipation or impaction. Forcing fluids (unless contraindicated) aids in hydration and ease of barium elimination. A laxative should be administered in most instances.

CHAPTER 53

Stomatitis

1. Primary stomatitis is usually a result of systemic disorders, while secondary stomatitis is generally the result of infection by opportunistic viral or bacterial organisms in clients who already have lowered host resistance.

2. c

3. b

4. a

5. d

6. a. bone marrow disorders
   b. allergy
   c. systemic disease
   d. drugs
   e. nutritional disorders
   f. emotional disturbance

7. b

8. c

9. a

10. c

11. c

12. Prevention is difficult because specific causative factors may be unidentifiable. Sequelae from the treatment of underlying systemic disorders may be unavoidable.

13. Onset of disease process; location and duration of symptoms; history of a similar problem; presence and location of pain and its nature; presence of systemic symptoms (fever, malaise, nausea, vomiting); disability resulting from condition; routine oral hygiene regimen; dentures or orthodontic appliances; effectiveness of any current treatment; nutritional habits; ability to chew and swallow; nutritional status; stress level; medications; psychosocial factors such as perception of current stressors, changes in lifestyle, emotional trauma, situational crises, coping patterns, perceived impact of oral lesions on self-concept

14. Oral cavity lesions, coating, cracking, fissures, odors; anterior lymphadenopathy; uvula displacement from midline; airway obstruction

15. a. avoidance of contact with the causative agent
    b. mental health practices that reduce stress levels and emotional tension
    c. maintenance of proper nutrition status
    d. routine oral hygiene

16. Submit the completed exercise to the clinical instructor for evaluation and feedback.

17. d

Tumors

18. b

19. c

20. d

21. a

22. a. lip
    b. buccal mucosa
    c. gingiva
    d. tongue
    e. floor of mouth
    f. hard palate
    g. tonsils
    h. tonsillar pillars

23. a. poorly fitting dentures
    b. broken or poorly repaired teeth
    c. cheek nibbling
    d. long-term malocclusion
    e. smoking
    f. exposure to excessive heat from foods
    g. poor nutrition
    h. poor oral hygiene

24. a. avoidance of tobacco products and alcohol

    b. good oral hygiene

    c. avoiding exposure to the sun

    f. good nutritional status

25. Occupation; exposure to known oral carcinogens or irritants (sunlight, heat, mechanical, alcohol, tobacco); family history of cancer or oral cancer; routine oral hygiene regimen; dentures or oral appliances; hemoptysis; nutritional status; appetite; problems with chewing or swallowing; weight loss; medications; psychosocial factors, including fear of cancer, support systems, coping mechanisms, impact on self-concept, comfort level, limitations to education or therapy

26. Lip color, texture, symmetry; pain; color of buccal mucosa, texture, presence of lesions; tongue movement; floor of mouth; speech; cervical nodes for enlargement or tenderness

27. b

28. a. ability to swallow without difficulty

    b. aspiration

    c. leakage of saliva or liquids from the suture line

Disorders of the Salivary Glands

29. a. acute sialadenitis

    b. postirradiation sialadenitis

    c. calculi

    d. tumors

30. c

31. a

Malocclusion

32. *Acute malocclusion* usually results from fractures of the teeth or mandible. *Chronic malocclusion* more commonly results from congenital facial deformity or a more long-term uncorrected malpositioning of the teeth.

33. a. motor vehicle accidents

    b. work accidents

    c. sports injuries

    d. assault

    e. falls

    f. osteoporosis

    g. biting on hard objects

    h. tooth decay

    i. poor nutrition

34. Complete dental history; onset of malocclusion symptoms; history of recent trauma especially to the head and neck; discomfort; change in sensory perception to the jaw; difficulty chewing; nutritional status and habits; drooling; psychosocial factors, including reactions to any facial fractures, body image, self-concept, recovery from trauma or assault, meaning of disability to lifestyle, educational level, and ability and desire to learn

35. Signs of facial structure deformity; abnormal movement; restriction of jaw movement; tenderness or pain on palpation; crepitus; presence of broken teeth; dentition status; condition of oral mucous membrane

36. b

37. a. require little or no chewing, reduce pain

    b. reduce stimulation of exposed tooth pulp or nerves

38. c

39. d

CHAPTER 54

Gastroesophageal Reflux Disease

1. a. location in the abdomen where the intra-abdominal pressure is higher that the intrathoracic pressure

   b. the acute angle of His formed where the lower portion of the esophagus enters the stomach

2. a. increased gastric contents

   b. elevated intra-abdominal pressure

   c. decreased LES tone

   d. inappropriate relaxation of the LES

3. c

4. Nighttime reflux results in increased exposure of the esophageal mucosa to acidic stomach contents because the person swallows less and is in a recumbent position. Decreased swallowing reduces esophageal peristalsis and recumbency impedes the action of gravity on esophageal emptying.

5. **Increased tone:** gastrin release; protein ingestion; cholinergic agents; antacids; metoclopramide

   Decreased tone: fatty meals; smoking; chocolate; xanthine beverages (tea, cola, coffee); beta-adrenergic agents; high estrogen or progesterone levels

6. Pain pattern (heartburn or pyrosis), including onset, frequency, duration, intensity, associated environmental or physical aggravating factors; regurgitation; water brash; dysphagia; odynophagia; ingestion of corrosive substances; radiation treatment to the head or neck region; frequent oral infections; dietary pattern; use of medications to relieve pain and their effect; work and leisure activities; psychosocial factors, including disruption in lifestyle and daily activities, knowledge about disorder, coping mechanisms used, resources available, support systems

7. Diagnosis of most (up to 80%) cases of GERD can be made with just the history of clinical manifestations of the disorder. This alleviates the need for a full diagnostic work-up, which is time-consuming, uncomfortable for the client, and costly both financially and emotionally.

8. General physical appearance; nutritional status, especially unplanned weight loss; ability to swallow and smoothness of laryngeal movement; auscultation for aspiration if regurgitation occurs; dysphagia; belching; flatulence; nausea or vomiting

9. e	14. d
10. c	15. b
11. b	16. c
12. f	17. d
13. a	18. c

Hiatal Hernia

19. *Sliding hernias* occur as a result of weakened hiatal muscle support structures and increases in intra-abdominal pressure. The esophagogastric junction and a portion of the stomach fundus move through the diaphragm into the thorax. *Paraesophageal hernias* result from an anatomical defect whereby the stomach is not securely anchored below the diaphragm. The gastroesophageal junction remains below the diaphragm, while portions of the stomach roll into the thorax.

20. Age; sex; weight; body build; daily work and leisure activities; dietary patterns; heartburn; regurgitation pattern; pain; dysphagia; belching; feeling of fullness after eating; breathlessness; feeling of suffocation; chest pain; psychosocial factors such as changes in lifestyle (work and leisure activities), knowledge of the disease and its treatment, self-care measures, ability to learn, coping mechanisms, support systems

21. General physical appearance; nutritional status; location of any pain; auscultation of chest for signs of aspiration or decreased lung sounds

22. c

Achalasia

23. Lack of esophageal peristalsis due to neuromuscular factors along with inadequate relaxation or spasm of the LES are likely to be involved

24. Dysphagia; pain; regurgitation; onset and duration of symptoms; aggravating factors; medications or home treatments and their effect; history of esophageal surgery or trauma; respiratory history; current respiratory difficulties; nutritional history and current status; psychosocial factors, including fear of malignancy, coping ability, support systems

25. Halitosis; current and previous weight

26. d

27. Refer to p. 1553 in the textbook for discussion.

Tumors

28. b

29. b

30. Race; culture; age; sex; alcohol consumption; tobacco use; history of esophageal problems (stricture, reflux); extreme weight loss; anorexia; dysphagia; pain pattern; dietary pattern; psychosocial factors, including fear of choking, reactions to the diagnosis of cancer, financial concerns

31. General physical appearance; weight; nutritional status; skin turgor; condition of mucous membranes; auscultation for signs of aspiration; palpation of cervical, neck, and axillary nodes; dysphagia; odynophagia; regurgitation; vomiting; foul breath; chronic hiccups; chronic cough; increased secretions; hoarseness

32. Altered Nutrition: Less than Body Requirements

33. c

34. a

35. c

Esophageal Diverticula

36. Diverticula are esophageal outpouchings in the mucosal lining. They result in blind pouches where food and liquids can be trapped and possibly regurgitated.

37. a

38. Dysphagia; regurgitation; fullness; halitosis; altered oral taste; symptom onset and duration; aggravating and relieving factors; history of previous esophageal surgery or trauma; respiratory history; current respiratory difficulty; nutritional history; psychosocial factors, including self-concept, lifestyle changes, coping ability, support systems

39. Lung assessment; halitosis; auscultation over the neck for gurgling

40. c

41. d

42. b

Esophageal Trauma

43. Blunt trauma or crush injury resulting from steering wheel injuries; stabbing; gunshot wounds; complications following esophageal surgery; chemical burns; swallowed foreign bodies

44. Sever episodes of vomiting related to excessive alcohol or food intake, chemotherapy, or hyperemesis gravidarum

45. Esophageal contents escape into the mediastinal area and expose those structures to digestive secretions. This exposure results in inflammation, edema, infection, respiratory difficulty, and shock.

46. Process of the injury; time injury occurred; respiratory difficulty; previous esophageal surgery; dysphagia; odynophagia; recent vomiting; nutritional status; swallowing ability; psychosocial factors, particularly history of suicidal behavior or previous suicide attempts

47. Signs of reddened, inflamed, or burned oral tissues; respiratory distress, including dyspnea, hyperpnea, or stridor; choking; hypotension; cervical crepitus and tenderness

48. a

49. b

CHAPTER 55

Gastritis

1. The gastric mucosa acts as a barrier and protects the stomach from acid autodigestion.

2. d	10. a
3. c	11. b
4. a	12. a
5. b	13. b
6. b	14. b
7. b	15. b
8. a	
9. a	

16. Age; sex; history of present and concurrent medical conditions (duodenal disease, autoimmune disease); history of radiation therapy; medications, including steroids or anti-inflammatory agents; lifestyle; health care practices; personal habits, including exposure to alcohol, coffee, drugs, tobacco; epigastric pain description, onset, duration, frequency, aggravating and relieving factors; reports of abdominal tenderness, cramps, indigestion, nausea, vomiting; anorexia; weight loss; interference with ADL; psychosocial factors, including stress tolerance and coping

17. General appearance; facial grimacing; restlessness; moaning; unkempt appearance; tense body posture; abdominal tenderness on palpation, guarding, distention, increased peristaltic waves, increased bowel sounds; nutritional status (weight, turgor, skin color, adipose tissue distribution); vomiting; hematemesis

18. c

19. a

20. d

Peptic Ulcer Disease

21. PUD is a break in the continuity of the gastrointestinal mucosa allowing contact with hydrochloric acid and pepsin.

22. a. **duodenum:** the most common location for peptic ulcers

    b. **stomach:** the second most common location for peptic ulcers

    c. **esophagus:** peptic ulcers rarely found in the lower portion

23. A global definition is misleading because there are differences in pathophysiology and causes for the two major types of peptic ulcers. Likewise, clients' subjective reports of pain episodes follow a variety of patterns.

24. Refer to Table 55-1 and pp. 1567–1570 in the textbook for discussion.

25. Refer to p. 1569 in the textbook for discussion.

26. *Intractability* refers to ulcer disease that is not relieved or cured by conservative management. Clients may become incapacitated or disabled or suffer life-threatening complications.

27. c

28. Age; sex; occupation; use of medications (especially corticosteroids, salicylates, indomethacin, phenylbutazone); diet history; eating patterns; daily stressors; smoking and alcohol use; caffeine consumption; any history of GI upset or symptoms; history of radiation treatment; occurrence and pattern of pain and its relationship to food ingestion, aggravating and relieving factors;

early satiety; anorexia; nausea; heartburn; psychosocial factors, particularly impact on lifestyle, stressors, income, educational levels, leisure activities

29. Nutritional status; pain location; posture; facial expression; dress; grooming; hygiene; abdominal tenderness, fullness or guarding to palpation; vomiting; melena; orthostatic change in vital signs and dizziness

30. a. diet therapy

   b. drug therapy

   c. rest and decreased physical activity

   d. mental rest and stress reduction

   e. stop smoking (if currently does so)

31. Submit the completed exercise to the clinical instructor for evaluation and feedback. Refer to pp. 1571–1574 and Chart 55-3 in the textbook for discussion.

32. b

33. Liquid antacids are more effective in neutralizing gastric secretions because they are already in suspension. If oral tablets must be taken, instruct the client to chew them carefully and completely to increase the amount of active surface area available for acid neutralization.

34. d

35. An administration schedule should consider and modifications to be made for laboratory or diagnostic tests. The following is suggested:

   Sucralfate at 7 a.m., 11:30 a.m., 4:30 p.m., 9 p.m.

   Maalox at 9 a.m., 11:00 a.m., 1:30 p.m., 3:30 p.m., 6:30 p.m., 8:30 p.m.

   Famotidine at 9 p.m.

   Breakfast at 8 a.m., lunch at 12:30 p.m., dinner at 5:30 p.m., snack at 8 p.m.

   This schedule requires delaying the lunch tray 15 minutes to accommodate the sucralfate administered at 11:30 a.m. Allowances are made to administer the sucralfate no sooner than 30 minutes after the Maalox dose prior to lunch and at least 30 minutes before and after the Maalox doses at 8:30 p.m. and 9:30 p.m.

36. c
37. d
38. a
39. d

Carcinoma of the Stomach

40. Spread within the gastric wall and into regional lymphatics; direct invasion of adjacent structures (liver, pancreas); hematogenous spread via the portal vein to the liver; systemic circulation to the lungs and bones; peritoneal seeding via the gastric serosa to the omentum, peritoneum, and ovary

41. b
42. d

43. Presences of risk factors, including history of gastric polyps, benign tumors, chronic gastritis, pernicious anemia, being male and over age 50; smoking history; dietary history for consumption of nitrates and salted foods or salted meat; unexplained weight loss; diet patterns; bowel habits; comfort level; changes in appetite, eating habits; food allergies; nausea; vomiting; discomfort; heartburn; eructation; indigestion; fullness; dysphagia; use of laxatives; pain symptoms with full details; psychosocial factors, including anxiety, depression, fear, coping mechanisms, support systems, family dynamics

44. Positive stool occult blood is often the only "early" physical finding. All other symptoms suggest advanced disease. Eructation; vomiting; weakness; weight loss; anemia; fatigue; epigastric mass; hepatomegaly; ascites; enlarged supraclavicular node; pallor; cachexia; acanthosis nigricans; recurrent phlebitis in the extremities

45. Symptoms are usually not evident until the gastric tumor is advanced and large enough to interfere with gastric motility or block the stomach lumen. Early symptoms are often vague.

46. c
47. b
48. d
49. a
50. d

51. a. hemorrhage

   b. obstruction

   c. gastric dilation (reflux gastritis)

   d. delayed gastric emptying

   e. anemia

   f. nutritional deficiency

   g. dumping syndrome

52. a. early satiety

   b. abdominal distention

   c. pain

   d. steatorrhea

53. TPN may be needed as a supplement to oral intake or for complete dietary management if a client cannot maintain adequate nutritional status. A major indicator for TPN is a weight loss of 10% or more of usual body weight.

CHAPTER 56

Irritable Bowel Syndrome

1. There is no inflammation present causing alteration in the bowel mucosa or intestinal wall.

2. a. anxiety
   b. depression
   c. fear
   d. food
   e. drugs
   f. toxins
   g. colonic distention

3. c

4. b

5. Sex; age; race; occupation; habits (cigarettes, alcohol, caffeine consumption); current stressors; dietary patterns; bowel patterns; past health problems; weight loss; nausea; belching; flatulence; anorexia; bloating; fatigue; anxiety; headaches; difficulty concentrating; psychosocial factors, including impact of the illness on individual, recent period of stress or emotional tension

6. Repeated episodes of diarrhea or constipation; abdominal cramps or pain; LLQ pain; fatigued appearance; normal bowel sounds; diffuse tenderness over abdomen

7. b

8. d

9. d

Herniation

10. a. pregnancy
    b. obesity
    c. heavy lifting or straining
    d. coughing

11. b

12. e

13. d

14. a

15. f

16. c

17. g

18. c

19. Sex; age; body build; weight; height; past or concurrent medical problems; medications; exercise patterns; occupation (any lifting); past herniation or symptoms; psychosocial factors including developmental stage, home situation, support systems

20. Abdominal bulging at rest or with straining; presence of bowel sounds; changes in inguinal ring with increased intra-abdominal pressure

21. Reduction attempts may result in perforation of the trapped loop of bowel, leading to peritonitis.

22. d

23. b

24. a

Colorectal Cancer

25. d, b, e, a, f, c

26. a. liver
    b. lung
    c. adrenal glands
    d. kidneys
    e. skin
    f. bone
    g. brain

27. Tumor seeding is a process that occurs when cancerous (malignant) cells break off from the primary tumor while it is being surgically removed. These cells then remain in the peritoneal cavity and become sources for further tumor growth.

28. a. bowel perforation and peritonitis
    b. abscess formation
    c. fistula formation to the urinary bladder or vagina
    d. frank bleeding
    e. gradual intestinal obstruction
    f. pressure on nearby organs

29. a

30. b

31. d

32. Age; sex; diet history; geographic location of residence; presence of risk factors, including family history of ulcerative colitis, polyposis, adenomas; recent weight loss; malaise; reports of abdominal pain or discomfort, tenesmus, fullness; change in bowel habits such as diarrhea or constipation; nausea; psychosocial factors, including fear, denial, guilt, loss of control, anger

33. Overall appearance (energy level, listlessness, weakness); cachexia; loose skin; muscle wasting; abdominal distention; abdominal guarding; palpable abdominal mass; rectal bleeding; vomiting; ascites

34. See p. 1603 in the textbook for discussion.

35. Submit the completed exercise to the clinical instructor for evaluation and feedback. Refer to p. 1603 in the textbook for discussion.

36. c

37. b

38. c

39. a

Intestinal Obstruction

40. h

41. g

42. d

43. f

44. a

45. c

46. b

47. e

48. See p. 1611 in the textbook for discussion

49. See p. 1611 in the textbook for discussion.

50. b

51. c

52. a

53. **Small intestine:** adhesions, hernias

    Large bowel: tumors, diverticulitis, volvulus

54. See Figure 56-6 on p. 1611 in the textbook.

55. Regulation of fluid and electrolytes; limited bowel manipulation during surgery; intubation and suction after abdominal surgery until function returns; maintaining NPO (nothing by mouth) status after abdominal trauma, surgery, spinal injury, acute diverticulitis, exacerbated Crohn's disease; education of high-risk clients (those having abdominal surgery, diverticular disease, Crohn's disease, ulcerative colitis, frequent constipation, hernias, abdominal radiation therapy); ongoing nursing assessment of elderly clients for effective bowel elimination

56. History of abdominal surgery, radiation therapy, or significant medical disorders (Crohn's disease, ulcerative colitis, diverticular disease, gallstones, hernias, tumors); diet history; nausea or vomiting; last bowel movement; family history of colorectal cancer; blood in the stool; change in bowel patterns; cramping; pain characteristics and location; psychosocial factors, including fear and anxiety

57. Peristaltic waves across abdomen; borborygmi; absent bowel sounds; abdominal distention and extent (if present); vomiting; characteristics of emesis; hiccups; absence of stool or gas per rectum; guarding; tenderness; low-grade fever; elevated pulse rate

58. d

59. c

60. b

61. b

62. c

63. a

Abdominal Trauma

64. a. blunt trauma (automobile accidents, assault, falls)

    b. penetrating trauma (gunshot or stab wounds)

65. a. delayed resuscitation due to time needed to transport client to a trauma center

    b. inadequate fluid volume replacement

    c. lack of a thorough evaluation of the client

    d. delayed surgical intervention

66. b

67. Fluid volume replacement needs are extensive. Blood replacement products, crystalloids, and isotonic saline are given, as well as intravenous antibiotics. All these interventions require multiple infusion ports and large-bore catheters to ensure a means of quick access. An upper extremity or central line is used to prevent fluid pooling in the abdominal cavity.

68. Serial blood work helps to identify true blood loss, whereas single samples may reflect hemo-concentration and volume loss.

69. Submit the completed exercise to the clinical instructor for evaluation and feedback.

70. Hemorrhage related to the trauma can occur weeks after blunt abdominal trauma. A client who is alerted about what to watch for can seek medical intervention immediately and possibly avoid further complications.

Polyps

71. b, c, f, g, h, j

72. b

Hemorrhoids

73. *Internal* hemorrhoids lie above the anal sphincter and cannot be seen on inspection of the perianal area. *External* hemorrhoids can be visualized during an inspection of the perianal area and lie below the anal sphincter.

74. a. straining at stool

 b. pregnancy

 c. portal hypertension

75. d

76. a. hemorrhage

 b. pain

 c. urinary retention

Malabsorption Syndrome

77. a. bile salt deficiency (fats, fat-soluble minerals)

 b. enzyme deficiency (lactase, vitamin B_{12})

 c. bacteria overgrowth (fats, vitamin B_{12})

 d. disrupted small bowel mucosa (most nutrients)

 e. altered lymphatic or vascular circulation (protein, minerals, vitamin B_{12}, folic acid, lipids)

 f. decreased absorptive surface area (vitamin B_{12}, bile salts, others)

78. Steatorrhea; weight loss; fatigue; decreased libido; easy bruising; anemia; bone pain; edema; hypovolemia; abdominal pain; bloating; abdominal distention

79. a. decreased mean corpuscular volume (MCV), mean corpuscular hemoglobin (MCH), mean corpuscular hemoglobin concentration (MCHC)

 b. increased MCV level, variable MCH level and MCHC

 c. low serum iron level

 d. low serum cholesterol level

 e. low serum calcium level

 f. low serum vitamin A level

 g. low serum albumin and total protein level

80. a

81. d

CHAPTER 57

Appendicitis

1. The appendix has no known function.

2. e, c, f, a, g, i, h, d, b

3. A *fecalith* is a stone-like mass of feces. Such "stones" are a common cause of obstruction of the appendix.

4. a

5. b

6. Age; sex; history of abdominal surgery (especially appendectomy); other medical conditions; recent barium intake; diet history including fiber intake; complete pain description (location, sequence related to other symptoms); pain localizing to RLQ; pain relief with flexion of right hip or knees; nausea or vomiting; anorexia; urge to defecate; urge to pass flatus; psychosocial factors, including ability to cope with an abrupt onset illness and surgery

7. Vomiting following pain onset; tenderness on palpation (varies with time related to symptom onset); tenderness or rebound tenderness over McBurney's point; muscle rigidity; elevated temperature; tachycardia

8. a. perforation

 b. abscess formation

 c. peritonitis

9. b

10. c

11. d

Peritonitis

12. c

13. a

14. *Primary* peritonitis is an acute bacterial infection unassociated with perforation of an abdominal organ. It may result from an infection located elsewhere within the body that travels to the peritoneum via the vascular system. *Secondary* peritonitis is a result of bacterial invasion following perforation or rupture of an abdominal organ or direct contamination by foreign bodies, surgical instruments, peritoneal catheters, or ascending reproductive tract infections.

15. Consuming a high-fiber diet; administering laxatives or enemas after barium ingestion; maintenance of treatment regimens for clients at risk of developing abdominal organ perforation; administering antibiotics to clients with reproductive or pelvic infections; reporting changes in abdominal pain and fever over 101°F; using aseptic technique when handling peritoneal trochars and catheters

16. History of abdominal pain (including whether localized or generalized); aggravating factors such as respiration or movement; reports of pain relief with knee flexion; abdominal distention; anorexia, nausea, vomiting, fever and chills, inability to pass flatus or feces; recent surgery; current or past medical conditions; last menstrual period (women); psychosocial factors, including fear, concerns related to the illness, coping ability, support systems

17. Lying still with knees flexed; abdominal guarding with cough or movement; location of pain; abdomen either rigid and distended (generalized) or localized tenderness and rebound tenderness (localized); high fever; tachycardia; dry mucous membranes; decreased turgor; decreased urinary output; hiccups; dry mouth; possible difficulty with respirations

18. a

19. d

20. c

21. b

Gastroenteritis

22. Gastroenteritis is an inflammation of the mucous membranes of the stomach and intestinal tract. It primarily affects the small bowel.

23. a. viral

    b. bacterial

24. An inflammatory response resulting in increased GI motility and loss of fluids and electrolytes via the feces

25. Alteration in normal intestinal flora allowing increased capability of invading organism to attach to the intestinal mucosa (client receiving antibiotics, malnourished, debilitated); alteration in intestinal pH (increased pH due to taking antacids; decreased intestinal motility increases risk of pathogens contacting the intestinal wall (immobility, inadequate dietary fiber or liquids, result of medication therapy)

26. The primary route of transmission of the infecting organisms is the fecal-oral route via contaminated food, water, or contact with infected animals or infants.

27. Children and the elderly are the most susceptible to shigellosis because they have depressed immune systems.

28. Avoid all water and food identified as possibly being contaminated; limit exposure to other people who have symptoms of gastroenteritis throughout the period of communicability; wash hands meticulously before and after eating, after contact with animals, after each defecation; symptomatic individuals should avoid contact with others

29. Acute onset of diarrhea; age; sex; recall of first symptoms of diarrhea; nausea or vomiting; other household members' health; outside contacts; recent travel and locations; sequence of symptoms' occurrence; abdominal pain; headache; myalgia; malaise; psychosocial factors, including fear of loss of bowel control and fear of being contagious

30. Diarrhea (amount and consistency); nausea or vomiting; fever; abdominal distention; hyperactive bowel sounds; diffuse tenseness to palpation; absence of rebound tenderness; dehydration (skin turgor, dry mucous membranes, orthostatic hypotension, oliguria)

31. a. stool culture

    b. Gram's stain of stool

32. Rapid weight gains and losses reflect an equivalent gain or loss of body fluids. Daily weight measurement assists the monitoring of the client's fluid balance as well as intake and output of all fluids.

33. Hypotonic solutions assist in replacing cellular fluid because these solutions are hypotonic compared with plasma. They also help replace free water lost via bowel elimination.

34. Once nausea and vomiting subside: clear liquids; dry crackers; toast with jelly; bland, regular foods as tolerated

35. c

36. b

Ulcerative Colitis

37. Loss of surface epithelium allows for ulceration and possible abscess formation. These changes result in an inability of the bowel to absorb nutrients and water, contributing to malnutrition, anemia, and dehydration.

38. Abscess formation; bowel stenosis; bowel perforation and peritonitis; fissures; fistula formation; increased risk of developing cancer of the bowel; anemia; coagulation defects; malnutrition; dehydration; debilitation

39. b

40. a

41. Sex; age; race; family history of inflammatory bowel disease; previous or current therapy for illness, including surgery; dietary history, including relationship of elimination patterns to intolerance of milk and milk products, greasy fried foods, spicy or hot foods; frequency, number, and characteristics of stools; medication history; recent travel; allergies; occupation; stressors; nausea or vomiting; psychosocial factors, including impact of the disease on lifestyle, events related to exacerbations, job-related stressors and symptoms, smoking or alcohol use and effect on bowels, sleep patterns, support systems, weight loss and change in body image, restrictions on activities especially outside the home, stage of development

42. Presence or absence of bowel sounds and their characteristics; presence of abdominal scars; skin turgor; areas of increased or localized abdominal tenderness; rebound tenderness; localized pain or cramping; rectal fissures or hemorrhoids; characteristics of stools, including presence of blood, pus, or mucus; presence of fever or tachycardia

43. a. viral or bacterial dysentery

    b. parasitic infection

44. c

45. a

46. d

Crohn's Disease

47. c

48. d

49. a

50. Data are similar to those for ulcerative colitis. Also include any current or past history of fistulas.

51. Initial discomfort in the RLQ; diarrhea; low-grade fever; tenderness; guarding; palpable mass in RLQ; periumbilical pain before or after bowel movements; steatorrhea; weight loss; anorexia

52. Altered Skin Integrity related to fistula formation

53. Nutritional status is at risk; GI secretions are composed of fluids, electrolytes, and digestive enzymes. Malnutrition, dehydration, and hypokalemia are common complications. Skin excoriation can occur, as well as abscesses and sepsis.

54. b

Diverticular Disease

55. See textbook Figure 57-7 on p. 1651 for an illustration of diverticula.

56. d

57. c

58. Age; sex; history of intermittent LLQ pain or constipation; presence of pain and its characteristics; changes in bowel function (constipation or diarrhea); known presence of diverticula and their location; dietary fiber intake and any changes; psychosocial factors, including anxiety and fear, concerns about the need for surgery

59. Abdominal tenderness with palpation; LLQ pain; signs of peritonitis (fever tachycardia); nausea or vomiting; constipation or diarrhea; abdominal distention; possible palpable colon; localized muscle guarding or spasm; rebound tenderness; blood in stool

60. The risk of perforation of an inflamed diverticulum or a localized abscess is high.

61. d

62. c

63. a. peritonitis

    b. pelvic abscess

    c. bowel obstruction

    d. fistula

    e. presence of a mass or tumor

    f. persistent fever or pain more than 4 days after treatment is initiated

    g. uncontrolled bleeding

64. c

Anorectal Problems

65. b

66. c

67. a

68. Sitz baths help promote circulation to the perianal area, are soothing, and help relax the anal sphincter, thereby decreasing spasm. The soaks also assist in cleaning the perianal skin area. These actions help to decrease pain and reduce risk of infection.

Parasitic Infection

69. Fecal-oral transmission via contaminated food or water is the most common mode.

70. d	76. f
71. f	77. b
72. b	78. c
73. a	79. e
74. c	80. a
75. e	81. d

82. Enteric precautions should be followed. Avoid splashing of stool outside of commode, toilet, or bedpan. Clean up spilled stool immediately with recommended product. Use meticulous hand washing after handling any stool or stool-contaminated items. Dispose of contaminated items and linens as recommended. Doublebag and clearly label laboratory specimens. Refer to specific agency protocol for additional measures.

83. Close, intimate contact increases risk of exposure to and transmission of parasites, particularly if bathroom facilities are shared and food is prepared without careful hand washing.

Food Poisoning

84. **Food poisoning:** not directly communicable person to person; has a relatively short incubation period (1 hour to 4 days depending on organism); does not result in acquired immunity because reinfection can occur; symptoms include diarrhea, nausea, and vomiting

    Gastroenteritis: readily transmitted person to person; period of communicability can range from days to weeks; does result in acquired immunity; symptoms include diarrhea, nausea, and vomiting

85. Botulism and salmonella

86. Botulism—it causes severe illness and can be life-threatening if paralysis and respiratory failure occur

CHAPTER 58

Cirrhosis

1. b
2. d
3. a
4. c
5. a
6. b
7. a
8. d
9. b
10. c

11. d
12. c
13. e
14. c
15. a
16. f
17. b
18. g
19. d

20. Laennec's cirrhosis—it is preventable with complete abstinence from alcohol

21. Age; sex; race; employment history (chemical toxin exposure); history of alcoholism in client or family; pattern of alcohol intake; past health problems related to the hepatobiliary system, viral infection, blood transfusion, heart failure, respiratory disorders; weight loss; generalized weakness; loss of appetite; early morning nausea or vomiting; dyspepsia; flatulence; bowel habit changes; psychosocial problems such as personality and behavior changes, emotional lability, sleep pattern disturbance, interruptions in work or family life, financial difficulties

22. Gastrointestinal bleeding; jaundice; ascites; spontaneous bruising; dry skin; rashes; purpuric lesions; palmar erythema; spider angiomas; hepatomegaly; peripheral edema; distended abdomen or bulging flanks; protruding umbilicus; caput medusae; orthopnea; dyspnea; problems with maintaining balance; inguinal hernia; increases in abdominal girth; presence of blood in emesis or stool; fetor hepaticus; amenorrhea or testicular atrophy; gynecomastia; impotence; mentation or personality changes; asterixis

23. a
24. d
25. c
26. e
27. a
28. c
29. b
30. c
31. a
32. b
33. See pp. 1673–1674 in the textbook for discussion.
34. c
35. a
36. These clients are susceptible to infection, disseminated intravascular coagulation (DIC), bleeding varices, and anesthesia reactions.
37. A peritoneovenous shunt drains ascitic fluid from the peritoneal cavity to the superior vena cava, thereby reducing fluid accumulation. The client is expected to improve by losing weight, decreasing the abdominal girth, increasing urinary output, and excreting renal sodium.
38. Fresh frozen plasma supplies serum proteins, platelets, and clotting factors. The serum proteins help increase the plasma colloid osmotic pressure to maintain intravascular fluid volume, whereas platelets and clotting factors reduce the risk of intraoperative bleeding and DIC. Vitamin K reduces risk of hemorrhage by helping to replenish prothrombin and other coagulation factor stores. Packed red cells supply immediately available hemoglobin for oxygen transport, as well as treat the anemia these clients frequently have from progressive blood loss. Whole blood is avoided because it increases vascular volume.
39. b
40. c
41. a. large crystalloid solutions
    b. colloids (plasma)
    c. packed red cells
    d. fresh frozen plasma
42. d
43. d

44. a
45. c
46. c
47. b
48. See Table 58-3 on p. 1668 in the textbook. Submit the completed exercise to the clinical instructor for evaluation and feedback.

Hepatitis

49. f, b, e, c, a, g, d
50. a. hepatitis A
    b. hepatitis b
    c. hepatitis C
    d. delta hepatitis
    e. hepatitis E
51. Hepatitis B

52. d	58. d
53. c	59. b
54. a	60. a
55. b	61. e
56. e	62. c
57. a	63. b

64. a. toxic or drug-induced hepatitis results in necrosis and fatty infiltration
    b. idiosyncratic toxic hepatitis is similar to viral hepatitis
65. b
66. a
67. c
68. Known exposure to a person with hepatitis; recent blood transfusions or hemodialysis; social activities, including sexual preference and intravenous drug use; recent ear piercing or tattooing; type of living accommodations; employment history; recent travel to areas of endemic hepatitis; fatigue; appetite loss; general malaise; weakness; myalgia; joint pain; headaches; irritability; depression; nausea or vomiting; psychosocial factors, including anger at being sick, anxiety about long-term effects of illness, guilt, social stigma, family member nonsupport
69. Liver tenderness, firmness; pain with jarring movement; jaundice; dark urine; clay-colored stools; rashes; fever
70. b
71. c
72. b
73. d

Other Liver Problems

74. b	80. a
75. a	81. c
76. c	82. a
77. b	83. b
78. c	84. c
79. a	

85. Esophagus, stomach, colon, rectum, breasts, lung, malignant melanoma
86. Hepatoma—originates in liver parenchymal cells; most common primary tumor form
87. a. cirrhosis
    b. viral hepatitis
    c. trauma
    d. nutritional deficiencies
    e. carcinogen exposure
    f. hepatotoxin exposure

Liver Transplantation

88. Candidates for liver transplantation include clients with end-stage liver disease that is nonresponsive to conventional medical or surgical intervention. Clients who are excluded from consideration are those with primary and malignant neoplasms and severe end-stage liver disease with life-threatening complications.
89. Between the fourth and tenth postoperative days
90. Organ rejection; infections; hemorrhage; abscess formation; fluid or electrolyte imbalance; pulmonary atelectasis; hepatic artery thrombosis; acute renal failure; hypothermia; psychological problems
91. a. changes in client's complaints of postoperative pain and pain relief
    b. changes in neurological status
    c. signs of continuous bloody oozing from tubes, drains, suture sites, or petechiae
    d. ecchymosis
92. a. cyclosporine (Cyclosporin A)
    b. prednisone (Orasone)
    c. azathioprine (Imuran)

CHAPTER 59

Biliary Disorders

1. *Acute* cholecystitis is usually a result of obstructed bile flow to the duodenum from a gallstone (or less commonly, bacterial invasion). This condition leads to edema, vascular congestion, and inflammation. The trapped bile is reabsorbed by the gallbladder and causes a chemical irritation. This irritation, coupled with the edema, leads to tissue ischemia, sloughing, necrosis, and gangrene. *Chronic* cholecystitis results from prolonged inefficient bile emptying and diseased muscle wall tissue. This condition may or may not be associated with gallstones.

2. c

3. d

4. Decreased blood flow to the gallbladder, which cause "gallbladder shock"

5. b

6. d

7. Sex; age; race; ethnic group; if female, obstetric history, menopausal state, use of birth control pills, estrogen, other hormones; food preferences and intolerances (include gastrointestinal symptoms); daily activity and exercise level; client or family history of gallbladder disease and its treatment; abdominal pain and its associated characteristics; anxiety; fears

8. Height; weight; tenderness with palpation; muscle guarding or rigidity; rebound tenderness; palpable mass in right upper quadrant below liver border; jaundice; clay-colored stools; dark urine; steatorrhea; possible fever, tachycardia, dehydration, pallor, diaphoresis, and prostration

9. None

10. b

11. d

12. d

13. c

14. d

15. c

16. a

17. b

18. Cholesterol, bilirubin, bile salts, calcium, various proteins

19. d

20. b

21. d

22. a

23. c

Acute Pancreatitis

24. *Autodigestion* is a process in which the pancreas lyses its own cells with the digestive enzymes it normally produces.

25. **Lipolytic process:** Lipase acts on pancreatic endocrine and exocrine cells, causing fatty acids to be released. These acids combine with calcium and result in a rapid decrease in serum calcium.

    Proteolysis: Trypsin activates proteolytic enzymes, which attack pancreatic parenchyma. Damage may be localized or involve the entire organ.

    Necrosis of blood vessels: Elastase is activated and acts on the elastic fibers of pancreatic blood vessels and ducts leading to bleeding. Kallikrein causes release of peptides, which contributes to increased vascular permeability, vessel destruction, and hemorrhage.

    Inflammatory stage: This last stage results when leukocytes converge around the hemorrhagic and necrotic pancreatic tissue. Lesions may become infected by bacteria, producing suppuration, or may become walled off and lead to an abscess.

26. a. bile reflux

    b. hypersecretion-obstruction

    c. alcohol induced

    d. reflux of duodenal contents

27. e   30. f

28. d   31. a

29. b   32. c

33. a. alcoholism

    b. biliary tract disease with gallstones

34. b

35. Reason for seeking treatment; presence of abdominal pain, characteristics and related details; alcohol intake and related details; family history of alcoholism, pancreatitis, or biliary tract disease; prior abdominal surgery or procedures; presence of other medical problems causative of pancreatitis; recent viral infections; recent drug consumption; stated weight loss; nausea; psychosocial factors such as excessive alcohol intake, recent traumatic loss

36. Weight loss; vomiting; jaundice; discoloration of abdomen and periumbilical area; bluish discoloration of flanks; absent or decreased bowel sounds; abdominal tenderness, rigidity, muscle guarding; palpable mass; dullness on percussion (ascites); possible fever, tachycardia, hypotension, adventitious breath sounds, dyspnea, orthopnea, changes in behavior and sensorium

37. a. serum amylase level

    b. serum lipase level

38. b

39. a

Chronic Pancreatitis

40. *Chronic calcifying pancreatitis* is alcohol induced and characterized by precipitates that plug the ducts, leading to obstruction, inflammation, and fibrosis of pancreatic tissue. Cysts may form, and the organ becomes hard and firm.

    Chronic obstructive pancreatitis is a result of obstruction of the sphincter of Oddi by gallstones, causing spasm and inflammation and leading to ductal erosion, inflammation, and autodigestion in the head of the pancreas.

41. b

42. b

43. a

44. b

45. a

46. a

47. Data are similar to those for acute pancreatitis. Ask specifically about alcohol intake, time and amount consumed, and its relationship to pain development; abdominal pain characteristics; psychosocial factors, especially use of opioid analgesics, use of street drugs, economic hardship on family

48. Abdominal tenderness; palpable mass in the left upper quadrant; dullness on abdominal percussion; adventitious breath sounds, dyspnea, orthopnea; steatorrhea; weight loss; muscle wasting; jaundice; dark urine; associated signs of diabetes mellitus

49. a. serum bilirubin level

    b. alkaline phosphatase level

    c. amylase level

    d. glucose level

50. The client may become or already be dependent on opioids. This problem complicates accurate assessment of pain episodes because the client may use manipulative behavior to obtain needed opioids. When the client is hospitalized, opioid or alcohol withdrawal may result, especially if the client is misleading about the quantity of either depressant substance he or she is accustomed to taking.

51. d

52. d

53. a

54. Submit the completed exercise to the clinical instructor for evaluation and feedback.

Pancreatic Carcinoma

55. Tumors are usually not found until in the last stages of development. They grow rapidly and metastasize easily via the lymphatic and vascular systems.

56. a. lung

    b. breast

    c. thyroid

    d. kidney

    e. skin melanoma

57. a. lung

    b. peritoneum

    c. liver

    d. spleen

    e. lymph nodes

58. b

59. c

60. a. chemical carcinogens

    b. cigarette smoking

    c. high-fat diet

61. Data are similar to those for acute and chronic pancreatitis. Also, past medical diagnoses, including diabetes mellitus or pancreatitis; ethnic origins; smoking history; coffee intake; exposure to environmental carcinogens in occupations; history of jaundice; anorexia; early satiety; nausea; weight loss; pruritis; pain characteristics; psychosocial factors, including anxiety or fear about appearance, fear of addiction, ability to cope with impending death

62. Jaundice; clay-colored stools; dark, frothy urine; signs of scratching; palpable, enlarged gallbladder or liver; thrombophlebitis; cachexia; vomiting; flatulence; dullness over abdomen due to ascites

63. a. serum amylase level

    b. serum lipase level

    c. alkaline phosphatase level

    d. bilirubin level

    e. carcinoembryonic antigen level

64. Endoscopic retrograde cholangiopancreatography (ERCP)

65. c

66. See pp. 1732–1733 in the textbook for discussion.

67. This route helps prevent reflux of feedings into the duodenum or pancreatic duct. Feedings are delivered in an amount and concentration that are more easily absorbed.

68. See pp. 1733–1734 in the textbook for discussion. Submit the completed exercise to the clinical instructor for evaluation and feedback.

CHAPTER 60

Anorexia Nervosa

1. a, d, e, g, h

2. a. actual weight 15% below expected weight for age and height

   b. morbid fear of fatness

   c. disturbed perception of body weight and shape

   d. amenorrhea (females) or decreased sexual interest and function (males)

3. These changes occur as a self-protective mechanism as the body attempts to protect itself and function on a limited food intake. There is an overall conservation of energy (e.g., decreases in enzyme production, circulating norepinephrine, amenorrhea), which is reflected in the observed clinical signs.

4. Individuals who are in a profession or who participate in sports that demand low weight are at increased risk of developing anorexia nervosa. Examples are ballet dancers, fashion models, jockeys, gymnasts, wrestlers, and actresses.

5. c

6. d

7. Demographic data (age, sex, socioeconomic status, education, occupation); medical problems; weight history, including onset of weight loss; sexual history; attitudes and behavior toward food and weight; activity level; history of psychiatric illness and treatment; use of addictive substances; family history

8. Obvious weight loss; amenorrhea; hypothermia; hypotension; orthostatic hypotension; bradycardia; bradypnea; acrocyanosis; loss of muscle mass and subcutaneous fat with prominent bone structure; lanugo hair; edema; parotid gland tenderness and swelling; discolored tooth enamel; possibly tetany or paresthesias; osteoporosis

9. Frequently middle to upper socioeconomic class, adolescent, Caucasian female; high achiever academically; high level of motivation and compliance exhibited; distortion of body image; low self-esteem; sense of ineffectiveness; family dynamics (strong parental control, conflict intolerance); altered mood state; altered level of consciousness; obsessions; compulsions; phobias; unusual ideas about food; ritualistic behaviors; poor sexual adjustment; decreased social interaction; client strengths such as motivation level, desire for success, effective communication skills

10. Return to a general state of health is desirable. Chronic conditions (e.g., anemia, organ dysfunctions) may develop if a starved state persists over a prolonged period. Establishing a lower weight that is acceptable to the client may result in the client's complying with the treatment regimen.

11. Presence of these individuals may increase the client's anxiety, which may interfere with eating. The client may try to enlist their sympathy and bargain to not eat what is on the tray.

12. c

13. b

14. c

15. d

16. b

17. a

18. c

Bulimia Nervosa

19. a, c, d, f, g

20. See Chart 60-6 on p. 1753 in the textbook for a list of the criteria.

21. b

22. a

23. See Table 60-4 on p. 1755 in the textbook for information to complete the chart.

24. Sequelae of vomiting and laxative abuse; history of or treatment for cardiac, renal, or gastrointestinal problems; any seizures; use of ipecac; weight history; sexual activity; attitudes and behaviors toward food and weight; details about binges and methods of purging; activity level; previous episodes of psychiatric illness or substance abuse; a legal history if indicated; family history; reports of weakness, tiredness, constipation, depression

25. Irregular pulse; seizures; peripheral paresthesias; dry mouth; swollen, tender parotid glands; loss of tooth enamel; gray or brown teeth, caries, periodontal disease; esophagitis; gastric dilation (abdominal distention, bowel sounds, abdominal pain); loss of bowel tone; rectal prolapse; dehydration; edema (rebound fluid retention); irregular menses; presence of scars on knuckles, calluses on abdomen

26. Caucasian, female, early to mid-20s; middle to upper socioeconomic class; extroversion; antisocial personality traits; traits such as hysteria or obsessiveness; prior or current treatment for depression or suicide attempts; social interaction; family dynamics

27. Bulimics may have borderline psychopathology features that put them at risk for harmful practices or acts of self-harm. A qualified, trained professional should be asked to evaluate the client carefully to determine whether the client is at immediate risk for self-harm.

28. b

29. Regular exercise will help the client use ingested calories, thereby allowing an increase in the amount of food permitted. It is not unusual for the bulimic client to be limited in the number of calories (1000–1200 per day), which contributes to a feeling of deprivation and an urge to binge and purge.

30. c

31. d

CHAPTER 61

Nutrition

1. Nutritional health includes the body's ability to use nutrients for growth, tissue repair, prevention of infection, and normal body functioning.

2. c

3. a

4. a. disease state

    b. infection

    c. psychological stress

5. a. disease

    b. eating behavior

    c. economic factors

    d. emotional stability

    e. cultural patterns

    f. medication

6. Diet history review; record of food and fluid intake; laboratory data; food–medication interactions; health history and physical examination; psychosocial assessment; anthropometric measurements

7. b

8. d

Malnutrition

9. Anorexia (disease related such as chronic illness, acute infection, or from treatment); impaired absorption, assimilation, or utilization of nutrients; increased demand on body's nutrients to fight infection; semistarvation from medical treatment regimens

10. a

11. d

12. Usual daily food intake; eating patterns; appetite change; recent weight changes; times of meals and snacks; types of foods usually consumed; change in eating habits or appetite; involuntary weight loss; change in taste; dysphagia; types of food avoided; nausea; vomiting; heartburn; discomfort with eating; dental problems; dentures worn; psychosocial factors such as economic status, educational level, living and cooking facilities, mental status, resources to buy and prepare food

13. Condition of hair, eyes, oral cavity, nails, musculoskeletal, and neurological systems; height; weight; skinfold thickness; noted difficulty chewing or swallowing; food and fluid intake

14. b

15. d

16. a

17. e

18. f

19. c

20. c

21. Refer to pp. 1770–1775 in the textbook for discussion.

22. b

23. c

24. b

25. Submit the completed exercise to the clinical instructor for evaluation and feedback.

Obesity

26. b

27. c

28. a

29. c

30. Economic status; usual food intake; eating behavior; cultural background; attitude toward food; appetite; chronic diseases; medications; physical activity level; 24-hour recall of food intake; frequency of food intake; psychosocial factors, including emotional and circumstantial status, self-perception of current weight, cause and duration of weight gain, family history of obesity, past attempts at weight reduction and results, current reason for desire to lose weight, current stressors, exercise patterns, current perception of self-worth

31. Height; weight; ideal body weight (IBW) and current percentage of IBW; body mass index; skinfold measurements; skin assessment for reddened or open areas

32. Morbid obesity (more than twice ideal weight); lack of response to traditional weight reduction methods; body mass index equal to or greater than 40; weight of more than 100 pounds (45.4 kg) above weight to height standards; no diseases of the liver, cardiac, or kidney or inflammatory bowel disease; emotionally stable

33. a

34. a. potential for drug abuse

    b. sleep disturbances

    c. heart palpitations

    d. increased blood pressure

    e. dry mouth

    f. depression

35. a. jaw wiring

    b. encircling the esophagus

    c. gastroplasty

    d. intestinal bypass

36. Adipose tissue has a relatively poor blood supply, compromising both the oxygen and nutrient supply. It is difficult to approximate wound edges adequately so that healing by first intention can occur. The obese abdomen is prone to higher intra-abdominal pressure from the excess tissue. All these factors interplay and put the obese client at greater risk for wound dehiscence and infection.

37. b

CHAPTER 62

Anatomy and Physiology Review

1.	k	14.	y
2.	o	15.	n
3.	i	16.	e
4.	m	17.	u
5.	w	18.	x
6.	p	19.	g
7.	t	20.	h
8.	d	21.	a
9.	z	22.	v
10.	b	23.	r
11.	l	24.	f
12.	j	25.	s
13.	q	26.	c

27. See Table 62-1 on p. 1787 in the textbook.

28. The feedback system involves the interaction of the hypothalamus and anterior pituitary with the thyroid, adrenal cortex, and gonads. See Figure 62-2 on p. 1787 in the textbook

29.	c	36.	b
30.	d	37.	a
31.	b	38.	b
32.	a	39.	a
33.	a	40.	a
34.	a	41.	b
35.	a		

42. a. bone

    b. kidney

    c. gastrointestinal tract

43. d

44. d

45. c

46. d

47. b

48. a. osteoporosis: decreased ovarian production of estrogen

    b. decreased glucose tolerance: decreased sensitivity of peripheral tissues to the effects of insulin

    c. impaired water excretion: decreased concentrating ability of the kidneys

    d. degenerative cellular metabolism: decreased overall metabolic rate

Subjective Assessment

49. Reason for seeking health care; nature of onset; previous treatment; any interference with activities of daily living; age; sex; family history of endocrine-related disorders; change in energy levels; change in elimination patterns; change in nutritional status or gastrointestinal disturbances; sexual and reproductive function such as menstrual cycle changes, male impotence, change in libido, or change in secondary sexual characteristics; change in hair texture or distribution; change in facial contour or body proportions; psychosocial factors such as coping skills, support systems, health beliefs, self-perception, ability to learn and manage self-care, socioeconomic status

50. Submit the completed exercise to the clinical instructor for evaluation and feedback.

Objective Assessment

51. Height; weight; body fat distribution; muscle mass; skin color; areas of hypo- or hyperpigmentation; edema of extremities or at base of spine; body hair distribution; nail thickness and strength; facial structure, features, and expression; visible thyroid enlargement; jugular vein distention; chest size and symmetry; truncal obesity; supraclavicular fat pads; buffalo hump; breast size, shape, symmetry, pigmentation, and any discharge; reddish striae on breasts or abdomen; size of external genitalia; distribution and quantity of pubic hair, irregular cardiac rate or rhythm; orthostatic change in pulse or blood pressure; bruit over thyroid; thyroid size, symmetry, shape, and nodularity

52. Submit the completed exercise to the clinical instructor for evaluation and feedback.

53. b

54. Simple measurement of hormonal levels does not always reveal variations in normal or abnormal levels. Some hormones have a wide range of normal serum or urine variation. Suppression/stimulation testing challenges the endocrine gland in question to see if it is capable of normal hormone production.

55. c

56. b

57. See p. 1799 in the textbook for discussion.

58. a. skull films

    b. computed tomography

    c. magnetic resonance imaging

    d. angiography and venography

    e. ultrasonography

CHAPTER 63

Disorders of the Anterior Pituitary Gland

1. a. *Primary* pituitary dysfunction is the result of a problem in the pituitary gland itself.

    b. *Secondary* pituitary dysfunction is the result of a dysfunction of the hypothalamus.

2. *Panhypopituitarism* is the partial or total failure (deficiency) of *all* of the anterior pituitary hormones.

3. b

4. d

5. b

6. Loss of secondary sexual characteristics such as facial and body hair, episodes of impotence, and decreased libido in the adult man; lack of development of secondary sexual characteristics in the adolescent boy such as inability to initiate or maintain erection; secondary amenorrhea, painful intercourse, decreased libido, or difficulty becoming pregnant in the adult woman; family history of chronic renal failure, pancreatic, liver or bone disease, diabetes mellitus, hypothyroidism, or need for gonadal hormones; nutritional defects (inadequate protein, carbohydrates, fats, vitamin D, calcium, phosphorus); malnutrition; gastrointestinal malabsorption syndromes; failure to thrive in infancy or childhood; psychosocial factors such as client's body image, feelings of self worth, self-esteem, interpersonal relationships, limitations in performing activities of daily living (ADL), sexual identity, emotional distress (depression, crying episodes, feeling hopeless or frustrated)

7. Visual disturbances (decreased acuity or peripheral vision); bilateral temporal headaches; diplopia; decrease or loss of facial or body hair, decreased muscle mass or tone, testicular atrophy in adult man; absence of secondary sexual characteristics, small gonad or penis size in adolescent boy; decrease or loss of axillary or pubic hair, dry skin, breast atrophy in adult woman; partial or complete absence of secondary sexual characteristics (breast size, axillary hair, pubic hair), decreased vaginal secretions; increased truncal fat and delayed secondary tooth development in child

8. a. T_3

    b. T_4

    c. testosterone

    d. estradiol

9. a and c

10. a

11. e and f

12. b and d

13. a. Body Image Disturbance

    b. Sexual Dysfunction

    c. Ineffective Individual Coping

14. b

15. c

16. d

17. a. somatotropic

    b. lactotropic

    c. adrenocorticotropic

18. GH

19. *Gigantism* results from GH overproduction during puberty prior to closure of the epiphyses. Rapid growth in length of all bones occurs. *Acromegaly* results from GH overproduction after puberty and epiphyseal closure. Onset is insidious, producing thickening of facial and skull bones, skeletal thickening, and enlargement of hands, feet, and visceral organs.

20. Prolactinomas are the most common; gonadotropin- and TSH-secreting tumors are the least common.

21. Age; sex; family history; change in hat, glove, ring, or shoe size; fatigue; lethargy; backache; arthralgia; visual changes; headaches; menstrual changes (amenorrhea, irregular menses), difficulty becoming pregnant, decreased libido, painful intercourse in woman; decreased libido or impotence in man; psychosocial factors such as changes in physical appearance, interpersonal relationships, fertility problems causing emotional distress (depression), irritability, hostility, anxiety

22. Changes in facial features (increased lip or nose size, prominent supraorbital ridge; enlarging head, hand, or foot size; jaw projection; thickened distal phalanges; cardiomegaly; hepatomegaly; hypertension; dysphagia; voice deepening; hypogonadism; galactorrhea

23. a. Body Image Disturbance

    b. Sexual Dysfunction

24. a

25. d

26. b

27. d

Disorders of the Posterior Pituitary Gland

28. c

29. *DI* is associated with ADH deficiency, or inability of the kidney to respond to ADH, resulting in excretion of large volumes of dilute urine. *SIADH* is associated with ADH excess, resulting in water retention, increase in ECF volume, and hyponatremia.

30. a

31. Tumors in hypothalamic-pituitary region; head trauma; infectious processes; hypophysectomy; metastatic tumors from the breast or lung; cerebrovascular hemorrhage or aneurysm; granulomatous disease; drug-related side effects; hypokalemia and hypercalcemia

32. Age; sex; report of increased frequency of urination; recent increase in fluid intake; recent onset of constipation; recent surgery, head trauma, or medication; presence of other medical conditions (e.g., diabetes mellitus, renal or heart disease,

hypothyroidism, adrenal insufficiency), fatigue from sleep disruption; report of discomfort from polyuria or polydipsia

33. Hypotension; tachycardia; increased respiratory rate; poor skin turgor; dry, cracked mucous membranes and skin

34. c

35. c

36. b

37. b

38. c

39. b

40. Age; sex; medical history especially of recent trauma, cerebrovascular disease, tuberculosis or other pulmonary disease, cancer; past and current medications; reports of appetite loss, nausea, vomiting; headaches; psychosocial factors such as irritability, anxiety, uncooperativeness reported by significant others

41. Vomiting; weight gain; absence of edema in extremities; lethargy; hostility; disorientation; change in level of consciousness; seizures; coma; decreased or sluggish deep tendon reflexes; tachycardia; hypothermia

42. d

43. a

44. a. Fluid Volume Excess

    b. High Risk for Injury

45. b

46. b

Adrenal Gland Hypofunction

47. a. inadequate secretion of ACTH

    b. dysfunction of the hypothalamic-pituitary control mechanism

    c. complete or partial destruction of the adrenal glands

48. Loss of adrenal cortex function is life-threatening because of the mineralocorticoid and glucocorticoid deficiencies. Loss of adrenal medulla function does not adversely affect homeostasis because other areas of the sympathetic nervous system can supply catecholamines.

49. a. *Cortisol* promotes glyconeogenesis in the liver and muscle tissues and maintains the glomerular filtration rate and gastric acid production. It helps maintain a normal range for serum glucose levels, serum urea nitrogen level, and gastric acid production.

    b. *Aldosterone* promotes renal clearance of potassium, sodium, and water. It helps prevent hyperkalemia, hyponatremia, hypovolemia, and metabolic acidosis.

c. *Androgens* help maintain body hair and serum testosterone levels, particularly in the female.

50. Addisonian crisis is an acute adrenal insufficiency and an emergency. The body's demand for glucocorticoids and mineralocorticoids exceeds supplies. Sodium levels fall, potassium levels rise rapidly, and intravascular volume depletion (collapse) occurs. Sever hypotension results.

51. d

52. c

53. Change in activity level; lethargy; headaches; fatigue; muscle weakness; salt craving and increased salt intake; anorexia; nausea; vomiting; diarrhea; abdominal pain; recent weight loss; menstrual changes; impotence; history of radiation to abdomen or head, tuberculosis, or intracranial surgery; use of steroid medications, anticoagulants, or cytotoxic drugs; psychosocial factors such as apathy, depression, confusion, emotional lability, or forgetfulness resulting in disrupted family relationships

54. Increased pigmentation; decreased body hair; sweating; tachycardia; tremors, postural hypotension; dry skin and mucous membranes; irregular apical pulse

55. Basal levels of cortisol and ACTH may be normal or low-normal in the absence of undue stress on the client. Stimulatory testing challenges the adrenal glands to produce cortisol level elevations, which a compromised gland is incapable of doing.

56. b

57. c

58. d

59. a

60. b

61. c

62. a

Adrenal Gland Hyperfunction

63. d

64. Age; sex; changes in activity or sleep patterns; fatigue; muscle weakness; bone pain; history of fractures, frequent infections, or easy bruising; amenorrhea; history of steroid use or alcohol abuse; psychosocial factors such as emotional lability, mood swings, irritability, confusion, depression, neuroses, psychoses, or changes in body image

65. Buffalo hump; truncal obesity; supraclavicular fat pads; round face; thin legs and arms; generalized muscle wasting; bruises; thin, translucent skin; nonhealing wounds; red-purple striae over abdomen or upper thighs; fine coat of hair over face and body; acne; hirsutism in a woman; clitoral hypertrophy; balding; elevated blood pressure

66. c

67. Cortisol levels vary throughout the day.

68. Refer to Chart 63-4 on p. 1819 and to pp. 1816–1820 and 1822–1824 in the textbook for discussion.

69. a. Fluid Volume Excess

b. Impaired Skin Integrity

c. Activity Intolerance

d. High Risk for Injury (fracture)

e. Body Image Disturbance

70. b

71. d

72. a

73. c

74. d

75. b

76. a

77. c

78. c

79. In case of client injury or episodes of unconsciousness, confusion, or other inability to communicate, health care providers should be made aware of the client's lack of endogenous cortisol and need for exogenous steroid replacement. Otherwise death may result.

80. d

81. Age; sex; reports of headache, fatigue, muscle weakness, nocturia, loss of stamina; increased thirst; increased urination; paresthesias, especially of the extremities; history of congestive heart failure, nephrosis, cirrhosis, edema, weight gain; interference with ADL, work, or relationships

82. Elevated blood pressure; vision changes (decreased visual acuity); decreased reflexes; muscle weakness; tetany; cardiac dysrhythmias

83. a. volume depletion test

b. saline load study

84. b

Pheochromocytoma

85. b

86. d

87. d

88. Paroxysmal hypertensive episodes resulting in palpitations, severe headaches, profuse

diaphoresis, flushing, feeling of impending doom; pain in chest or abdomen; nausea; vomiting; known precipitating factors (e.g., increased abdominal pressure, micturition); reports of heat intolerance; weight loss; tremors; polyuria; polydipsia; current and past medications; psychosocial factors such as anxiety and impact of hypertensive episodes on ability to function

89. Baseline blood pressure; orthostatic hypotension; hyperreflexia; presence of hand tremors; sweating; fever; flushing; tachycardia; dysrhythmias; tachypnea; dyspnea; baseline weight; weight loss; weakness; pallor; vomiting

90. 24-hour urine collection for

   a. vanillylmandelic acid

   b. metanephrine

   c. free catecholamines

91. b

92. a. phentolamine (Regitine)

   b. phenoxybenzamine (Diabenzyline)

   c. prazosin (Minipress)

93. c

CHAPTER 64

Hyperthyroidism

1. a

2. d

3. b

4. Refer to p. 1834 in the textbook for discussion.

5. b

6. *Thyroid storm* (or *crisis*) is uncontrolled hyperthyroidism due to Graves' disease. It is life-threatening because signs and symptoms of crisis develop suddenly, often triggered by a major stressor such as infection. The crisis symptoms include systolic hypertension, confusion, psychosis, seizures, and coma.

7. a. maintaining airway patency

   b. providing adequate ventilation

   c. maintaining hemodynamic stability

8. Signs and symptoms are due to the increased metabolic rate and include fever, tachycardia, systolic hypertension, abdominal pain, nausea, vomiting, diarrhea, agitation, tremors, anxiety, restlessness, confusion, psychosis, seizures, and coma.

9. c

10. c

11. a

12. d

13. b

14. Age; sex; weight; usual weight; recent weight loss; increased appetite; change in bowel habits (diarrhea); heat intolerance; palpitations; chest pain; change in breathing patterns; changes in vision (blurring, diplopia, fatigue); difficulty performing ADL because of insomnia; change in menses (female); increase in libido; history of thyroid surgery or radiation therapy to neck; use of medications; psychosocial factors such as emotional lability, irritability, decreased attention span, manic behavior, change in mental or emotional status, mood fluctuation

15. a

16. Lid retraction; lid lag; globe lag; exophthalmos; thyroid gland enlargement; bruits over lobes of thyroid; fine, smooth hair; smooth skin; tachycardia; systolic hypertension; wide pulse pressure; tachypnea; dysrhythmias; diarrhea; tremors; seizures; fever; hyperactive deep tendon reflexes

17. b

18. d

19. a. Decreased Cardiac Output

   b. Altered Nutrition: Less than Body Requirements

   c. Sensory/Perceptual Alterations (Visual)

20. d

21. b

22. a. hemorrhage

   b. respiratory distress

   c. parathyroid gland injury (hypocalcemia, tetany)

   d. laryngeal nerve damage

23. b

Hypothyroidism

24. c

25. *Goiter* is the term used to describe the noncancerous enlargement of the thyroid gland that results when thyroid hormone production is insufficient.

26. a. deficiency of iodine in local soil or water resulting in inadequate iodine in the diet

   b. genetic defects preventing iodine metabolism

   c. diets consisting mainly of goitrogenic foods

   d. medications that contain large amounts of iodine

27. Refer to pp. 1844–1845 in the textbook for discussion.

28. d

29. b

30. a

31. c

32. Changes in sleep habits (increased time spent sleeping); generalized weakness; anorexia; muscle aches; paresthesias; constipation; cold intolerance; decrease in libido; fertility problems; use of medications such as lithium; history of treatment for hyperthyroidism; psychosocial factors such as depression, mania, apathy, withdrawal, decreased attention span or memory, paranoia, agitation

33. Coarse facial features; periorbital edema; blank facial expression; slow movements; hypotension; bradycardia; hearing loss; slowed deep tendon reflexes; hypothermia; bradypnea; lethargy; bruises

34. Ineffective Breathing Pattern: first priority for the nurse because the airway must be maintained to prevent acidosis, narcosis, and respiratory failure

    Decreased Cardiac Output: second priority to treat to prevent cardiovascular collapse from hypovolemia, hyponatremia, and dysrhythmias

    Altered Thought Processes: third priority for intervention by implementing measures to prevent further cerebral edema, acidosis, and hypoglycemia

35. Refer to Chart 64-6 in the textbook and p. 1845 for discussion.

36. a

37. c

38. d

Hyperparathyroidism

39. c

40. Refer to pp. 1850–1851 in the textbook for discussion.

41. b

42. c

43. d

44. a

45. b

46. a

47. Family history of primary hyperparathyroidism (e.g., associated with multiple endocrine neoplasia); family history of ulcer disease, bone disease, kidney stones, other endocrine disorders; drugs taken such as diuretics and vitamin D; headache; drowsiness; lethargy; flank pain; muscle weakness; GI problems; depression; past bone fractures; recent weight loss; arthritis; radiation to the head or neck; psychosocial factors such as personality changes, emotional lability, recent memory loss

48. Minimal physical manifestations. Waxy pallor of skin; bone deformities of back and extremities; vomiting; weight loss; mental confusion; decreased deep tendon reflexes

49. Decreased Cardiac Output related to cardiac dysrhythmias

50. Refer to pp. 1851–1853 in the textbook for discussion.

51. c

52. b

Hypoparathyroidism

53. d

54. Neck surgery or radiation therapy to the head or neck; perioral tingling of hands or feet; severe muscle cramps; irritability; seizures

55. Flexion of metacarpals, phalangeals, wrists, elbows; positive Chvostek's or Trousseau's sign; carpopedal spasms; convulsions; psychosis; cataracts; dental enamel hypoplasia; in pseudo-hypoparathyroidism may see short stature, round face, short thick neck, obesity, mental retardation, shortened metacarpals and metatarsals

56. a. IV calcium (calcium chloride, calcium gluconate)

    b. oral elemental calcium (lactate, gluconate, or carbonate)

    c. vitamin D (ergocalciferol)

    d. magnesium sulfate

57. a

CHAPTER 65

Pathophysiology Review

1. Diabetes mellitus is a subgroup of disease processes characterized by a deficiency or lack of insulin. The lack of insulin affects metabolism of carbohydrates, proteins, and fats and leads to long-term complications throughout the body.

2. a. type I, or IDDM

   b. type II, or NIDDM

   c. other, including gestational diabetes and several categories of glucose intolerance

3. c

4. b

5. a. glucagon

 b. epinephrine

 c. norepinephrine

 d. growth hormone

 e. cortisol

6.	b	16.	a
7.	c	17.	b
8.	a	18.	c
9.	d	19.	a
10.	c	20.	b
11.	c	21.	a
12.	b	22.	c
13.	d	23.	b
14.	d	24.	c
15.	c	25.	c

26. a. infection

 b. gangrene

 c. amputation

27. b

28. a

29. a

30. b

31. b

32. a

33. b

34. c

35. b

36. a. diabetic ketoacidosis: not enough insulin

 b. hypoglycemia: too much insulin

 c. hyperglycemic hyperosmolar nonketotic coma: inadequate amount of insulin but enough to suppress ketosis

37. Refer to Table 65-3 on p. 1862 and to pp. 1861–1862 in the textbook for discussion.

38. c

39. d

40. a

41. a

42. d

43. b

44. c

45. a

46. b

Collaborative Management

47. Age; sex; race; usual weight; height; dietary intake for 3 days; previous diagnosis of diabetes and which type; how long symptoms have been present; taking any diabetes medications (name, dose, strength, last dose); sites used for insulin injections; history of hypoglycemia, symptoms, and treatment; current stressors; presence of concurrent illness; use of other medications; type of glucose monitoring used; past illnesses, surgery, immunizations; family history of diabetes mellitus, heart disease, stroke, obesity; level of exercise; fatigue or lethargy; visual changes; intermittent claudication; extremity coolness, tingling, or pain; delayed wound healing; itchy skin; diarrhea with incontinence; urinary retention or urinary tract infections; postprandial fullness or bloating; a history of stillbirth, miscarriage, or large babies in women; psychosocial factors such as depression and impaired self-perception or self-concept, ability to function and interact with others, ability to understand and perform self-care techniques, support systems

48. Periodontal disease; cavities; dental extractions; skin turgor; dry skin; level of consciousness; vital signs; fruity breath odor; signs of retinopathy (tortuous vessels or pinpoint hemorrhages or exudates); neuropathy (depressed tendon reflexes, vibratory sense, and perception of sharp versus dull); decreased vascular flow (decreased peripheral pulses and cool skin)

49. d

50. a

51. BUN level and serum creatinine levels are indicators of renal function, specifically glomerular filtration. In diabetic nephropathy, nephrons are damaged, glomerular filtration decreases, and BUN and serum creatinine levels rise.

52. c

53. *Renal threshold* is the point at which blood glucose is filtered out of the blood into the urine. It varies among individuals and rises with the aging process and with kidney damage. Consequently, measurements of urine glucose levels are inaccurate and underestimate the true levels of blood glucose, resulting in periods of untreated hyperglycemia.

54. Urine test results can be altered by the amount of fluid ingested; the client may make errors in timing when reading results; a number of medications that the client may be taking interfere with accurate results; some tests are more accurate that others; and there is controversy about whether a first or second voided urine specimen should be used for testing.

55. d

56. c

57. b

58. c

59. b

60. Refer to Table 65-10 on p. 1880, Table 65-11 on p. 1882, Chart 65-5 on p. 1885, and Chart 65-6 on p. 1886 in the textbook for discussion. Submit the completed exercise to the clinical instructor for evaluation and feedback.

61. a. lack of insulin during the night, resulting in hyperglycemia

    b. dawn phenomenon, in which blood glucose levels rise between 5 and 6 a.m. due to hormone secretions

    c. the Somogyi effect, in which hormone secretions cause a rapid rise in blood glucose levels despite hyperglycemia

62. d

63. d

64. a. usual dietary intake

    b. weight to height ratio

    c. cultural norms

    d. daily schedule

65. d

66. a. bread

    b. vegetable

    c. fruit

    d. meat

    e. fat

    f. milk

67. b

68. b

69. b

70. d

71. a. anorexia nervosa

    b. bulimia nervosa

72. a

73. Exercise increases the body's ability to utilize calories and decreases the need for insulin. The combined effect of these two actions is that the diabetic client may have a hypoglycemic episode due to having too much exogenous insulin or insufficient glycogen stores. Simple sugars provide a ready supply of useable glucose to meet the body's needs during these episodes.

74. c

75. d

76. a

77. d

78. a. fear of loss

    b. fear of having a severe hypoglycemic reaction

    c. fear of being different

    d. fear of losing control

79. b

80. c

CHAPTER 66

Anatomy and Physiology Review

1. a. aging process

   b. emotional stress

   c. injury

   d. disease

2. c

3. b

4. a

5. b

6. c

7. a

8. a

9. c

10. c

11. b

12. b

13. a

14. c

15. b

16. b

17. c

18. a

Subjective Assessment

19. Age; race; nationality; occupation; hobbies; prior or current medical illness or surgery; family tendency toward chronic skin problems; recent skin problems in the family; recent exposure to prescription and over-the-counter drugs; diet history (weight, height, body build, food preferences); recent travel; exposure to sun or use of tanning salons; living conditions; bathing facilities; availability of running water in home; specific details about any rashes; associated problems (itching, burning, numbness, pain, fever, nausea, vomiting, sore throat, stiff neck, aggravating and relieving factors); psychosocial factors such as alterations in body image, self-concept, social isolation, rejection

20. b

21. d

22. Submit the completed exercise to the clinical instructor for evaluation and feedback.

Objective Assessment

23. Color; lesions (primary or secondary, color, size, location, isolated changes or grouped in a pattern, generalized or localized); edema (pitting or nonpitting); moisture; dryness; scaling; vascular markings (petechiae, ecchymoses, birthmark, cherry angioma, spider angioma, venous star); intactness (abrasions, tears, needlemarks); cleanliness; consistency of lesions (flat or raised, associated tenderness); tenderness on palpation; nature of any secretions; skin temperature; texture (rough or smooth, thickness, elasticity); turgor; hair (cleanliness, distribution, quantity, quality); dandruff; patches of hair loss; hirsutism; nail color, shape, thickness, texture, and presence of lesions; nail ridges; nail blanche response; nail be angle; nail hardness

24. Submit the completed exercise to the clinical instructor for evaluation and feedback.

25. c   38. g
26. b   39. e
27. c   40. f
28. b   41. e
29. d   42. c
30. h   43. b
31. f   44. a
32. a   45. d
33. j   46. d
34. c   47. c
35. b   48. b
36. d   49. d
37. i

CHAPTER 67

Minor Irritations

1. b
2. a. central heating
   b. air conditioning
   c. wind
   d. cold
   e. sunlight
   f. frequent bathing with harsh soap and hot water
3. e
4. a

5. Implementing measures to lubricate the skin; keeping the fingernails trimmed short and smooth; keeping the room cool and humidified; administering antihistamines at bedtime; using distraction or relaxation techniques; wearing mittens or splints at night; taking therapeutic baths with colloidal oatmeal or tar extract in cool or tepid water; applying cool compresses

6. b
7. a
8. d
9. c
10. a. exposure to a specific noxious stimulus
    b. histamine is released in dermal tissue
    c. vasodilation occurs
    d. plasma proteins leak into the dermal layer to form wheals
11. b

Trauma

12. b
13. c
14. a
15. a, f, i, m, g, c, d, h, b, j, e, l, k
16. b
17. c

Pressure Ulcers

18. a. pressure
    b. friction
    c. shear
19. b
20. Underlying cause if known (e.g., chronic skin ulcers, history of delayed healing); associated factors such as diabetes mellitus, prolonged bed rest, immobility, incontinence, inadequate nutrition or hydration; psychosocial factors such as perceived body image, ineffective coping patterns, compliance with prescribed treatment, cost of treatment, fear of disfigurement, availability of assistance with wound care if needed, modifications necessary in ADL
21. *Partial-thickness wound:* bulla formation; crusting or scab formation over a denuded area; stripping of skin (tape burns); presence of cellulitis; fever; increase in size or depth of wound

    Full-thickness wound: presence or absence of necrotic tissue; eschar; increased wound exudate; granulation tissue; hypertrophic granulation; soft-tissue hardness; sinus tracts; necrotic cavities

22. b

23. a. removing unwanted debris from wound surface

    b. protecting exposed viable tissues

    c. re-establishing a temporary barrier between the body and the environment until wound closure is complete

24. Amount of necrotic material or exudate present

25. a. physical therapy (mechanical débridement)

    b. drug therapy (topical antibacterial agents)

    c. diet therapy (nutrients necessary for tissue repair)

26. a

27. c

28. d

29. a. avoid direct contact with wound secretions (wear gloves, use forceps)

    b. avoid cross-contamination between clients (wash hands before and after dressing changes, dispose of soiled dressings according to protocol)

Common Infections

30. d

31. Recent history of skin trauma; past or current problems with a specific infecting organism (e.g., *Staphylococcus* or *Streptococcus*); location of lesions; history of similar lesions in the same location; prodromal signs of burning, tingling, or pain; recent stressors; previous exposure to chickenpox; contact with an infected individual; poor personal hygiene practices; frequent contact with animals; type and frequency of sport activities; factors contributing to decreased host resistance (e.g., immunosuppressive drug therapy, antibiotics, diabetes mellitus, cancer, nutritional deficits, obesity); psychosocial factors such as intimate contact with others, changes in body image and self-esteem

32. Refer to Chart 67-4 on p. 1951 in the textbook.

33. d

34. c

35. a

36. b

Parasitic Disorders

37. c

38. b

Common Inflammations

39. b

40. c

41. a

42. a

43. b

44. c

45. a

46. Present or past problems with allergies; past of recent exposure to potential irritants or allergens; occupation; hobbies; hygiene practices; aggravating and relieving factors; personal or family history of the problem; history of asthma or allergic rhinitis; recent medication history; severe pruritus; fever; psychosocial factors such as self-concept, fear of contagion, interference with ADL

47. Refer to Chart 67-6 on p. 1956 in the textbook.

48. b

49. e

Psoriasis

50. b

51. Family history of psoriasis; age of onset; description of disease progression; pattern of recurrences; description of the current flare-up; associated symptoms (fever, pruritus); possible precipitating factors (recent skin trauma, upper respiratory tract infection, recent surgery; menopause; medications; recent stressors); previous treatment modalities; psychosocial factors such as self-perception, self-concept, fear of contagion

52. b

53. a

54. c

55. a

56. b

57. a

58. c

59. b

60. a. topical corticosteroids

    b. topical tar and anthralin preparations

    c. ultraviolet light

61. c

62. d

63. d

64. b

Benign Tumors

65. b

66. e

67. c

68. a

69. f

70. d

71. a

72. d

73. e

74. c

75. f

76. b

Skin Cancer

77. a

78. b

79. Change in color of lesion (darkening, spreading); change in size of lesion (rapid growth); change in shape of lesion (borders or elevation); redness or swelling around a lesion; change in sensation in lesion (itching, tenderness); change in character of lesion (oozing, crusting, bleeding, scaling)

80. Age; race; family history of skin cancer; past surgery for removal of skin growths; recent changes in size, color, sensation of any lesion or scar; geographic locations where client has lived and where currently living; occupational and recreational activities; exposure to chemical carcinogens; skin lesions subject to chronic irritation; itching; tenderness; psychosocial factors such as fear, anxiety, hopelessness

81. Location, size, color, and surface characteristics of any lesions; see also Table 67-10 on p. 1962 in the textbook for further discussion.

82. b

83. c

84. e

Plastic and Reconstructive Surgery

85. a. correct functional defects

    b. alter physical appearance

86. Client's description of the problem; why the problem is bothersome; what is expected as a result of the change; previous surgeries and client's reaction to them; history of medical problems; psychosocial factors such as the client's perceived emotional investment in the surgery

87. c

88. b

89. Alteration in appearance ranging from significant to mild; asymmetry of anatomical features; wrinkling of skin; skin redundance; scars; disfiguring skin marks; obvious skin lesions

90. d

91. c

Other Disorders of the Skin and Nails

92. a, b, f, g, h, j, m, o

CHAPTER 68

Pathophysiology

1. a

2. b

3. Maintain internal constancy for fluids and electrolytes; maintain temperature homeostasis; prevent invasion of internal environment by harmful organisms; act as an organ of excretion through perspiration; serve as a sensory input channel for pain, pressure, temperature, touch; produce vitamin D; contribute to the individual's identity through variations in unique individual form and character

4. c

5. a. first-degree (superficial): epidermis; painful, red, swollen, increased sensitivity to heat; heals on its own

    b. second-degree (superficial partial): upper dermis and deep dermis; painful, red, wet, increased sensitivity to heat; heals on its own in 10–14 days

    c. second-degree (deep partial): deep dermis; cherry red or white; swelling, painful; heals in 3–6 weeks

    d. third-degree (full): entire dermis and subcutaneous fat; eschar is ivory, brown, gray, black, cherry red; swelling, sometimes painful; heals after grafting

6. a

7. b

8. d

9. a. dry heat

    b. moist heat

    c. contact with hot surface

    d. chemicals

    e. electricity (high voltage)

    f. ionizing radiation

10. d

11. b

12. c

13. a. turn down hot water heater temperature to below 120°F

    b. install an adjustable water-mixing valve on shower heads and faucets

    c. supervise children and elderly or disabled adults during baths and showers

14. a. slowed response time

    b. existence of preexisting chronic conditions (e.g., arthritis, stroke)

    c. presence of physical disabilities

Collaborative Management

15. c

16. a

17. d

18. b

19. c

20. d

21. Time of injury; source of heat or injurious agent; detailed description of how the burn occurred; whether alcohol or drugs may have been a factor; the physical surroundings in the immediate area where the burn was sustained; the events occurring from the time of the burn to admission in the health care facility

22. Age; height; weight; presence of chronic illness, physical disability, or organ pathology; specific medications including over-the-counter drugs; allergies; history of smoking or excessive use of alcohol; sex; race; religious preference; dietary habits; cultural background; occupation; family history; social history; financial history

23. History of abuse, neglect, unsafe environment; drug use; unusual habits; guilt feelings; grieving; loss of memory or gaps in recall; incongruent affect; unstable employment history; cultural beliefs about coping with pain and crisis; fears, especially of death

24. Assessment of coping mechanisms used by the client and family may indicate how they can be expected to cope during the present situation. The care plan can use previously successful coping styles. The presence of support systems for the client is vital to survival.

25. Appearance and function of mouth, nose, pharynx, trachea, pulmonary mechanisms; presence of burns on head, face, neck, upper thorax; presence of facial injury, singed hair on head, eyebrows, eyelids, nasal mucosa; blisters or soot on lips or oral mucosa; evidence of carbon particles in sputum; progressive hoarseness; presence of sound with respirations (wheezes, crowing, stridor); disappearance of wheezes once present; headache; nausea; drowsiness; confusion; stupor; coma; moist breath sounds; crackles; shortness of breath; increased dyspnea when supine; tight eschar around thorax, neck, or throat

26. b

27. Presence and strength of peripheral pulses and central pulses; hypotension; slow peripheral capillary refill; presence of edema; following resuscitation, pulses are stronger, diastolic blood pressure increases, edema and weight increase, capillary refill improves in the early postburn period

28. d

29. b

30. Decreased urinary output; high urine specific gravity; hematuria; presence of particulate matter in urine; foamy urine

31. c

32. c

33. a. size and depth of burn injury

    b. estimate of total body surface area involved in burn injury

    c. change in skin color or appearance

34. b

35. a. absent bowel sounds

    b. hypoactive bowel sounds

    c. nausea

    d. vomiting

    e. abdominal distention

    f. blood in stool or emesis

36. c

37. a. low core body temperature

    b. increased pulse rate

    c. polyuria

    d. polydipsia

    e. polyphagia

    f. fruity breath

38. b

39. a

40. a. extent of active and passive ROM in all joints, including neck, on admission

    b. any limitations

41. b

42. To prevent shock by maintaining adequate circulating fluid volume

43. a. 14,000 mL

    b. 7000 mL in the first 8 hours and 7000 mL in the next 16 hours; the first 8-hour period ends at 5 p.m.

44. a. brain

    b. heart

    c. kidneys

45. Submit the completed exercise to the clinical instructor for evaluation and feedback.

46. c

47. b

48. a

49. a

50. *Débridement* is the removal of eschar and other cellular waste materials from the burn wound. It can be done mechanically, with enzymes, or by surgical excision.

51. c

52. a

53. b

54. c

55. a

56. c

57. b

58. c

59. a. posttraumatic stress

b. sexual dysfunction

c. severe depression

60. c

61. b

62. a. age

b. extent of burn injury

c. presence of inhalation burn injury

d. wife's death

CHAPTER 69

Anatomy and Physiology Review

1. a. kidneys

b. ureters

c. urinary bladder

d. urethra

2. n

3. o

4. b

5. q

6. g

7. r

8. i

9. t

10. u

11. e

12. p

13. d

14. v

15. w

16. m

17. a

18. s

19. j

20. f

21. l

22. c

23. h

24. x

25. k

26. Refer to Figure 69-3 on p. 2014 in the textbook.

27. a. removal of nitrogenous waste products

b. regulation of fluid, electrolyte, and acid–base balance

c. regulation of blood pressure

28. b

29. a

30. c

31. e, c, f, a, d, b

32. c

33. d

34. a

35. a. active vitamin D: necessary for gastrointestinal absorption of calcium; promotes renal and bone reabsorption of calcium

b. erythropoietin: stimulates bone marrow to produce red blood cells

c. kinins: influence arteriole dilation and capillary permeability

d. prostaglandins: promote vasoconstriction or vasodilation; counteract effects of ADH, promoting urinary loss of water and sodium

e. renin: assists in regulation of blood pressure

36. j

37. i

38. d

39. m

40. c

41. l

42. n

43. a

44. g

45. f

46. h

47. e

48. b

49. k

50. Refer to pp. 2021–2022 for discussion and Chart 69-1 on p. 2022 in the textbook

Subjective Assessment

51. Age; sex; race; personal and family history of kidney disease (including Bright's disease, nephritis, nephrosis, polycystic kidney disease); urinary tract infection, tumors, or stones; urinary surgery; diabetes mellitus; hypertension; medication history; history of protein in urine; renal-associated problems in pregnancy; exposure to environmental or chemical toxins of infectious organisms; recent physical trauma; sexual contact; diet history (including recent changes, excessive intake of milk or dairy products, fluid intake, appetite, change in taste sensation, weight reduction dieting); socioeconomic data

(including whether income is sufficient or lacking for health care, ability to comply with a prescribed medical regimen, knowledge level); current health status; change noted in odor, color, or clarity of urine; urinary patterns (frequency, nocturia, quantity of voidings) ability to turinate or control urination; oliguria; anuria polyuria; hesitancy; dysuria; urgency; retention; hematuria; nausea; anorexia; vomiting; diarrhea; muscle cramps or twitching; itching; flank pain, especially radiating to lower abdomen, perineum, groin, or genitals

52. Emotional response including embarrassment, fear, anxiety, anger, guilt, sadness; childhood experiences with toilet training, bed wetting; anxiety about body image; fear of sexual dysfunction; fear of death

53. f
54. h
55. e
56. i
57. a
58. c
59. j
60. b
61. g
62. d

63. Submit the completed exercise to the clinical instructor for evaluation and feedback

Objective Assessment

64. General appearance; yellow skin color; rashes, ecchymoses, or discolorations; edema; lung sounds; weight; blood pressure; level of consciousness, including deficit in concentration, thought processes, memory, dysarthria, alertness; gait; coordination; flank asymmetry or discoloration; abdominal bruit; bruit over renal artery; bladder distension (dull to percussion); palpable right or left kidney; tenderness upon blunt percussion over costovertebral angle; urethral discharge, blood, mucus, or purulent drainage; perineal lesions, rashes, or other abnormality

65. Submit the completed exercise to the clinical instructor for evaluation and feedback

66. d
67. c
68. b
69. d
70. a
71. a. antibiotics such as the aminoglycosides
    b. nonsteroidal anti-inflammatory agents
    c. radiopaque contrast material
72. d
73. b

74. a. intravenous pyelography
    b. nephrotomography
    c. computed tomography with contrast material
    d. renal arteriography

CHAPTER 70

Infectious Disorders

1. c
2. b
3. c
4. a
5. Mucin helps prevent urothelial inflammation and damage; usual acid pH of urine helps control bacteria reproduction; downward and outward flow of urine helps flush bacteria from bladder and urethra
6. External opening via the urethra to external body surface provides a point of entry for contaminating bacteria; proximity of urethral meatus to vagina and rectum in women as well as urethra's short length increases risk of contamination from normal body flora in vagina and GI tract; prostatic enlargement in men restricts outflow of urine and bacteria present in prostate gland is a source of contamination.
7. c
8. Age; sex; medication history; identification of risk factors such as prior urinary tract infection (UTI) or other renal or urologic problems; chronic health problems such as diabetes mellitus, neurogenic bladder, urinary reflux; past or current exposure to sexually transmitted disease; dysuria; urgency; hesitancy; expressed feeling of incomplete bladder emptying; urinary frequency; urethral or vaginal discharge; presence of abdominal or back discomfort; psychosocial factors such as guilt or embarrassment about sexual activity, fear of having a sexually transmitted disease, fears about sexual functioning or impotence, level of understanding about basic anatomy
9. Inability to urinate or empty bladder completely; urine characteristics (color change, turbidity, foul odor, presence of blood or mucus); bladder distention; inflammation of urethral meatus; skin lesions of perineum; prostatic enlargement or tenderness; confusion in elderly client
10. d
11. a. complete the prescribed medication regimen
    b. consume a liberal fluid intake
    c. obtain adequate rest, sleep, and nutrition
    d. avoid known irritants
    e. practice proper hygiene

f. keep follow-up appointments

g. seek prompt medical care if recurrence is suspected

12. b

Urinary Incontinence

13. d

14. e

15. b

16. a

17. c

18. c

19. Age; sex; voiding patterns and any changes; whether incontinence occurs during sleep or intermittently during day; nature of onset (brief or long term); contributing factors such as coughing, sneezing; feelings of bladder fullness; presence of warning signals (bladder spasm); history of pregnancies or surgical procedures; menopause; medications, current perceived stressors in life; past urological surgical procedure; spinal cord trauma; diabetes mellitus; neurological disease (e.g., Parkinson's, Alzheimer's, multiple sclerosis); psychosocial factors, including embarrassment, self-concept, body image, self-esteem, and interpersonal relationships

20. Bladder distention; tenderness on palpation; dullness on percussion; urine leakage with pressure over bladder urethral or uterine prolapse, cystocele; secretions from genitourinary orifices; tight rectal sphincter; presence of fecal impaction; prostate enlargement

21. a. Social Isolation

b. High Risk for Impaired Skin Integrity

c. Body Image Disturbance

22. c 29. c

23. a 30. c

24. a 31. a

25. b 32. c

26. b 33. b

27. b 34. c

28. b

35. Intermittent self-catheterization decreases the chance of induced bladder infection as opposed to having an in-dwelling catheter. An in-dwelling catheter provides a means of direct access for external pathogens into the bladder, particularly from vaginal or rectal sources. Intermittent catheterization following adequate cleaning of the perineum is less likely to introduce contaminants into the bladder.

Urolithiasis

36. c

37. a

38. b

39. Supersaturation of the filtrate with a particular element (e.g., calcium, phosphate, oxalate, uric acid, struvite, or cystine crystals); urinary pH promotes or inhibits calculus formation by providing a medium for stone formation; urinary stasis resulting from stones that lodge in the ureteropelvic angle, aortoiliac bend, or ureterovesicle angle and block urine flow; presence of other substances that may promote crystallization

40. *Hydroureter:* enlargement of the ureter, usually due to obstruction of urinary flow

Hydronephrosis: enlargement of the kidney, usually due to persistent blockage of urine flow

41. Previous personal or family history of kidney or bladder stones; diet history; surgical, invasive, or noninvasive treatments for stone removal; known results of stone analysis; presence of pain (especially flank pain or pain radiating to abdomen or perineum); nausea; changes in urination patterns; psychosocial factors such as anxiety about pain control, interference with work or other personal goals, fear of kidney failure

42. Vomiting; chills; fever; ureteral colic; hematuria; oliguria or anuria; turbidity; bladder distention; pale, ashen, diaphoretic skin; tachycardia; tachypnea; elevation of blood pressure

43. Presence in urine of RBCs, WBCs, bacteria, and crystals; elevation of serum WBC count with increased number of immature cells; increased serum calcium, serum phosphate, and uric acid levels

44. d

45. a. Pain

b. High Risk for Infection

c. High Risk for Injury

46. d

47. b

48. Urine may leak around the drainage tubes that are placed in the urinary tract to maintain patency. Prompt changing of wet dressings keeps the skin dry, prevents excoriation, and maintains skin integrity against bacterial invasion.

49. Refer to pp. 2069–2072 and Table 70-5 on p. 2067 in the textbook for discussion.

Urothelial Cancer

50. Active and passive consumption of cigarette smoke; dyes; metals; paints; rubber by-products; organic chemicals; coffee; artificial sweeteners; chronic infections; bladder stones; exposure to cyclophosphamide

51. Age; sex; race; exposure to cigarette smoke; occupation; noted change in urine color or patterns; abdominal discomfort; burning with urination; dysuria; frequency; urgency; psychosocial factors such as emotional response, anxiety, fear, sadness, anger, guilt, coping mechanisms, support systems

52. Skin color, general nutritional status; asymmetry of abdomen; tenderness on abdominal palpation or percussion; bladder distention; hematuria

53. e
54. d
55. b
56. f
57. a
58. c
59. d

CHAPTER 71

Congenital Disorders

1. a. the disorder is inherited, not acquired
   b. these clients are at increased susceptibility to infection
   c. increased risk of developing renal failure
2. c
3. a
4. b
5. Family history especially of parents and their current health status; age that parent developed polycystic kidney disease, and his or her symptoms; other family history of kidney disease or sudden death from "stroke"; problem with constipation or abdominal discomfort; change in color or frequency of urination; hypertension; headaches; flank pain; anorexia; nausea; vomiting; pruritus; fatigue; psychosocial factors such as feelings of anger, resentment, hostility, futility, sadness, anxiety, guilt, and concern
6. Distended abdomen; readily palpable kidneys; tenderness of kidney to palpation; bright red or cola-colored urine; cloudy, foul-smelling urine; hypertension; edema
7. d

8. a. Pain
   b. Fluid Volume Excess
   c. Anxiety
   d. Constipation
9. c
10. d
11. b

Infectious Disorders

12. c
13. a
14. b
15. a
16. Previous occurrence of pyelonephritis; history of urinary tract infection; diabetes mellitus; previous renal stone formation; known structural or functional abnormality of the urinary system; pregnancy; presence of flank or abdominal discomfort; feelings of malaise or fatigue; chills; reports of frequency, urgency, or burning with urination; psychosocial factors such as anxiety, embarrassment, guilt
17. Hematuria; cloudy urine; fever; malaise; flank asymmetry; flank or costovertebral tenderness on palpation or percussion; flank edema or erythema
18. a. pyelolithotomy
    b. nephrectomy
    c. ureteral diversion
    d. reimplantation of ureters
19. c
20. *Hydroureter:* enlargement of the ureter, usually due to obstruction of urinary flow in the lower urinary tract

    Hydronephrosis: enlargement of the kidney, usually due to persistent blockage of urine flow from the pelvis and calyceal system
21. a. urethral stricture
    b. tumors
    c. stones
    d. trauma
    e. congenital structural defects
    f. retroperitoneal fibrosis

Immunologic Disorders

22. b
23. History of recent infection of skin or upper respiratory tract; recent travel or exposure to pathogens; recent illnesses, surgery, or other

invasive procedures; known systemic diseases (e.g., lupus erythematosus); change in pattern of urination (color); dysuria; decreased amount of urine; dyspnea, especially nocturnal or with exertion; orthopnea; fatigue; anorexia; nausea; malaise; psychosocial factors such as anxiety, fear, sadness, grief, support systems

24. Presence of skin lesions; edema; systolic and diastolic hypertension; dark-colored urine; weight; crackles; presence of S_3 heart sound; neck vein engorgement; vomiting

25. a. red blood cells

    b. protein

    c. red blood cell casts

    d. leukocytes

    e. white blood cell casts

    f. granular casts

    g. waxy casts

26. a

27. End-stage renal disease

28. a. change in memory or ability to concentrate

    b. frequent interruption of conversation

    c. irritability

29. a. jaundice

    b. ecchymoses or rashes

    c. dry skin

    d. breaks in skin integrity from scratching

    e. slurred speech

    f. ataxia

    g. tremors or asterixis

30. a

31. c

32. c

Degenerative Disorders

33. b

34. d

35. b

Tumors

36. d

37. c

38. b

39. d

40. a

41. Age; sex; presence of known risk factors such as smoking, environmental exposure; history of

weight loss; change in urine color; abdominal or flank discomfort; fever; psychosocial factors such as anxiety, fear, guilt, fear of death or kidney failure, anxiety about treatment

42. Flank asymmetry; abdominal mass; renal bruit; skin pallor; increased areolar pigmentation; gynecomastia; muscle wasting; weakness; weight loss; hematuria

43. d

44. b

45. b

Trauma

46. Minor: one or both kidneys sustain contusions, small lacerations, or forniceal disruption (parenchyma or calyceal) that result in bruising or small blood vessel tears. Localized hematomas are the consequence.

    Major: injury is to the cortex, medulla, or a branch of the renal artery or vein. Resulting hematomas may be intracapsular or disrupt the capsule and bleeding is extensive.

    Pedicle: injury involves laceration or disruption of the renal artery or vein with extensive, rapid hemorrhage

47. a

48. b

49. a

50. b

51. b

52. a

53. History of renal or urological disease; past urinary system surgical intervention; systemic health problems (e.g., diabetes mellitus, hypertension); time and nature of the trauma; flank or abdominal pain and its nature; psychosocial factors such as anxiety, fear, coping abilities, and support systems

54. Blood pressure; apical and peripheral pulses; respirations; temperature; flank asymmetry, evident bruising, or obvious penetrating injury; ecchymoses; abdominal distention; bleeding from the urethra

55. Altered (Renal) Tissue Perfusion

56. c

57. Bladder trauma is more common than ureteral trauma. The bladder is closer to the surface of the abdomen and more subject to compression injury or penetrating injury. The ureters are located deep within the abdomen and protected by layers of tissue.

CHAPTER 72

Chronic Renal Failure

1. Chronic renal failure: gradual onset; pathology not reversible; nitrogen waste buildup not present in early stages but occurs increasingly as disease progresses; dialysis is required for end-stage renal disease (ESRD)

   Acute renal failure: rapid onset; pathology is reversible; buildup of nitrogenous waste occurs rapidly from the onset of the disease process; dialysis may be needed for short-term management but it is not always necessary

2. c
3. a
4. b
5. a
6. b
7. c
8. c
9. d
10. d
11. b
12. b
13. b
14. c
15. d

16. a. renal dialysis

    b. peritoneal dialysis

    c. renal transplantation

17. c

18. Age; sex; changes in weight (loss or gain); current and past medical conditions (sore throat, influenza, prostate enlargement, hypertension, diabetes mellitus, lupus, cancer, tuberculosis); family history of renal disease; past and current medications; diet history; report of change in taste of food; excessive intake of fluids or salt; nausea; vomiting; anorexia; hiccups; diarrhea; constipation; current energy level; recent injury or bleeding; weakness; drowsiness; shortness of breath; urinary patterns (frequency, hesitancy, appearance); changes necessary in daily routine; psychosocial factors such as understanding of diagnosis, implications of disease process on diet, medications, need for dialysis, anxiety, coping mechanisms used, family relationships, social activity, work patterns, body image, sexual activity

19. Weakness; lassitude; alternating periods of extreme drowsiness and excitement or insomnia; decreased attention span; peripheral neuropathies (hand); headaches; muscle twitching; seizures; coma

20. Hypertension; pulmonary and peripheral edema; congestive heart failure; shortness of breath with exertion; paroxysmal nocturnal dyspnea; S_3; pericardial friction rub; jugular venous distension; crackles

21. Breath smells of urine; deep sighing; yawning; shortness of breath; Kussmaul's breathing; pulmonary edema; hilar pneumonitis (thick sputum, decreased coughing, increased respiratory rate, fever); pleural friction rub

22. Anemia; abnormal bleeding; fatigue; pallor; weakness; lethargy; shortness of breath; dizziness; easy bruising; bleeding from mucous membranes; vaginal bleeding; GI bleeding (melena)

23. Anorexia; nausea; vomiting; constipation or diarrhea; breath smells like urine; metallic taste in mouth; mouth inflammation; melena; sever GI bleeding

24. Change in urine amount, frequency; hematuria; proteinuria; cloudy urine with much sediment; change in urine to clear and dilute

25. Pale yellow color; crystal crust on face and eyebrows (uremic frost); severe itching; ecchymosis; purpura; rashes; decreased turgor; dry skin

26. b

27. a. Fluid Volume Excess

    b. Altered Nutrition: Less than Body Requirements

28. a. regulation of protein intake

    b. limitation of fluid intake

    c. restriction of potassium, sodium, and phosphorus

    d. appropriate vitamin and mineral supplements

    e. adequate caloric intake

    f. individualized nutritional needs

29. d

30. Individuals on peritoneal dialysis lose more protein with the dialysate exchange than do clients on hemodialysis.

31. c

32. b

33. Hemodialysis removes excess fluids and waste products from the body that the kidneys usually remove. Hemodialysis also restores chemical and electrolyte balance. It involves circulating the client's blood through a semipermeable membrane that acts as an artificial kidney.

34. e

35. h

36. d

37. a

38. g

39. c

40. f

41. b
42. a. amount of metabolic waste to be removed
    b. clearance capacity of the dialyzer
    c. amount of fluid to be removed
43. a
44. Protamine sulfate
45. c
46. c
47. d
48. a. hepatitis B
    b. human immunodeficiency virus
49. c
50. a. changes in the peritoneal membrane's permeability caused by infection or irritation
    b. changes in peritoneal capillary blood flow result from vasoconstriction, vascular disease, or decreased perfusion
51. b
52. a. intermittent peritoneal dialysis
    b. continuous ambulatory peritoneal dialysis (CAPD)
    c. continuous cycle peritoneal dialysis
    d. multiple-bag CAPD
    e. automated peritoneal dialysis

53. b	61. d
54. b	62. d
55. c	63. d
56. a	64. b
57. d	65. b
58. c	66. d
59. a	67. d
60. a	

68. Refer to Table 72-9 on p. 2144 and to pp. 2143–2144 in the textbook for discussion.
69. b
70. Refer to p. 2146 in the textbook for discussion. The stages are honeymoon, discouragement and disillusionment, and acceptance of the chronic sick role.

Acute Renal Failure

71. Refer to Table 72-10 on p. 2148 and to pp. 2147–2148 in the textbook for discussion.
72. Refer to Table 72-11 on p. 2149 and to p. 2147 in the textbook for discussion.
73. c
74. d

75. d
76. b
77. Exposure to nephrotoxins; recent surgery, trauma, transfusions; renal or systemic diseases (diabetes mellitus, systemic lupus erythematosus, chronic hypertension); recent acute illnesses (influenza, colds, gastroenteritis, sore throat, or pharyngitis); hemorrhage; shock; burn injury; congestive heart failure; volume depletion from bowel preparations and nothing by mouth status; hesitancy; change in amount or appearance of urine; stream force; nocturia; urgency; kidney stones; malignant carcinoma; psychosocial factors including anxiety, coping ability, and family reactions
78. Hypotension; tachycardia; decreased urinary output; decreased cardia output; decreased central venous pressure; lethargy
79. Oliguria; anuria; edema; hypertension; elevated central venous pressure; tachycardia; shortness of breath; crackles; weight gain; anorexia; vomiting; varying level of consciousness
80. Oliguria; intermittent anuria; severe uremia; lethargy; hesitancy; change in urine stream force
81. Fluid Volume Deficit
82. Because of the varying time table for the phases that the client goes through, the client's status may change quickly. The plan of care should be updated to reflect this.
83. c
84. a. hyperalimentation (total parenteral nutrition and intralipids)
    b. enteral nutrition supplement or replacement
85. a. femoral vein
    b. subclavian vein
    c. internal jugular vein
86. d

CHAPTER 73

Anatomy and Physiology Review

1. t	10. k
2. x	11. u
3. y	12. s
4. h	13. w
5. n	14. j
6. v	15. q
7. o	16. f
8. r	17. d
9. b	18. p

19. m
20. e
21. a
22. i
23. l
24. c
25. g
26. b
27. a. The uterus has an extensive blood supply.

b. Lymphatic networks in all three layers of the uterus and cervix provide communication to the abdomen and gastrointestinal tract.

28. c	47. b
29. a	48. c
30. d	49. a
31. b	50. d
32. b	51. d
33. c	52. d
34. b	53. d
35. b	54. g
36. a	55. i
37. b	56. b
38. a	57. e
39. a	58. h
40. c	59. d
41. c	60. f
42. c	61. c
43. a	62. a
44. b	63. b
45. a	64. d
46. c	

65. a. axillary hair growth

b. vocal cords lengthen and thicken

c. increased sebaceous gland activity

d. increase in muscle mass and body size

66. c	73. e
67. j	74. g
68. i	75. k
69. m	76. h
70. b	77. f
71. l	78. d
72. a	79. a

Subjective Assessment

80. Cultural influences; religious beliefs; race; age; age at which secondary sexual characteristics developed; health habits (diet high in fat, amount of sleep, and exercise); use of alcohol, tobacco, or drugs; history of rubella (females), mumps or smallpox (males), orchitis, endocrine disorders, chronic diseases, pelvic inflammatory disease, ruptured appendix, gonorrhea (women); prolonged use of medications such as steroids or hormones; past surgery; injury; allergies; current medication; family history (puberty onset, chronic diseases, cancer, pregnancy complications); type of leisure activities; exposure to teratogenic substances; educational level; daily routines; pain associated with reproductive system and its characteristics; bleeding from genital tract and its characteristics; genital discharge; lesions, bleeding, itching, or pain in any body orifices related to sexual intercourse

81. Age of menarche; cycle frequency and duration; amount of flow; any spotting; dysmenorrhea; premenstrual syndrome; last menstrual period; if menopausal, date of last menstrual period and any climacteric symptoms; vaginal discharge; history of sexually transmitted diseases (STDs); date and results of last Pap smear; breast self-examination practices; breast mass or changes and relationship to menstrual cycle; douching practices; obstetric history; complications during pregnancy or labor and delivery; perinatal data; sexual activity as well as satisfaction of sexual response; pain or bleeding with intercourse contraceptive use and type; maternal use of diethylstilbesterol; age of first intercourse; number of sex partners

82. Testicular changes; practice of testicular self-examination; breast changes; problems with urination; penile discharge; rectal problems; history of STDs; hernia; sexual functioning; past fertility; contraceptive use and type; current problem or change in sexual response; occurrence of impotence

83. Sources of support; personal history of childhood or adulthood sexual trauma; punishment for masturbatory practices; perception of reproductive organs; anxiety; inability to cooperate with examination; fear; satisfaction with own sexuality and body image

84. Use of

a. alcohol

b. tobacco

c. hallucinogenic drugs

85. a. corticosteroids

b. antihypertensives

c. chemotherapeutic agents

86. b

87. b

88. a, b, d, g, h, i, j, k, m, n, o, p, r, s

89. Submit the completed exercise to the clinical instructor for evaluation and feedback.

Objective Assessment

90. Breast examination; abdominal examination; pubic hair color, distribution, and presence of infestation; vulva skin and mucosa for symmetry, lesions, inflammation, swelling, discharge, urethral discharge; Bartholin's gland discharge, inflammation, tenderness; perineal support; vaginal wall strength; cervix size, consistency, dilation, shape, and color, integrity of external os; cervical discharge, bleeding, masses, lesions; vaginal wall lesions or inflammation; posterior vaginal wall masses or tenderness; uterus size, shape, consistency, mobility, tenderness, masses, position; ovary and adnexa size, shape, consistency, mobility, masses; stool for occult blood

91. Distribution pattern and color of pubic hair, presence of infestation; penile skin for intactness, prominent dorsal vein, lesions or ulcers; phimosis; glans penis for inflammation, fungal infection, chancres, other lesions, smegma, placement of urinary meatus; discharge from meatus; penile tenderness, hard areas, inflammation; scrotum shape and contour, presence of lesions, nodules, pain, edema; inguinal and femoral areas for bulging; testes size, shape, symmetry, tenderness, nodules, consistency; epididymis size, shape, tenderness; spermatic cord for nodules, swelling, varicocele; anal area for lesions, ulceration, masses, fissures; prostate for size of lateral lobes, contour, consistency, mobility, tenderness; seminal vesicles if palpable; stool for occult blood

92. Submit the completed exercise to the clinical instructor for evaluation and feedback.

93. c

94. b

95. d

96. Within normal limits: absence of atypical or abnormal cells

Inflammatory atypia: mild atypical cytology, no evidence of malignancy

CIN grade I: suggestive of but not conclusive for malignancy

CIN grade II: Strongly suggestive of malignancy

CIN grade III: Conclusive for malignancy

97. e

98. c

99. g

100.	d	110.	g
101.	f	111.	m
102.	a	112.	f
103.	b	113.	d
104.	c	114.	b
105.	n	115.	i
106.	h	116.	a
107.	k	117.	o
108.	e	118.	j
109.	l	119.	c

CHAPTER 74

Breast Self-Examination

1. Early detection of breast cancer

2. a

3. b

4. a

5. c

6. d

Benign Breast Disorders

7.	c	15.	a
8.	a	16.	c
9.	d	17.	a
10.	b	18.	c
11.	d	19.	c
12.	b	20.	a
13.	a	21.	b
14.	c	22.	d

23. a. application of heat or ice

    b. antiestrogens (e.g., danazol)

    c. diuretics and limiting premenstrual salt intake

    d. mild analgesics

    e. supportive bra

24. c

25. d

26. b

27. c

Breast Cancer

28. d

29. b

30. a. bone

    b. lungs

    c. brain

    d. liver

31. b

32. a

33. Age; sex; race; marital status; weight; height; personal and family history of breast cancer; hormonal history (symptoms of menopause, age at first menarche, age at menopause, age at first child's birth, number of children); if mass present, how, when, and by whom discovered; interval between mass discovery and seeking care; review of body systems including common sites of metastases; knowledge, practice, and regularity of BSE; mammograms; diet history; medications, especially hormonal supplements; psychosocial factors such as fear, anxiety, knowledge of anyone with breast cancer, types of experiences with cancer in general, feelings about cancer, its treatment, recovery, and ability to learn, support systems, financial concerns

34. a. fear of cancer

    b. threat to body image, sexuality, and intimate relationships

35. a. psychological distress (inability to cope)

    b. physiological distress (pain)

    c. relational distress (support from others)

36. Evaluate mass for location, shape, size, consistency, fixation; skin changes (dimpling, peau d'orange, increased vascularity, nipple retraction, ulceration); axillary and supraclavicular areas for enlarged nodes; pain or tenderness with palpation

37. b

38. d

39. a

40. a. Anxiety

    b. High Risk for Altered Tissue Perfusion

41. b

42. a. type of surgery planned

    b. specific postoperative care (e.g., drainage device)

    c. location of incision

    d. permitted postoperative activity level

    e. length of hospital stay

    f. whether additional therapy is planned

43. In a modified-radical mastectomy, the pectoralis muscles and nerves are left intact.

44. a. taking blood pressure

    b. giving injections

    c. drawing blood specimens

45. a

46. b

47. a

48. a. stage of disease

    b. age of the client

    c. menopausal status

    d. client's preference

    e. hormone receptor status of tumor

    f. pathological examination

49. a. to decrease risk of recurrence or metastases

    b. to prolong survival after metastases occur

50. c

51. d

CHAPTER 75

Menstrual Cycle Disorders

1.	c	9.	a
2.	f	10.	c
3.	a	11.	a
4.	e	12.	d
5.	d	13.	c
6.	b	14.	c
7.	c	15.	d
8.	d		

16. It is expensive and may cause undesirable side effects such as acne, hirsutism, weight gain, decreased breast size, and hot flashes.

17. b

18. Complete menstrual history; illnesses; weight change; change in diet, exercise; drugs taken; pain, psychosocial factors such as anxiety, fear, and threat to sexual identity

19. Pelvic examination; anemia; systemic diseases (renal, liver, obesity, undernutrition); abnormal hair growth; abdominal mass

20. a. medroxyprogesterone

    b. combined oral contraceptives

    c. progesterone

    d. danazol

21. b
22. e
23. d

Inflammation and Infections

24. b
25. d
26. e
27. a
28. h
29. g
30. f
31. c
32. a. front-to-back perineal cleaning
    b. wearing cotton underwear
    c. avoiding strong douches and feminine hygiene sprays
    d. avoiding tight-fitting pants or pantyhose

Pelvic Support Problems

33. d
34. c
35. e
36. a
37. b
38. d

Benign Neoplasms

39. b
40. g
41. f
42. c
43. d
44. a
45. e
46. a. bed rest and analgesics
    b. oral contraceptives
    c. cystectomy
    d. oophorectomy
    e. salpingo-oophorectomy and hysterectomy

47. b	52. c
48. d	53. a
49. b	54. c
50. a	55. b
51. c	

Malignant Neoplasms

56. d
57. c
58. Presence of risk factors (obesity, diabetes mellitus, uterine polyps, sterility, nulliparity, polycystic ovary disease, estrogen stimulation, late menopause, postmenopausal bleeding, family history of uterine cancer); low back, low pelvic, or abdominal pain; psychosocial factors such as fears about cancer, disbelief, anger, anxiety, withdrawal, support systems, body image concerns
59. Postmenopausal bleeding; watery, serosanguinous vaginal discharge; palpable uterine mass or polyp
60. a. lungs (chest x-ray)
    b. ureters (intravenous pyelography)
    c. sigmoid colon, rectum, and anal canal (barium enema)
    d. pelvis (ultrasound, computed tomographic scan)
    e. lymph nodes (lymphangiogram)
    f. liver and bone (radioactive scans)
61. a. High Risk for Altered Tissue Perfusion
    b. Body Image Disturbance
62. The position of the uterine applicator must be confirmed by radiography for correct placement to allow for maximal exposure of the tumor to the radiation. Inserting the radioactive isotope either in surgery or in the radiology department would needlessly expose others to radiation as the client is transported back to her room. Dislodgement of the isotope during transport is also a dangerous possibility.
63. d
64. a. antiemetics
    b. broad-spectrum antibiotics
    c. tranquilizers
    d. analgesics
    e. heparin
    f. antidiarrheals

65. a	74. b
66. b	75. a
67. c	76. d
68. b	77. b
69. d	78. b
70. d	79. b
71. d	80. a
72. a	81. c
73. c	82. d

83. It is a laparoscopy or laparotomy performed a year or so after chemotherapy for ovarian cancer. It is done to confirm the absence or presence of tumor and to remove any residual tumor

84. d

85. d

86. c

87. a

88. b

89. b

90. a. repeated pregnancies

    b. sexually transmitted diseases

    c. prior radiation therapy

91. d

92. a

CHAPTER 76

Benign Prostatic Hyperplasia

1. b

2. d

3. Age; urinary frequency; nocturia; hesitancy; intermittency; diminished urine stream force or caliber; sensation of incomplete bladder emptying; postvoid dribbling; hematuria; psychosocial factors such as concerns with self-image and sexuality

4. a

5. Edema; pruritus; pallor; ecchymoses; distended bladder after voiding; expressed feeling of urgency with suprapubic pressure over the bladder; uniform, elastic, nontender enlargement of gland to palpation

6. b

7. d

8. High Risk for Injury related to urinary obstruction

9. c

10. b

11. d

12. b and c

13. a

14. c

15. a

16. a

17. b

18. d

19. d

20. d

21. a

22. a

23. b

24. a. fear of an automatic loss of sexual functioning ability

    b. fear of permanent urinary incontinence

25. b

26. c

27. d

28. c

29. d

30. b

31. c

Prostate Cancer

32. d

33. a

34. b

35. a. estrogens

    b. gonadotropin-releasing hormone analogs

Impotence

36. b

37. a. anxiety

    b. fatigue

    c. boredom

    d. depression

    e. guilt

    f. pressure to perform well sexually

38. a. injury (spinal cord damage, pelvic fracture)

    b. disease (diabetes mellitus, arteriosclerosis)

    c. hormonal imbalance (disorders of the thyroid, adrenals, hypothalamus or pituitary, decreased testosterone)

    d. surgery (prostatectomy, cystectomy, abdominoperineal resection)

39. Specific nature of the impairment (e.g., inability to obtain or maintain an erection during intercourse; does penis become firm at all, slightly firm but insufficient to achieve penetration); life events occurring at the time dysfunction first appeared; is dysfunction constant or related to certain circumstances; history of underlying disease process known to affect penile erection; medications taken; personal habits such as smoking, alcohol use, illicit drug use; family history of erectile dysfunction; psychosocial factors such as relationship difficulties, problems related to employment or financial concerns, presence of nervousness, anxiety, depression

40. Psychological: acute onset, selectivity, periodicity; presence of nocturnal erections and emissions; ability to masturbate successfully; ability to have an erection and function under certain circumstances; retention of testicular sensitivity

Physical: gradual onset; degree of erectile dysfunction in all sexual circumstances; absence of nocturnal erections and emissions; history of normal erectile function; has maintained sexual desire, interest, and libido; decreased testicular sensitivity

41. d

42. c

43. Symptoms of diabetes mellitus (particularly decreased sensation is testes and penis); hypertension

44. c

45. d

46. b

47. a

Testicular Cancer

48. a

49. b

50. Age; race; history of undescended testis; family history of testicular cancer; current family situation; future plans to have children; psychosocial factors such as feeling sexually handicapped, disturbed body image, rejection, strained interpersonal relationships

51. Inspection and palpation of testes for presence of masses, induration, nodularity, irregularity; femoral lymph node enlargement or tenderness; abdominal mass; gynecomastia; signs of pulmonary metastasis

52. b

53. b

54. d

Other Problems Affecting Male Reproductive Structures

55. e		64. d	
56. i		65. d	
57. h		66. e	
58. g		67. b	
59. c		68. g	
60. b		69. a	
61. j		70. c	
62. f		71. f	
63. a			

CHAPTER 77

Infections Associated with Ulcers

1. d

2. f

3. h

4. g

5. b

6. e

7. c

8. a

9. Primary

　　a. 10–90 days

　　b. localized

　　c. chancre

　Secondary

　　a. 6 weeks to 6 months

　　b. systemic

　　c. rash

　Late Latent

　　a. 1 year or longer

　　b. systemic

　　c. none; only to fetus in a pregnant woman

　Late

　　a. 4–20 years

　　b. systemic

　　c. gummas

10. c

11. b

12. d

13. c

14. Submit the completed exercise to the clinical instructor for evaluation and feedback

15. d

16. b

17. d

Infections of Epithelial Surfaces

18. a	23. a
19. d	24. c
20. c	25. c
21. b	26. b
22. d	27. d

28. a. urethral Gram's stain and culture

    b. tissue culture (endocervix and urethra)

    c. Chlamydiazyme

    d. MicroTrak

29. c

Pelvic Inflammatory Disease

30. Pelvic inflammatory disease (PID) is an infectious process involving one or more pelvic structures, especially the fallopian tubes. It is the leading cause of infertility and ectopic pregnancy in the United States.

31. a

32. a

33. Complete medical, family, menstrual, obstetric, and sexual history; history of previous episodes of PID or other infections; contraceptive use and type of device used; history of surgery to the reproductive tract; reported onset of symptoms concurrent or following menstruation; lower abdominal pain and tenderness; reported chills, fever, malaise, purulent vaginal discharge, tachycardia, dysuria, or irregular vaginal bleeding; psychosocial factors such as anxiety, fear, embarrassment, guilt

34. Lower abdominal tenderness; abdominal rigidity; rebound tenderness; tenderness with uterine or cervical manipulation; swollen adnexa

35. a. Anxiety

    b. Pain

36. c

37. b

38. A sexual partner may also be infested with the organism, causing a sexually transmitted disease. Repeated exposure for the client will result in reinfestation.